ORAL AND MAXILLOFACIAL SURGERY

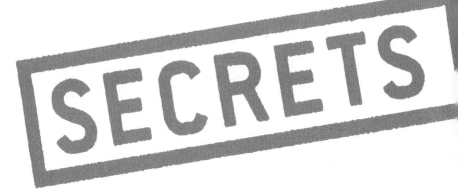

ORAL AND MAXILLOFACIAL SURGERY

SECRETS

THIRD EDITION

A. OMAR ABUBAKER, DMD, PhD
Professor and S. Elmer Bear Chair
Department of Oral and Maxillofacial Surgery
VCU School of Dentistry and VCU Medical Center
Virginia Commonwealth University
Richmond, Virginia

DIN LAM, DMD, MD
Private Practice
Charlotte, North Carolina

KENNETH J. BENSON, DDS
Private Practice - Central Carolina Oral and Maxillofacial Surgery
Oral and Maxillofacial Surgery
Apex, North Carolina

ELSEVIER

ELSEVIER

3251 Riverport Lane
St. Louis, Missouri 63043

ORAL AND MAXILLOFACIAL SURGERY SECRETS, THIRD EDITION   ISBN: 978-0-323-29430-0
Copyright © 2016, Elsevier Inc. All Rights Reserved.

Notices

Knowledge and best practice in this field are constantly changing. As new research and experience broaden our understanding, changes in research methods, professional practices, or medical treatment may become necessary.

Practitioners and researchers must always rely on their own experience and knowledge in evaluating and using any information, methods, compounds, or experiments described herein. In using such information or methods they should be mindful of their own safety and the safety of others, including parties for whom they have a professional responsibility.

With respect to any drug or pharmaceutical products identified, readers are advised to check the most current information provided (i) on procedures featured or (ii) by the manufacturer of each product to be administered, to verify the recommended dose or formula, the method and duration of administration, and contraindications. It is the responsibility of practitioners, relying on their own experience and knowledge of their patients, to make diagnoses, to determine dosages and the best treatment for each individual patient, and to take all appropriate safety precautions.

To the fullest extent of the law, neither the Publisher nor the authors, contributors, or editors, assume any liability for any injury and/or damage to persons or property as a matter of products liability, negligence or otherwise, or from any use or operation of any methods, products, instructions, or ideas contained in the material herein.

Previous editions copyrighted 2007, 2001.

ISBN: 978-0-323-29430-0

Executive Content Strategist: Kathy Falk
Professional Content Development Manager: Jolynn Gower
Senior Content Development Specialist: Courtney Sprehe
Publishing Services Manager: Hemamalini Rajendrababu
Senior Project Manager: Divya KrishnaKumar
Design Direction: Ryan Cooke

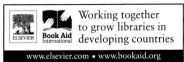

Working together
to grow libraries in
developing countries

www.elsevier.com • www.bookaid.org

Printed in India

Last digit is the print number: 9   8   7   6

CONTRIBUTORS

Shelly Abramowicz, DMD, MPH
Assistant Professor
Department of Oral and Maxillofacial Surgery
School of Medicine
Emory University
Associate Chief, Section of Dentistry/Oral and
    Maxillofacial Surgery
Children's Healthcare of Atlanta
Atlanta, Georgia

A. Omar Abubaker, DMD, PhD
Professor and S. Elmer Bear Chair
Department of Oral and Maxillofacial Surgery
VCU School of Dentistry and VCU Medical Center
Virginia Commonwealth University
Richmond, Virginia

Ravi Agarwal, DDS
Assistant Program Director and Chairman
Department of Oral and Maxillofacial Surgery
Medstar Washington Hospital Center
Washington, DC

David M. Alfi, DDS, MD
Department of Oral and Maxillofacial Surgery
Houston Methodist Hospital
Houston, Texas

Fahad M. Alsaad, DDS
Chief Resident
Department of Oral and Maxillofacial Surgery
School of Dentistry and Medical Center
Virginia Commonwealth University
Richmond, Virginia

Ludmils Antonos, Jr., DMD
Resident
Department of Oral and Maxillofacial Surgery
School of Dentistry
Virginia Commonwealth University
Richmond, Virginia

Shahid R. Aziz, DMD, MD, FACS
Professor
Department of Oral and Maxillofacial Surgery
School of Dental Medicine
Rutgers, The State University of New Jersey
Newark, New Jersey

Shahrokh Bagheri, DMD, MD, FACS
Chief, Division of Oral and Maxillofacial Surgery
Department of Surgery, Northside Hospital
Georgia Oral and Facial Surgery, and Eastern
    Surgical
Associates and Consultants
Atlanta, Georgia
Clinical Associate Professor
Department of Oral and Maxillofacial Surgery
Georgia Health Sciences University
Augusta, Georgia
Clinical Assistant Professor
Department of Surgery, School of Medicine
Emory University
Atlanta, Georgia
Adjunct Assistant Professor of Surgery
School of Medicine, University of Miami
Miami, Florida

Kenneth J. Benson, DDS
Private Practice - Central Carolina Oral and
    Maxillofacial Surgery
Oral and Maxillofacial Surgery
Apex, North Carolina

Behnam Bohluli, DMD, OMFS
Associate Professor
Oral and Maxillofacial Surgery
Azad University
Tehran, Iran

Lauren G. Bourell, DDS, MD
Former Chief Resident of Oral and Maxillofacial
    Surgery
Bellevue Hospital Center
New York University
New York, New York
Private Practice - Western Lake Erie Oral &
    Maxillofacial Surgery
Toledo, Ohio

Hani F. Braidy, DMD, FRCD(C)
Associate Professor
Department of Oral and Maxillofacial Surgery
School of Dental Medicine
Rutgers, The State University of New Jersey
Newark, New Jersey

Tuan Bui, MD, DMD
Affiliate Assistant Professor
Department of Oral and Maxillofacial Surgery
School of Dentistry
Oregon Health and Sciences University
Private Practice - Head and Neck Surgical
Associates
Portland, Oregon

Srinivasa Chandra, MD, BDS, FDS, FDSRCS
Clinical Assistant Professor
Department of Oral and Maxillofacial Surgery
School of Dentistry
University of Washington
Seattle, Washington

Ray Cheng, DDS, MD
Resident
Department of Oral and Maxillofacial Surgery
College of Dentistry
New York University
New York, New York

Matthew Cooke, DDS, MD, MPH
Assistant Professor
Departments of Anesthesiology and Pediatric
Dentistry
School of Dental Medicine
University of Pittsburgh
Pittsburgh, Pennsylvania
Assistant Adjunct Professor
Departments of Pediatric Dentistry and Oral and
Maxillofacial Surgery
School of Dentistry
Virginia Commonwealth University
Richmond, Virginia

Renie Daniel, MD, DMD, MS
Private Practice - Charleston Area Medical Center
Charleston, West Virginia

George R. Deeb, DDS, MD
Associate Professor and Director of Graduate and
Undergraduate Implant Programs
Department of Oral and Maxillofacial Surgery
School of Medicine
Virginia Commonwealth University
Richmond, Virginia

Dean M. DeLuke, DDS, MBA
Associate Professor and Director of Predoctoral
Oral and Maxillofacial Surgery
Department of Oral and Maxillofacial Surgery
School of Dentistry and Medical Center
Virginia Commonwealth University
Richmond, Virginia

Bhavik S. Desai, DMD, PhD, Dip ABOM
Assistant Professor
Division of Oral Medicine
Department of Diagnostic Sciences
School of Dental Medicine
Tufts University
Boston, Massachusetts

Jasjit Dillon, DDS, MBBS, FDSRCS, FACS
Program Director, Department of Oral and
Maxillofacial Surgery
Clinical Assistant Professor, Oral and Maxillofacial
Surgery Department at Harborview Medical
Center
University of Washington
Seattle, Washington

Richard D'Innocenzo, DMD, MD
Clinical Professor and Director of Pre-doctoral
Education, Department of Oral and Maxillofacial
Surgery
Vice Chairman, Dentistry and Oral and Maxillofacial
Surgery, Boston Medical Center
Henry M. Goldman School of Dental Medicine
Boston University
Boston, Massachusetts

Lisa Marie Di Pasquale, DDS, MD
Resident
Division of Oral and Maxillofacial Surgery
School of Dental Medicine
University of Connecticut
Farmington, Connecticut

T.J. Dyer, DDS
Resident
Department of Oral and Maxillofacial Surgery
Henry M. Goldman School of Dental Medicine
Boston University
Boston, Massachusetts

Harry Dym, DDS
Chair, Dentistry and Oral and Maxillofacial Surgery
The Brooklyn Hospital Center
Brooklyn, New York

Siavash Siv Eftekhari, DMD, MD
Faculty/Fellow
Head and Neck Oncologic and Reconstructive
Surgery
Department of Oral and Maxillofacial Surgery
John Peter Smith Hospital
Fort Worth, Texas
Resident
Department of Oral and Maxillofacial Surgery
School of Dentistry
Oregon Health and Science University
Portland, Oregon

Vincent Carrao, DDS., MD
Chief of the Division of Oral Maxillofacial Surgery
The Mount Sinai Hospital
One Gustave L. Levy Place
New York, New York

Sidney Eisig, DDS
George Guttmann Professor of Clinical Craniofacial
    Surgery
Division Director of Oral and Maxillofacial Surgery
Chair of Hospital Dentistry
College of Dental Medicine
Columbia University
New York, New York
Chief, Hospital Dental Service
New York-Presbyterian Hospital/Columbia
    University Medical Center
New York, New York

Ariel Farahi, MPH
USC Master of Public Health Program (MPH)
Doctoral (DMD) Candidate (2016)
School of Dental Medicine
University of Pennsylvania
Philadelphia, Pennsylvania

Tirbod Fattahi, MD, DDS, FACS
Chair and Associate Professor
Department of Oral and Maxillofacial Surgery
College of Medicine
University of Florida
Jacksonville, Florida

Rui Fernandes, DMD, MD
Associate Professor
Department of Surgery
College of Medicine - Jacksonville
University of Florida
Jacksonville, Florida

Ruben Figueroa, DMD, MS
Clinical Associate Professor
Department of Oral and Maxillofacial Surgery
Henry M. Goldman School of Dental Medicine
Boston University
Boston, Massachusetts

Joel M. Friedman, DDS, BA
Associate Professor of Clinical Surgery
Weill Cornell Medical College
Associate Attending Surgeon
New York-Presbyterian/Weill Cornell Medical Center
New York, New York
Clinical Associate Professor of Surgery (Dentistry,
    Oral and Maxillofacial Surgery)
Weill Cornell Medical College
Cornell University
Ithaca, New York

Helen Giannakopoulos, DDS, MD
Associate Professor
Department of Oral and Maxillofacial Surgery
School of Dental Medicine
University of Pennsylvania
Philadelphia, Pennsylvania

James A. Giglio, DDS, MEd
Retired Professor
Department of Oral and Maxillofacial Surgery
School of Dentistry
Retired Professor of Surgery
Department of Surgery, Division of Oral and
    Maxillofacial Surgery
School of Medicine
Virginia Commonwealth University
Richmond, Virginia

Steven G. Gollehon, DDS, MD, FACS
Director, Piedmont Facial Cosmetic and
    Reconstructive Surgery
Private Practice - Piedmont Oral and Maxillofacial
    Surgery Center
Greensboro, North Carolina

Michael J. Grau Jr., DMD
Assistant Program Director, Oral and Maxillofacial
    Surgery Training Program
Department of Oral and Maxillofacial Surgery
Naval Medical Center
San Diego, California

Arin K. Greene, MD, MMSc
Department of Plastic and Oral Surgery
Boston Children's Hospital
Associate Professor of Surgery
Harvard Medical School
Boston, Massachusetts

Bradley A. Gregory, DMD
Private Practice - Center for Oral and Maxillofacial
    Surgery
Findlay, Ohio

Alden H. Harken, MD, FACS
Professor and Chairman
Department of Surgery
University of California-San Francisco, East Bay
Chief of Surgery
Department of Surgery
Alameda County Medical Center
Oakland, California

Tabetha R. Harken, MD, MPH
Associate Professor
Division of General Obstetrics and Gynecology
School of Medicine
University of California, Irvine
Irvine, California

David L. Hirsch, DDS, MD, FACS
Clinical Assistant Professor
Department of Oral and Maxillofacial Surgery
College of Dentistry
New York University
New York, New York

Jason A. Jamali, DDS, MD
Assistant Professor
Department of Oral and Maxillofacial Surgery
College of Dentistry
University of Illinois at Chicago
Chicago, Illinois

Michael Jaskolka, DDS, MD
Cleft and Craniomaxillofacial Surgery
New Hanover Regional Medical Center
Wilmington, North Carolina
Adjunct Assistant Professor
Department of Oral and Maxillofacial Surgery
University of North Carolina Hospitals
Chapel Hill, North Carolina

Tong Ji, DDS, MD, PhD
Professor
Oral Maxillofacial Surgery-Head and Neck Oncology
Shanghai Jiao Tong University
Shanghai, China

Amber Johnson, DO, DMD
Resident
Department of Oral and Maxillofacial Surgery
School of Dentistry
Virginia Commonwealth University
Richmond, Virginia

Lewis Jones, DMD, MD
Assistant Professor
Department of Oral and Maxillofacial Surgery
University of Louisville
School of Dentistry
Louisville, Kentucky

Alia Koch, DDS, MD
Assistant Professor
Department of Oral and Maxillofacial Surgery
College of Dental Medicine
Columbia University
New York, New York
Attending, Oral and Maxillofacial Surgery
New York Presbyterian Hospital
Columbia University Medical Center
New York, New York

Deepak G. Krishnan, DDS
Assistant Professor of Surgery
Residency Program Director
Division of Oral Maxillofacial Surgery
School of Medicine
University of Cincinnati
Cincinnati, Ohio

Din Lam, DMD, MD
Private Practice
Charlotte, North Carolina

Robert C. Lampert, DMD
Resident
Department of Oral and Maxillofacial Surgery
School of Dental Medicine
Rutgers, The State University of New Jersey
Newark, New Jersey

Regina Landesberg, DMD, PhD
Associate Professor
Division of Oral and Maxillofacial Surgery
School of Dental Medicine
University of Connecticut
Farmington, Connecticut

Stuart Lieblich, DMD
Clinical Professor
Department of Oral and Maxillofacial Surgery
University of Connecticut
Farmington, Connecticut
Private Practice - Avon Oral and Maxillofacial
  Surgery
Avon, Connecticut

Sapna Lohiya, DDS
Resident
Department of Oral and Maxillofacial Surgery
School of Dentistry
University of Washington
Seattle, Washington

David W. Lui, DMD, MD
Private Practice - Yardley Oral Surgery
Yardley, Pennsylvania

Renato Mazzonetto, DDS, PhD
Associate Professor
Department of Oral and Maxillofacial Surgery
Piracicaba Dental School
University of Campinas
Piracicaba, São Paulo, Brazil

Daniel J. Meara, MS, DMD, MD, FACS
Chair, Department of Oral and Maxillofacial Surgery
  and Hospital Dentistry
Director, Research and Simulation Training, Oral
  and Maxillofacial Surgery
Christiana Care Health System
Wilmington, Delaware

Andrew T. Meram, DDS, MD
Chief Resident
Department of Oral and Maxillofacial Surgery/Head
  and Neck Surgery
Louisiana State University Health Sciences
  Center – Shreveport
Shreveport, Louisiana

Roman G. Meyliker, DMD
Private Practice - Shore Oral and Maxillofacial
    Surgery
Galloway, New Jersey

Naveen Mohan, DDS
Resident
Department of Oral and Maxillofacial Surgery
The Brooklyn Hospital Center
Brooklyn, New York

Sarah Naghibi, DMD
Resident
Department of Oral and Maxillofacial Surgery
School of Dental Medicine
Case Western Reserve University
Cleveland, Ohio

Gregory M. Ness, DDS
D.P. Snyder Professor of Oral Surgery
Division of Oral and Maxillofacial Surgery and
    Anesthesiology
College of Dentistry
The Ohio State University
Columbus, Ohio

Joe Niamtu, III, DMD, FAACS
Private Practice - Cosmetic Facial Surgery
    Richmond
Richmond, Virginia

Emery Nicholas, DMD
Resident
Department of Oral and Maxillofacial Surgery
New York-Presbyterian Hospital/Weill Cornell
    Medical Center
New York, New York

George Obeid, DDS
Chairman and Director of the Residency Training
    Program
Department of Oral and Maxillofacial Surgery
Medstar Washington Hospital Center
Washington, DC

Mark A. Oghalai, DDS
Private Practice - Bailey, Peoples and Oghalai: Oral
    Maxillofacial Surgery
Winston-Salem, North Carolina

Esther S. Oh, DDS, MD
Clinical Assistant Professor
Department of Oral and Maxillofacial Surgery
College of Dentistry
University of Florida
Gainesville, Florida

HuiShan Ong, BDS, MD
Department of Oral Maxillofacial-Head and Neck
    Oncology
Shanghai Ninth People's Hospital
Shanghai Jiao Tong University
Shanghai, China

Zachary S. Peacock, DMD, MD, FACS
Assistant Professor
Department of Oral and Maxillofacial Surgery
Massachusetts General Hospital and Harvard
    School of Dental Medicine
Boston, Massachusetts

Vincent J. Perciaccante, DDS
Adjunct Associate Professor of Surgery
Division of Oral and Maxillofacial Surgery
Department of Surgery
School of Medicine
Emory University
Atlanta, Georgia
Private Practice - SouthOMS
Fayetteville and Peachtree City, Georgia

Faisal A. Quereshy, MD, DDS, FACS
Associate Professor and Residency Program
    Director
Department of Oral and Maxillofacial Surgery
School of Dental Medicine
Case Western Reserve University
Cleveland, Ohio

Bashar Rajab, DDS, MD
Head of Oral and Maxillofacial Surgery Department
Al-Adan Medical Center, Kuwait
Kuwait City, Kuwait

Sonali A. Rathore, BDS, MS
Assistant Professor
Department of Oral Diagnostic Sciences
School of Dentistry
Virginia Commonwealth University
Richmond, Virginia

Noah Sandler, DMD, MD
Private Practice - Midwest Oral & Maxillofacial
    Surgery, PA
Savage, Minnesota

Samir Singh, DMD
Chief Resident
Department of Oral and Maxillofacial Surgery
School of Dentistry
Virginia Commonwealth University
Richmond, Virginia

Christos A. Skouteris, DMD, PhD
Clinical Assistant Professor
Department of Surgery
School of Medicine
Clinical Assistant Professor and Predoctoral
 Clinic Director
Department of Oral and Maxillofacial Surgery
School of Dentistry
University of Michigan
Ann Arbor, Michigan

Osama Soliman, DMD
Private Practice
Toronto, Ontario, Canada

Daniel B. Spagnoli, DDS, PhD
Private Practice – Brunswick Oral and Maxillofacial
 Surgery
Southport, North Carolina
Chairman (retired)
Department of Oral and Maxillofacial Surgery
School of Dentistry
Louisiana State University
New Orleans, Louisiana

Robert A. Strauss, DDS, MD
Professor and Director
Residency Training Program
Department of Oral and Maxillofacial Surgery
School of Dentistry
Virginia Commonwealth University
Richmond, Virginia

David Webb, DDS
Attending Surgeon
Department of Oral Maxillofacial/Head and Neck
 Surgery
David Grant Medical Center
Travis Air Force Base
Fairfield, California

John Wessel, DMD, MD
Fellow
Carolinas Center for Oral and Facial Surgery
Charlotte, North Carolina

Graham H. Wilson, DDS
Chief Resident
Department of Oral and Maxillofacial Surgery
School of Dentistry
Virginia Commonwealth University
Richmond, Virginia

Jennifer E. Woerner, DMD, MD
Assistant Professor
Fellowship Director of Craniofacial and Cleft
 Surgery
Department of Oral and Maxillofacial Surgery
Louisiana State University Health Sciences
 Center-Shreveport
Shreveport, Louisiana

Andrew Yampolsky, DDS, MD
Resident
Department of Oral and Maxillofacial Surgery
School of Dental Medicine
Rutgers, The State University of New Jersey
Newark, New Jersey

Melvyn S. Yeoh, DMD, MD
Assistant Professor
Department of Oral and Maxillofacial Surgery/Head
 and Neck Surgery
Louisiana State University Health Sciences
 Center – Shreveport
Shreveport, Louisiana

Jacob Yetzer, DDS, MD
Consultant
Mayo Clinic
Rochester, Minnesota

Yedeh Ying, DMD, MD
Resident
Massachusetts General Hospital
Boston, Massachusetts

Joseph Zeidan, DMD
Resident
Department of Oral and Maxillofacial Surgery
The Brooklyn Hospital Center
Brooklyn, New York

Chen Ping Zhang, DDS, MD, PhD
Professor
Department of Oral Maxillofacial-Head Neck
 Oncology
Faculty of Oral and Maxillofacial Surgery
Ninth People's Hospital
Shanghai Jiao Tong University School of Medicine
Shanghai Key Laboratory of Stomatology
Shanghai, China

Vincent B. Ziccardi, DDS, MD, FACS
Professor, Chair, and Residency Director
Department of Oral and Maxillofacial Surgery
School of Dental Medicine
Rutgers, The State University of New Jersey
Newark, New Jersey

PREFACE

It has been almost eight years since the publication of the last edition, and in a rapidly expanding specialty such as oral and maxillofacial surgery, that is a long time. The third edition of *Oral and Maxillofacial Surgery Secrets* contains a large number of new chapters, so the readers (including dental students, oral and maxillofacial residents, and clinicians) will find the entire breadth of knowledge relevant and abundant. Also, because the new chapters cover the expanded scope of the specialty, fellows, and those who are preparing for fellowship, will have in this edition a readily available reference. Once again, in keeping with the style of the last edition, and still believing that the best way to teach is to question, this book uses this effective teaching approach to help guide students, residents, and clinicians in acquiring and retaining the significant knowledge in the field.

As with the previous two editions, this edition is intended not only to answer questions residents and student are being asked, but also to provide a quick source of knowledge that an oral and maxillofacial surgery clinician, resident, or dental student needs to take better care of patient problems, whether they be local or systemic in nature. We have also tried, as much as possible, to include only factual information rather than opinion and to have adequate but brief answers to the questions, recognizing that in some instances these goals are not all achievable. With the help of our contributors, we have updated the contents of the previous edition, covered new topics that were not previously covered, and in many instances, combined updated contents and added entirely new questions and answers. Notably, a number of entirely new chapters cover completely new topics. It should be noted that some of the changes in this edition were based on feedback the senior editor of this edition has received in person and in writing from readers of the previous editions, and for that we sincerely thank our readers. Finally, we would like to mention that we recognize that with the continuous expansion of the field, some areas may still not be fully covered. This emphasizes the fact that no one book (including this one) can be the only source of all the knowledge and all the information that a good practitioner needs to know. We do hope this new and updated edition can continue to be the fastest, most concise, and to-the-point way of finding the answers to most questions that students, residents, and clinicians find themselves in need of on a daily basis.

A. Omar Abubaker

Din Lam

Kenneth J. Benson

ABOUT THE THIRD EDITION

NEW TO THIS EDITION

FIFTEEN CHAPTERS

Chapter 9: Anesthesia for Difficult Patients
Chapter 13: Introduction to Mechanical Ventilation and ICU Care
Chapter 24: Wound Healing
Chapter 29: Diagnosis and Management of Dentoalveolar Injuries
Chapter 35: Craniofacial Syndromes
Chapter 36: Oromandibular Dysostosis
Chapter 40: Distraction Osteogenesis
Chapter 45: Cancer of the Oral Cavity
Chapter 47: Vascular Anomalies
Chapter 48: Osteoradionecrosis/Osteonecrosis of the Jaws
Chapter 49: Neck Mass
Chapter 50: Bone Grafting to Facilitate Dental Implant Placement
Chapter 51: Local and Regional Flaps
Chapter 52: Reconstruction of the Facial Subunits
Chapter 53: Microvascular Surgery

CHAPTERS DEALING WITH COSMETIC SURGERY

Chapter 54: Evaluation of the Aging Face
Chapter 55: Cosmetic Blepharoplasty
Chapter 56: Rhytidectomy
Chapter 57: Rhinoplasty
Chapter 58: Minimal-Invasive Cosmetic Procedures

KEY FEATURES

- Core knowledge is presented in the popular and trusted Secrets® question-and-answer format.
- Over 2,300 questions and answers provide valuable pearls, tips, memory aids, and secrets from experts in the field.
- Chapters are written by internationally recognized experts in the field, making this an authoritative resource for the safe and effective practice of OMS.

CONTENTS

IV MANAGEMENT CONSIDERATIONS FOR THE MEDICALLY-COMPROMISED PATIENTS

V ORAL AND MAXILLOFACIAL SURGERY

VI COSMETIC SURGERY

TOP 100 SECRET QUESTIONS

1. Basal function of most organ systems remains unchanged due to the aging process; however, the functional reserve and ability to compensate for physiological stress are reduced.

2. Patients who are on beta blockers should take them on the day of surgery and continue them perioperatively. Abrupt interruption of the regimen can lead to withdrawal symptoms: rebound hypertension, tachycardia, and myocardial ischemia.

3. Blood transfusion should not be based solely on hemoglobin or hematocrit level. The decision should be individualized to the clinical situation and take into consideration the patient's health status.

4. Forced vital capacity (FVC), forced expiratory volume in 1 second (FEV_1), the FEV_1/FVC ratio, and the flow between 25% and 75% of the FVC (mean maximal flow [MMF_{25-75}]) are the most clinically helpful indices obtained from spirometry.

5. Propofol is the least likely of all induction agents to result in nausea and vomiting. Termination of the effects of intravenous anesthetics is by redistribution, not biotransformation and breakdown.

6. The systolic blood pressure in the radial artery may be as much as 20 to 50 mm Hg higher than the pressure in the central aorta.

7. Cocaine sensitizes the cardiovascular system to the effects of endogenous catecholamine. Ketamine potentiates the cardiovascular toxicity of cocaine and should be avoided.

8. Physiologic alterations in patients during pregnancy include increases in cardiac output, heart rate, plasma volume, minute ventilation, and oxygen consumption; decreases in SVR; dilutional anemia; loss of functional residual capacity (FRC); and a hypercoagulable state.

9. In the pacemaker coding system, the first letter refers to the chamber paced, the second letter to the chamber in which sensing occurs, the third letter to the responses to sensing in chambers, and the fourth letter to rate responsiveness.

10. Patients with diabetes have a high incidence of coronary artery disease with an atypical or silent presentation.

11. When in doubt, remember that a p value less than 0.05 is generally considered statistically significant, and the finding by chance alone is 1 in 20.

12. In febrile patients, a white blood cell or band count is rarely useful in differentiating between bacterial and viral illnesses.

13. A septal hematoma must be ruled out in the setting of nasal bone fracture. Failure to drain a septal hematoma may result in a septal abscess, septal perforation, and/or saddle nose deformity.

14. *Streptococcus pneumoniae*, *Haemophilus influenzae*, and *Moraxella catarrhalis* are the most common causes of acute bacterial sinusitis.

15. Surgical treatment of TMD is reserved for internal derangement of the TMJ and not for musculoskeletal disorders.

16. The facial nerve is capable of regeneration. The degree of return to normal is mostly dependent on the degree of initial injury. The single most important factor is whether the nerve lost function slowly over days or immediately at the time of the trauma.

17. A positive ANA, RF, SS-a, and SS-b and an elevated erythrocyte sedimentation rate are suggestive of Sjögren's syndrome, but the definitive diagnosis is made by a minor salivary gland biopsy in the lower lip, which will show glandular atrophy with an abundance of lymphocytes and histiocytes.

18. The most common parotid viral infection is mumps. Less common are cytomegalovirus, coxsackievirus, and Epstein-Barr viruses. Bacterial sialadenitis is commonly associated with coagulase-positive *Staphylococcus aureus*, but *S. pneumoniae*, *Escherichia coli*, *H. influenzae*, and oral anaerobe infections may also occur.

19. Infection of the danger space between the alar fascia and the prevertebral space can lead to mediastinitis and death if not appropriately treated.

20. The most common landmark for identification of the facial nerve during parotidectomy is the tympanomastoid suture line.

21. Biopsies of the possible primary sites should be obtained, including the nasopharynx, tongue base-valleculae, pyriform sinus, and tonsils, during diagnostic work-up in patients with unknown primary with malignant lymph node in the neck.

22. Radiotherapy is more effective when given concomitantly with chemotherapy in treatment of head and neck squamous cell carcinomas.

23. Phenol, when used as a skin-resurfacing chemical agent, can be cardiotoxic, hepatotoxic, and nephrotoxic. Steps must be taken to minimize the risk for these toxicities.

24. When using carbon dioxide laser in skin resurfacing, a yellow-chamois color indicates that one has reached the reticular dermis.

25. Rhytidectomy can only correct wrinkling in the lower two-thirds of the face and the neckline.

26. A patient with a glasgow coma scale (GCS) score of 8 or less requires intubation.

27. Forced duction testing is a simple and direct method to detect extraocular muscle entrapment, which may occur with orbital blowout fractures.

28. If given in the setting of mononucleosis, amoxicillin or penicillin can cause a salmon-colored rash.

29. Erb's point is on the side of the neck where applied pressure on the roots of the fifth and sixth cervical nerves causes paralysis of the brachial muscles. Muscles involved are of the upper arm (e.g., deltoid, biceps, brachialis anterior).

30. The level of reduced hemoglobin at which a patient becomes cyanotic is 5 g/dL.

31. Anisocoria refers to inequality of the pupils. It is a common normal variation of pupil size but can be an indication of pathology.

32. Amide local anesthetics are metabolized mainly by the liver (microsomal enzymes), whereas the ester types are metabolized by the plasma (pseudocholinesterase). An easy way to remember how the most commonly used local anesthetic is metabolized is *l*idocaine and *l*iver.

33. The lipid solubility determines the potency of a local anesthetic. A greater lipid solubility produces a more potent local anesthetic. The degree of protein binding of a local anesthetic agent determines the duration of a local anesthetic. A greater degree of protein binding at the receptor site will create a longer duration of action. The pKa of a local anesthetic determines its speed of onset. The closer the pKa of a local anesthetic is to the pH of tissue (7.4), the more rapid the onset.

34. Morphine, codeine, and meperidine (Demerol) cause histamine release, resulting in vasodilation and possible hypotension. Fentanyl, sufentanil, and alfentanil do not stimulate histamine release.

35. Plasma cholinesterase is produced in the liver and metabolizes succinylcholine (SCh) as well as ester local anesthetics and mivacurium, a nondepolarizing neuromuscular

blocker (NMB). A reduced quantity of plasma cholinesterase, such as occurs with liver disease, pregnancy, malignancies, malnutrition, collagen vascular disease, and hypothyroidism, may prolong the duration of blockade with SCh.

36. Fluid resuscitation is preferable with 5% dextrose in water (D_5W) over lactated Ringer's solution for symptomatic hypernatremia. Otherwise D_5W is rarely indicated because the glucose load may induce osmotic diuresis.

37. In pediatric patients younger than ages 10 to 12, tracheostomy is the preferred emergency surgical airway. The small 3-mm-wide cricothyroid membrane and poorly defined anatomic landmarks make cricothyrotomy all but impossible in children.

38. Malignant hyperthermia (MH) is a hypermetabolic state involving skeletal muscle that is precipitated by certain anesthetic agents in genetically susceptible individuals. The incidence of MH is <0.5% of all patients who are exposed to anesthetic agents. The major clinical characteristics of MH are (1) acidosis, (2) rigidity, (3) fever, (4) hypermetabolism, and (5) myoglobinuria.

39. Creatinine is used as a sensitive, indirect measurement of glomerular filtration rate (GFR) because it is filtered by the glomeruli, but it is minimally secreted or reabsorbed.

40. Analysis of human data shows that fetuses of <16 weeks who had an acute exposure of 0.5 Gy had a higher risk of growth restriction, microcephaly, and mental retardation. During the fetal period, the fetus becomes less sensitive to radiation but retains CNS sensitivity that may lead to growth restriction at term. Diagnostic radiographs that deliver <0.05 to 0.1 Gy are not believed to be teratogenic. Virtually all plain film and CT scan irradiation delivers <0.01 Gy to the fetus.

41. Fresh frozen plasma (FFP) is used for replacement of deficiencies of factors II, V, VII, IX, and XI when specific component therapy is not available or desirable. In an average-size adult, each unit of FFP increases the level of all clotting factors by 2% to 3%, and most bleeding can be controlled by transfusion of FFP at a dose of 10 mL/kg of body weight.

42. *Cis*-atracurium is the best choice muscle relaxant to use in a patient with liver dysfunction because it is eliminated by Hofmann elimination and is independent of liver function.

43. *Staphylococcus aureus* and *Staphylococcus epidermidis* are most commonly cultured from infected prosthetic joints because the majority of infections involving prosthetic joints are caused by staphylococcal contamination during the placement of the prosthesis. The bacteria that have been identified in cases of infected prosthetic joints arising by hematogenous spread of infection to the prosthesis from oral sites of infection are *Streptococcus viridans* and *Streptococcus sanguis*.

44. Ludwig's angina is bilateral, brawny, boardlike induration of the submandibular, sublingual, and submental spaces due to infection of these spaces. The term *angina* is used because of the respiratory distress caused by the airway obstruction. This obstruction can occur suddenly owing to the possible extension of the infection from the sublingual space posteriorly to the epiglottis, causing epiglottic edema.

45. Erysipelas is a superficial cellulitis of the skin that is caused by beta-hemolytic streptococcus and by group B streptococcus. It usually presents with warm, erythematous skin and spreads rapidly from release of hyaluronidase by the bacteria. It is associated with lymphadenopathy and fever and has an abrupt onset with acute swelling. It may affect the skin of the face. Treatment consists of parenteral penicillin.

46. Vertical maxillary excess (VME) can be treated with orthodontic intervention early in life (8 to 12 years) with high-pull head gear or open bite Bionater to control vertical growth of the maxilla. If successful, such treatment may resolve the skeletal abnormalities, and ultimately the soft tissues and other facial structures grow accordingly. However, when an adult presents with this condition, it usually is treated with Le Fort I osteotomy and superior repositioning of the maxilla. Recently, with use of skeletal anchorage, skeletal open bite can be closed with orthodontic treatment alone through intrusion of the posterior teeth.

47. Neurosensory deficits of the inferior alveolar nerve following bilateral saggital split osteotomy (BSSO) is one of the most significant concerns with this procedure. Complications occur in 20% to 85% of surgeries. However, the incidence is only 9% at 1 year after surgery. This complication is more common in patients older than age 40 and in patients who undergo simultaneous genioplasty.

48. Transverse expansion of the maxilla is the most unstable orthognathic procedure. The greatest relapse is seen in the second molar region with an average of 50% loss of surgical expansion. After 1 year, inferior maxillary positioning and mandibular setbacks were also found to be less predictable than in other surgical techniques.

49. Mandibular prognathism may be present in the following syndromes: basal cell nevus syndrome (Gorlin's syndrome), Klinefelter's syndrome, Marfan's syndrome, osteogenesis imperfecta, and Waardenburg's syndrome. The following syndromes may be associated with midface deficiency: achondroplasia, Apert's syndrome, cleidocranial dysplasia, Crouzon's syndrome, Marshall's syndrome, Pfeiffer's syndrome, and Stickler's syndrome.

50. Surgical repair of cleft lip is generally carried out at 10 to 14 weeks of age. However, the time of repair of cleft lip often is based on the Rule of Tens. According to this rule, cleft lip can be closed when the infant is 10 weeks old, the hemoglobin is 10 g/dL, and the infant's weight is 10 lb.

51. Rapid tumor growth or a sudden growth acceleration in a long-standing salivary mass, pain, and peripheral facial nerve paralysis are some of the signs and symptoms suggestive of salivary gland malignancy. However, it has been reported that peripheral facial nerve paralysis can be associated with acute suppurative parotitis, nonspecific parotitis with inflammatory pseudotumor, amyloidosis, and sarcoidosis of the parotid.

52. Sialoliths in the early stage of development are small and not adequately mineralized to be visible radiographically. It has also been reported in the literature that 30% to 50% of parotid and 10% to 20% of submandibular sialoliths are radiolucent. These radiolucent sialoliths can be visualized indirectly by the imaging defect that they produce on sialography, or directly through sialoendoscopy.

53. Fine-needle aspiration (FNA) biopsy is an efficacious modality in the diagnosis of salivary gland pathology. The specificity of the procedure ranges from 88% to 99% and the sensitivity is 71% to 93%.

54. Sublingual salivary gland tumors comprise <1% of all salivary gland neoplasms. These tumors are predominantly malignant (>80%) and are usually adenoid cystic or mucoepidermoid carcinomas.

55. Syndromes that can affect the salivary glands are primary Sjögren's syndrome, which is usually characterized by parotid and lacrimal gland enlargement, xerostomia, and xerophthalmia; secondary Sjögren's syndrome, which involves autoimmune parotitis that occurs with rheumatoid arthritis, lupus, systemic sclerosis, thyroiditis, primary biliary cirrhosis, and mixed collagen disease; and sarcoidosis, which may involve the parotid gland. Sarcoidosis of the parotid gland along with fever, lacrimal adenitis, uveitis, and facial nerve paralysis is called Heerfordt's syndrome. Recently, a sicca syndrome-like condition has been recognized in HIV-positive children. This condition presents with parotid gland enlargement, xerostomia, and lymphadenopathy.

56. The most common benign tumor of minor and major salivary glands is pleomorphic adenoma.

57. The most common malignant tumors of minor and major salivary glands are mucoepidermoid carcinoma in the parotid gland and adenoid cystic carcinoma in the submandibular, sublingual, and minor salivary glands.

58. The methods that have been used for the surgical management of drooling include bilateral submandibular duct relocation to the posterior tonsillar pillar (most preferred); bilateral parotid duct relocation to the posterior tonsillar pillar; bilateral parotid duct diversion with autogenous venous grafts; bilateral submandibular duct relocation

plus parotid duct ligation; bilateral submandibular and parotid duct ligation; bilateral submandibular gland excision with parotid duct ligation, if the problem is very severe; and chorda tympani neurectomy (only as an adjunct procedure in carefully selected cases).

59. The incidence of development of cystic lesions around retained, asymptomatic, impacted mandibular third molars is 0.3% to 37%.

60. Thyroglossal duct, dermoid, and epidermoid cysts are the most common soft tissue cysts in children. The most common benign soft tissue tumor in children is hemangioma. Odontoma is the most common benign odontogenic intraosseous tumor in children; ossifying fibroma is the most common nonodontogenic tumor in children.

61. A Sistrunk procedure is a surgical procedure used for the excision of thyroglossal duct cysts. In this operation, the central portion of the hyoid bone is always excised. The retrohyoid cyst tract is dissected and excised at the base of the tongue together with the area of the foramen cecum.

62. The most common anatomic sites for oral cancer are the tongue and floor of the mouth. Other sites might be more common in different parts of the world because of certain predisposing ethnic, cultural, or other factors.

63. The sentinel node is any lymph node receiving direct lymphatic drainage from a primary tumor site.

64. The most common laser used in the OMS practice is the carbon dioxide (CO_2) laser. Because of their high affinity for tissue water found in the epidermis and dermis, the CO_2 and Er:YAG lasers are the most common lasers used for skin resurfacing techniques.

65. Wound infections from human bites are frequently caused by *Streptococcus* and *Staphylococcus* organisms. Serious infections may also be associated with *Eikenella*. Prophylactic antibiotic coverage with penicillin or amoxicillin-clavulanic acid is recommended. Unlike human bites, 50% to 75% of infections in animal bites are caused by *Pasteurella multocida*. Amoxicillin-clavulanic acid is recommended for prophylaxis in animal bites. Tetanus immunization is required for all bites, and rabies prophylaxis may be required when animals exhibit suspicious behavior.

66. In general, for most oral and maxillofacial bony defects, 10 mL of noncompacted corticocancellous bone is required for every 1 cm of defect to be reconstructed.

67. The seven anatomic structures that attach to the anterior iliac crest are the fasciae latae, inguinal ligament, tensor fasciae latae, sartorius, iliacus, and internal and external abdominal oblique muscles.

68. Defects of approximately one-third of the lower lip and one-quarter of the upper lip can be closed primarily without resulting in a significant microstomia.

69. The location of the oral defect determines where a tongue flap is based (whether it should be an anteriorly based or posteriorly based flap). For defects of the soft palate, retromolar region, and posterior buccal mucosa, a posteriorly based flap is used. Anteriorly based flaps are used for hard palate defects, defects of the anterior buccal mucosa, anterior floor of the mouth, or lips.

70. The incidence of osteoradionecrosis (ORN) ranges from 1% to 44.2% with an overall incidence of 11.8% in most studies published before 1968. Recent studies showed incidences of 5% to 15% with an overall incidence of 5.4%. ORN has a bimodal incidence, peaking at 12 months and again at 24 to 60 months. However, it can occur as late as 30 years later. It is often related to traumatic injuries such as preirradiation extraction (4.4%), postirradiation extraction (5.8%), and denture trauma (<1%). ORN may occur spontaneously (albeit rarely) owing to progression of periapical or periodontal disease.

71. Hyperbaric oxygen therapy is an administration of 100% oxygen via head tent, mask, or endotracheal tube within a special chamber at 2.4 atmospheric absolute (ATA) pressure for 90 minutes each session. The treatment should be delivered once a day, five times (dives) a week.

72. Submental liposuction is performed at the supraplatysmal plane, a distinct layer of subcutaneous fatty tissue located below the dermis at which the procedure is safely performed in a near bloodless field. The area treated from the submental incision is bounded by the anterior border of the sternocleidomastoid muscle, inferior border of the mandible, and superior border of the thyroid.

73. The chemical properties and interface chemistry of dental implants are determined by the oxide layer and not by the metal of the implant. Therefore the dense oxide film of a titanium implant, for example, is about 100 angstroms (Å) thick. This is considered a normal space between implant and bone in an osseointegrated titanium implant.

74. Torque testing can be done to check for osseointegration at the time of implant uncovering. Ideally, one should be able to place a force of 10 to 20 N/cm without unscrewing an implant if it is successfully osseointegrated. Other clinical subjective signs of integration are percussion and immobility when placing a fixture mount or impression coping on the implant. When a lateral force of 5 lb is applied, no movement should be seen. Horizontal mobility of >1 mm or movement <500 g of force indicates a failed implant.

75. The most useful radiographic sign of implant failure is loss of crestal bone. Early crestal bone loss is a sign of stress at the permucosal site. At least 40% of the trabecular bone must be lost to be detected radiographically. Rapid progressive bone loss indicates failure. This will usually be accompanied by pain on percussion or function.

76. Magnetic resonance imaging (MRI) and CT scans are not contraindicated in patients with pure titanium implants. Most CT scanners can subtract titanium and other metals from the image and eliminate the scatter images.

77. The average size of the maxillary sinus is 14.75 mL, with a range of 9.5 to 20 mL. On average, the width is 2.5 cm; height, 3.75 cm; and depth, 3 cm.

78. Split-thickness skin grafts (STSGs) can be of varying thickness. An STSG is composed of the epidermis layer and part of the dermis layer. The STSG can be classified as thin, intermediate, or thick, based on the amount of dermis included. STSGs are between 0.010 and 0.025 inch.

79. The thinner a skin graft, the more the contraction. A thin STSG contracts more than an intermediate STSG, which contracts more than a thick STSG. Full-thickness skin grafts hardly contract at all. Primary contraction is caused by elastic fibers in the skin graft as soon as it has been cut. This can be overcome when a graft is sutured in place. Secondary contraction begins about postoperative day 10 and continues for up to 6 months.

80. Plasmic imbibition is the process by which a skin graft absorbs a plasma-like fluid from its underlying recipient bed. It is absorbed into the capillary network by capillary action. This process is the initial means of survival for a skin graft and continues for approximately 48 hours.

81. Obstructive sleep apnea (OSA) is characterized by repetitive, discrete episodes of decreased airflow (hypopnea) or frank cessation of airflow (apnea) for at least a 10-second duration in association with >2% decrease in oxygen hemoglobin saturation. Obstructive events occur during stages III and IV and the rapid eye movement (REM) stage, which are the deeper stages of sleep. Pharyngeal wall collapse is more common during these stages because the muscles are most relaxed.

82. Respiratory disturbance index (RDI) represents the number of obstructive respiratory events/hr of sleep. The RDI, along with oximetry, is the primary clinical indicator in the diagnosis of obstructive sleep apnea syndrome (OSAS). RDI is calculated as $RDI = apnea + hypopnea/total\ sleep\ time \times 60$. An RDI of 5 is the upper limit of normal.

83. For every 1° C rise in body temperature, there is a corresponding 9 to 10 beats/min increase in the patient's heart rate.

84. The most common cause of dysuria in the immediate postoperative period is related to the agents incorporated in the administration of general anesthesia that can inhibit the micturitic reflex, and the patient can suffer bladder distention, which itself may inhibit the ability to micturate. Treatment of postoperative dysuria should begin simply by having the patient stand by or sit on the toilet while running water in the sink. If this does not help and there is no evidence of a hypovolemic state, then the patient should be catheterized. If the residual measures >300 mL, then the catheter should be left in overnight.

85. A surgical wound infection or *surgical site infection* (SSI) is an infection that occurs typically 12 hours to 7 days postoperatively but can occur within 30 days of surgery unless a foreign body is left in situ. In the case of implanted foreign material, 1 year must elapse before surgery can be excluded as causative.

86. The four conditions other than asystole that can lead to a flat line tracing on electrocardiogram (ECG) are (1) fine ventricular fibrillation, (2) loose electrode leads, (3) no power, and (4) signal gain is turned down.

87. Drugs that can be administered through the endotracheal tube are lidocaine, epinephrine, atropine, and Narcan (L-E-A-N). Administer all tracheal medications at 2 to 2.5 times the recommended IV dosage, diluted in 10 mL of normal saline or distilled water. Tracheal absorption is greater with distilled water as the diluent than with normal saline, but distilled water has a greater adverse effect on PaO_2.

88. Kiesselbach's plexus of septum arterioles is the source of 90% of nosebleeds. Four anastomosed arteries make up this plexus: the sphenopalatine, anterior ethmoidal, greater palatine, and superior labial arteries. The nasopalatine branch of the descending palatine artery anastomoses with septal branches of the sphenopalatine artery, the anterior ethmoidal artery, and superior lateral branches of the superior labial branch of the facial artery. Traumatic nasal bleeding can be caused by laceration of the nasal mucosa, and any of the nasal vessels can be the source of the bleeding.

89. The nasolacrimal duct lies within the thin, bony wall between the maxillary sinus and the nasal cavity. The duct ends at the inferior nasal meatus through the valve of Hasner. The position of the nasolacrimal duct beneath the inferior turbinate is 11 to 14 mm posterior to the piriform aperture and 11 to 17 mm above the nasal floor.

90. The sebaceous glands of the eyelid are called the glands of Zeis. The sweat glands of the eyelid are called the glands of Moll.

91. Crocodile tears is a condition that results after injury to the fibers of the facial nerve carrying parasympathetic secretory fibers that normally innervate the salivary gland. The injury causes the fibers to heal in contact with fibers supplying the lacrimal gland, leading to crying when the patient eats.

92. All facial muscles except the mentalis, levator angularis superioris, and buccinator receive their innervation along their deep surfaces. However, because these three muscles are located deep within the facial soft tissue and lie deep to the plane of the facial nerve, they receive their innervation along their superficial surfaces. All other facial muscles of expression are located superficial to the plane of the facial nerve and, thus, receive their innervation along their deep or posterior surfaces.

93. The anulus of Zinn, or common tendinous ring in the orbit, is the fibrous thickening of the periosteum from which the rectus muscles originate.

94. Tenon's capsule is a fascial structure that subdivides the orbital cavity into two halves—an anterior (or precapsular) segment and a posterior (or retrocapsular) segment. The ocular globe occupies only the anterior half of the orbital cavity. The posterior half of the orbital cavity is filled with fat, muscles, vessels, and nerves that supply the ocular globe and extraocular muscles and provide sensation to the soft tissue surrounding the orbit.

95. The inferior alveolar nerve is most often located buccal and slightly apical to the roots of a mandibular third molar. The root of the tooth that is most often dislodged into

the maxillary sinus during an extraction procedure is the palatal root of the maxillary first molar. The most reliable signs of a potential nerve injury during extraction of an impacted mandibular third molar are diversion of canal, interruption of canal borders, and darkening of roots.

96. Tinel's sign is a provocative test of regenerating nerve sprouts in which light percussion over the nerve elicits a distal tingling sensation. It is used as a sign of small fiber recovery but is poorly correlated with functional recovery and easily confused with neuroma formation.

97. The incidence of inferior alveolar, lingual, and, less frequently, long buccal nerve injury during mandibular third molar removal ranges between 0.6% and 5.0%. In general, the incidence of inferior alveolar nerve (IAN) injuries is higher than that of the lingual nerve. Factors such as age, surgical technique, and proximity of the nerve to the tooth influence the incidence of these injuries. More than 96% of patients with lingual nerve injuries recover spontaneously.

98. The average rate of an injured axon's forward growth is approximately 1 to 2 mm/day.

99. The sural nerve graft is the best donor site for an interpositional graft for an inferior alveolar nerve defect of approximately 25 mm. The sural nerve can provide up to 30 mm of graft harvest. It provides sensation to the posterior and lateral aspect of the leg and foot. It also has up to 50% fewer axons and smaller axonal size than the inferior alveolar nerve. Because of primary contracture, the length of the harvested nerve should be at least 25% longer than the defect.

100. More than 50% of mandibular fractures are multiple. For this reason, if one fracture is noted along the jaw, the patient should be examined closely for evidence of additional fractures. Radiographic films must be scrutinized carefully for discrete fracture lines. Also, associated injuries are present in 43% of all patients with mandibular fracture, most of whom were involved in vehicular accidents. Cervical spine fractures were found in 11% of this group of patients. It is imperative to rule out cervical neck fractures, especially in patients who are intoxicated or unconscious.

I

PATIENT EVALUATION

CHAPTER 1

ARE YOU READY FOR YOUR SURGERY ROTATION?*

Tabetha R. Harken, Alden H. Harken

Surgery is a participatory, team, and contact sport. Present yourself to patients, residents, and attendings with enthusiasm (which covers a multitude of sins), punctuality (type A people do not like to wait), and cleanliness (you must look, act, and smell like a doctor). Make sure to knock on the door (or ask for permission) to come into the room, and introduce everybody with you (who may not have introduced themselves) and what status they are (attendings, residents, or students). *Remember that taking care of a patient is a privilege—to you and not to the patient.*

1. **Why should you introduce yourself to each patient and ask about his or her chief complaint?**
   Symptoms are perception, and perception is more important than reality. To a patient, the chief complaint is not simply a matter of life and death—it is much more important. Patients routinely are placed into compromising, uncomfortable, embarrassing, and undignified predicaments. Patients are people, however; they have interests, concerns, anxieties, and a story. As a student, you have an opportunity to place your patient's chief complaint into the context of the rest of his or her life. This skill is important, and the patient will always be grateful. You can serve a real purpose as a listener and translator for the patient and his or her family.

   Patients want to trust and love you. This trust in surgical therapy is a formidable tool. The more a patient understands about his or her disease, the more the patient can participate in getting better. Recovery is faster if the patient helps. Similarly, the more the patient understands about his or her therapy (including its side effects and potential complications), the more effective the therapy is (this principle is not in textbooks). You can be your patient's interpreter. This is the fun of surgery (and medicine).

2. **What is the correct answer to almost all questions?**
   Thank you. Gratitude is an invaluable tool on the wards.

3. **Are there any simple rules from the trenches?**
   - **Get along with the nurses.** The nurses do know more than the rest of us about the codes, routines, and rituals of making the wards run smoothly. They may not know as much about pheochromocytomas and intermediate filaments, but about the stuff that matters, they know a lot. Acknowledge that, and they will take you under their wings and teach you a ton!
   - **Help out.** If your residents look busy, they probably are. So, if you ask how you can help and they are too busy even to answer, asking again probably would not be very high yield. Always leap at the opportunity to shag X-rays, track down lab results, and retrieve a bag of blood from the bank. The team will recognize your enthusiasm and reward your contributions.
   - **Get scutted.** We all would like a secretary, but one is not going to be provided on this rotation. Your residents do a lot of their own scut work without you even knowing about it. So if you feel like scut work is beneath you, perhaps you should think about another profession.
   - **Work hard.** This rotation is an apprenticeship. If you work hard, you will get a realistic idea of what it means to be a resident (and even a practicing doc) in this specialty. (This has big advantages when you are selecting a type of internship.)
   - **Stay in the loop.** In the beginning, you may feel like you are not a real part of the team. If you are persistent and reliable, however, soon your residents will trust you with more important jobs.
   - **Educate yourself, and then educate your patients.** Here is one of the rewarding places (as indicated in question 1) where you can soar to the top of the team. Talk to your patients about everything (including their disease and therapy), and they will love you for it.

---

*Reprinted from Harken TR, Harken AH, Swift UMB, Harken AH: Are you ready for your surgery rotation? In Harken AH, Moore EE, editors: *Abernathy's surgical secrets,* ed 6, Philadelphia, 2009, Elsevier.

- **Maintain a positive attitude.** As a medical student, you may feel you are not a crucial part of the team. Even if you are incredibly smart, you are unlikely to be making the crucial management decisions. So what does that leave? Attitude. If you are enthusiastic and interested, your residents will enjoy having you around, and they will work to keep you involved and satisfied. A dazzlingly intelligent but morose complainer is better suited for a rotation in the morgue. Remember, your resident is likely following 15 sick patients, gets paid less than $2/hour, and has not slept more than 5 hours in the last 3 days. Simple things such as smiling and saying thank you (when someone teaches you) go an incredibly long way and are rewarded on all clinical rotations with experience and good grades.
- **Have fun!** This is the most exciting, gratifying, rewarding, and fun profession—and is light years better than whatever is second best (this is not just our opinion).

4. What is the best approach to surgical notes?

   Surgical notes should be succinct (Box 1-1). Most surgeons still move their lips when they read. With the advent of EMR, copy and paste are as unoriginal as thinking that most patients and most diseases are the same or similar. In some instances, it even may be against the institution's policies. Write every note, as many people will read this note and judge your care by the quality of your note.

Box 1-1. Best Approach to Surgical Notes

Although since the initial publication of this chapter most notes have become electronic in nature and may even follow a specific template, the following guidelines for notes are still valid in helping develop a sequence of how to approach documentation.

Admission Orders

Admit to 5 West (attending's name)

Condition:	Stable
Diagnosis:	Abdominal pain; r/o appendicitis
Vital signs:	q4h
Parameters:	Please call HO for:
	T > 38 °C
	160 < BP < 90
	120 < HR < 60
Diet:	NPO
Fluids:	1000 LR w 20 mEq KCl @ 100 mL/h
Med[ication]s:	ASA 650 mg PR prn for T > 38.5 °C

Thank you.

   Sign your name/leave space for resident's signature.

   (your beeper number)

   Key: r/o = rule out, q = every, HO = house officer, T = temperature, BP = systolic blood pressure, HR = heart rate, NPO = nothing by mouth (this includes water and pills), ASA = aspirin, PR = per rectum, prn = as needed. Other useful abbreviations: OOB = out of bed, BRP = bathroom privileges.

   Note: You cannot be too polite or too grateful to patients or nurses.

History and Physical Exam (H&P)

Mrs. O'Flaherty is a 55 y/o w/w [white woman] admitted with a cc [chief complaint]: "My stomach hurts." Pt [patient] was in usual state of excellent health until 2 days PTA [before admission] when she noted gradual onset of crampy midepigastric pain. Pain is now severe (7/10 = 7 on a scale of 10) and recurring q5min. Pt described + vomiting (+ bile, − blood) [with bile, without blood].

PMH [Past Medical History]

Hosp[italizations]:	Pneumonia (1991)
	Childbirth (1970, 1972)
	Surg[ery]—splenectomy for trauma (1967)
Allergies:	Codeine, shellfish
ETOH [alcohol]:	Social
Tobacco:	1 ppd [pack per day] × 25 years

Box 1-1. Best Approach to Surgical Notes—(Continued)

ROS [Review of Systems]

Resp[iratory]:	Productive cough
Cardiac:	ō chest pain [ō = not observed, noncontributory, or not here]
	ō MI [myocardial infarction]
Renal:	ō dysuria
	ō frequency
Neuro[logic]:	WNL [within normal limits]

Physical Exam (PE)

BP: 140/90	*HR:* 100 (regular)
RR [respiratory rate]: 16 breaths/min	*Temp:* 38.2 °C

WD [well developed], WN [well nourished], mildly obese, 55 y/o in moderate abdominal distress.
      HEENT [head, eyes, ears, nose, and throat]: WNL.

Resp:	Clear lungs bilat[erally]
	ō wheeze
Heart:	ō m [murmur]
Abdomen:	RSR [regular sinus rhythm]
	Mildly distended, crampy, midepigastric pain
	High-pitched rushes that coincide with crampy pain
	Tender to palpation (you do not need to hurt the patient to find this out)
	ō rebound
Rectal:	(Always do; never defer the rectal exam on your surgical rotation)
	Hematest—negative for blood
	No masses, no tenderness
Pelvic:	No masses
	No adnexal tenderness
	No chandelier sign (if motion of cervix makes your patient hit the chandelier)
	No pelvic inflammatory disease (PID; gonorrhea)
Extremities:	Full ROM [range of motion]
	ō edema
	Bounding (3+) pulses
Imp[ression]:	Abdominal pain
	r/o SB [small bowel] obstruction 2° [secondary] to adhesions
Rx (Treatment/Plan):	NG [nasogastric] tube
	IV fluids
	Op[erative] consent
	Type and hold
	[Signature]

Notes on the Surgical H&P

- A surgical H&P should be succinct and focused on the patient's problem.
- Begin with the chief complaint (in the patient's words).
- Is the problem new or chronic?
- PMH: Always include prior hospitalizations and medications.
- ROS: Restrict review to organ systems (lung, heart, kidneys, and nervous system) that may affect this admission.
- PE: Always begin with vital signs (including respiration and temperature); that is why these signs are vital.
- Rebound means inflammatory peritoneal irritation or peritonitis.

Preoperative Note

The preoperative note is a checklist confirming that you and the patient are ready for the planned surgical procedure. Place this note in the Progress Notes:

Preop dx [diagnosis]:	SB obstruction 2° to adhesions
CXR [chest X-ray]:	Clear
ECG [electrocardiogram]:	NSR w/ST-T wave changes
Blood:	Type and crossmatch x 2 u
Consent:	In chart

Continued

Box 1-1. Best Approach to Surgical Notes—(Continued)

Operative Note

The operative note should provide anyone who encounters the patient after surgery with all the needed information:

Preop dx:	SB obstruction
Postop dx:	Same, all bowel viable
Procedure:	Exp[loratory] Lap[arotomy] with lysis of adhesions
Surgeon:	Name him/her
Assistants:	List them
Anesthesia:	GEA [general endotracheal anesthesia]
I&O [intake and output]:	In: 1200 mL Ringer's lactate (r/L)
	Out: 400 mL urine
EBL [estimated blood loss]:	50 mL
Specimen:	None
Drains:	None
	[Sign your name]

CHAPTER 2

PREOPERATIVE EVALUATION

Harry Dym, Naveen Mohan, Joseph Zeidan, A. Omar Abubaker

1. **Which components of the preoperative evaluation are obtained from the patient?**
   Chief complaint, history of present illness, past medical history, family history, surgical history, personal/social history, and review of systems.

2. **What are the goals of the preoperative evaluation?**
   The preoperative evaluation consists of gathering information about the patient and formulating an anesthetic and surgical plan. The overall objective is reduction of perioperative morbidity and mortality.
   Ideally (and through an interview, physical exam, and review of pertinent current and past medical records), the patient's physical and mental status is determined. All recent medications are recorded, and a thorough drug allergy history is taken. The patient should be questioned about use of cigarettes, alcohol, and illicit drugs. The patient's prior anesthetic experience is of particular interest, specifically if there is a history of any anesthetic complications, problems with intubation, delayed emergence, malignant hyperthermia, prolonged neuromuscular blockade, or postoperative nausea and vomiting. From this evaluation, a decision can be made whether any preoperative tests or consultations are indicated, and an anesthetic care plan can be formulated. If done well, the preoperative evaluation establishes a trusting doctor-patient relationship that significantly diminishes patient anxiety and measurably influences postoperative recovery and outcome.

3. **What is the difference between a physical sign and a symptom?**
   In general, a symptom is an abnormal sensation felt by the patient, whereas a sign can be seen, felt, or heard by the examiner.

4. **What is an informed consent?**
   Informed consent is communication with the patient so he or she understands the procedures and the possible intraoperative and postoperative complications, including postoperative pain. The alternatives, potential complications, and risks vs. benefits are discussed, and the patient's questions are answered.

5. **How do you calculate body mass index (BMI)?**
   The BMI is calculated by dividing the weight by height in centimeters (weight in kg/height in cm). The normal BMI is 18.5 to 25, a BMI of 25 to 30 is overweight, and a BMI of >30 is obese.

6. **What is the importance of calculating the BMI for a patient?**
   Being overweight or obese are proven risk factors for diabetes, heart disease, stroke, hypertension, osteoarthritis, and some forms of cancer.

7. **What are the vital signs?**
   Pulse, blood pressure, temperature, and respirations.

8. **Are vital signs really "vital"?**
   Yes. For example, if heart rate and blood pressure are on the wrong side of 100 (heart rate is >100 beats/min, systolic blood pressure is <100 mm Hg), watch out! Also, tachypnea (respiratory rate >16) reflects either pain or systemic acidosis. Temperature, however, is less reliable. Fever may develop late, particularly in the immunosuppressed patient who may be afebrile even in the presence of infection.

9. **What are macules, papules, and nodules?**
   Macules are localized changes in skin color that occur in various shapes, sizes, and colors and are not palpable. Papules are solid and elevated, with a diameter of less than 5 mm. Nodules are also solid and elevated but extend deeper into the skin than papules and usually have diameters greater than 5 mm.

15

10. Which ribs are referred to as "floating" ribs?
   The eleventh and twelfth ribs.

11. Where is the angle of Louis?
   The angle of Louis is located at the junction between the manubrium and the body of the sternum; it marks the articulation of the second rib on the sternum. It is also known as the angle of Ludwig.

12. Where is the intercostal angle?
   The inferior margins of the seventh, eighth, and ninth costicartilages meet in the midline (at the infrasternal notch) to form the intercostal angle. It normally measures less than 90 degrees and is increased in obstructive lung disease.

13. Where on the abdomen is the liver percussed?
   On the upper right quadrant. A liver span of 6 to 12 cm in the midclavicular line is considered normal.

14. What is rebound? What is the significance of rebound tenderness during an abdominal exam?
   Because the peritoneum is well innervated and exquisitely sensitive, pressure on the abdomen of a patient with an inflamed peritoneum can elicit a distinctive tenderness. During an abdominal exam, if you depress the abdomen gently and release and the patient winces, it is an indication that the peritoneum is inflamed (rebound tenderness).

15. What is the significance of abdominal distention?
   Abdominal distention may arise from either intraenteric or extraenteric gas or fluid, or from blood. Abdominal distention is always significant and concerning.

16. Is abdominal palpation important?
   Yes. Tenderness to palpation leads the examiner to the anatomic zone of the diseased area. It is best to start palpation in an area that does not hurt and proceed toward the painful (tender) region.

17. What is the significance of bowel sounds?
   Not unlike other parts of the body, if the part hurts, the patient tends not to use it. Inflamed bowel is less functional and therefore is quiet. Bowel contents squeezed through a partial obstruction produce high-pitched tinkles. However, bowel sounds are not always reliable.

18. What is the Hering-Breuer reflex?
   When the lungs become overly inflated, stretch receptors activate an appropriate feedback response to limit further inspiration. These stretch receptors are located in the walls of the bronchi and bronchioles throughout the lungs that, when overstretched, transmit inhibitory signals through the vagus nerve in the inhibitory center. It seems to be a protective mechanism to prevent overinflation rather than normal control of ventilation.

19. What is a pterygium?
   A raised, yellow plaque, termed the pinguecula, is normal and found on a horizontal plane between the canthus and limbus of the eye. In response to chronic irritation, the pinguecula will grow to extend a vascular membrane, termed pterygium, over the limbus toward the center of the cornea. Vision may become obstructed.

20. What is anisocoria?
   Anisocoria refers to inequality of the pupils. It is a common, normal variation of pupil size but can be an indication of pathology.

21. What are the components of the corneal reflex?
   - Sensory limb: fifth cranial nerve (V2)
   - Motor response: seventh cranial nerve; look for eye blinking

22. What is the oculocardiac reflex?
   The trigeminal-vagal reflex. Pressure applied to the globe or stretching of the extraocular muscles results in 10% to 15% reduction in heart rate. It also can cause junctional rhythm and possible premature ventricular contractions (PVCs). Atropine is not useful in treating this situation.

23. What is the direct light reflex?
   The direct light reflex occurs when a light is shone into the eye to the retina and the pupil constricts (retina-optic nerve-optic tract).

24. **What is the consensual light reflex?**
    The consensual light reflex occurs when a light is shone into the eye to the retina and the pupil of the opposite eye constricts.

25. **What is nystagmus?**
    Nystagmus is an involuntary, rapid, rhythmic movement of the eyeball, which may be horizontal, vertical, rotatory, or mixed. There are various forms of nystagmus, some of which may be indicative of certain diseases of the vestibular system.

26. **What is strabismus?**
    Strabismus is a deviation of the eye that the patient cannot overcome. The visual axis deviates from that required by the physiologic conditions. There are many forms of strabismus, depending on the direction of the strabismus, whether the condition is affecting one eye or both, and the cause of the condition.

27. **What are important features to be aware of during an otoscopic exam?**
    Scaling, cerumen, discharge, lesions, erythema, foreign bodies, and bleeding.

28. **What important anatomic feature is noted just beyond the canal hair in an otoscopic exam?**
    The junction between the lateral cartilaginous canal and the medial bony canal.

29. **When examining the ear, where is the light reflex normally located and what conditions will alter its location or appearance?**
    The light reflex is normally noted at about the five o'clock position. Conditions that can alter its appearance include retracted drumhead, serous otitis, bulging drumhead, air bubbles in serous otitis, and a perforated drumhead.

30. **What is Darwin's tubercle?**
    Darwin's tubercle is a fusiform swelling that occasionally develops on the surface of the pinna above the midpoint of the helix on the ear.

31. **What is the difference between bone conduction and air conduction when applied to tuning fork tests of hearing?**
    Air conduction implies sound transmission through the ear canal, tympanic membrane, and ossicle, to the cochlea, and finally to the eighth, or auditory, nerve. Bone conduction relies on the transmission of sound through the skull to the cochlea and to the auditory nerve.

32. **What is the difference between the Rinne and Weber tests of auditory function?**
    The Rinne test makes use of air conduction and bone conduction, whereas the Weber test makes use of bone conduction. A Rinne test is considered normal or positive when sound is heard better by air conduction than by bone conduction. In a Weber test of hearing, a conductive deafness will cause sound to be referred to the side of the deaf ear. The Weber test checks lateralization.

33. **Where is Erb's point?**
    On the side of the neck where applied pressure on the roots of the fifth and sixth cervical nerves causes paralysis of the brachial muscles. Muscles of the upper arm are involved (e.g., deltoid, biceps, brachialis anterior).

34. **What is the difference between a remittent fever and an intermittent fever?**
    A remittent fever has a diurnal variation of more than 2°F but has no normal readings. Intermittent fever refers to episodes of fever separated by days of normal temperature.

35. **What is quotidian fever?**
    A daily recurring fever often associated with hepatic abscess or acute cholangitis.

36. **What fever pattern is associated with Hodgkin's disease?**
    Pel-Ebstein fever. This pattern describes several days of continuous remittent fever followed by remissions for an irregular number of days.

37. **What are Korotkoff sounds?**
    The sounds produced by the turbulence created when the inflated blood pressure cuff disrupts normal arterial laminar blood flow.

38. **What is the result of using a blood pressure cuff that is too large or too small for the diameter of the patient's arm?**
Too large a cuff will result in an erroneously low pressure recording, whereas too small a cuff will result in an erroneously high measurement.

39. **What standardized screening exam is most often used to evaluate mental status and cognition?**
The Mini-Mental State Examination (MMSE) takes approximately 10 minutes to administer and is used to screen for dementia. The exam measures orientation, registration, attention and calculation, recall, and language. Typically a score greater than 26 indicates normal cognitive function.

40. **What is the difference between Broca and Wernicke aphasias?**
Broca aphasia is an expressive aphasia. The patient's reading and word comprehension are intact; however speech and writing are impaired. Wernicke aphasia is a receptive aphasia. The patient can have fluent speech, however it may be incomprehensible. Reading comprehension and writing are impaired. It is also possible for a patient to have global aphasia, a combination of both types.

41. **What are some of the key differences between delirium and dementia?**
Delirium typically has a sudden onset, symptoms can increase and decrease throughout the day, and can potentially be reversible. It can often have a clear etiology such as medication, alcohol withdrawal, infections, or organ failure. Dementia has a slow onset, symptoms are typically stable, and it is a progressive condition. It is caused by structural diseases of the brain.

42. **If a patient has a Marcus-Gunn pupil, how would the affected pupil respond to light shined in the contralateral pupil?**
The affected pupil would constrict. The swinging light test is used to rule out Marcus-Gunn pupil, or relative afferent pupillary defect. It is most often caused by a lesion of the optic nerve. The efferent limb of the light reflex relayed by the oculomotor nerve is intact. Light sensed by the unaffected eye would result in bilateral pupillary constriction.

43. **In a patient with known trauma to the periorbital region, what is the likely cause of an intraocular pressure of 43 mm Hg?**
The patient likely has orbital compartmental syndrome, possibly caused by a retrobulbar hematoma. A lateral canthotomy would be indicated. The normal IOP range is between 10 and 21 mm Hg. A ruptured globe can cause an abnormally low IOP. Other causes of a high IOP include glaucoma and hyphema.

44. **How are deep tendon reflexes graded?**
0 = no response
1+ = diminished; low normal
2+ = normal
3+ = more brisk than average
4+ = hyperactive

45. **How is the Babinski sign elicited?**
Babinski testing is done by lightly stroking the lateral aspect of the sole of the foot vertically from the heel to the base of the toes. The course of stimulation is changed as you approach the toes by medially directing the path of stimulation along the base of the toes toward the great toe. Normal response is plantar flexion, whereas abnormal response is dorsiflexion of the toe, fanning of the other toes, and dorsiflexion of the ankles.

46. **What is Homans' sign?**
Pain in the calf when the toe is dorsiflexed. This is an early sign of deep venous thrombosis.

47. **What are the ocular manifestations of hypertensive retinopathy?**
Retinal arteriolar narrowing, arteriovenous nicking, opacity of arteriolar wall, hemorrhage, cotton-wool spots, hard exudates, and microaneurysms.

48. **What descriptors are important in a lymph node exam?**
Examination of the lymph nodes should note size, tenderness, shape, and consistency of palpable nodes. It is also important to note if the nodes are fixed, matted, or discrete.

49. **What are the major lymph node groups of the head and neck region?**
Occipital, postauricular, preauricular, parotid/retropharyngeal, submandibular, submental, superficial cervical, posterior cervical, deep cervical, and supraclavicular nodes.

50. **What are the classic symptoms of cardiac disease?**
Chest pain, dyspnea, palpitations, syncope, and edema.

51. **A patient with heart failure typically exhibits what type of edema?**
Edema associated with heart failure is typically pitting edema. The edematous area remains depressed upon palpation with a finger. Peripheral edema is one of the signs of right-sided heart failure.

52. **What are the common locations for detection and evaluation of a pulse? Which pulse is most representative of the aortic pulse?**
Common locations include the carotid, radial, brachial, femoral, popliteal, posterior tibial, and dorsalis pedis. The carotid pulse is the most illustrative of the aortic pulse. The carotid pulse should be the only pulse utilized in detecting cardiovascular anomalies.

53. **At what percent of arterial oxygen saturation will a patient become cyanotic?**
Patients will begin becoming cyanotic around 85% arterial oxygen saturation.

54. **At what level of reduced hemoglobin does a patient become cyanotic?**
$5\,g/dL$.

55. **Which side of the stethoscope is used for high-frequency sounds?**
High-frequency sounds such as such as S_1 and S_2, the murmurs of aortic and mitral regurgitation, and pericardial friction rub are better heard with the diaphragm, while low-frequency sounds such as S_3, S_4, and the diastolic murmur of mitral stenosis are best heard with the bell.

56. **What is the difference between hyperventilation and hyperpnea?**
Hyperventilation is an increase in both rate and depth of respiration, whereas hyperpnea is an increase in depth only.

57. **What is Cheyne-Stokes breathing?**
Cheyne-Stokes breathing is alternating hyperpnea, shallow respiration, and apnea.

58. **What is stridor?**
A high-pitched respiratory sound, such as the inspiratory sound heard often in acute laryngeal obstruction.

59. **When evaluating the pulmonary valve of the heart, where is it best to auscultate?**
The left second intercostal space. The aortic valve is best heard in the right second intercostal space. The tricuspid valve is best heard in the left fourth intercostal space.
    The mitral valve is best heard at the cardiac apex or the point of maximal impulse. This is the location where the cardiac apex, specifically the left ventricle, abuts the chest wall. It is located at the intersection of the midclavicular line and the fourth or fifth intercostal space on the left side.

60. **What is the diaphragmatic effect on the heart?**
During inspiration, the diaphragm descends, stretching the heart from its anchorage in the fascia surrounding the aorta and pulmonary artery. The vertical cardiac axis becomes elongated, the transverse direction narrowed, and filling of the right ventricle is delayed.

61. **When does blood from the coronary arteries perfuse the heart muscle?**
During diastole.

62. **What is the PMI?**
The *point* of *maximum impulse* of the heart. At the beginning of systole, the heart is rotated forward toward the chest wall, where the impulse can be felt. The PMI is normally felt at the fifth interspace between the ribs, 1 to $2\,cm$ medial to the left midclavicular line.

63. **What causes the heart sounds?**
At the beginning of systole, the ventricles contract, increasing the ventricular pressure and causing the mitral and tricuspid valves to close. Blood rebounds in the ventricles, transmitting vibrations to the chest wall, which can be heard with the stethoscope as S_1. Blood then courses silently through

the aorta and pulmonary arteries. The second sound occurs when the ventricles relax in diastole, ventricular pressure decreases, and the aortic and pulmonary valves close. The backflow of blood against these valves sets up another series of vibrations audible as the second heart sound, S_2.

64. **What is the difference between a physiologic and an organic heart murmur?**
Heart murmurs are caused by disruption of the normal laminar flow of blood. Causes include regurgitation of blood, blood flow through narrowed or stenotic valves or vessels, shunting of blood, increased rate of blood flow, and decreased blood viscosity. An organic murmur is pathologic and caused by some intrinsic cardiac disease or defect, such as deformed or stenotic heart valves, ventricular septal defects, or a patent ductus arteriosus. Physiologic murmurs are not pathologic and usually result from an altered metabolic state, such as in pregnancy or early childhood.

65. **What is a flow murmur?**
A flow murmur is induced when the velocity of normal blood is increased as it courses through a normal heart.

66. **What is pulse pressure?**
Pulse pressure is the numeric difference between the systolic and diastolic blood pressures. The normal pulse pressure is in the range of 30 to 40 mm Hg. Causes of an increased or widening pulse pressure include hyperkinetic states (anxiety, fever, exercise, hyperthyroidism), aortic regurgitation, and increased aortic rigidity (aging, atherosclerosis). A decrease or narrowing of the pulse pressure can be caused by obstructed ventricular output, as in aortic stenosis, or decreased stroke volume from shock or heart failure.

67. **What are the grades of intensity of heart murmurs?**
Intensity of heart murmur is graded on a scale of 1 to 6. The subjectivity of this scale is minimized by the following guidelines:
- Grade 1: Very faint and heard only when paying close attention
- Grade 2: Faint, but unmistakably present
- Grade 3: Clearly louder than faint, but not associated with a thrill
- Grade 4: Loud and associated with a thrill
- Grade 5: Very loud but requiring a stethoscope partly on the chest to be heard
- Grade 6: Able to be heard with stethoscope off the chest

68. **What maneuvers or special positions are used to accentuate abnormalities of heart sounds?**
For accentuation of aortic regurgitation, ask the patient to sit up, lean forward, exhale completely, and hold breath in expiration. For accentuating mitral murmurs or S_3, ask the patient to roll onto his or her left side, then listen at the apical area.

69. **What is the difference between stable and unstable angina? How can one differentiate between pain associated with angina versus an acute myocardial infarction?**
Angina pectoris, or chest pain, is a common symptom of obstructive coronary artery disease. Reversible myocardial ischemia causes episodes of angina that are often triggered by physical exertion or stress. Symptoms typically last 2 to 10 minutes and resolve with rest or nitroglycerin administration. Patients with stable angina oftentimes "know their limits" regarding the amount of exertion until symptoms arise. Physical or emotional stress elicits similar symptoms repeatedly. Patients experiencing unstable angina have changes to the pattern of stable angina. Symptoms become more frequent or severe. Symptoms may also arise with lesser exertion or even at rest.
 Pain associated with myocardial infection is typically more severe and longer lasting than angina.

70. **What is pulsus paradoxus?**
Normally, systolic pressure will decrease up to 10 mm Hg on inspiration due to negative pressure in the thorax. Pulsus paradoxus is a condition in which there is a greater decrease with inspiration. This is seen in pericardial tamponade, obstructive pulmonary disease, hypovolemic shock, and pregnancy.

71. **When evaluating a patient's pulse, what are some of the signs of aortic coarctation, aortic stenosis, and aortic regurgitation?**
Coarctation, or narrowing, of the aorta is most commonly found along the aortic arch. To evaluate a patient for this condition, the brachial and femoral pulse must be palpated simultaneously. A clear delay in the peak of the pulse will occur between the brachial pulse and the femoral pulse.

Patients with pronounced aortic stenosis will have a delayed carotid pulse with a small volume. Often there is also a palpable thrill.

Severe aortic regurgitation produces a pulse with a high amplitude. The pulse may abruptly collapse, in turn; this pattern is also known as a "water hammer pulse." This pulse pattern and a high pulse pressure together are highly suggestive of severe aortic stenosis. A slight splitting of the peak of the pulse, or bisferiens pulse, is common in aortic regurgitation also.

72. **What are the heart sounds, and what physiologic event do they correlate with?**
    - S_1: Closure of the atrioventricular valves
    - S_2: Closure of the aortic and pulmonary valves
    - S_3: Oscillation of blood in the ventricles during mid-diastole. Usually associated with heart failure
    - S_4: Abnormal turbulence of blood associated with stiff ventricular walls

73. **What is the STOP-Bang Questionnaire?**
    It is a screening tool developed by anesthesiology for Obstructive Sleep Apnea (OSA). It is a questionnaire about risk factors: snoring, feeling tired, observed apnea, BMI >35, age >50, neck circumference >17″ for males and >16″ for females, and male gender.

74. **What are some complications of OSA?**
    1. Patients with OSA have increased rates of diabetes, hypertension, atrial fibrillation, stroke, heart failure, pulmonary hypertension, and CAD.
    2. Ventilation via mask, direct laryngoscopy, endotracheal intubation, and fiberoptic visualization of the airway are more difficult in patients with OSA.
    3. Such patients are likely to have perioperative airway obstruction, hypoxemia, atelectasis, ischemia, pneumonia, and prolonged hospitalizations.

75. **What time period of smoking cessation reduces the relative risk of cardiac events?**
    Eight weeks. Surprisingly, those who stop smoking for less than 8 weeks have a higher risk than those who continue to smoke.

76. **How long after an acute respiratory illness should elective surgery be delayed?**
    Enough time needs to be permitted to allow recovery of the tracheobronchial mucosa; generally this is 2 to 6 weeks. Mild URIs in adult patients undergoing elective surgeries that do not involve the chest or abdomen do necessitate postponing surgery due to minimal risk.

77. **What information should be gathered in evaluating an asthmatic patient?**
    1. Number of hospitalizations and emergency room visits in the past 2 years related to asthma
    2. Amount of daily inhaler usage
    3. History of steroid or other medication
    4. Aggravating symptoms

78. **What are the lung sounds on auscultation?**
    1. Vesicular: soft or low pitched. Heard through inspiration, continue without pause through expiration, and then fade away about one-third of the way through expiration.
    2. Bronchovesicular: inspiratory and expiratory sounds equal in length, at times separated by a silent interval. Differences in pitch and intensity are often more easily detected during expiration.
    3. Bronchial: louder and higher in pitch, with a short silence between inspiratory and expiratory sounds. Expiratory sounds last longer than inspiratory.

79. **What is egophony?**
    Egophony is heard when asking the patient to say "ee" and is heard as "ay" (E-to-A change), seen in a lobar consolidation from pneumonia.

80. **What is pectoriloquy?**
    Pectoriloquy is increased resonance of the lungs. Whispered sounds are heard louder and clearer.

81. **What is Kussmaul breathing?**
    Kussmaul breathing is a deep and labored breathing often associated with severe metabolic acidosis such as diabetic ketoacidosis (DKA). Hyperventilation by increased rate or depth attempts to reduce carbon dioxide in the blood.

82. **What is visceral pain?**
Visceral pain occurs when hollow abdominal organs such as the intestine or biliary tree contract forcefully or when they are distended or stretched. Solid organs such as the liver can become painful when their capsules are stretched. Visceral pain may be difficult to localize and varies in quality. It may be gnawing, burning, cramping, or aching.

83. **What is parietal pain?**
Parietal pain originates in the parietal peritoneum and is caused by inflammation. It is a steady aching pain that is usually more severe than visceral pain and more precisely localized over the involved structure.

84. **What is a positive Murphy's sign?**
Tenderness in palpating the right upper quadrant while the patient is deeply inspiring, which is a sign of acute cholecystitis.

85. **What are the indications for a definitive airway in a patient who has sustained severe trauma?**
Unconsciousness, maxillofacial injuries, aspiration risk, obstruction risk, apnea, poor respiratory effort, closed head injury, and GCS <8.5.

86. **What are the 5 P's of compartment syndrome?**
    1. Pulselessness
    2. Pallor
    3. Poikilothermia
    4. Pain
    5. Paresthesia

87. **What is the definition of anemia?**
A hemoglobin concentration of less than 14 g/dL in males and 12.3 g/dL in females.

88. **What factors influence the decision to transfuse a surgical patient?**
    1. Estimated blood loss of the procedure
    2. Underlying risk factor for ischemic heart disease

89. **Define each class of hemorrhage and describe symptoms associated with each class.**
    - Class I hemorrhage: Less than 15% of total blood volume has been lost. There are no changes in blood pressure or heart rate. Typically, no treatment is indicated.
    - Class II hemorrhage: Approximately 15% to 30% of total blood volume is lost. Typical signs include tachypnea, tachycardia, and an increased diastolic blood pressure (narrowing of pulse pressure). Urine output may be affected. Resuscitation with crystalloid fluids is recommended.
    - Class III hemorrhage: Approximately 30% to 40% of total blood volume is lost. Significant tachycardia and tachypnea is present. The patient is hypotensive and pulse pressure is decreased. Hypoperfusion is evident including delayed capillary refill, decreased urine output, and changes in mental status. Blood transfusion and/or crystalloid resuscitation is indicated.
    - Class IV hemorrhage: Approximately 40% or greater total blood volume is lost. The patient is severely hypotensive with tachycardia and tachypnea. Signs of class III are magnified. Rapid transfusion of blood is indicated along with emergent surgery to identify and address the source of bleeding.

90. **The American Society of Anesthesiologists (ASA) suggests that the preanesthesia visit include the following:**
    1. An interview with the patient or guardian to establish a medical, anesthesia, and medication history
    2. An appropriate physical examination
    3. Indicated diagnostic testing
    4. Review of diagnostic data (laboratory, ECG, radiographs, consultations)
    5. Assignment of an ASA status score
    6. A formulation and discussion of anesthesia plans with the patient or responsible adult before obtaining informed consent

91. **What is included in the preanesthetic evaluation?**
    1. Examination of airway, heart, lungs
    2. Review of vital signs including oxygen saturation
    3. Measurement of height and weight

92. **What are the two key features of the airway exam?**
They are the oropharynx and mental space.
    The *oropharynx* is examined with the patient in the sitting position, with the neck extended, tongue out, and phonating. The four classes of oropharynx, originally described by Mallampati, are grouped according to visualized structures (Fig. 2-1).
    The **Mallampati** classification of the oropharynx
    - Class I: Soft palate, fauces uvula, anterior and posterior tonsillar pillars
    - Class II: Soft palate, fauces, uvula
    - Class III: Soft palate, base of uvula
    - Class IV: Soft palate only
    The *mental space* is the distance from the thyroid cartilage to the inside of the mentum, measured while the patient sits with the neck in the sniff position. A correlation is found between higher oropharyngeal class and decreased glottic exposure at laryngoscopy. The higher oropharyngeal class combined with a mental space <2 fingerbreadths better predicts increased difficulty with intubation. Other features include diminished neck extension, decreased tissue compliance, large tongue, overbite, large teeth, narrow, high-arched palate, decreased temporomandibular joint mobility, and a short, thick neck.

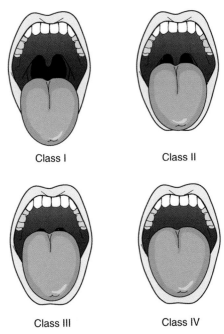

Class I   Class II

Class III   Class IV

Figure 2-1. Mallampati classification of the oropharynx. *(From Phillips N: Berry and Kohn's operating room technique, ed 12, St Louis, 2013, Mosby.)*

93. **What are the recommendations for taking home medications prior to surgery?**
    1. Generally all regular medications are continued.
    2. Beta blockers should be continued for patients who use them to treat angina, symptomatic arrhythmias, or hypertension.
    3. Hold oral hypoglycemic agents 8 hours preoperatively or AM dose.
    4. Hold diuretics AM dose unless prescribed for CHF.
    5. Hold ACE/ARB AM dose unless prescribed for CHF.
    6. Hold insulin AM dose.

94. **What comprises the preoperative evaluation of a diabetic patient?***

How long has the patient had diabetes mellitus? How good is the glycemic control? Patients with frequent insulin reactions and episodes of ketoacidosis (i.e., "brittle" diabetics) are more likely to be metabolically unstable perioperatively. Diabetics with a long history of poor control are also more likely to have end-organ disease. Specifically, the anesthesiologist should look for evidence of coronary disease (often "silent"), hypertension, autonomic neuropathy (check for orthostatic changes in vital signs), renal insufficiency, cardiomyopathy, and gastroparesis (ask about reflux and early satiety). Find out what medications the patient takes for the diabetes, the most recent dose, and current blood sugar. Some diabetics may have diminished neck extension owing to atlantooccipital involvement with the stiff joint syndrome.

Serious preoperative metabolic derangements are seen more often in insulin-dependent diabetic patients, especially in the setting of trauma or infection. Look for high or low glucose levels, electrolyte abnormalities, ketoacidosis, hypovolemia, and hyperosmolarity.

Preoperative testing should include, at a minimum, glucose, electrolytes, blood urea nitrogen, creatinine, urinalysis, and electrocardiogram. Additional lab work might include arterial blood gas, ketones, osmolarity, calcium, phosphorus, and magnesium.

95. **What are the recommendations for diabetic patients?**
    1. Type 1 and type 2 diabetics should discontinue intermittent short-acting insulin.
    2. Patients with insulin pumps continue their lowest basal rate.
    3. Type 1 diabetics take a small amount (⅓ to ½) of their intermediate to long-acting morning insulin on the day of surgery to avoid ketoacidosis.
    4. Type 2 diabetics take none or up to ½ dose of intermediate to long-acting insulin the day of the operation.
    5. Ultrashort-acting insulin such as glargine insulin can be taken as scheduled.
    6. Metformin does not need to be discontinued before the day of surgery and will not cause hypoglycemia during fasting periods of 1 to 2 days. There is no risk for lactic acidosis in patients with functioning liver and kidneys.
    7. Oral hypoglycemic drugs are generally withheld on the day of surgery to avoid hypoglycemia.

96. **What are some of the cardiac assessments for preoperative evaluation?**

For predicting perioperative events, poor exercise tolerance has been defined as the inability to walk four blocks, climb two flights of stairs, or meet four METS (carrying 15 to 20 lbs) due to dyspnea, angina, or fatigue.

97. **What are the definitions for risk stratification?**
    1. Surgical risk:
       a. Low risk: Endoscopic procedure, superficial procedure, cataract surgery, breast surgery
       b. Intermediate risk: Peritoneal/thoracic surgery, carotid endarterectomy, head and neck surgery, orthopedic surgery, prostate surgery
       c. High risk: Emergent, aortic/major vascular, peripheral vascular, anticipated prolonged procedure associated with large fluid shifts and/or blood loss
    2. Patient risk:
       a. Low risk: Health with no medical problems (ASA I) or well-controlled chronic conditions (ASA II)
       b. High risk: Multiple medical comorbidities not well controlled (ASA III) or extremely compromised function secondary to comorbidities (ASA IV)

98. **Which tests are needed prior to surgery?**
    1. Patients who are scheduled for outpatient surgery or low-risk surgery generally do not require any preoperative testing.
    2. For patients scheduled for low or intermediate risk surgery:
       a. Hb/HCT only if there are clinical signs of anemia or anticipated major intraoperative blood loss (>500 cc)
       b. Urine pregnancy test the morning of surgery on any menstruating female
       c. ECG on any patient with the following history: ischemic heart disease, compensated or prior heart failure, diabetes mellitus, renal insufficiency, and cerebrovascular disease, and the patient is having intermediate- or high-risk surgery
       d. No CXR unless a history of significant pulmonary dysfunction with no previous CXR for one year
       e. No PT/PTT unless a history of bleeding, easy bruising, or known liver disease

*Reprinted from Role PA, Galloway FM: The preoperative evaluation. In Duke J, editor: *Anesthesia secrets*, ed 2, Philadelphia, 2000, Hanley & Belfus.

99. **What is the American Society of Anesthesiologists (ASA) Classification?**
    - ASA I: Healthy patient
    - ASA II: A patient with mild systemic disease
    - ASA III: A patient with severe systemic disease
    - ASA IV: A patient with severe systemic disease that is a constant threat to life
    - ASA V: Moribund, not expected to live >24 hours regardless of the operation
    - ASA VI: A declared brain-dead patient whose organs are being removed for donor purposes

100. **Which conditions identified at preoperative evaluation most commonly result in changes in the anesthetic care plan?**
    The conditions identified at preoperative evaluation that most commonly result in changes in the anesthetic care plan are gastric reflux, Type 1 diabetes mellitus, asthma, and suspected difficult airway.

101. **Which patients are at higher risk for aspiration?**
    Higher risk patients are those with any degree of gastrointestinal obstruction, a history of gastroesophageal reflux, diabetes (gastroparesis), recent solid-food intake, abdominal distention (obesity, ascites), pregnancy, depressed consciousness, or recent opioid administration (decreased gastric emptying). In addition, nasooropharyngeal or upper gastrointestinal bleeding, airway trauma, and emergency surgery are high-risk settings.

102. **How are patients with Gastroesophygeal Reflex Disease (GERD) managed?**
    - NPO 6 to 8 hours prior
    - Careful anesthesia planning to avoid aspiration
    - Poorly controlled GERD should be delayed until better control
    - Preanesthesia H2 blockers
    - Rapid sequence intubation with cricoid pressure
    - Postoperative suctioning with an NG tube

103. **What is the role of renal disease in perioperative management of the patient?**
    Renal disease is associated with hypertension, cardiovascular disease, excessive intravascular volume, electrolyte disturbances, and metabolic acidosis, and oftentimes the amount and type of drugs administered must be altered.

104. **When should dialysis be performed in elective cases?**
    Dialysis should be performed within 24 hours of surgery, but not immediately before to avoid acute volume depletion and electrolyte alterations.

105. **What are the perioperative considerations for diabetic patients?**
    1. Diabetic patients are at risk for multiorgan dysfunction, with renal insufficiency, strokes, peripheral neuropathies, visual impairment, and cardiovascular disease.
    2. Chronically poor control increases comorbid conditions such as vascular disease, heart failure, and infections.
    3. Targeting control in the immediate perioperative period likely will not have a substantial impact on outcomes in a diabetic having surgery.
    4. Diabetic ketoacidosis and hypoglycemia are the only conditions that absolutely warrant perioperative intervention.

106. **What is the significance of runny nose and postnasal drip in a child before an elective surgery with general anesthesia or deep sedation? Should you postpone surgery?**
    It has been shown that viral upper respiratory tract infections (URIs) are associated with intraoperative and postoperative bronchospasm, laryngospasm, and hypoxia because of their effect on the quality and quantity of airway secretions and increased airway reflexes to mechanical, chemical, or irritant stimulation. In addition, there is evidence that the risk of pulmonary complications may remain high for at least 2 weeks, and possibly 6 to 7 weeks, after a URI. Accordingly, some recommend avoiding anesthesia whenever possible for at least several weeks after a URI. However, in most children, it is generally agreed that chronic nasal discharge poses no significant anesthesia risk. In contrast, children with severe URI or lower respiratory tract infections almost always have their elective surgery postponed. Probably most anesthesiologists will proceed to surgery with a child with a resolving, uncomplicated URI, unless the child has a history of asthma or other significant pulmonary disease.

107. What particular medical and anesthetic problems are associated with obesity?*
Obesity is defined as excess body weight >20% over the predicted ideal body weight. Obese patients have a higher incidence of diabetes, hypertension, and cardiovascular disease. There is a higher incidence of difficulty with both mask ventilation and intubation. They have a decreased functional residual capacity, increased O_2 consumption and CO_2 production, and, often, diminished ventilation ranging from mild ventilation-perfusion mismatch to actual obesity-hypoventilation and obstructive sleep apnea (pickwickian syndrome). These changes result in more rapid apneic desaturation. If the patients are pickwickian, they may have pulmonary hypertension with or without right ventricular failure. Increased intraabdominal pressure is associated with hiatal hernia and reflux. Because of their higher gastric volume and lower pH, obese patients are at greater risk for aspiration. Pharmacokinetics for many anesthetic agents are altered in them. Finally, regional anesthesia is more difficult and more often unsuccessful.

108. How long should a patient fast before surgery?
Current guidelines for adults with no risk factors for aspiration include no solid food for 6 to 8 hours; oral preoperative medications may be taken up to 1 to 2 hours before anesthesia with sips of water. Current fasting guidelines for pediatric patients are:
- Clear liquids up to 2 hours preoperatively in newborns to age 6 months
- Solid foods, including milk, up to 4 hours preoperatively in newborns to age 6 months; up to 6 hours in children ages 6 months to 3 years; and up to 8 hours in children older than age 3

BIBLIOGRAPHY

Abrams J: Physical examination of the heart and circulation. In Rosendorff C, editor: *Essential cardiology: principles and practice*, ed 2, Totowa, NJ, 2005, Humana Press.
Awtry EH, Loscalzo J: Evaluation of the patient with cardiovascular disease. In Andreoli TE, Carpenter CCJ, Griggs RC, Loscalzo J, editors: *Cecil essentials of medicine*, ed 6, Philadelphia, 2004, Saunders.
Barber HD, Matheson JD, Fonseca R: *Oral and maxillofacial surgery*, ed 2, St. Louis, 2009, Saunders Elsevier.
Bates B, Bickley L, Hoekelman R: *A guide to physical examination and history taking*, ed 6, Philadelphia, 1995, J.B. Lippincott.
Bickley L: *Bates guide to physical examination & history taking*, ed 8, Philadelphia, 2003, Lippincott Williams & Wilkins.
Giglio JA, Abubaker AO: Preoperative evaluation. In Abubaker AO, Benson KJ, editors: *Oral and maxillofacial surgery secrets*, ed 2, St Louis, Missouri, 2007, Mosby/Elsevier.
Handler B: History and physical examination. In Kwon PH, Laskin DM, editors: *Clinician's manual of oral and maxillofacial surgery*, ed 2, Carol Stream, Ill, 1997, Quintessence.
Longo D, Fauci A, et al.: *Harrisons Principles of internal medicine*, ed 18, New York, 2011, McGraw-Hill Professional.
Miller RD, Pardo M: *Basics of anesthesia*, ed 6, Philadelphia, 2011, Elsevier Saunders.
Powell J, Moe J, Steed MB: Surgical ophthalmologic examination, *Oral Maxillofac Surg Clin North Am* 24:557–572, 2012.
Role PA, Galloway FM: The preoperative evaluation. In Duke J, editor: *Anesthesia secrets*, ed 2, Philadelphia, 2000, Hanley & Belfus.
Sarin EL, Moore JB: Initial assessment. In Harken AH, Moore EE, editors: *Abernathy's surgical secrets*, ed 5, Philadelphia, 2005, Mosby.
Seidel HM, Ball JW, Dains JE, et al.: *Mosby's guide to physical examination*, ed 7, St. Louis, 2011, Mosby Elsevier.
Seidel HM, Ball JW, Dains JE, et al.: *Mosby's guide to physical examination*, ed 6, St Louis, 2006, Mosby.
Swank KM: Preoperative evaluation. In Duke J, editor: *Anesthesia secrets*, ed 3, Philadelphia, 2006, Mosby.

---

*Reprinted from Role PA, Galloway FM: The preoperative evaluation. In Duke J, editor: *Anesthesia secrets*, ed 2, Philadelphia, 2000, Hanley & Belfus.

ELECTROCARDIOGRAM

Richard D'Innocenzo, Ruben Figueroa, T.J. Dyer

1. **What are the components of an electrocardiogram (ECG)? How do they relate to the physiology of the myocardium?**

   The ECG tracing is a recording of the summed electrical vectors produced during depolarization and repolarization of the heart. Electrical forces directed toward an electrode are represented as positive forces (upward deflections), whereas forces directed away from an electrode are represented as negative forces (downward deflections).

   The standard representation of the cardiac cycle is seen in the ECG as the P wave, the QRS complex, and the T wave. These waves and complexes are separated by regularly occurring intervals.

   The **P wave** represents atrial depolarization and contraction. It originates in the sinoatrial (SA) node. Usually, depolarization is noted on an ECG with repolarization usually too small or obscured by other waves. Normal is <0.12 seconds. The **PR interval** represents conduction of an impulse through the atrioventricular (AV) node. Normal is <0.2 seconds. The **QRS complex** represents the electrical activity of ventricular depolarization and contraction. Normal is <0.12 seconds. The **ST segment** represents the maintenance depolarization of the ventricles. The **T wave** represents electrical repolarization of the ventricles and is not associated with any physical event (Fig. 3-1).

2. **How does the ECG pattern relate to the cardiac cycle?**

   The electrical impulse that is generated precedes the myocardial contraction that it stimulates (Fig. 3-2).

   S1: Closure of the mitral valve

   S2: Closure of the aortic valve

   S3: In older adults, usually indicates a change in ventricular compliance that is pathologic

   S4: Usually not heard but marks atrial contraction in normal healthy patients. It can also represent a pathologic change in ventricular compliance.

   P wave: Atrial depolarization

   QRS complex: Ventricular depolarization

   T wave: Ventricular repolarization

3. **What is the function of the sinus node (SA), atrioventricular node (AV), and conduction fibers?**

   The SA node is the main pacemaker of the heart. The SA node fires at the beginning of the P wave in the ECG, and we assume that atrial contraction begins at the peak of the P wave. The intrinsic SA node rate is 60 to 100 beats/min. The atrial electrical conduction reaches the AV node and is insulated from the rest of the ventricles.

   The AV node provides the necessary electrical conduction delay to give time for the ventricles to fill with blood before ventricular contraction. The AV node fires intrinsically at about 60 beats/min.

   From the AV node and bundle of His, the electrical current reaches the left and right bundle branches within the ventricular septum and then to the Purkinje system, depolarizing the entire ventricle. Ventricles depolarized intrinsically around 30 to 40 beats/min (Fig. 3-3).

4. **When analyzing ECGs, what are the five factors to consider?**
   - Rate
   - Rhythm
   - Axis
   - Hypertrophy
   - Infarction

5. **What are the markings of an ECG?**

   1 small square (light lines) = 1 mm = 1 mV = 0.04 seconds

   1 large square (dark lines) = 5 mm = 5 mV = 0.2 seconds

   Normal paper speed = 25 mm/s

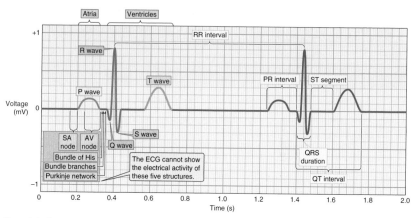

Figure 3-1. Components of the electrocardiogram (ECG) recording. AV, atrioventricular; SA, sinoatrial. *(From Boron WF: Medical physiology, updated ed 2, Philadelphia, 2011, Saunders.)*

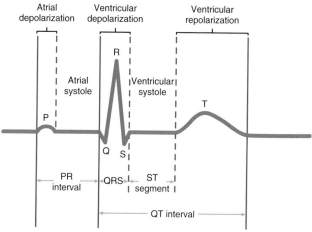

Figure 3-2. Normal EKG waveforms, intervals, and correlation with events of the cardiac cycle. The P wave represents atrial depolarization, followed immediately by atrial systole. The QRS represents ventricular depolarization, followed immediately by ventricular systole. The ST segment corresponds to phrase 2 of the action potential, during which time the heart muscle is completely depolarized and contraction normally occurs. The T wave represents ventricular repolarization. The PR interval, measured from the beginning of the P wave to the beginning of the QRS, corresponds to atrial depolarization and impulse delay in the atrioventricular (AV) node. The QT interval, measured from the beginning of the QRS complex to the end of the T wave, represents the time from initial depolarization of the ventricles to the end of ventricular repolarization. *(From Urden LD, Stacy KM, Lough ME: Critical care nursing: diagnosis and management, ed 7, St Louis, 2014, Mosby.)*

6. **How do I determine the heart rate from an ECG?**
   The distance between the heavy lines represents 1/300 min. So two 1/300-min units = 2/300 min = 1/150 min (or 150/min rate), and three 1/300 units = 3/300 min = 1/100 min (or 100/min rate). So, to determine the actual rate, find the R wave nearest the dark line and then count the dark lines until the next R wave. If the R wave falls on the next dark line, the rate is 300; if it falls on the second dark line, the rate is 150; if it falls on the third dark line, the rate is 100, and so on (Fig. 3-4).

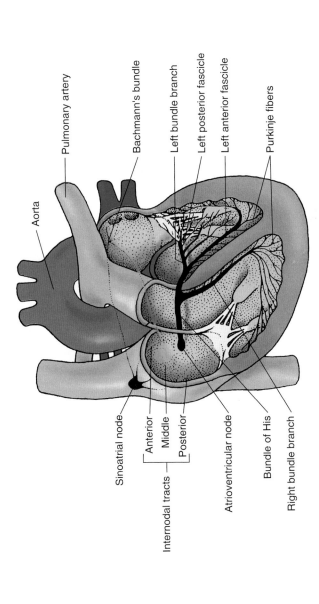

Figure 3-3. Conduction system of the heart. *(From Ignatavicius DD, Workman ML: Medical-Surgical Nursing: Critical Thinking for Collaborative Care, ed 5, St. Louis, 2006, Saunders.)*

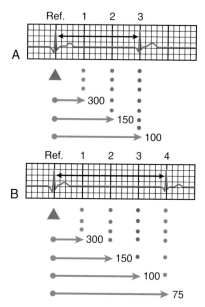

Figure 3-4. Determining heart rate-sequence method. To measure the ventricular rate, find a QRS complex that falls on a heavy dark line. Count 300, 150, 100, 75, 50 until a second QRS complex occurs. This will be the heart rate. **A,** Heart rate = 100 beats/min. **B,** Heart rate = 75 beats/min. *(From Crawford MV, Spence MI: Commonsense approach to coronary care, rev ed 6, St Louis, 1994, Mosby.)*

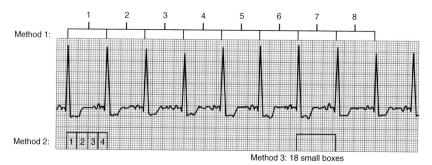

Figure 3-5. Calculating heart rate. Method 1: Number of R-R Intervals in 6 seconds × 10 (e.g., 8 × 10 = 80/min). Method 2: Number of large boxes between QRS complexes divided into 300 (e.g., 300 divided by 4 = 75/min). Method 3: Number of small boxes between QRS complexes divided by 1500 (e.g., 1500 divided by 18 = 84/min). *(From Urden LD, Stacy KM, Lough ME: Critical care nursing: diagnosis and management, ed 7, St Louis, 2014, Mosby.)*

Alternatively, the rate can be determined by multiplying the number of beats in 6-second strips (two 3-second marks) by 10, or through another method in which the number of small boxes between QRS complexes is divided by 1500 (Fig. 3-5).

7. **How do I determine the axis of the heart's electrical impulse?**
   Lead I and aVF are perpendicular to each other and are used to determine axis. Lead I flows from right to left, and lead aVF flows from superior to inferior. Remember, the more positive the deflection in each lead indicates the axis following in the same direction. A normal axis (−30 to +90 degrees) will have positive defections in both leads I and aVF. Left axis deviation (−30 to −90 degrees)

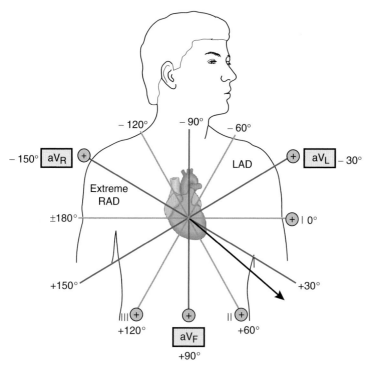

Figure 3-6. Determination of electrical axis. *(From Beachey W:* Respiratory Care Anatomy and Physiology: Foundations for Clinical Practice, *ed 2, St. Louis, Mosby, 2007.)*

demonstrates positive deflection in lead I and negative deflection in aVF. Differentials for left axis deviation may include left ventricular hypertrophy or bundle branch block. Right axis deviation (+90 to ±180 degrees) demonstrates negative deflection in lead I and positive deflection in aVF. Differentials for right axis deviation may include right ventricular hypertrophy, lateral wall MI, or left posterior fascicular block. Extreme right axis deviation is negative in both leads I and aVF and is rare (Fig. 3-6).

8. **Can the ECG provide information about the contractility of the myocardium?**
   No. To determine the effectiveness of the heart's mechanical activity, the patient's blood pressure and pulse need to be assessed.

9. **What do the various types of PR intervals indicate?**
   The *normal* PR interval (<0.2 seconds) represents the lag in electrical conduction through the AV node. It allows time for ventricular filling. A *narrow* PR interval (<0.12 seconds) may reveal accelerated AV conduction (as in Wolff-Parkinson-White syndrome) or premature junctional complexes. *Wide* PR intervals (>0.2 seconds) indicate first-degree AV block. *Progressively lengthening* PR intervals indicate second-degree AV block or multifocal atrial tachycardia.

10. **If the AV junction paces the heart, how will the P wave appear on the ECG?**
    The electrical impulse that is produced will travel in a retrograde direction to activate the atria. In leads II, III, and aVF, the P wave will be inverted if present, and it will be seen before the QRS complex if the atria depolarize before the ventricles. If the ventricles and atria depolarize at the same time, the P wave will not be visualized, as it will be buried in the QRS complex. If the atria depolarize after the ventricles, the P wave will appear after the QRS complex or can present as a distortion of the end of the QRS complex (Fig. 3-7).

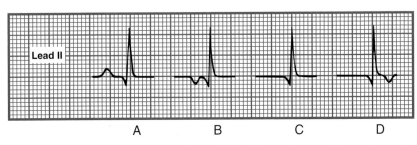

A   B   C   D

Figure 3-7. A, With a sinus rhythm, the P wave is positive (*upright*) in lead II because the wave of depolarization is moving toward the positive electrode. The P wave associated with a junctional beat (in lead II) may be **B,** inverted (*retrograde*) and appear before the QRS; **C,** be hidden by the QRS; or **D,** appear after the QRS. *(From Grauer K: A practical guide to ECG interpretation, ed 2, St Louis, 1998, Mosby.)*

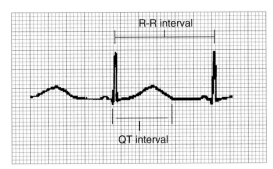

Figure 3-8. Measuring the QT, and R-R intervals. *(From Jenkins D, Gerred SJ: ECGs by Example, ed 3, Edinburgh, 2011, Churchill Livingstone.)*

11. **What is a corrected QT interval?**
    Due to the variability of the QT interval with the patient's heart rate, the QT interval can be measured more accurately if it is corrected for the patient's heart rate. The corrected QT interval is calculated as the measured QT interval divided by the square root of the R-R interval and is noted as QTc. It is considered prolonged if it is 0.45 seconds or longer in men, and 0.46 seconds or longer in women. A QTc of 0.50 seconds or longer is associated with a higher risk of ventricular dysrhythmias.

12. **How can one determine if the QT interval is prolonged, and what is the significance of a prolonged QT interval?**
    The QT interval represents ventricular depolarization through repolarization.
    The QT interval is measured from the Q wave to the end of the T wave. If the Q wave is not present, then measure from the beginning of the R wave. The QT interval will shorten when the heart rate increases and lengthen when the heart rate slows. To quickly estimate the QT interval, measure the interval between two consecutive R waves. If the measured QT interval is less than half of the R-R interval of that QRS complex and the R wave of the following complex, it is most likely normal, as long as the heart rate is less than 95 beats/min. If the QT interval is more than half the R-R interval, it is probably prolonged. A prolonged QT interval is associated with a greater risk of ventricular dysrhythmias, such as torsades de pointes (Figs. 3-8 and 3-9).

13. **What is the meaning of narrow and wide QRS complexes?**
    The width of the QRS complex could be used to categorize tachycardia on the electrocardiogram. Narrow QRS complex arrhythmias (<80 ms) means rapid activation of the ventricles via the His-Purkinje system, suggesting supraventricular arrhythmia (e.g., supraventricular tachycardia). Wide QRS complex (>80 ms) is secondary to slow ventricular activation.

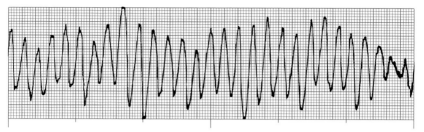

Figure 3-9. Polymorphic ventricular tachycardia. *(From Aehlert B: ECGs made easy, ed 5, St Louis, 2013, Elsevier.)*

The arrhythmia originates below the His bundle (e.g., ventricular tachycardia). The impulse originates from an ectopic site within the ventricle and takes longer to activate the entire mass of the ventricle.

There are exceptions like aberrant supraventricular tachycardia, which can produce a widened QRS if there are either preexisting or rate-related abnormalities within the His-Purkinje system (e.g., supraventricular tachycardia with aberrancy) or if conduction occurs over an accessory pathway. Thus, wide QRS complex tachycardias may be either supraventricular or ventricular in origin.

14. **What is a Q wave, and when is it significant?**
   The Q wave is the first downward stroke of the QRS complex. An insignificant Q wave is less than 0.04 seconds and represents mid-septal depolarization. A significant Q wave indicates necrosis and is diagnostic for an infarction. For a Q wave to be significant, it must be at least 0.04 seconds or one-third of the entire QRS amplitude.

15. **What medications can cause a prolonged QT interval?**
   Medications are a common cause of a prolonged QT interval. The major classes of drugs include:
   - Antiarrhythmics (e.g., quinidine, sotalol, dofetilide, amiodarone, disopyramide)
   - Certain antihistamines (terfenadine, astemizole)
   - Certain antibiotics (fluoroquinolones, macrolides, metronidazole)
   - Certain psychotropic medications (some antipsychotics, some SSRIs, and tricyclic antidepressants)
   - Analgesics/sedatives: methadone, oxycodone, chloral hydrate
   - Certain gastric motility agents (cisapride)

   There are many drugs that cause prolonged QT interval, and the list is constantly expanding. All medications should be carefully scrutinized for potential QT interval prolongation as a side effect.

16. **What is a U wave, and when is it clinically significant?**
   A U wave represents repolarization of the Purkinje fibers, and it may be occasionally seen following the T wave on an ECG. When seen, the amplitude of a normal U wave should be approximately 11% of the preceding T wave amplitude. Tall U waves may be caused by CNS disease, electrolyte imbalances, hyperthyroidism, long QT syndrome, or certain medications (e.g., amiodarone, digitalis, procainamide, phenothiazines). Inverted U waves in leads V2 to V5 are abnormal and may be seen in ischemic heart disease. In hypokalemia, as serum potassium continues to drop below normal levels, the T waves on an ECG flatten or become inverted, and a U wave may appear.

17. **What is the J point on an ECG, and can you explain its significance?**
   The J point on an ECG is the point where the QRS complex and ST segment meet. The J point is significant in the identification of ST elevation or depression. To evaluate for ST elevation or depression, first identify the J point. Then use the TP segment to evaluate its position in relation to the isoelectric line. ST depression of more than 0.5 mm in leads V2 and V3, or more than 1.0 mm in all other leads, is suggestive of MI. ST elevation for acute injury can vary from 0.5 to 2.5 mm, depending on age, gender, and ECG lead (Fig. 3-10).

18. **What disorders can be evaluated perioperatively by the ECG?**
   Preoperative ECG, when indicated, can be used to evaluate and help diagnose the following conditions:
   - Conduction abnormalities (AV blocks, premature atrial contractions [PACs], premature ventricular contractions [PVCs])

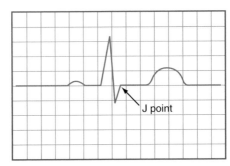

Figure 3-10. Normal position of the J point. *(Modified from Urden LD, Stacy KM, Lough ME:* Critical care nursing: diagnosis and management, *ed 7, St Louis, 2014, Mosby.)*

- Myocardial ischemia
- Myocardial infarctions
- Ventricular and atrial hypertrophy
- Pacemaker function
- Preexcitation (e.g., Wolff-Parkinson-White syndrome)
- Drug toxicity (digitalis, antiarrhythmics, tricyclic antidepressants)
- Electrolyte abnormalities (e.g., disturbances in calcium, potassium)
- Various medical conditions (e.g., pericarditis, hypothermia, pulmonary emboli, cor pulmonale, cerebrovascular accidents, increased intracranial pressure)

19. **Who should have a preoperative 12-lead ECG?**
    For the most part, this depends on many factors, including the clinical presentation of the patient and the individual hospital regulations. However, it is generally agreed that the following patients may benefit from a preoperative 12-lead ECG to fully assess the surgical and anesthetic risks of these patients:
    - Any patient older than age 50, or any patient older than age 40 when risk factors are present
    - Any other patient who has signs or symptoms of cardiac disease
    - Patients with prior history of cardiac ischemia, dysrhythmias, or pacemaker placement
    - Patients with history of cocaine use who are to undergo a procedure under general anesthesia

20. **Why is lead II used for monitoring intravenous sedation?**
    Lead II is good for monitoring P waves, dysrhythmias, and inferior ischemia. Lead II is appropriate for monitoring ASA I and ASA II patients.

21. **What are some of the causes of intraoperative artifact on ECG monitoring?**
    Artifact can mimic cardiac dysrhythmias. It can be caused by loose electrodes, poor electrical contact, broken lead wires, patient movement, shivering, and 60-cycle interference.

22. **What are tachycardia and bradycardia?**
    Sinus tachycardia indicates a rate >100 beats/min, and bradycardia is a rate <60 beats/min.

23. **What are typical ECG signs of ischemia, injury, and infarction?**
    Ischemia shows inverted T waves in the leads nearest the part of the affected myocardium most easily identified in the chest leads. ST depression may also be seen. *Injury* to heart muscle is indicated by ST elevation and tall, positive T waves. *Infarction* shows Q waves that are 0.04 seconds or longer or greater than one-third the size of the entire QRS complex. Location can be determined from the lead. Anterior leads show Q waves in V1 and V2; inferior leads in II, III, and aVF; and lateral leads in I, aVL, V5, and V6 (Table 3-1).

24. **How do potassium and calcium affect the ECG?**
    Hypokalemia causes U waves (small, positive deflections following T waves). Hypokalemia may also be seen as ST depression and flat T waves. Hyperkalemia causes tall, narrow, peaked T waves, QRS widening, and P wave flattening and can progress to ventricular fibrillation. Hypocalcemia causes prolonged QT intervals. Finally, hypercalcemia causes shortened QT intervals, with or without ST segment elevation (Figs. 3-11 to 3-15).

Table 3-1. Localization of a Myocardial Infarction

LOCATION OF MI	LEAD CHANGES	AFFECTED CORONARY ARTERY
Anterior	V3, V4	Left coronary artery
		*LAD: diagonal branch
Anteroseptal	V1, V2, V3, V4	Left coronary artery
		*LAD: diagonal branch
		*LAD: septal branch
Anterolateral	I, aVL, V3, V4, V5, V6	Left coronary artery
		*LAD: diagonal branch
		*Circumflex branch
Inferior	II, III, aVF	Right coronary artery
		*Posterior descending branch
		Left coronary artery
		*Circumflex branch
Lateral	I, aVL, V5, V6	Left coronary artery
		*LAD: diagonal branch
		*Circumflex branch
		Right coronary artery
Septum	V1, V2	Left coronary artery
		*LAD: septal branch
Posterior	V7, V8, V9	Right coronary or circumflex artery

Modified from Aehlert B: *ECGs made easy,* ed 5, St Louis, 2013, Elsevier.

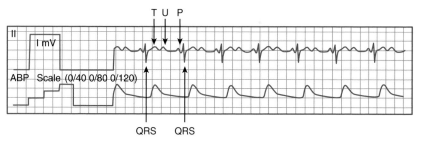

Figure 3-11. ECG tracing from a patient with hypokalemia. *(Modified from Urden LD, Stacy KM, Lough ME: Critical care nursing: diagnosis and management, ed 7, St Louis, 2014, Mosby.)*

25. **What is Wolff-Parkinson-White (WPW) syndrome?**
    WPW presents an abnormal ECG pattern caused by the presence of an accessory pathway that bypasses the AV node. Early depolarization of the ventricles produces the following ECG characteristics (Fig. 3-16):
    - Wide QRS complex
    - Shorter PR interval, as a result of early depolarization of the ventricles
    - Delta wave, which is seen in the upstroke of the QRS complex

26. **How is digitalis toxicity seen on ECG?**
    Digitalis toxicity has several ECG manifestations, including SA and AV node blocks, tachycardia, PVCs, ventricular tachycardia, atrial fibrillation, and possible sloping of the ST segment.

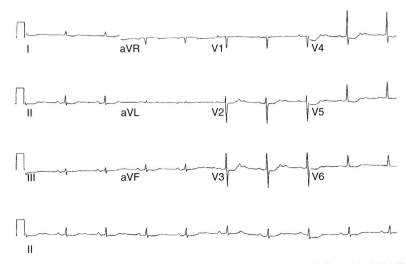

Figure 3-12. ECG of a patient presenting with hypokalemia. Note the prominent U wave after the T wave in leads V2 to V6. *(From Duke JC, Keech BM: Anesthesia secrets, ed 5, Philadelphia, 2016, Saunders.)*

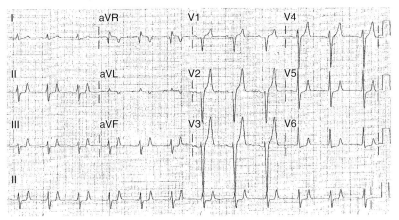

Figure 3-13. ECG of a patient presenting with hyperkalemia. Note the peaked T waves. *(From Duke JC, Keech BM: Anesthesia secrets, ed 5, Philadelphia, 2016, Saunders.)*

27. **What is the ECG manifestation of hypothermia?**
    Hypothermia is seen on ECG as sinus bradycardia, AV junctional rhythm, or ventricular fibrillation. Typically, there is an elevated J point, and there may be an intraventricular conduction delay and prolonged QT interval.

28. **What are some of the common causes of PVCs?**
    Caffeine ingestion, anxiety, acid-base imbalance, ischemic heart disease, hypoxia, valvular heart disease, heart failure, electrolyte imbalance, smoking, drug toxicity, cardiomyopathy, and medications.

29. **What is the significance when the R wave of a PVC falls on the T wave of the preceding beat?**
    There is a possibility that the PVC can precipitate VT or VF if it occurs during this period of the cardiac cycle, associated with the relative refractory period. This is referred to as the R-on-T phenomenon.

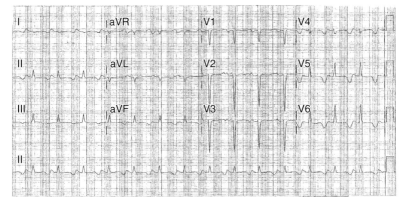

Figure 3-14. ECG of a patient presenting with hypocalcemia. The QT interval is prolonged. *(From Duke J: Anesthesia secrets, ed 4, Philadelphia, 2011, Mosby.)*

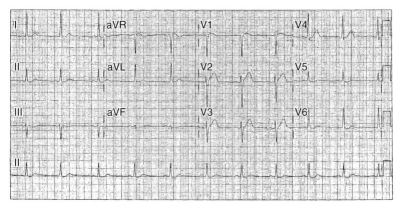

Figure 3-15. ECG of a patient presenting with hypercalcemia. The QT interval is shortened, and the ST-T segment is elevated. *(From Duke J: Anesthesia secrets, ed 4, Philadelphia, 2011, Mosby Elsevier.)*

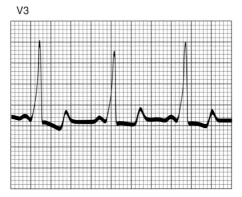

Figure 3-16. Typical Wolff-Parkinson-White (WPW) syndrome pattern showing the short PR interval, delta wave, wide QRS complex, and secondary ST segment and T wave changes. *(From Surawicz B, Knilans TK: Chou's electrocardiography in clinical practice: adult and pediatric, ed 6, Philadelphia, 2008, Saunders.)*

30. **What are some of the causes of ST segment elevation?**
    All of the following can lead to ST segment elevation: normal variant, acute ST segment elevation myocardial infarction, early repolarization pattern, hypercalcemia, hyperkalemia, pericarditis, Brugada syndrome, left bundle branch block, and left ventricular hypertrophy.

31. **What is Brugada syndrome?**
    Brugada syndrome is a hereditary condition caused by dysfunctional cardiac sodium channels responsible for nearly one-half of sudden death in healthy individuals without structural heart disease. It is characterized by a right bundle branch block (RBBB) and ST elevation in leads V1 to V3, with a peaked downsloping shape in the elevated ST segments.

32. **Can you describe bundle branch block?**
    Bundle branch block is impairment of conduction in either the left or right bundle system that leads to a wide QRS interval. With complete bundle branch block, the QRS interval would be >0.12 seconds. Incomplete bundle branch block is between 0.10 and 0.12 seconds. The orientation of the QRS vector is usually in the direction of the myocardial area where depolarization is delayed. In RBBB, the QRS vector is oriented to the right and anteriorly. Note the presence of a secondary R wave (R′) in V1 and slurred S wave in lead V6. In left bundle branch block (LBBB), the QRS vector is directed to the left and posteriorly. LBBB generates predominantly negative QS complexes in lead V1 and positive R complexes in lead V6 (Fig. 3-17).

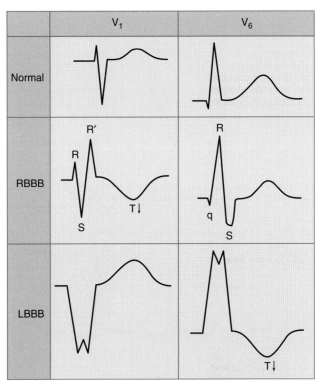

Figure 3-17. Comparison of typical QRS-T patterns in right bundle branch block (RBBB) and left bundle branch block (LBBB) with the normal pattern in leads V1 and V6. Note the secondary R wave (R′) in V1 and slurred S wave in V6 with RBBB. Note the secondary T wave inversions (*arrows*) in leads with an rSR′ complex with RBBB and in leads with a wide R wave with LBBB. *(From Goldberger AL, Goldberger ZD, Shvilkin A:* Goldberger's clinical electrocardiography: a simplified approach, *ed 8, Philadelphia, 2013, Saunders.)*

33. How can you determine left ventricular hypertrophy using a 12-lead ECG?

Add the depth of the S wave in V1 to the height of the R wave in V5 in mm. If the total is greater than 35 mm, then left ventricular hypertrophy is present. The T wave in V5 and V6 often show inversion and asymmetry. Left axis deviation will be present.

34. What ECG changes may be seen in a patient who develops a pulmonary embolus?

Lead I: Large S wave
Lead II: ST segment depression
Lead III: Large Q wave with T wave inversion
T wave inversion may be seen in leads V1 to V4, along with an RBBB.

35. What rhythm is shown in Figure 3-18?

Sinus rhythm. This normal regular rhythm originates in the SA node, with a normal rate of 60 to 100 beats/min. The PR interval is 0.12 to 0.2 seconds. The QRS complex is 0.04 to 0.12 seconds.

36. What rhythm is shown in Figure 3-19?

Premature atrial contractions. PACs originate when an irritable atrial automaticity focus suddenly fires, producing an early, ectopic P wave. The rate varies depending on the number of these contractions. This ectopic P wave will appear premature and will be unusually shaped when compared to the normal P waves; it may fall coincidently on the T wave and present as a taller T wave. A shortened PR interval may be evident. The QRS complex is usually normal but may appear slightly widened due to aberrant ventricular conduction in that premature cycle.

37. What rhythm is shown in Figure 3-20?

Sinus tachycardia. This rhythm originates from the SA node and occurs when the SA node paces the heart at a rate greater than 100 beats/min. The P waves, PR intervals, and QRS complexes are normal. The rhythm is regular.

38. What rhythm is shown in Figure 3-21?

Supraventricular tachycardia. Generally, the rate is 150 to 250 beats/min. The P waves differ from normal, and the rate may be so rapid that the P waves may be coincident with the previous T waves, with a noticeable lack of PR interval. Certain conditions may widen the QRS complex in SVT.

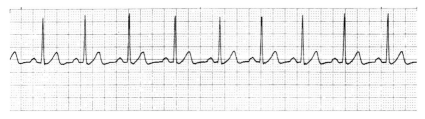

Figure 3-18. Normal sinus rhythm. *(From Linton AD:* Introduction to Medical-Surgical Nursing, *ed 5, St. Louis, 2012, Saunders.)*

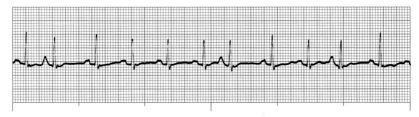

Figure 3-19. Sinus tachycardia with three premature atrial complexes (PACs). From the left, beats 2, 7, and 10 are PACS. *(From Aehlert B:* ECGs made easy, *ed 5, St Louis, 2013, Elsevier.)*

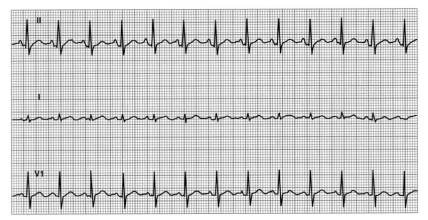

Figure 3-20. Sinus tachycardia at 120 beats/min. *(From Aehlert B:* ECGs made easy, *ed 5, St Louis, 2013, Elsevier.)*

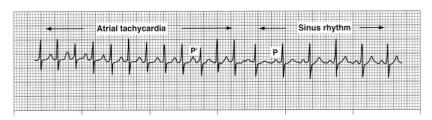

Figure 3-21. Supraventricular tachycardia that ends spontaneously with the abrupt resumption of sinus rhythm. The P waves of the tachycardia are superimposed on the preceding T waves. *(From Goldberger AL, Goldberger ZD, Shvilkin A:* Goldberger's clinical electrocardiography: a simplified approach, *ed 8, Philadelphia, 2013, Saunders.)*

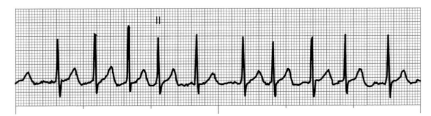

Figure 3-22. Atrial fibrillation. *(From Aehlert B:* ECGs made easy, *ed 5, St Louis, 2013, Elsevier.)*

39. What rhythm is shown in Figure 3-22?
    Atrial fibrillation. It is caused by the continuous rapid firing of multiple parasystolic atrial foci, producing a rapid "irregularly irregular rhythm." The rate is usually 300 to 500 beats/min, with a ventricular capture rate of 150 to 180 beats/min. P waves are usually unidentifiable, and PR intervals are virtually impossible to distinguish. The QRS complexes are normal.

40. What rhythm is shown in Figure 3-23?
    Atrial flutter. P waves appear in a "sawtooth pattern" known as flutter or F waves. The atrial rate averages 220 to 350 beats/min and ventricular rate ranges around 100 to 220 beats/min. This rhythm is a reentrant arrhythmia in the atria or an endless electrical loop. PR intervals are usually regular and the QRS complexes normal.

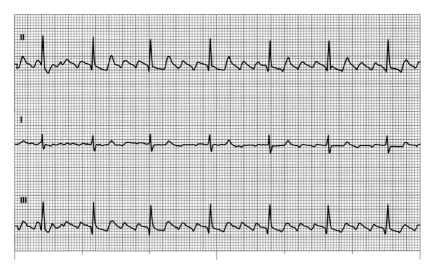

Figure 3-23. Atrial flutter. *(From Aehlert B: ECGs made easy, ed 5, St Louis, 2013, Elsevier.)*

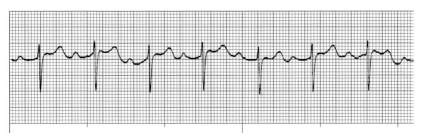

Figure 3-24. Sinus rhythm with a first-degree atrioventricular (AV) block. *(From Aehlert B: ECGs made easy, ed 5, St Louis, 2013, Elsevier.)*

41. **What rhythm is shown in Figure 3-24?**
First-degree AV block. This rhythm presents with a prolonged PR interval, >0.2 seconds.

42. **What rhythm is shown in Figure 3-25?**
Second-degree AV block, Mobitz Type 1 (Wenckebach). The atrial rate is usually fixed, but the ventricular rate is slower. The PR interval prolongs until the point that it no longer conducts to the ventricles and there is no QRS complex.

43. **What rhythm is shown in Figure 3-26?**
Second-degree AV block, Mobitz Type II. The atrial rate and P waves are normal, but the ventricular rate is slower by a factor of two (2:1) or three (3:1) The PR interval is usually normal, but there are missed QRS complexes for P waves.

44. **What rhythm is shown in Figure 3-27?**
Third-degree AV block: complete heart block. Atrial contractions are normal, but there is complete electrical conduction dissociation with the ventricles. The ventricles generate a signal through an escape mechanism. The ventricular escape beats are usually "slow" at a rate of 20 to 60 beats/min. The P waves and QRS complexes are regular, but they do not coincide.

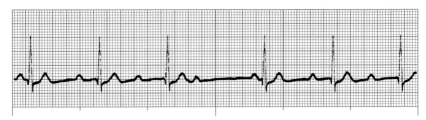

Figure 3-25. Second-degree atrioventricular (AV) block type I. *(From Aehlert B:* ECGs made easy, *ed 5, St Louis, 2013, Elsevier.)*

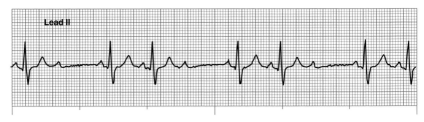

Figure 3-26. Second-degree atrioventricular (AV) block type II. *(From Aehlert B:* ECG study cards, *St Louis, 2004, Mosby.)*

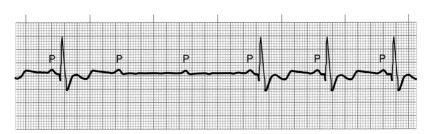

Figure 3-27. Third-degree atrioventricular block. *(From Monahan FD, Sands JK, Neighbors M et al:* Phipps' medicalsurgical nursing: health and illness perspectives, *ed 8, St Louis, 2006, Mosby.)*

45. What rhythm is shown in Figure 3-28?
    Premature ventricular contractions. The overall rate is normal. However, the fourth and sixth beats do not have preceding P waves, and a PR interval cannot be measured. The QRS complexes are wide (>0.12 seconds).

46. What rhythm is shown in Figure 3-29?
    Ventricular tachycardia. P waves and PR intervals are not seen. The rate is usually greater than 100 beats/min, and the QRS complexes are 0.12 seconds or greater (wide).

47. What rhythm is shown in Figure 3-30?
    Ventricular fibrillation. The rate cannot be determined, and there are no discernible P waves, PR interval, or QRS complexes.

48. What rhythm is shown in Figure 3-31?
    Asystole. No discernible waves present. It is a total absence of ventricular activity. There is no ventricular rate or rhythm, no pulse or cardiac output. It may also be known as cardiac standstill or flat line.

II

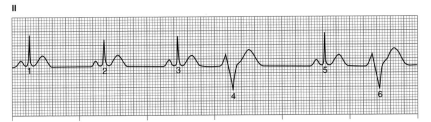

Figure 3-28. Sinus rhythm with premature ventricular complexes (PVCs). The fourth and sixth complexes are very different in appearance from the normally conducted beats. They are PVCs and are not preceded by P waves. *(From Grauer K: A practical guide to ECG interpretation, ed 2, St Louis, 1998, Mosby.)*

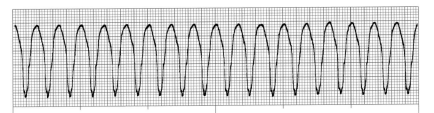

Figure 3-29. Ventricular tachycardia. *(From Aehlert B: ECGs made easy, ed 5, St Louis, 2013, Elsevier.)*

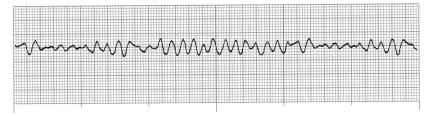

Figure 3-30. Ventricular fibrillation. *(From Aehlert B: ECGs made easy, ed 5, St Louis, 2013, Elsevier.)*

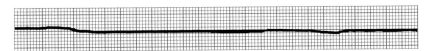

Figure 3-31. Asystole. *(From Goldberger AL, Goldberger ZD, Shvilkin A: Goldberger's clinical electrocardiography: a simplified approach, ed 8, Philadelphia, 2013, Saunders.)*

BIBLIOGRAPHY

Aehlert B: *ECGs made easy*, ed 5, St Louis, 2013, Elsevier.

Baker WA, Lowery CM: Cardiac dysrhythmias. In Duke J, editor: *Anesthesia secrets*, ed 4, Philadelphia, 2011, Mosby Elsevier.

Baker WA, Lowery CM: Electrocardiography. In Duke J, editor: *Anesthesia secrets*, ed 4, Philadelphia, 2011, Mosby Elsevier.

Becker DE: Fundamentals of electrocardiography interpretation, *Anesth Prog* 53:53–64, 2006.

Berul CI, Seslar SP, Zimetbaum PJ, Josephson ME: Acquired long QT syndrome. From UpToDate, Post TW, editor: *Waltham*. Accessed on July 25, 2014.

Bickley LS: *Bates' guide to physical examination and history taking*, ed 11, Philadephia, 2013, Wolters Kluwer Health.

Bisognano JD, Beck GR, Connell RW: *Manual of outpatient cardiology*, London, 2012, Springer.

Davies A, Scott A: *Starting to read ECGs: the basics*, London, 2014, Springer.

Dubin D: *Rapid interpretation of EKG's*, ed 6, Fort Myers, 2000, Cover.

Gomella L, Haist S: *Clinician's pocket reference*, ed 11, New York, 2007, McGraw-Hill.

Khan MG: *Rapid ECG interpretation*, ed 3, Totowa, 2008, Humana Press.

Longo D, Fauci A, Kasper D, Hauser S: *Harrison's principles of internal medicine*, ed 18, New York, 2012, McGraw-Hill.

Podrid P, Ganz LI: *Approach to the diagnosis and treatment of wide QRS complex tachycardias*. From UpToDate, Literature review current through: July 2014.

Strauss R: Interpretation of the electrocardiogram. In Laskin DM, editor: *Clinician's handbook of oral & maxillofacial surgery*, Hanover Park, 2010, Quintessence.

CHAPTER 4

LABORATORY TESTS

Joel M. Friedman, Emery Nicholas

1. **What is included in a complete blood count (CBC), and how are the results charted?**
   The CBC, or heme 8, typically includes the items described in Table 4-1 and Figure 4-1.

2. **What information does a white blood cell (WBC) differential provide?**
   The total WBC count is made up of neutrophils (50% to 70%), lymphocytes (20% to 40%), monocytes (0% to 7%), eosinophils (0% to 5%), and basophils (0% to 1%). Most labs provide the absolute number of each cell type as well as percentage. Differentials for alterations in the WBC fractions are described in Box 4-1.

3. **What is a left shift, and how is it significant?**
   Polymorphonuclear neutrophils (PMNs) are subdivided morphologically on the blood smear into segmented neutrophils (segs or polys) and band forms (bands), based on the nuclear lobes and their chromatin connections. The segs are more mature neutrophils, having two to five nuclear lobes and thin strands of chromatin and comprising 50% to 70% of total PMNs. The bands are immature neutrophils, make up 0% to 5% of total PMNs, and have a thick band of chromatin connecting one to two nuclear lobes. On the early manual neutrophil counting machines, the keys that represented the bands were on the left side and the keys representing segs were on the right. If the bands increased to more than 20% of the WBC total, or the PMNs were more than 80% of the WBC total, the result was said to have a left shift. This shift increases the likelihood of bacterial infection, sepsis, or hemorrhage as the etiology of an elevated WBC count.

4. **How are the red blood cell (RBC) indices used clinically?**
   The indices are used to diagnose and classify anemia, which is defined as either a decreased RBC mass or hemoglobin (Hgb) content below physiologic needs. The mean corpuscular volume (MCV) and mean corpuscular hemoglobin concentration (MCHC) are the most useful in determining the etiology of the anemia.
   - MCV = (Hematocrit [Hct] × unit constant)/RBC
   - Macrocytic (>100 fL): megaloblastic (pernicious) anemia (B12 or folate deficiency), chronic liver disease, alcoholism, reticulocytosis, physiologic in the newborn
   - Microcytic (<80 fL): iron deficiency, thalassemia, chronic disease (cancer, renal, infection), or lead toxicity

$$MCH = Hgb/RBC$$

   The mean corpuscular hemoglobin (MCH) helps to diagnose chromaticity of cells because cells with increased Hgb content will have more pigment (hyperchromic) and will be hypochromic in the reverse situation. Increased MCH suggests hyperchromic cells while decreased MCH suggest hypochromic cells. This parallels changes in MCV in that macrocytic cells are hyperchromic and microcytic cells are hypochromic.
   The MCHC increases with prolonged severe dehydration, heavy smoking, intravascular hemolysis, and spherocytosis. It will be decreased in over-hydration, iron deficiency anemia, thalassemia, and sideroblastic anemia.

5. **What does the reticulocyte count mean?**
   Reticulocytes are immature RBCs. These cells are larger, continue Hgb synthesis, and are bluer in color on smears than mature erythrocytes. Reticulocytes constitute approximately 1% of total RBCs but can increase when the need for erythrocytes rises. A corrected count is made by multiplying the reticulocyte count by the measured Hct divided by 45; the result should be <1.5%. If the count is increased, then erythropoiesis is usually caused by bleeding, hemolysis, and correction of iron, folate, or B12 deficiencies. Decreased reticulocyte counts are often the result of transfusions or aplastic anemia.

Table 4-1. Complete Blood Cell Count

	DEFINITION	NORMAL RANGE
White blood cell count		$4\text{-}11 \times 10^3$ cells/mm^3
RBC count		$4.5\text{-}6 \times 10^6$ cells/mm^3
Hgb		Men: 14-18 g/dL
		Women: 12-16 g/dL
Hematocrit	Percentage of RBC mass in blood volume	Men: 40%-54%
		Women: 37%-47%
Platelets		$150\text{-}400 \times 10^3$/mm^3
RBC indices:		
Mean corpusclular volume	Average RBC volume in fL	80-100 fL
Mean corpuscular hemoglobin	Estimates weight of Hgb in average RBC	27-31 pg
Mean corpuscular hemoglobin concentration	Estimates average concentration of Hgb in average RBC	32%-36%

fL, Femtoliters; *Hgb*, hemoglobin; *RBC*, red blood cell.

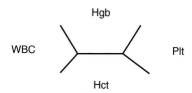

Figure 4-1. Demonstrates method of recording values in patient chart. The charting method allows universal communication with the patient progress notes.

Box 4-1. Differentials for Alterations in the White Blood Cell Fractions

Polymorphonuclear Neutrophils (PMNs)

Increased	Decreased
Bacterial infection	Aplastic anemia
Tissue damage (myocardial infarction, burn, or crush injury)	Viral infection drugs
Leukemia	Radiation
Uremia	Kidney dialysis
Diabetic ketoacidosis (DKA)	
Acute gout	
Eclampsia	
Physiologic:	
Severe exercise	
Late pregnancy	
Labor	
Surgery	
Newborn	

Lymphocytes (Lymphs)

Increased (lymphocytosis)	Decreased
Viral infections	Uremia
Acute or chronic lymphocytic leukemia	Stress
Tuberculosis (TB)	Burns

Box 4-1. Differentials for Alterations in the White Blood Cell Fractions—(*Continued*)

Increased (lymphocytosis)	Decreased
Mononucleosis	Trauma
	Steroids
	Normal in 20% of population

Monocytes

Increased (monocytosis)	Decreased
Subacute bacterial endocarditis	Aplasia of bone marrow
TB	
Protozoal infection	
Leukemia	
Collagen disease	

Basophils

Increased (basophilia)	Decreased
Chronic myeloid leukemia	Acute rheumatic fever
Polycythemia	Lobar pneumonia
After recovery of infection or hypothyroidism (rarely)	Steroid treatment
	Stress
	Thyrotoxicosis

Eosinophils

Increased (eosinophilia)	Decreased
Allergy	Steroids
Parasite	Stress (infection, trauma, and burn)
Malignancy	Increased adrenocorticotropic hormone (ACTH)
Drugs	Cushing's syndrome
Asthma	
Addison's disease	
Collagen vascular diseases	

6. **What information is obtained from the Hgb and Hct values?**

The Hgb concentration is an indicator of oxygen-carrying capacity of blood. It is dependent primarily on the number of RBCs and much less significantly (or treatably) on the amount of Hgb per cell. Additionally, Hgb is known to vary by as much as 1 g/dL diurnally, with peaks in the morning. Studies have also shown a 1 g/dL variation between Hgb values drawn on admission and those taken following one night of bed rest. The relation between Hgb and Hct is given by:

$$\text{Hgb} \times 3^* = \text{Hct}$$
$$\text{RBC (millions)} \times 3 = \text{Hgb}$$
$$\text{RBC} \times 9 = \text{Hct}$$

Increased Hgb and Hct values may result from polycythemia, dehydration, heart disease, increased altitude, heavy smoking, or birth physiology. Decreased levels may indicate anemia, hemorrhage, dilution, alcohol, drugs, or pregnancy.

*This varies between 2.7 and 3.2 based on the MCHC.

7. **Are Hgb and Hct primary indicators of blood loss and the need for transfusion?**

No! These are poor early measures of bleeding because plasma and RBCs are lost in equal measures. It takes 2 to 3 hours after fluid resuscitation for Hgb/Hct to reflect blood loss. Today most patients are transfused for Hgb <7 g/dL, but the best guidelines are the vital signs and symptoms such as shortness of breath and exercise intolerance. Initially low Hct values suggest chronic blood loss, which should be supported by low MCV and a high reticulocyte count.

8. What are some common terms and significant morphologic changes on smears?
   - Poikilocytosis: Irregularly shaped RBCs
   - Anisocytosis: Irregular RBC size
   - Sickled cells: Crescent or sickle-shaped RBCs seen with decreased oxygen (O_2) tension
   - Howell-Jolly bodies: Large RBC basophilic inclusions (megaloblastic anemia, splenectomy, hemolysis)
   - Basophilic stippling: Small RBC blue inclusions (lead poisoning, thalassemia, heavy metals)
   - Spherocytes: Spherical RBCs (autoimmune hemolytic anemia, hereditary)
   - Burr cells: Spiny RBCs (liver disease, anorexia, ↑ bile acids)
   - Schistocytes: Helmet RBCs (severe anemia, hemolytic transfusion reaction)
   - Döhle's inclusion bodies: PMNs (burns, infection)
   - Toxic granulation: PMNs (burns, sepsis, fever)
   - Auer bodies: Acute myelogenous leukemia
   - Hypersegmentation: PMNs with six to seven lobes (megaloblastic anemia, liver disease)

9. What is clinically useful about the platelet count?
   - A normal platelet count is 150,000 to 440,000/mm^3. *Thrombocytopenia* is defined as a count of <150,000/mm^3 and is a *quantitative platelet disorder*. Intraoperative bleeding can be severe with counts of 40,000 to 70,000/mm^3, and spontaneous bleeding usually occurs at counts <20,000/mm^3. The minimal recommended platelet count before surgery is 75,000/mm^3 and it is safe to operate provided platelet function is normal. Thrombocytopenia (low platelet count) that is <50,000/mm^3 is an absolute contraindication to elective surgical procedures because of the possibility of significant bleeding.
   - Possible etiologies for low platelet counts are idiopathic thrombocytopenic purpura (ITP), disseminated intravascular coagulation (DIC), marrow invasion or aplasia, hypersplenism, drugs, cirrhosis, transfusions, and viral infections (mononucleosis).
   - Although prophylactic preoperative platelet transfusion is generally advocated to treat preexisting thrombocytopenia, the methods of evaluating clinical need are imprecise. Qualitative differences in platelet function make it unwise to rely on platelet number as the sole criterion for transfusion. Thrombocytopenic patients with accelerated destruction but active production of platelets have relatively less bleeding than patients with hypoplastic disorders at a given platelet count.

10. How are platelet abnormalities categorized?
    Platelet disorders can be either quantitative or qualitative in nature:
    - **Quantitative platelet disorders**: In these, the platelet count is decreased (thrombocytopenia) or increased (thrombocytosis). They can be hereditary or, more often, acquired and include thrombocytopenia; dilution, as after massive blood transfusion; decreased platelet production as a result of malignant infiltration (aplastic anemia, multiple myeloma); drugs (chemotherapy, cytotoxic drugs, ethanol, hydrochlorothiazide); radiation exposure; or bone marrow depression after viral infection. Other examples are increased peripheral destruction due to hypersplenism, DIC, extensive tissue and vascular damage after extensive burns, or immune mechanisms (ITP, drugs such as heparin, autoimmune diseases).
    - **Qualitative platelet disorders**: In this type of abnormality, the platelet count may be normal, but the platelets do not function normally. Therefore, increased bleeding can result. This abnormality can also be an inherited (e.g., von Willebrand disease) and/or acquired (uremia; cirrhosis, particularly after ethanol; drugs, such as aspirin, NSAIDs) disorder.

11. What is bleeding time, and how does it assess platelet function?
    Bleeding time is a screening test that assesses platelet function. The test is performed by inflating a blood pressure cuff to 40 mm Hg, making a standard incision in the patient's forearm, and recording the time until the bleeding stops (Ivy method). Normal bleeding time ranges from 4 to 9 minutes, and a bleeding time >1.5 times normal (>15 minutes) is considered significantly abnormal. It has been recommended that this test be used to diagnose specific hemorrhagic diseases and to monitor therapy of these diseases, but not to screen preoperative patients who have no history of bleeding or abnormal coagulation studies. Assessment of preoperative platelet function is complicated by a lack of correlation between bleeding time and any other test of platelet function and a tendency to increase intraoperative bleeding.

    The bleeding time is increased by platelet counts <100,000; by the presence of drugs such as aspirin, NSAIDs, and antibiotics (synthetic penicillins); and conditions such as uremia, alcoholism, chronic liver disease, vasculitis, Ehlers-Danlos syndrome, and von Willebrand disease. There is an undefined risk of bleeding with elevated test times until about double the control time.

12. **How do aspirin and NSAIDs affect platelet function and bleeding time?**
Primary hemostasis is controlled by the balance between the opposing actions of two prostaglandins: thromboxane A2 and prostacyclin. Depending on the dose, salicylates (aspirin) produce a differential effect on prostaglandin synthesis in platelets and vascular endothelial cells. Lower doses preferentially inhibit platelet cyclooxygenase, impeding thromboxane A2 production and inhibiting platelet aggregation irreversibly; as platelets lack a cell nucleus and cannot produce protein, the effect lasts for their 7- to 10-day life span. The effect begins within 2 hours of ingestion. Because approximately 10% of platelets are replaced each day, it takes an average of 2 to 3 days for bleeding time to normalize, but most experts recommend allowing 7 days without aspirin before surgery.
    Other nonsteroidal antiinflammatory drugs (NSAIDs) reversibly inhibit the activity of cyclooxygenase, and therefore they will alter platelet function only temporarily, usually <24 hours. NSAIDs have a similar but more transient effect than aspirin, lasting for only 1 to 3 days after cessation of use.

13. **Which clotting factors are synthesized in the liver?**
Four clotting factors are synthesized in the liver: factors II, VII, IX, and X.

14. **Which vitamin deficiency can affect coagulation and extrinsic pathway coagulation lab values?**
Vitamin K deficiency. Vitamin K is required for the synthesis of coagulation factors II, VII, IX, and X, as well as anticoagulants protein C and protein S.

15. **What are the differences between the coagulation tests?***
The basic difference between the intrinsic and extrinsic pathways is the phospholipid surface on which the clotting factors interact before union at the common pathway. Either platelet phospholipid (for the intrinsic pathway) or tissue thromboplastin (for the extrinsic pathway) can be added to the patient's plasma, and the time taken for clot formation is measured. Less than 30% of normal factor activity is required for the tests to be sensitive enough to detect decreased levels. The tests are also prolonged in cases of decreased fibrinogen concentration (<100 mg/dL−1) and dysfibrinogenemias.

Measurement of the Intrinsic and Common Pathways

1. Partial thromboplastin time (PTT)
   - PTT measures the clotting ability of all factors in the intrinsic and common pathways except factor XIII.
   - Partial thromboplastin is substituted for platelet phospholipid and eliminates platelet variability.
   - Normal PTT is about 40 to 70 seconds.

2. Activated PTT (aPTT)
   - An activator is added to the test tube before addition of partial thromboplastin; this activator speeds up the clotting time, and a smaller and more consistent range of values results.
   - Normal aPTT is 25 to 35 seconds.
   - This test is more sensitive than the PTT and therefore used often to monitor patients on heparin therapy.

3. Activated clotting time (ACT)
   - Fresh whole blood (providing platelet phospholipid) is added to a test tube already containing an activator.
   - The automated ACT is widely used to monitor heparin therapy in the operating room.
   - Normal range is 90 to 120 seconds.

Measurement of the Extrinsic and Common Pathways

1. Prothrombin time (PT)
   - Tissue thromboplastin is added to the patient's plasma.
   - Test varies in sensitivity and response to oral anticoagulant therapy whether measured as PT in seconds or simple PT ratio (PT patient/PT normal) (normal = the mean normal PT value of the lab test system).
   - Normal PT is 11 to 13 seconds.

---

*Reprinted from Katz JJ: Coagulation. In Duke J, editor: *Anesthesia secrets*, ed 2, Philadelphia, 2000, Hanley & Belfus.

2. International normalized ratio (INR)
    - It was developed to standardize the interpretation of coagulation tests, which can vary widely based on testing method.
    - This converts the PT ratio to a value that would have been obtained using a standard PT method.
    - INR is calculated as (PT patient/PT normal) ISI. (ISI is the international sensitivity index assigned to the test system.)
    - The recommended therapeutic ranges for standard oral anticoagulant therapy and high-dose therapy, respectively, are INR values of 2.0 to 3.0 and 2.5 to 3.5.

16. What are the most common indications of use of warfarin?
    The most common indications of warfarin therapy are:
    - Prophylaxis and treatment of deep venous thrombosis and its extension, pulmonary embolism (PE)
    - Prophylaxis and treatment of thromboembolic complications associated with atrial fibrillation (AF) and/or cardiac valve replacement
    - Reduction in the risk of death, recurrent myocardial infarction (MI), and thromboembolic events such as stroke or systemic embolization after myocardial infarction, and congestive heart failure

17. What are the current indications for transfusion of fresh frozen plasma (FFP)?*
    A task force of the American Society of Anesthesiologists (ASA) recommends the use of FFP in the following circumstances:
    - Urgent reversal of warfarin therapy
    - Correction of known anticoagulation deficiencies for which specific concentrates are unavailable
    - Correction of microvascular bleeding in the presence of elevated (>1.5 times normal) PT or PTT
    - Correction of microvascular bleeding secondary to coagulation factor deficiencies in patients transfused with more than one blood volume, when a PT or PTT cannot be obtained in a timely fashion
    The dose given should be calculated to achieve a minimum of 30% of plasma factor concentration (usually about 10 to 15 mL/kg of FFP).

18. What are the indications for the use of platelets?*
    The ASA recommends the following:
    - Prophylactic platelet transfusion is ineffective and rarely indicated when thrombocytopenia is caused by increased platelet destruction.
    - For surgical patients with thrombocytopenia caused by decreased platelet production and surgical and obstetric patients with microvascular bleeding, platelet transfusion is rarely indicated when the count is >100 × 109/L and usually indicated if the count is <50 × 109/L. With intermediate values, platelet therapy should be based on the risk of bleeding.

19. What is DIC?*
    DIC is not a disease entity, but rather a manifestation of disease associated with various well-defined clinical entities:
    - Obstetric conditions (amniotic fluid embolism, placental abruption, retained fetus syndrome, eclampsia, saline-induced abortion)
    - Intravascular hemolysis (hemolytic transfusion syndromes, minor hemolysis, massive transfusion)
    - Septicemia (gram-negative: endotoxin; gram-positive: mucopolysaccharides)
    - Viremias (cytomegalovirus, hepatitis, varicella, HIV)
    - Disseminated malignancy
    - Leukemia
    - Burns
    - Crush injury and tissue necrosis
    - Liver disease (obstructive jaundice, acute hepatic failure)
    - Prosthetic devices (LeVeen shunt, aortic balloon)
    DIC usually is seen in clinical circumstances in which the extrinsic or intrinsic coagulation pathway (or both) is activated by circulating phospholipid, leading to generation of thrombin; however, the usual mechanisms preventing unbalanced thrombus formation are impaired. After systemic deposition of intravascular fibrin thrombi, consumption of factors V and VIII, and loss of platelets, the resulting circulating level of clotting factors and platelets represents a balance between depletion and production. The fibrinolytic system is activated, and plasmin begins to cleave fibrinogen and fibrin into fibrinogen and fibrin degradation products (FDPs). Recognition and understanding of the syndrome are made difficult by the occurrence of both acute and chronic forms and by a clinical spectrum varying from diffuse thrombosis to diffuse bleeding or both.

20. What tests are used for the diagnosis of DIC?*

There is no one pathognomonic test for the diagnosis of DIC. In acute DIC, the PT is elevated in about 75% of patients, whereas PTT is prolonged in 50% to 60%. Platelet count is typically greatly reduced and hypofibrinogenemia is common. The D-dimer test is a newer diagnostic test. The D-dimer is a neoantigen formed by the action of thrombin in converting fibrinogen to cross-linked fibrin. It is specific for fibrin degradation products formed from the digestion of cross-linked fibrin by plasmin. In 85% to 100% of patients with DIC, FDPs are elevated. Elevated levels are not diagnostic of DIC but indicate the presence of plasmin and plasmin degradation of fibrinogen or fibrin.

21. What is the treatment for DIC?*

The treatment for DIC is case-dependent and controversial. The triggering process should be identified and treated accordingly. Heparin is the first-line treatment used to stop bleeding and the consumption process before administration of specific coagulation products. If these measures fail, specific blood components may be depleted and should be replaced after identification. If bleeding still continues, antifibrinolytic therapy with epsilon aminocaproic acid should be considered, but only if the intravascular coagulation process is shown to have stopped and residual fibrinolysis to continue.

22. What factors increase and decrease PT?

PT will be increased by warfarin, vitamin K deficiency, fat malabsorption, liver disease, DIC, and artificially increased tourniquet time. Warfarin blocks vitamin K use, whereas broad-spectrum antibiotics elevate PT by killing normal bowel flora, which decreases vitamin K absorption. Heparin in high doses also will increase PT by altering factor X. FFP will reverse warfarin effects immediately, whereas vitamin K requires 12 to 24 hours to begin decreasing the PT. For most minor oral surgical procedures, INR <3.5 is unlikely to produce significant peri-operative bleeding episodes.

23. How does heparin work?

Heparin's primary effect is to activate antithrombin III, which blocks coagulation by inhibiting mostly factors IX and X. Antithrombin III amounts are significantly decreased in severe malignancy, severe liver disease, nephrotic syndrome, deep venous thrombosis (DVT), septicemia, major surgery, malnutrition, and DIC. Low molecular weight heparin (enoxaparin) also works on antithrombin III. Heparin's peak effect is at 30 minutes to 1 hour after intravenous use and 3 to 4 hours after subcutaneous dose; its duration of effect is approximately 3 to 4 hours when given intravenously and 6 hours subcutaneously.

24. Why are FDPs and fibrin split products (FSPs) important?

The result of the clotting cascade is an insoluble polymeric fibrin meshwork. Naturally occurring fibrinolysin (plasmin) attacks and breaks down fibrinogen and fibrin, leaving split products behind. Physiologically, this occurs after trauma or surgery and is quickly regulated. Pathologically, plasmin may be activated in DIC, DVT, malignancy, emboli, infections (especially gram-negative sepsis), necrosis, or infarctions. This will result in an elevated fibrin split product assay. Fibrinogen assays will be decreased (<150 mg/dL) in DIC, burns, surgery, neoplasia, severe acute bleeding, snakebites, and some hematologic diseases. Protamine sulfate and D-dimer (a specific FSP) are other tests that look for abnormal clotting activity. Though not very specific, the D-dimer assay is used to screen for DVT in the emergency department because a normal value virtually excludes the possibility of this clotting problem.

25. What is measured in a blood chemistry test (also called basic metabolic, chem 7, or SMA 7), and how is it charted?

The basic electrolytes, renal function evaluation, and blood glucose are tested (Fig. 4-2).

		Normal Ranges
1.	Sodium (Na)	136-145 mEq/L
2.	Potassium (K)	3.5-5.2 mEq/L
3.	Chloride (Cl)	95-108 mEq/L
4.	Carbon dioxide (CO_2)	24-30 mEq/L
5.	Blood urea nitrogen (BUN)	6-20 mg/dL
6.	Creatinine	0.7-1.4 mg/dL
7.	Glucose	65-110 mg/dL (fasting)

*Reprinted from Katz JJ: Coagulation. In Duke J, editor: *Anesthesia secrets*, ed 2, Philadelphia, 2000, Hanley & Belfus.

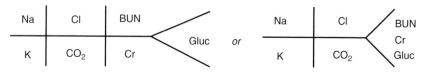

Figure 4-2. Demonstrates method of recording values in the patient chart. This charting method allows universal communication within the patient progress notes.

Box 4-2. Common Causes of Basic Electrolyte Disturbances

	Increase	Decrease
Sodium (Na)	Dehydration	Diuretics
	Glycosuria	CHF
	Diabetes insipidus	Renal failure
	Cushing's syndrome	Vomiting
	Excessive sweating	Diarrhea
		Liver failure
		Nephrotic syndrome
		SIADH
		Hypothyroidism
		Pancreatitis
		Hyperlipidemia
		Multiple myeloma
		Hyperglycemia—corrected
		Na = 1.6 x 1/100 g glucose over 100 g/dL
Potassium (K)	Factitious (sample hemolysis,	Diuretics
	probably most common cause)	Nasogastric suctioning
	Dehydration	Alkalosis
	Renal failure	Mineral corticoid excess
	Acidosis	Zollinger-Ellison syndrome
	Addison's disease	Vomiting
	Iatrogenic	Excessive sweating
Chloride (cl)	Dehydration	CHF
	Metabolic acidosis (nonanion gap)	Chronic renal failure
	Diarrhea	Diuretics
	Diabetes insipidus	DKA
	Medications	SIADH
	Aldosterone deficiency	Aldosterone excess
Carbon dioxide (CO_2)	Dehydration	Metabolic acidosis
	Respiratory acidosis	Respiratory alkalosis
	Vomiting	Renal failure
	Emphysema	Diarrhea
	Metabolic alkalosis	Starvation

CHF, Congestive heart failure; *DKA*, diabetic ketoacidosis; *SIADH*, syndrome of inappropriate secretion of diuretic hormone.

26. What are common causes of basic electrolyte disturbances (Box 4-2)?

27. What tests are used as markers for liver function or disease?
    Serum albumin, total protein, bilirubin, aspartate aminotransferase (AST = SGOT), alanine aminotransferase (ALT = SGPT), alkaline phosphatase (ALP), gamma-glutamyl transferase (GGT), lactate dehydrogenase (LDH), PT, bile acids, and blood ammonia.

28. How is the synthetic function of the liver evaluated?
    Serum levels of albumin, total protein, PT, bile acids, conjugated bilirubin, BUN, and ammonia are used to examine liver function. Although not widely used, the most sensitive test for liver or bile tract

abnormality is for bile acids. Bile acids are water-soluble compounds produced from cholesterol metabolism in the liver. Bile acid tests are best done 2 hours after eating and will show abnormalities in inactive cirrhosis and resolving hepatitis when other tests are normal. A more commonly used liver function test is albumin level, which is decreased with liver damage as well as starvation, inflammatory bowel disease, hemolysis, nephrotic syndrome, leukemia, and hemorrhage or burns. Albumin is produced almost exclusively by the liver and makes up almost 75% of the total protein in serum, so these tests usually parallel each other. Prothrombin is synthesized by the liver using vitamin K and will be abnormal in severe, most often end-stage, and chronic liver disease. The absence of conjugated bilirubin in the blood with severely elevated unconjugated bilirubin could indicate severely decreased liver function. The ammonia level is used to diagnose and follow hepatic encephalopathy when failure of the liver is already known.

29. **What is the clinical significance of liver enzymes?**
Any increase of hepatic enzymes indicates cellular damage. AST is made in the liver, heart, skeletal muscle, and RBCs, so elevations may be due to liver disease, acute myocardial infarction (AMI), pancreatitis, muscle trauma, hemolysis, congestive heart failure (CHF), surgery, burns, or renal infarction. Increased specificity for liver damage occurs with elevation of ALT, GGT, or 5′-nucleotidase. ALP is found in liver cells, bile duct epithelium, and osteoblasts. Therefore, elevations of ALP should be confirmed to involve the liver or bile ducts by checking a liver specific fraction (GGT, ALT, or 5′-nucleotidase level). These tests will help rule out bone diseases, bone growth, healing of fractures, pregnancy, or childhood physiology as the cause of ALP elevation. Last, LDH is also increased in liver cell damage with the LDH5 subfraction showing about the same sensitivity and somewhat greater specificity as AST.

30. **What are the causes of bilirubin abnormalities?**
Bilirubin is produced by the breakdown of hemoglobin in the reticuloendothelial system. This newly formed bilirubin (indirect or unconjugated) circulates through the bloodstream bound to albumin. Hepatocytes extract the bilirubin and convert it to a water-soluble pigment via a process called conjugation; the pigment, called direct or conjugated bilirubin, is subsequently excreted in bile. Elevations of total bilirubin in the blood cause jaundice (yellowing of skin and sclera, and pruritus) and may be caused by bile obstruction or excessive hemolysis. Elevation of unconjugated bilirubin occurs with obstruction and hepatocellular disease, hemolytic anemia, and physiologically in newborns. The conjugated bilirubin increases primarily with obstruction to bile flow and should be associated with an increase in ALP.

31. **What are common lab trends in liver disorders (Table 4-2)?**

32. **What tests monitor calcium (Ca) in the body?**
Ca is the fourth most common extracellular cation and plays a vital role in membrane permeability. The metabolically active Ca in the body is the ionized Ca^{2+} portion, which represents approximately 50% of total serum Ca. The range that is considered normal covers only 0.44 mg/dL, an indication of its physiologic importance. The other half of serum Ca is bound by albumin (45%) and complexed with anions. Total Ca level will be lowered by decreases in albumin such that for each 1 mg/dL drop of albumin, Ca will decrease by 0.8 mg/dL. That is, corrected total Ca = 0.8 × (normal albumin − measured albumin) + measured Ca. Possible causes of hypercalcemia include hyperparathyroidism, Paget's disease, metastatic bone tumor, hyperthyroidism, hypervitaminosis D, multiple myeloma, osteoporosis, immobilization, thiazide drugs, and parathyroid-secreting tumors (lung, breast). Causes of hypocalcemia include hypoparathyroidism (commonly after thyroid surgery), insufficient vitamin D, chronic renal failure, hypomagnesemia, seizures, acute pancreatitis, and inaccurate reading as a result of hypoalbuminemia.

33. **What two body elements are commonly linked to Ca metabolism?**
Magnesium (Mg) and phosphorus (P) play important nutritional roles in the body and are associated with Ca metabolism (Box 4-3). Mg is the second most abundant intracellular cation and is found mostly in muscle, soft tissues, and bones (50%). Less than 5% of Mg circulates in the blood, and 30% of this is bound to albumin. P, the most common intracellular anion, is used interchangeably with phosphate because much of the body's store is as the anion compound. About 80% to 85% of P is found in bones and 10% in muscle.

34. **What blood tests are used to follow renal function?**
BUN (normal: 6 to 20 mg/dL) and creatinine (normal: 0.7 to 1.4 mg/dL) blood levels are the products of protein and muscle metabolism, respectively, that are excreted by the kidneys. Decreased levels of creatinine are rarely significant, whereas drops in BUN may be due to liver failure (site of urea production), starvation, protein deficiency, over-hydration, nephrotic syndrome, or late pregnancy. Elevations

Table 4-2. Lab Trends in Liver Disorders

	AST	ALT	ALP	BILIRUBIN TOTAL	CONJUGATED	UNCONJUGATED	GGT	BILE ACID
Acute viral hepatitis	↑↑↑↑	↑↑↑↑	↑	↑ varies	↑↑	↑	↑-↑	↑↑↑
Chronic-resolving hepatitis	N-↑	N-↑	N-↑	N	—	—	N-↑	↑↑
Cirrhosis (active)	↑↑↑	↑↑	↑	N-↑	—	—	↑↑	↑↑↑
Cirrhosis (inactive)	N-↑	N-↑	N-↑	N-↑	—	—	N-↑	↑↑↑
ETOH hepatitis	↑↑↑	↑-↑↑	↑	N-↑	—	—	↑↑↑	↑↑↑
Obstruction (intrahepatic)	↑↑	N-↑↑	↑↑-↑↑↑	↑↑	↑↑	↑↑	↑↑↑	↑↑↑
Obstruction (extrahepatic)	N-↑	N-↑	↑↑↑	↑↑↑	↑↑↑	N-↑	↑↑↑	↑↑
Metastatic disease	N	N	↑↑	±↑	—	—	↑↑	↑↑

ETOH, Ethyl alcohol.

Box 4-3. Common Causes of Calcium Metabolism Abnormalities

	Increased Levels	Decreased Levels
Magnesium (Mg)	Renal failure	Alcoholism
	Mg antacid overdose	Malnutrition
	Specimen hemolysis	Severe diarrhea
	DKA	Hypercalcemia
	Lithium intoxication	Hemodialysis
	Hypothyroidism	Loop/thiazide diuretics
		Hypoalbuminemia
		Nasogastric suction
		Pancreatitis
		Acidosis compensation
Phosphorus (P)	Hypoparathyroidism	Hyperparathyroidism
	Chronic renal failure	Alcoholism
	Bone diseases	Vitamin D deficiency
	Healing fracture	Glucose or insulin administration
	Childhood	Hypomagnesemia
	Hemolysis	Diuretics
		Antacids
		Nasogastric suction
		Alkalosis
		Hypokalemia
		Gram-negative sepsis

DKA, Diabetic ketoacidosis.

of these compounds indicate severely decreased glomerular or tubular function. This can be the result of reduced blood volume to kidneys (dehydration, shock, and pump failure), increased protein intake, or catabolism. It can also be the result of direct parenchymal damage (glomerulonephritis, chronic pyelonephritis, acute tubular necrosis, and acute glomerular damage) or obstruction of urine flow (stones, strictures, tumor). These etiologies are often grouped as prerenal, renal, and postrenal, respectively, and may be responsible, separately or in combination, for elevations of the BUN or creatinine.

35. **Are there more sensitive indicators of kidney dysfunction?**
   Yes. Urine clearance of creatinine, specific gravity, osmolality, electrolyte excretion, and free water clearance are tests used to evaluate kidney function. Clearance studies are most sensitive at defining mild-to-moderate, diffuse glomerular disease by providing an estimate of glomerular filtration rate (GFR). Creatinine is most often used because it estimates GFR with approximately 90% accuracy, whereas urea only approximates to 60%. These studies are very difficult to perform because they require a 24-hour collection, and all urine needs to be obtained accurately. In addition, the creatinine clearance must be corrected for variation in muscle mass, age, and sex. Urine specific gravity and osmolality tests measure the renal tubules' ability to concentrate urine and involve protracted preparation and collection times. All the above tests give more sensitive information regarding both glomerular and tubular function than BUN or creatinine; however, all are more expensive and difficult to obtain.

36. **What information is obtained from a urinalysis?**
   - **pH** (4.5 to 8.0): Provides little useful information
   - **Specific gravity** (1.001 to 1.035): This provides a spot view of kidney tubule concentrating ability.
   - **Osmolality** (500 to 1200 mOsm/L): It provides similar information as specific gravity.
   - **Blood or hemoglobin:** Results may indicate stone, trauma, tumor, infection, or menstruation.
   - **Glucose/acetone:** Positive results may indicate diabetes mellitus, pancreatitis, tubular disease, or shock.
   - **Bilirubin:** Normal is negative; positive results may indicate hepatitis or obstructive jaundice.
   - **Protein:** Normal is negative; positive results might indicate fever, hypertension, glomerulonephritis, nephrotic syndrome, myeloma, or heavy exercise.

- **Nitrite:** Normal is negative; positive results indicate infection.
- **Leukocyte esterase:** Normal is negative; positive results indicate infection.
- **Ketones:** Normal is negative; positive results may indicate starvation, diabetic ketoacidosis (DKA), vomiting, diarrhea, or pregnancy.
- **Microscopic:**
  - Squamous epithelial cells: Normal is none; any may indicate contamination.
  - RBC: Normal is none; any may indicate tumor, stone, or pyelonephritis.
  - WBC: Count <5/hpf indicates infection.
  - Casts indicate tubular kidney disease or crystals/stones.

37. What lab studies are used to evaluate the pancreas?

    Because the production of enzymes in the pancreas is vital for digestion and maintenance of homeostasis, the effects of pancreatic disease are seen in many tests. However, serum levels of amylase (starch digestion), lipase (fat digestion), and trypsin (protein digestion) allow a direct indication of pancreatic cell damage. Amylase levels peak about 29 hours after the onset of acute pancreatitis, as does lipase; however, once active cell damage has stopped, the amylase returns to normal within 72 hours, whereas lipase does not normalize for 7 to 10 days. Amylase levels also may be elevated because of common bile duct lithiasis, cholecystitis, tumor, peritonitis, peptic ulcer, intraabdominal hemorrhage, intestinal obstruction or infarction, acute salivary gland disease, DKA, pregnancy, burns, and renal failure. Lipase shows an increased specificity to the pancreas because lipase levels are elevated in pancreatitis, pancreatic duct obstruction, renal failure, and, much less significantly, intestinal obstruction or infarction and cholangitis. Trypsin is the most pancreatic-specific exocrine enzyme, but this assay is not widely available. Last, Ca levels also are followed in acute pancreatitis because calcium levels decrease with lipase's digestion of peritoneal fat (fat necrosis), which can provide prognostic information.

38. How is blood glucose regulation monitored by the lab?

    Glucose is regulated primarily by the liver in response to hormones released from structures such as the pancreas (insulin, glucagon), adrenal medulla (epinephrine), and adrenal cortex (cortisol/cortisone). Blood glucose is used most commonly to diagnose diabetes mellitus and to explain altered mental status. A fasting level above 140 mg/dL or non-fasting glucose >200 mg/dL is indicative of diabetes. A glucose tolerance test provides a more accurate assessment of the patient's ability to process glucose but may be inaccurate in cases of fever, stress, afternoon testing, inactivity, advancing age, trauma, or MI. Glycosylated hemoglobin or HgbA1c is used to monitor patient compliance and treatment effectiveness and should be below 5.7%. An HgbA1c level above 6.5% indicates diabetes. The amount of Hgb glycosylated is a function of degree and duration of RBC exposure to glucose and illustrates average blood glucose over a 2- to 4-month period.

    An *increase* in glucose levels may indicate diabetes mellitus (type I or II), acute pancreatitis, hyperthyroidism, Cushing's syndrome, acromegaly, epinephrine (e.g., exogenous, pheochromo, stress, burn), advancing age, or sample drawn above intravenous access.

    A *decrease* in glucose levels may indicate oral hypoglycemics or exogenous insulin, pancreatitis, starvation, liver disease, sepsis, hypothyroidism, or postprandial reactive hypoglycemia (after gastric surgery).

39. What is measured by a blood gas?

    This test is conducted by drawing blood from an artery (usually radial or femoral) and then sending the sample to the lab in ice with the patient's temperature and current oxygen supplementation recorded (Table 4-3). Blood gas tests are used to determine the carbon dioxide and oxygen concentrations in the blood and can therefore be used to measure the pH of blood.

40. What components of the blood gas are used in determining acid–base status?

    The essential test values are the pH, PCO_2, HCO_3^-, base difference, and anion gap (AG) from a basic metabolic formula with a normal value of 8 to 12 mEq/L. The major buffering system of the blood is bicarbonate-carbonic acid with the normal $HCO_3^-/CO_2 = 20$.

    The lungs are the major regulator of PCO_2 with an increase of 10 mm Hg in hypoventilation corresponding to a pH drop of 0.08 U. The kidney regulates $[HCO_3^-]$ with response to acid–base abnormalities, but is much slower than the lungs and takes 1 to 2 days for correction. Hemoglobin accounts for 75% of nonbicarbonate-based buffering of blood, while phosphate and other extracellular proteins account for the rest.

Table 4-3. Blood Gas Measurements

	DEFINITION	NORMAL RANGE
pH	Negative logarithm of hydrogen ion concentration	7.35-7.45
PCO_2	Partial pressure of CO_2 gas in blood that is proportional to the amount of dissolved CO_2	34-45 mm Hg
HCO_3^-	Concentration of bicarbonate in serum	20-28 mEq/L
Base difference or excess/deficit	The normal base amount is calculated using measured Hgb and normal values for pH and HCO_3^-, then this is compared with measured amount of blood base	+2-2
PO_2	Blood oxygen tension or dissolved O_2 content of plasma	80-95 mm Hg If patient is younger than age 60, the lower limit is dropped 1 mm Hg/year until age 60 is reached
$\%SaO_2$	Amount of Hgb bound with O_2 compared with the amount of Hgb available	Should be >90%

Hgb, Hemoglobin.

41. **How are acid–base abnormalities determined and classified?**
    The first step is to evaluate pH. If pH <7.35, then the finding is **acidosis**. A pH >7.45 indicates **alkalosis**. Any pH changes beyond 6.8 to 7.8 are incompatible with life. The next step uses PCO_2 and HCO_3^- to classify the primary abnormality as **respiratory** or **metabolic**, respectively. Metabolic acidosis is then further classified as an AG or nonanion gap problem. There will be a response to the primary disturbance by the opposite component in an attempt to compensate or normalize the pH. If the blood gas does not match the calculated compensation, then a mixed acid–base disorder should be suspected; that is, a respiratory acidosis and metabolic acidosis occurring simultaneously.

42. **What are the common causes and compensations in the primary acid–base disorders?**
    - Respiratory acidosis (hypoventilation): PCO_2 >45 mm Hg; HCO_3^- increase = change $PCO_2/10$ (acute) or $4 \times DPCO_2/10$ (chronic 2 to 5 days). Possible etiology: chronic obstructive pulmonary disease (COPD), asthma, cardiac arrest, severe pulmonary edema or pneumonia, injury to airway or chest wall, cerebrovascular accident (CVA), drugs (narcotics, sedatives), foreign body, muscular dystrophy, or myasthenia gravis.
    - Respiratory alkalosis (hyperventilation): PCO_2 <35 mm Hg; HCO_3^- decrease = $2 \times DPCO_2/10$ (acute), $5 \times DPCO_2/10$ (chronic). Possible etiology: anxiety, pain, fever, pulmonary embolus, mechanical overventilation, head injury, hypoxia, increased altitude, interstitial lung disease, pregnancy, hyperthyroidism, hepatic insufficiency, aspirin overdose, or early sepsis.
    - Metabolic acidosis: HCO_3^- <20 mEq/L; PCO_2 decrease = $8 + (1.5 \times HCO_3^-)$. Possible etiology:
      - AG normal: diarrhea, fistula, renal tubular acidosis
      - AG increased = extra acid
        - Exogenous: aspirin, methanol, ethylene glycol, ETOH ketoacidosis, hyperalimentation
        - Endogenous: lactic acidosis, DKA or starvation ketoacidosis, uremia, severe dehydration
    - Metabolic alkalosis: HCO_3^- >28 mEq/L, CO_2 increase = $0.6 \times D[HCO_3^-]$. Possible etiology: nasogastric suction, vomiting, diuretics, cystic fibrosis, posthypercapnia, Cushing's syndrome, hyperaldosteronism, exogenous steroids, or hypoparathyroidism.

43. What components of the blood gas evaluate oxygenation?

The PO_2 and $\%SaO_2$ are used to monitor oxygenation. The PO_2 gives an estimate of the alveolar gas exchange with inspired air, so that the patient likely has normal ventilation if the PO_2 is normal. The amount of oxygen available to cells is given by the $\%SaO_2$, which may also be obtained using pulse oximetry. The *pulse ox* has been shown to measure Hgb O_2 saturation accurately between 70% and 100%, or PO_2 >35 to 40 mm Hg. The oxygen saturation is influenced by temperature, pH, level of 2,3-diphosphoglycerate (2,3-DPG), and PO_2 as seen on the sigmoid-shaped O_2 dissociation curve. Hgb's affinity for O_2 is decreased by acidosis, fever, elevated 2,3-DPG, and hypoxia, which causes a shift of the curve to the right, and is increased with alkalosis, hypothermia, decreased 2,3-DPG, and banked blood, which causes a shift to the left.

44. How is an AMI ruled in or ruled out by the lab?

Much like the liver and pancreas, the heart has enzymes and proteins that are released from its cells in damage or death. A single measure alone of these substances is not adequate to rule out an AMI, and they should be checked at least twice in a 12-hour timeframe.

AST (SGOT) is found to increase in 90% to 95% of AMIs, begins elevation in 8 to 12 hours, peaks at 1 to 2 days, and is normal in 3 to 8 days. There is a rough correlation between degree of elevation and extent of damage to the heart but low specificity for heart muscle.

LDH levels are elevated in 92% to 95% of AMIs with slightly increased sensitivity over AST. LDH begins to rise at 24 to 48 hours, peaks at 2 to 3 days, and is normal at 5 to 10 days. Fractionating of isoenzymes shows improved specificity. LDH1/LDH2 >1 is seen in 80% to 85% of AMIs. LDH1 is found in RBCs, the heart, and the kidney, and normal values at 24 and 48 hours effectively rule out AMI.

Creatine kinase (CK) is increased in 90% to 93% of AMIs. Levels begin to rise in 3 to 6 hours, peak at 12 to 24 hours, and are normal in 1 to 2 days. Fractionated isozymes are MM (skeletal muscle, 94% to 100% of total), BB (brain and lung, usually 0% of total), and MB (heart fraction, usually <6% of total) and allow greater test specificity. There is a rough correlation with size of increase and amount of heart infarcted. Levels are usually checked at 0, 12, and 24 hours or 0, 8, 16, and 24 hours.

Troponin-T is an antibody that detects the cardiac-specific regulatory proteins. It has approximately the same specificity and sensitivity as CK-MB but rises in 4 to 6 hours, peaks at 11 hours, and is normal in 4 days.

Troponin-I is the same as troponin-T, but its timing is different; it begins to rise after 4 to 6 hours, peaks at 10 to 24 hours, and is normal after 10 days or more.

45. What tests are used to evaluate possible collagen vascular diseases?

Several nonspecific lab tests are used to help diagnose these enigmatic diseases:
- **Rheumatoid factor:** Positive in collagen vascular diseases, rheumatoid arthritis (RA), systemic lupus erythematosus (SLE), Sjögren's syndrome, scleroderma, polyarteritis nodosa, infections, CHF, inflammation, subacute bacterial endocarditis, MI, and lung disease
- **Lupus erythematosus (LE) preparation:** No cells = normal; positive in SLE, RA, scleroderma, and drug-induced lupus
- **Antinuclear antibody (ANA):** Negative result = normal; positive in SLE, scleroderma, drug-induced lupus, mixed connective tissue disease, RA, polymyositis, and juvenile RA
- **Antimicrosomal:** Detects Hashimoto thyroiditis
- **Anticentromere:** Tests for scleroderma, Raynaud disease, calcinosis, Raynaud phenomenon, esophageal involvement, sclerodactyly, and telangiectasia (CREST) syndrome
- **Anti-SCL 70:** Detects scleroderma
- **Anti-DNA:** Detects SLE, mononucleosis, chronic active hepatitis.

46. What are C-reactive protein (C-RP) and erythrocyte sedimentation rate (ESR) tests used to evaluate?

The C-RP and ESR are nonspecific but very sensitive markers for infections and inflammatory diseases. The ESR measures changes in plasma proteins (mainly fibrinogen) and is evaluated using several scales (zeta sedimentation ratio, Wintrobe method, Westergren method). The ESR is increased by any infection, inflammation, rheumatic fever, endocarditis, neoplasm, or AMI. The C-RP is a glycoprotein produced by acute inflammation and tissue destruction. Its levels are noted to begin elevating 4-6 hours after onset of inflammation and should be normal 5-7 days postoperatively or at least decreasing by day 3 after surgery; otherwise, an infection is likely. Other than inflammation or infection, the C-RP is also increased by pregnancy, oral contraceptives, and malignancies.

47. **What tests are used to screen for thyroid disease?**
    The most sensitive screening test for thyroid disease is the thyroid stimulating hormone (TSH) level, which is elevated in hypothyroidism and low in hyperthyroidism. The thyroxine total (T4 Tot) screens for hyperthyroidism with 95% sensitivity but is less accurate for hypothyroidism. Triiodothyronine (T3) resin uptake (RU) is an indirect measurement of T4. The test measures the protein thyroid-binding sites that are unbound and is elevated in hyperthyroidism, as a result of low thyroid-binding globulin (TBG), or if the patient is taking medications that bind TBG (e.g., phenytoin, aspirin, steroids, heparin). The T3 RU is 80% sensitive for hyperthyroidism but only 40% for hypothyroidism. The free thyroxine index (FTI) is determined by multiplying the T4 Tot by the T3 RU and has a 95% sensitivity for hyperthyroidism and 90% to 95% sensitivity for hypothyroidism. The FTI attempts to balance the TBG effects on T4 measurement. TBG is elevated in pregnancy, estrogen use, liver disease, and hypothyroidism. Total serum T3 (T3-RIA) is also measured in some labs and is equivalent to T4 Tot measurements.

48. **What tests can be used to evaluate possible bone disease?**
    The Ca and P levels (discussed previously). Alkaline phosphatase also can be used and is elevated in hyperparathyroidism, Paget's disease, osteoblastic bone tumors, osteomalacia, rickets, pregnancy, childhood, healing fractures, hyperthyroidism, and liver disease. The liver disorders may be ruled out using fractionated enzyme levels or checking GGT or 5′-nucleotidase.

49. **What procedures are done to evaluate body fluids and pathology specimens for organisms?**
    The most definitive test to isolate infectious agents is culturing, but this requires 24 hours at minimum. Staining allows for rapid screening identification to assist in selecting empiric antibiotics. The most common stains are:
    - **Gram:** Positive organisms turn a violet color because the microorganisms' thick cell walls of peptidoglycan and teichoic acid resist decolorization. Negative organisms have a thin cell wall and outer lipoprotein or lipopolysaccharide coat that decolorize in alcohol and pick up the counterstain (red).
    - **Acid-fast:** These organisms do not decolorize in strong acid and are usually *Mycobacterium* species.
    - **Potassium hydroxide (KOH):** 10% KOH dissolves most cellular elements except for fungus species.
    - **Wayson:** Used for general bacteria screening
    - **India ink:** Identifies mostly fungi in cerebrospinal fluid (CSF)
    - **Giemsa:** Stains intracellular organisms (*Chlamydia*, malaria) and viral inclusion bodies
    - Newer technology with DNA/polymerase chain reaction (PCR) probes and enzyme-linked immunosorbent assay (ELISA) tests allows rapid detection of organisms (e.g., Gonozyme, Streptozyme) or monospot tests

50. **What tests are used to evaluate viral hepatitis?**
    Hepatitis A: Oral/fecal hepatitis is usually self-limited. Acute infection tests positive for immunoglobulin M (IgM) ± IgG. Old infection or convalescence tests negative for IgM but positive for IgG. The antigen may be detected in stool but usually is gone before symptoms appear.
    Hepatitis B: Blood-borne disease with 1% acute fatality; 5% to 15% develop chronic disease, and 3% develop hepatocellular carcinoma.
    - HBsAg: Surface antigen from viral outer envelope indicates current or active hepatitis B virus (HBV) infection; DNA PCR probe is most accurate indicator of activity, infectivity, and progression to chronicity.
    - Anti-HBs: This indicates immunity and end of acute HBV.
    - Anti-HBcAg (presence of antibody to core viral protein): Indicates a recent or acute infection and is present during core window while HBsAg and anti-HBs are negative; drops out after 3 to 6 months.
    - Anti-HBc Tot: Stays positive for life; shows old infection if HBsAg and HBc-IgM are negative.
    - HBeAg/Anti-HBe: Indicate infectivity, because as anti-HBe increases, the infectivity decreases.
    - Chronic hepatitis B states:
      - Carrier-positive HBsAg but negative biopsy and liver function tests (LFTs)
      - Persistent hepatitis B: As above, with negative biopsy and abnormal LFTs
      - Active hepatitis B: As above, with positive biopsy and abnormal LFTs

Hepatitis C: Post-transfusion transmission; low severity acutely but 60% for chronic disease. Hepatitis C virus (HCV) nucleic probe shows current infection, but this is still investigational, and anti-HC indicates current, convalescing, or old HCV infection.

Hepatitis D: Requires HBV infection to be present, parenteral transmission, 5% acute fatality, 5% chronic. HDAg indicates infection; may follow with antibody levels.

51. **What tests are used to detect and monitor HIV infection?**

HIV antigen detection is used by blood banks because they may detect viral presence as early as 1 to 2 weeks. Antibodies are used to detect core proteins p24 or p55 and envelope glycoproteins gp41, 120, or 160. They are about 80% to 90% sensitive if patients have symptoms but 60% to 65% without. Nucleic acid probe with PCR amplification is also being used with 98% sensitivity at 3 months but 40% to 60% at 1 to 2 weeks. More commonly, patients are screened for the presence of antibodies in their serum, which take an average of 6 to 10 weeks to develop or seroconvert. The ELISA test screens the patient's blood for antibodies. A positive ELISA test is confirmed by Western blot, which looks for the most specific antibodies to gp41 and p24 or group-specific antigen (gag) core protein. Once HIV infection is determined, the CD4 T-cell count, viral load, and beta-2-microglobulin levels are followed for infection severity, prognosis, and activity and to direct therapy. The CD4 count (normal 600 to 1600 cells/mm^3) is a useful indicator of immune system damage and ability to respond effectively to pathogens. Immune suppression occurs with counts below 500 cells/mm^3 denoting an advanced risk of opportunistic infections and need for prophylactic antibiotics. Viral load assays appear to be the best prognostic marker for a patient's long-term clinical outcome and are used in conjunction with CD4 counts to direct antiviral therapy. Beta-2-microglobulin is a soluble marker for immune system activation and can be used to evaluate disease progression or exacerbation.

52. **What tests screen for or assist in the diagnosis of cancer?**

Alpha-fetoprotein (AFP): Elevated in hepatocellular carcinoma, testicular tumors, occasionally benign hepatic disease (hepatitis, alcoholic cirrhosis) and in pregnancy: neural tube defects, multiple gestation, or fetal death.

Cancer antigen 19-9 (CA 19-9): Elevated in 80% to 85% pancreatic adenocarcinoma, 40% to 50% gastric adenocarcinoma, 30% to 40% colorectal cancer, 50% hepatocellular carcinoma, 16% to 20% lung cancer, and 14% to 27% breast cancer.

CA 125: Increased in ovarian, endometrial, and colon cancers; also in endometriosis, inflammatory bowel disease, pelvic inflammatory disease, pregnancy, breast lesion, and teratomas.

Carcinoembryonic antigen (CEA): Not used to screen but is a good monitor of recurrence and response to treatment (if checked before started). Elevated in colon, pancreas, lung, and stomach cancers, as well as in smokers and those with Crohn's disease, liver disease, and ulcerative colitis.

Prostate specific antigen (PSA): Good for screening and monitoring after treatment. Levels above 10 mg/dL are associated with cancer >90%. Also, a velocity of 0.75 mg/mL/year indicates high suspicion for cancer. Differential diagnosis for elevation includes prostate cancer, acute prostatitis, benign prostate hypertrophy, prostate surgery, and vigorous prostate massage. Normal rectal exam has no influence.

53. **What basic tests are used to evaluate CSF?**

Opening pressure: Normal is 100 to 200 mm Hg; most significantly elevated in bacterial infections (meningitis) and subarachnoid hemorrhage (SAH).

Color or appearance: Normal is clear and colorless, but bloody or xanthochromic (yellow from Hgb breakdown) after 2 to 8 hours in SAH and white or cloudy in bacterial infections.

Glucose: Normal is 0.5 serum glucose (45 to 80 mg/dL) but will be <20 mg/dL in meningitis and between 20 and 40 mg/dL in granulomatous infection (tuberculosis or fungal).

Protein: Normal range is 15 to 45 mg/dL, but the upper limit is debated. Levels will be 50 to 1500 mg/dL in meningitis and will be increased but <500 mg/dL in granulomatous disease.

Cell count: Normal is up to 5/mm^3 with all being lymphocytes; any condition that affects the meninges will cause CSF leukocytosis, the degree being determined by type, duration, and severity of irritation. The highest counts are seen in meningitis with PMNs dominating, whereas viral and granulomatous disease causes elevations to 10 to 500 cells, with lymphocytes predominant. SAH and traumatic taps will have increased cell counts made up of RBCs and WBCs in a ratio about equal to blood (1 WBC per 500 to 1000 RBCs). However, no good formulas exist to confirm that the WBC elevation is an artifact from a traumatic tap versus infective or inflammatory increase. Gram stain and culture are performed in all suspected infective taps.

54. **What tests can be done to verify or exclude a CSF leak in craniofacial trauma?**
    Confirmation of CSF otorrhea or rhinorrhea in trauma can be challenging. Typically, one looks for a colorless fluid, glucose about 45 mg/dL (nasal secretions <30 mg/dL and blood >80 usually), and low protein and potassium compared with nasal secretions or serum. Trauma patients, however, often exhibit a complex mixture of these body fluids, blocking chemical analysis. The most sensitive and specific test requires about 2 to 10 mL of fluid, protein electrophoresis, and about 3 hours to complete in a modern lab. The beta-2-transferrin isozyme will be isolated correctly in the presence of any mixture of fluid, and a beta-1 subset allows reduction of cirrhotic false-positive results. This test helps prevent the need for more invasive radiologic studies to rule out CSF leak.

55. **Is a CBC of value in making a diagnosis?**
    Yes, but mostly in certain diagnoses. For example, if the Hct is high (>45%), the patient is most likely dehydrated or may have COPD (emphysema). If it is low (<30%), the patient may have a more chronic disease associated with blood loss.
    Similarly, for WBC count, it takes hours for inflammation to release cytokines and cause elevation of the WBC count. Accordingly, a normal WBC count is not entirely inconsistent with infection.

56. **How is urinalysis useful?**
    WBCs in the urine should direct attention to the diagnosis of pyelonephritis or cystitis, complications of urinary tract infections. Hematuria may indicate renal or ureteral stones. RBCs and WBCs may be found in the urine of patients with appendicitis.

BIBLIOGRAPHY

Aziz N, Detels R, Fahey JL, et al.: Prognostic significance of plasma markers of immune activation, HIV viral load and CD4 T-cell measurements, *AIDS* 12:1581–1590, 1998.
Brinser P: Laboratory tests. In Abubaker AO, Benson KJ, editors: *Oral and maxillofacial surgery secrets*, ed 2, Philadelphia, 2007, Mosby Elsiever.
Burns ER, Lawrence C: Bleeding time. A guide to its diagnostic and clinical utility, *Arch Pathol Lab Med* 113:1219–1224, 1989.
Fauci A, editor: *Harrison's principles of internal medicine*, ed 14, New York, 1997, McGraw-Hill.
Gomella LG, editor: *Clinician's pocket reference*, ed 8, Stamford, Conn, 1997, Appleton & Lange.
Harken AH: Priorities in evaluation of the acute abdomen. In Harken AH, Moore EE, editors: *Abernathy's surgical secrets*, ed 5, St Louis, 2005, Mosby.
Harken AH, Moore EE, editors: *Abernathy's surgical secrets*, ed 5, St Louis, 2005, Mosby.
Jacobs DS, DeMott WR, Grady HJ, et al.: *Laboratory test handbook*, ed 4, Hudson, Ohio, 1996, Lexi-Corp.
Kaiser R, Kupfer B, Rockstroh JK, et al.: Role of HIV-1 phenotype in viral pathogenesis and its relation to viral load and CD4+ T-cell count, *J Med Virol* 56:259–263, 1998.
Krutsch JP: Coagulation. In Duke J, editor: *Anesthesia secrets*, ed 3, Philadelphia, 2006, Mosby.
Kwon P, Laskin D, editors: *Clinical manual of oral and maxillofacial surgery*, ed 2, Chicago, 1997, Quintessence.
Little JW, Falace DA, Miller CS, et al.: *Dental management of the medically compromised patient*, ed 6, St Louis, 2002, Mosby.
Malley WJ: *Clinical blood gases: assessment and intervention*, ed 2, Philadelphia, 2005, Saunders.
Keane M, O'Toole MT: *Miller-Keane encyclopedia & dictionary of medicine, nursing, & allied health*, ed 7, Philadelphia, 2005, Saunders.
Patton LL, Shugars DC: Immunologic and viral markers of HIV-1 disease progression: implications for dentistry, *J Am Dent Assoc* 130:1313–1322, 1999.
Peacock MK, Ryall RG, Simpson DA: Usefulness of beta2-transferrin assay in the detection of cerebrospinal fluid leaks following head injury, *J Neurosurg* 77:737–739, 1992.
Ravel R: *Clinical laboratory medicine*, ed 6, St Louis, 1995, Mosby.
Schwarz SI, Shires GT, Spencer FC, editors: *Principles of surgery*, ed 7, New York, 1998, McGraw-Hill.
Wu AHB: *Tietz clinical guide to laboratory tests*, ed 4, St Louis, 2006, Saunders.
Zaret DL, Morrison N, Gulbranson R, et al.: Immunofixation to quantify beta2-transferrin in cerebrospinal fluid to detect leakage of cerebrospinal fluid from skull injury, *Clin Chem* 38:1908–1912, 1992.

CHAPTER 5

DIAGNOSTIC IMAGING FOR THE ORAL AND MAXILLOFACIAL SURGERY PATIENT

Sonali A. Rathore, A. Omar Abubaker

1. **What are the basic units of radiation?**
   The units of absorbed radiation:
   - Gray (Gy)
   - Rads
   The units of biologically effective radiation:
   - Rem
   - Sieverts (Sv)
   Conversion between units:
   - 1 Gy = 100 rad
   - 1 mSv = 0.001 Gy

2. **What are the radiographic patterns of disease on an X-ray exam of the chest?**
   The patterns of disease on a chest radiograph are limited. The three most common patterns are:
   1. **Alveolar.** Pulmonary alveolar disease is the most common pattern and appears as a localized, homogeneous, fluffy density. It can represent water, blood, pus, or tumor within the alveoli.
   2. **Interstitial.** The interstitial pattern may be reticular (linear), nodular, or a combination of the two (reticulonodular). The reticular pattern usually is bilateral and diffuse.
   3. **Nodular.** The nodular pattern of disease appears as discrete, well-circumscribed, radiopaque masses in the lung field.

3. **What is the diagnostic value of posteroanterior (PA) chest films?**
   A PA chest film (Fig. 5-1) is taken by directing an X-ray beam from posterior to anterior on the chest. This radiograph is useful to evaluate the soft tissue and bony tissues of the chest, the diaphragm, the heart and mediastinum, the hila of the lungs, and the entire PA view of the lung fields.

4. **What are the main uses of a lateral chest film (Fig. 5-2)?**
   - Localizing lesions to a specific area of the lungs or mediastinum
   - Diagnosing small pleural effusions (blunting of the posterior costophrenic angles)
   - Diagnosing vertebral and sternal abnormalities

5. **What is the chest X-ray appearance of a pneumothorax (Fig. 5-3)?**
   Pneumothorax is usually represented by a thin, linear density that parallels the chest wall. No long markings should be seen peripheral to this line. In tension pneumothorax, a shift in the mediastinum is seen, especially with a large tension pneumothorax.

6. **What radiographic changes are associated with chronic obstructive pulmonary disease (COPD)?**
   - Hyperexpanded lung fields
   - A large, radiolucent zone behind the sternum
   - Flattening of the diaphragm
   - Elongated heart

7. **What radiographic changes are associated with chronic bronchitis?**
   Chest radiographs of chronic bronchitis show increased bronchovascular markings at the base of the lungs. In patients with emphysema, chest radiographs show overdistension of the lungs, flattening of the diaphragm, and emphysematous bullae.

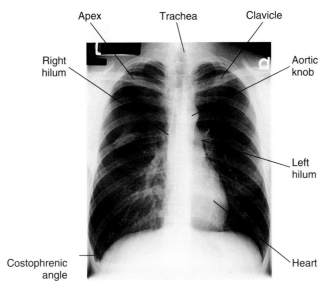

Figure 5-1. Posteroanterior chest projection. *(From Long BW, Frank ED, Ehrlich RA: Bony thorax, chest, and abdomen. In Long BW, Frank ED, Ehrlich RA, editors:* Radiography essentials for limited practice, *ed 2, St Louis, 2006, Saunders.)*

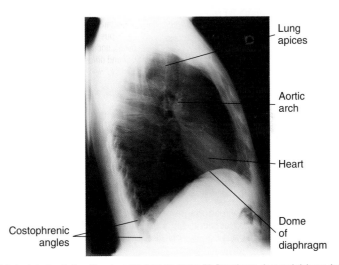

Figure 5-2. Lateral chest projection. *(From Long BW, Frank ED, Ehrlich RA: Bony thorax, chest, and abdomen. In Long BW, Frank ED, Ehrlich RA, editors:* Radiography essentials for limited practice, *ed 2, St Louis, 2006, Saunders.)*

8. How do lung masses show up on chest films?
   Lung masses usually follow the nodular pattern of disease. Masses within the lung fields can be divided into cavitary and noncavitary lesions and represent either tumor or infection. Other causes of masses include vascular malformations, but these are far less common than tumor and infection.

9. What is a lordotic chest radiograph used for?
   A lordotic chest radiograph permits better visualization of the apices of the lung. This view should be obtained when a questionable lesion is seen in these areas on a standard chest radiograph.

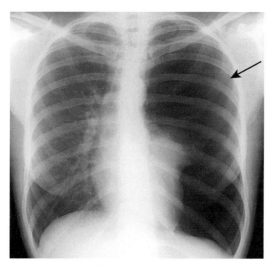

Figure 5-3. Posteroanterior chest film showing a left pneumothorax (arrow). *(From Bosker JI, Powers MP, Bosker H: Management of nonpenetrating chest trauma. In Fonseca RJ, Walker RV, Betts NJ, editors:* Oral and maxillofacial trauma, *ed 3, St Louis, 2005, Saunders.)*

10. **What is the common chest radiographic finding in AIDS patients?**
    Infectious pulmonary disease. *Pneumocystis carinii* pneumonia, the most common infection, usually has the pattern of a fine, diffuse reticular process.

11. **Which views are included in an acute abdominal series? When are they used?**
    - Supine and upright abdominal films (to view the kidneys, ureter, and bladder)
    - Chest radiograph
    These views are used for the initial evaluation of acute abdominal pain or trauma.

12. **What is a KUB?**
    A KUB is a radiographic view to evaluate the *k*idneys, *u*reters, and *b*ladder. The series, which is also known as a supine abdominal radiograph, is useful in the initial work-up of abdominal pain, distention of the bowel, and change of bowel habits. It also is used for evaluation of urinary tract problems. Renal stones and 10% to 20% of gallstones are visualized by a KUB. Evaluation of the KUB views involves examining the bowel gas pattern and looking for calcifications and radiopaque foreign bodies. The psoas; renal, liver, and splenic shadows; flank stripes; vertebral bodies; and pelvic bones also are examined.

13. **What is a barium swallow (esophagram)?**
    An esophagram, usually performed with barium, a water-soluble contrast agent, is used to evaluate the swallowing mechanism and to look for esophageal lesions or abnormal peristalsis. No preparation is required for this study.

14. **What is the upper gastrointestinal series (UGI)?**
    UGI, which includes an esophagram, is used to study the stomach and duodenum. This double-contrast study uses barium and air and is useful for detection of gastritis, ulcers, masses, hiatal hernias, and gastrointestinal reflux. It is also an important part of the work-up of heme-positive stools and upper abdominal pain.

15. **What is an intravenous pyelogram (IVP)?**
    This imaging technique uses intravenous (IV) contrast to evaluate the kidneys, ureters, and bladder. This test is indicated for patients with hematuria, kidney stones, urinary tract infection, and suspected malignancy of the kidney or bladder and is used for the work-up of patients with flank pain.

16. **What are the different nuclear scans and their uses?**
In nuclear scans, or nuclear medicine studies, radionuclides are injected intravenously, and results are based on detection of the tissue uptake of these radionuclides, specifically the degree of uptake, the time intervals between the studies, and the injection of the radionuclides.

   A bone scan is a nuclear scan study that uses radioactive tracers, such as technetium 99, to detect areas of increased or decreased bone metabolism (turnover). Areas that absorb little tracer appear as dark or "cold" spots, which may indicate a lack of blood supply to the bone or the presence of certain types of cancer. Areas of rapid bone growth or repair absorb increased amounts of the tracer and show up as bright or "hot" spots in the pictures, which indicate the presence of a tumor, a fracture, or an infection. Bone scans are used in metastatic work-ups, especially in patients with cancer that has a predilection to metastasize to bone (e.g., breast, prostate, kidney, lung, thyroid). They are also used as screening tests for primary tumors, osteomyelitis, avascular necrosis, and stress fractures.

   A gallium scan is used to locate abscesses that are more than 5 to 10 days old. When used in combination with a bone scan, the gallium scan is very specific for osteomyelitis. Indium 111 white blood cell scans can be substituted for gallium scanning to detect osteomyelitis.

   The cardiac scan has become increasingly popular in recent years and is used for many purposes, including detection of myocardial infarction and ischemia, stress testing, and evaluation of ejection fractions, cardiac output, and ventricular aneurysms.

   A liver-spleen scan is used to estimate parenchymal disease, abscess, tumors, and cysts in these organs. The current preference for computed tomography (CT) scanning has significantly decreased the use of the liver-spleen scan.

   The ventilation-perfusion lung scan is used principally for the evaluation of pulmonary emboli. Although not as sensitive or specific as a pulmonary angiogram or spiral CT, the ventilation-perfusion scan is less invasive and often is obtained following a chest radiograph when the diagnosis of pulmonary embolus is suspected.

17. **What (plain film) views are included in a facial series, and what are they used for?**
A facial series usually includes Caldwell's view, Waters' view, lateral skull view, and submentovertex view (view of the zygomatic arches). These studies are used for the initial work-up of facial trauma.

18. **What plain film views are included on a mandibular series, and what are they used for?**
A mandibular series includes a Towne's view, a PA skull view, both oblique views of the mandible, and a panoramic view. This series is used mainly for evaluation of the mandible following facial trauma.

19. **What views are included in a nasal bone series?**
A nasal bone series includes an anteroposterior (AP) skull view and both lateral views of the nasal bones. This series is used for evaluation of trauma to the nose.

20. **What are the normal anatomic radiographic landmarks on a panoramic image?**
See Figure 5-4.

21. **What is a sinus series?**
A sinus series is used for evaluating the paranasal sinuses, including the frontal, ethmoid, maxillary, and sphenoid sinuses. The views taken usually include a Caldwell's, Waters', lateral, and submentovertex. This series is used for the initial evaluation of sinusitis or sinus masses.

22. **What views are included in the cervical spine series?**
The cervical spine series usually includes PA and lateral views, both oblique views, and odontoid views of the cervical spine. This series is useful for evaluating traumatic injury, neck pain, and neurologic symptoms referable to the upper extremities. All seven cervical vertebrae must be seen for the exam to be considered acceptable.

23. **What views are included in airway films?**
Airway films include AP and lateral views of the neck to provide good visualization of the airways and adjacent soft tissues. They are used as the initial step in the work-up of masses, foreign bodies, and infections of the airway.

24. **What are the uses and advantages of plain film tomography?**
With the advent of CT, plain film tomography now has only limited utility in the evaluation of problems within the head and neck. Its principal advantage is that it does not show the metallic artifact that

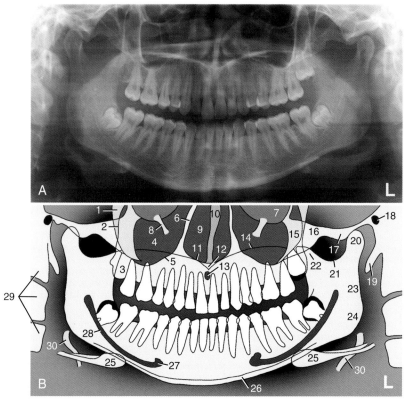

Figure 5-4. Panoramic radiograph showing numbered anatomic landmarks. *(From White SC, Pharoah MJ, Oral Radiology: Principles and Interpretation, ed 7, St. Louis, Mosby, 2014.)*

1. Pterygomaxillary fissure	11. Floor of the nasal cavity	22. Coronoid process
2. Posterior border of maxilla	12. Anterior nasal spine	23. Posterior border of ramus
3. Maxillary tuberosity	13. Incisive foramen	24. Angle of mandible
4. Maxillary sinus	14. Hard palate/floor of the nasal cavity	25. Hyoid bone
5. Floor of the maxillary sinus	15. Zygomatic process of the maxilla	26. Inferior border of mandible
6. Medial border of maxillary sinus/	16. Zygomatic arch	27. Mental foramen
lateral border of the nasal cavity	17. Articular eminence	28. Mandibular canal
7. Floor of the orbit	18. External auditory meatus	29. Cervical vertebrae
8. Infraorbital canal	19. Styloid process	30. Epiglottis
9. Nasal cavity	20. Mandibular condyle	
10. Nasal septum	21. Sigmoid notch	

often obscures the CT evaluation of postoperative patients. It also has the advantage of allowing three-plane evaluation of bony structures, which can only be accomplished with CT scans by reconstruction of axial views. In evaluating temporomandibular joints (TMJs), sagittal tomography frequently provides more information about the bony architecture of these joints than axial CT scans do.

25. **When are CT scans of the head and neck indicated?**
    - Head CT: Head trauma to rule out intracranial injury or pathology and to evaluate for skull fractures
    - MaxFace CT: Head or facial trauma to evaluate midface and/or orbital fractures
    - MaxFace CT with extension through the mandible: Head or facial trauma to evaluate midface and/or orbital fractures, with suspected mandible fracture also
    - Neck CT: To evaluate the mandible and/or airway for trauma and/or infection
    - C-spine CT: When a cervical spine series is deemed inadequate

26. **When is contrast indicated/contraindicated for head and neck CT scans?**
    Contrast agents are used in CT exams and in other radiology procedures to improve visualization of structures. Some contrasts are natural, such as air or water. Iodine or barium sulfate oral or rectal contrast is usually given when examining the abdomen or cells, but not when scanning the brain or chest. Iodine is the most widely used IV contrast agent and is given through an IV needle. Iodine in contrast medium has a large atomic number and thus effectively absorbs X-rays.
    Indications: To illuminate anatomy, malignant facial tumors (more vascularized), enlarged lymph nodes containing metastatic carcinoma.
    Contraindications: Allergic reaction, renal failure, elevated creatinine.

27. **What prophylactic measures may be taken for patients who have a previous allergy to IV contrast?**
    Anaphylactic reactions to contrast agents used during endoscopic retrograde cholangiopancreatography (ERCP) are rare. Nevertheless, a history of sensitivity to iodine contrast or drug should always be considered in the preprocedure assessment and in the informed consent process. In patients with prior allergy to contrast media, prophylactic measures adopted by most endoscopists include:
    * Use of nonionic/low osmolarity contrast media.
    * Premedication with oral steroids starting the day before ERCP, or IV steroids when allergy is discovered just before the procedure. Some endoscopists also give an IV antihistamine in combination with the steroids.

28. **What is sialography?**
    Sialography is an imaging study used for the radiographic demonstration of the salivary gland ductal system. It is accomplished by cannulating the ducts of the submandibular and parotid glands and injecting a radiopaque contrast medium.

29. **When is sialography indicated?**
    * To detect or confirm small radiopaque or radiolucent sialoliths or foreign bodies
    * To evaluate damage secondary to recurrent inflammation
    * To provide a more detailed evaluation of suspected neoplasms, such as size, location, and extension into adjacent tissues
    * To evaluate fistulas, strictures, and diverticula of the ductal system, especially in posttraumatic cases
    * To detect chronic sialadenitis and chronic stricture (rarely used)

30. **When is sialography contraindicated?**
    * In patients with known sensitivity to iodine compounds
    * In acute salivary inflammation

31. **What does the obstructive form of salivary gland disease look like on a sialogram?**
    In the acute form of obstructive salivary gland disease and acute sialadenitis, sialography is rarely performed and mostly contraindicated. However, a sialogram performed during a clinically quiescent period of the disease in a patient with the obstructive form of the disease usually shows a focal narrowing (stricture) of the main duct and a central dilatation (sialectasia), with these ducts tapering dramatically to normal peripheral ducts. If the acini are compressed and destroyed by the cellular infiltrate, the peripheral ducts and acini are not visualized, even on a technically good sialogram.

32. **What is the appearance of Sjögren's syndrome on a sialogram?**
    Sjögren's syndrome initially involves only the peripheral intraglandular ducts and acini. Accordingly, the early stages of the disease are manifested on a sialogram as a normal central duct system and numerous, uniform, peripheral punctate collections of contrast material throughout the gland. These changes are the earliest sialographic features and are diagnostic of the disease. As the disease progresses, the sialogram is said to resemble a leafless fruit-laden tree or a mulberry tree. The advanced form of the disease is seen on a sialogram as dilatation of the central ducts and, eventually, a large peripheral collection of the contrast material and the associated changes of sialadenitis superimposed on the punctate and globular findings of Sjögren's syndrome.

33. **What is the best imaging technique to diagnose TMJ disc displacement (Fig. 5-5)?**
    Currently, magnetic resonance imaging (MRI) is the imaging of choice to show disc displacement with and without reduction. Dynamic MRI techniques are also used to enhance the diagnostic quality of the

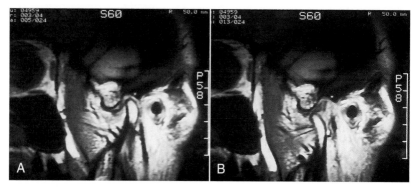

Figure 5-5. Magnetic resonance imaging of open (A) and closed (B) views of right temporomandibular joint with early anterior disc displacement with reduction. *(From Quinn PD: Diagnostic imaging of the temporomandibular joint. In Quinn PD, editor:* Color atlas of temporomandibular joint surgery, *St Louis, 1998, Mosby.)*

image. Although an arthrogram was used in the past to make such a diagnosis, it is currently rarely used for such purpose.

34. **How are disc perforations of the TMJ diagnosed?**
Although MRI is usually the first choice for soft tissue imaging of the TMJ in most clinical situations, the best imaging modality available to diagnose disc perforations is arthrography. Because of the recent decrease in use of arthrography, diagnosis of disc perforation currently is based on clinical exam.

35. **What are the advantages and disadvantages of MRI for the diagnosis of TMJ pathology?**
Advantages
- Provides an image of both hard and soft tissue structures of the TMJ in multiple planes
- Does not use radiation
- Is not technically demanding
Disadvantages
- Is expensive for patients
- Is not well tolerated by patients suffering from claustrophobia

36. **What are the indications and contraindications for MRI?**
Magnetic resonance images are based on proton density and proton relaxation dynamics due to magnetic fields. These vary according to the tissue under examination and reflect its physical and chemical properties. There is no radiation exposure during MRI.
In the detection, localization, and treatment planning of head and neck tumors, MRI offers an advantage over CT because of its multiplanar capabilities, the tissue characterization potential, and the absence of bone and teeth artifacts. MRI affords ready distinction of vessels from lymph nodes. MRI also depicts the contents of the orbit. MRI is absolutely contraindicated in patients with cerebral aneurysm clips and cardiac pacemakers. However, it should be noted that titanium in bone plates and dental implants do not affect the MRI exam. Remember that MRI machines are large magnets that never turn off!

37. **How do you differentiate between T1 and T2 weighted images?**
As a rule of thumb, if you see fluid darker than solids, then it is a T1 or proton density image. If the fluid such as CSF is white, then you are dealing with a T2 weighted image.

In a T1 weighted image:	DARK = water, cerebrospinal fluid (CSF), edema, calcium
	LIGHT = lipid, gadolinium
In a T2 weighted image:	DARK = calcium, bone
	LIGHT = water, CSF, edema

38. **What is cone beam computed tomography?**
Cone beam computed tomography (CBCT) is a medical image acquisition technique based on a cone-shaped X-ray beam centered on a two-dimensional (2D) detector. The technology gets its name from use of a divergent pyramidal or cone-shaped source of ionizing radiation. Imaging is accomplished

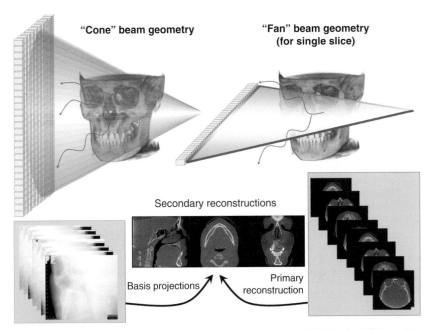

Figure 5-6. Difference in acquisition geometry in "cone" beam CT and "fan" beam of MDCT. *(From Scarfe W, Farman A: What is cone-beam CT and how does it work?* Dental Clin N Am *52:707–730, 2008.)*

by using a rotating gantry to which an X-ray source and detector are fixed. The X-ray source and detector rotate around a rotation fulcrum fixed within the center of the region of interest. The images are reconstructed in a three-dimensional (3D) data set using a modification of the original cone beam algorithm developed by Feldkamp et al.

39. **What is the basic difference between cone beam CT and traditional medical CT?**
    In a cone beam CT, the X-ray source and detector rotate around a rotating fulcrum, which is fixed within the center of the region of interest. During rotation, multiple (from 150 to more than 600) sequential planar projection images of the field of view (FOV) are acquired in a complete, or sometimes partial, arc. Only one rotational sequence of the gantry is necessary to acquire enough data for image reconstruction. This procedure varies from a traditional medical CT, which uses a fan-shaped X-ray beam in a helical progression to acquire individual image slices of the FOV and then stacks the slices to obtain a 3D representation. Each slice requires a separate scan and separate 2D reconstruction (Fig. 5-6).

40. **What imaging modality is used for dental implant treatment planning?**
    The position statement of the American Academy of Oral and Maxillofacial Radiology (AAOMR) was released in June 2012 with regard to dental implants. The paper states that panoramic radiography supplemented with intraoral radiographs should be used for the initial evaluation of the dental implant patient. However, any potential implant site evaluation should include cross-sectional imaging orthogonal to the site of interest. Conventional tomography provides cross-sectional information but is technique sensitive and images are more difficult to interpret than CBCT. The AAOMR recommends CBCT imaging as the current method of choice for cross-sectional imaging in that it provides the greatest diagnostic yield at an acceptable radiation dose risk. CBCT helps in dental implant planning by providing information on the morphologic characteristics and orientation of the residual alveolar ridge (RAR). It also helps in identification of local anatomic or pathologic conditions restricting implant placement.

41. **What are the applications of cone beam CT in dentistry?**
    Cone beam CT has found various clinical applications in dentistry. The most common clinical applications are impacted teeth and implantology. It has also found applications in specialized dentistry

(orthodontics, endodontics, periodontics, and forensic dentistry). It has been found to be very promising in endodontics, especially to look for apical lesions, root fractures, canal identification, and characterization of internal and external root resorption. In periodontics, it is used to visualize bone topography and lesion architecture. Current research has found it no more superior than 2D imaging in caries detection, especially in the presence of beam-hardening artifacts.

42. **What are the dose considerations with cone beam CT?**
Any radiographic procedure should consider the trade-off between diagnostic benefits to dose detriment for the patient. Dental CBCT is recommended as a dose-sparing technique for the common oral and maxillofacial radiographic imaging tasks compared to the alternative standard medical CT scans. Effective doses from a standard dental protocol scan MDCT are in the range of 1.5 to 12.3 times greater than comparable medium FOV dental CBCT scans. The effective doses can vary for various CBCT devices, ranging from 29 to 477 mSv, depending on the type and model of CBCT equipment and FOV selected. If we compare these doses with multiples of a single panoramic dose or background equivalent radiation dose, CBCT provides an equivalent patient radiation dose of 5 to 74 times that of a single film-based panoramic X-ray, or 3 to 48 days of background radiation.

43. **What are the different cone beam CT artifacts?**
Artifacts are distortions or errors that reduce the diagnostic quality of the resultant image.
The different types of artifacts are:
- Beam-hardening artifacts: These can occur as cupping artifacts, seen as distortions of metallic structures, or streaking artifacts, where streaks and dark bands appear between two dense objects.
- Patient-related artifacts: These can occur due to patient motion, which can cause unsharpness in the resultant image.
- Scanner-related artifacts: These can occur due to poor calibration and appear as circular or ring shapes in the image.
- Cone beam artifacts: These are grouped together as partial volume averaging, undersampling, and cone beam effect.
- Image noise and poor soft tissue contrast

44. **What are the advantages and limitations of cone beam CT compared to multi-detector CT (MDCT)?**
Advantages: The biggest advantages of cone beam CT compared to MDCT are low radiation dose and reduced cost. It offers a real-size data set with multiplanar cross-sectional and 3D reconstructions based on a single scan. It has potential for generating 2D images such as panoramic radiographs, lateral cephalograms, and TMJs. It has user-friendly postprocessing and viewing software. It offers energy saving compared to medical CT.
Disadvantages: The most important disadvantage of CBCT imaging is the low contrast resolution and limited capability of visualizing the internal soft tissues. Some of its other limitations are a small detector size, which limits the field of view, and the resulting scanned volume. It cannot be used for estimation of Hounsfield units as compared to MDCT.

45. **How is diagnostic and interventional angiography used by the oral and maxillofacial surgeon?**
Diagnostic and interventional angiography assists the oral and maxillofacial surgeon in the diagnosis and delineation of uncontrollable hemorrhage and vascular tumors in the maxillofacial region. When coupled with CT and MRI exams, the surgical approach and definitive treatment can be planned. The use of interventional angiography for embolization of vascular tumors before or instead of surgical resection has become a popular modality in the management of these tumors.

46. **What is the role of radionuclide scintigraphy in oral and maxillofacial surgery?**
Oral and maxillofacial surgeons use radionuclide scintigraphy to evaluate bone and joint diseases because it provides more sensitive bone imaging than conventional radiologic techniques. Specifically, scintigraphy or bone scanning can assist in the evaluation of arthritic changes to the TMJ, condylar hyperplasia, idiopathic condylar resorption (active and inactive), metabolic disorders, viability of bone grafts, trauma, dental disorders, osteomyelitis, and malignancies. However, it should be noted that scintigraphy has a low specificity for abnormal findings, and 20% to 50% of patients referred for routine bone scan may have abnormal activity in the mandible or face.

47. What diagnostic imaging modalities are useful for the diagnosis of cysts and benign odontogenic tumors of the jaw?

Most pathologies in the oral and maxillofacial region can be demonstrated through conventional radiographs. The panoramic radiograph is still the primary screening film for the oral and maxillofacial surgeon. Traditionally, multiplanar views were obtained primarily with multidetector CT (MDCT) and magnetic resonance imaging (MRI). With the introduction of CBCT, all three dimensions are recorded by multiplanar (axial, coronal, and sagittal planes) imaging of CBCT. Such multiplanar views provide important information on the presence and extent of bone resorption, sclerosis of neighboring bone, cortical expansion and internal or external calcifications, and proximity to other vital anatomy. With newer CBCT units, slice thicknesses are as small as 0.1 mm; these thin slices allow better visualization of the bony margins of the lesion. MDCT is extremely helpful for illustrating cysts and tumors of the mandible and maxilla, especially if the lesion extends beyond the bony cortex with encroachment on the adjacent soft tissue structures. MRI is useful in differentiating cysts from solid tumors and differentiating fluid within the cystic lumen from other cystic components such as keratin and blood degradation products. However, compared to MDCT and MRI, CBCT units are preferred in the OMFS office due to smaller physical dimension, lower cost, and easier operation.

48. What diagnostic imaging modalities are used for evaluation of malignant diseases of the jaws?
    - CT
    - CBCT
    - MRI
    - Radionuclide scanning techniques
    - Panoramic radiography

Radiologic evaluation of jaw lesions requires an image that accurately differentiates bone and soft tissue. CT permits the accurate assessment of tumor size, location, and extent of spread and detects subtle bony involvement and calcifications. If a malignancy is suspected to involve osseous components, cross-sectional imaging with either MDCT or CBCT can reliably predict bone invasion by the malignant lesion. However, CBCT images are not useful in analyzing soft tissue tumors. In this case, MRI or soft tissue window MDCT is a better diagnostic tool. MRI provides high-resolution, thin tomographic images with superior soft tissue contrast. In addition, MRI allows visualization of blood vessels without IV contrast agents and some information regarding tissue composition.

In most cases of a suspicious malignant lesion, a complete diagnostic work-up of the patient will include multiple examinations using CBCT, MDCT, MRI, or nuclear medicine.

49. What are the uses of the different imaging techniques for mandibular fractures?

Initial assessment of complex jaw fractures can be achieved with periapical or panoramic radiographs. In addition, AP, lateral skull, Waters', and Towne's views also can be helpful. However, for diagnosing root fractures, multiple jaw fractures with bone displacement, and interarticular fractures of the condylar head, CBCT may be a valuable imaging tool. However, the role of CBCT in fracture diagnosis is limited to fractures of teeth, sports-related injuries, or minor assault. MDCT with or without MRI is a better imaging choice in automobile or industrial accidents that involve jaws along with other parts of the body.

50. Which imaging modalities are used to diagnose midfacial fractures?

The initial radiographic survey of patients with midface trauma should include Waters', Towne's, AP, lateral skull, and submentovertex views. However, because the facial bone diverges in a posterior-to-anterior direction, AP views distort bone anatomy and produce magnified and overlapping structural images. Hence, CT or CBCT is the definitive means of imaging midfacial trauma. CBCT has been found to be very useful to study fractures of the zygomatico-maxillary complex, in particular with regard to surgical navigation, localization of bony fragments, and evaluation of screw anchorage. The coronal and sagittal CBCT images are also very useful in patients with fractures of the cribriform plate, nose, orbital floor, and orbital roof. However, when clinical examination reveals potential intracranial, skull base, or cranial nerve damage, MDCT or MRI examination is recommended. Other instances such as epidural or subdural hematoma, cerebral concussion, and intraorbital or globe lesions also necessitate an MDCT or MRI examination.

51. What imaging techniques are used for evaluation of maxillary sinus pathology?

Traditionally, a routine sinus examination consisted of Waters' sinus view along with Caldwell, lateral skull, and submento-vertex views. However, these plain film views are considered inadequate in detecting maxillary sinus opacification and "very poor" in detecting masses in the ethmoid, frontal, and sphenoid sinuses. In recent years, both ENT practitioners and oral and maxillofacial surgeons have been using CBCT as an efficient in-house examination tool. CBCT images are helpful in identification of mucus retention phenomena, antral polyps, sinonasal polyposis, oroantral fistula, or displacement of an implant into the sinus. Low-dose imaging such as CBCT is crucial as inflammatory sinus disease is often recurring and can sometimes result in repetitive imaging requests. Another major advantage of CBCT is that images have the same quality in all possible planes. One major disadvantage of CBCT is poor contrast resolution. MRI is the imaging modality of choice in patients with suspect malignancy or in patients presenting with neurologic signs and/or deficits. MRI is useful as it is not affected by the beam-hardening artifacts from dental amalgam or dense cortical bone. CT is performed in instances to allow visualization of the extent of bone destruction and soft tissue reactions to disease including infiltrations.

52. **What imaging modalities are used for diagnosis of inflammatory disorders of the jaw?**
Most inflammatory disorders of the jaw can be evaluated by plain radiographs, but plain films may require supplementation by CT, CBCT, MRI, or radionuclide scanning techniques. Both inflammation and malignancy can have similar radiographic features, which necessitate cross-sectional imaging for further evaluation. Oral and maxillofacial surgeons rely on occlusal radiographs to identify periosteal reactions of the bone. However, wrong angulation or exposure factors can limit the utility of an occlusal radiograph. With CBCT images, the thin layer of periosteal bone can be seen in the multiplanar slices. In addition, bony sequestra can be better identified with cross-sectional imaging. Also in evaluating BRONJ, CBCT is more useful than panoramic radiography. Scintigraphy or radionuclide imaging is the most definitive way of demonstrating bone changes and clinical activity caused by inflammation or suspected osteomyelitis.

53. **Which imaging techniques will reveal soft tissue infection in the head and neck regions (Fig. 5-7)?**
The primary imaging modalities to evaluate infection in the head and neck are CT and MRI. CT and MRI both differentiate abscess from cellulitis, indicate the presence of venous thrombosis and airway

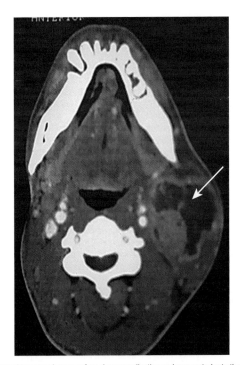

Figure 5-7. Computed tomography scan of an abscess collection and gas posterior to the mandible (*arrow*).

compromise, and show the exact location and extent of the infectious process. CT is better than MRI in evaluating the integrity of cortical bone, and CT takes less time, costs less, and is more readily available than MRI. MRI, on the other hand, allows imaging in the sagittal, coronal, and axial planes with the patient supine, does not use radiation, and is not affected or degraded by artifacts from dental amalgam. Overall, CT with contrast with a very high diagnostic quality in all stages of oral and facial infections is most commonly used for this purpose.

BIBLIOGRAPHY

Abrams JJ: CT assessment of dental implant planning, *Oral Maxillofac Surg Clin North Am* 4:1–18, 1992.
Ahmad M, Jenney J, Downie M: Application of cone beam computed tomography in oral and maxillofacial surgery, *Aust Dent J* 57(Suppl 1):82–94, March 2012.
Barsotti JB, Westesson PL, Ketonen LM: Diagnostic and interventional angiographic procedures in the maxillofacial region, *Oral Maxillofac Surg Clin North Am* 4:35–50, 1992.
Casselman JW, Gieraerts K, et al.: Cone beam CT: non-dental applications, *JBR–BTR* 96, 2013.
Conway WF: Diagnostic imaging. In Kwon PH, Laskin DM, editors: *Clinical manual of oral and maxillofacial surgery*, ed 2, Chicago, 1996, Quintessence.
De Vos W, Casselman J, Swennen GRJ: Cone beam computerized tomography of the oral and maxillofacial region: a systematic review of the literature, *Int J Oral Maxillofac Surg* 38(6):609–625, June 2009.
Doddarayapete U, Viswanath D, Kumar M: Application of cone-beam computed tomography in oral and maxillofacial surgery, *J Indian Aca Oral Med Radiol* 25(3):192–195, 2013.
Dolan KD, Ruprecht A: Imaging of mandibular and temporomandibular joint fractures, *Oral Maxillofac Surg Clin North Am* 4:113–124, 1992.
Dolan KD, Ruprecht A: Imaging of midface fractures, *Oral Maxillofac Surg Clin North Am* 4:125–152, 1992.
Hashimoto K, Arai Y, Iwai K, et al.: A comparison of a new limited cone beam computed tomography machine for dental use with a multidetector row helical CT machine, *Oral Surg Oral Med Oral Pathol Oral Radiol Endod* 95:371–377, 2003.
Holliday RA, Prendergast NC: Imaging inflammatory processes of the oral cavity and suprahyoid neck, *Oral Maxillofac Surg Clin North Am* 4:215–240, 1992.
Little JW, Falace DA, Miller CS, et al.: *Dental management of the medically compromised patient*, ed 6, St Louis, 2002, Mosby.
Ludlow JB, Davies-Ludlow LE, Brooks SL, et al: Dosimetry of 3 CBCT devices for oral and maxillofacial radiology: CB Mercuray, NewTom 3G and i-CAT., *Dentomaxillofac Radiol* 35(4):219–226, Jul 2006.
Ludlow JB, Davies-Ludlow LE, Mol A: Dosimetry of recently introduced CBCT units for oral and maxillofacial radiology. In: *Proceedings of the16th international congress of dentomaxillofacial radiology, Beijing, China*, 26–30 June, 2007, p 97.
Ludlow JB, Ivanovic M: Comparative dosimetry of dental CBCT devices and 64-slice CT for oral and maxillofacial radiology, *Oral Surg Oral Med Oral Pathol Oral Radiol Endod* 106:106–114, 2008.
Miles DA: Imaging inflammatory disorders of the jaw: simple osteitis to generalized osteomyelitis, *Oral Maxillofac Surg Clin North Am* 4:207–214, 1992.
Miracle AC, Mukherji SK: Conebeam CT of the head and neck, part 2: clinical applications, *AJNR* 30:1285–1292, August 2009.
O'Mara RE: Scintigraphy of the facial skeleton, *Oral Maxillofacial Surg Clin North Am* 4:51–60, 1992.
Scaf G, Lurie AG, Mosier KM, et al.: Dosimetry and cost of imaging osseointegrated implants with film-based and computed tomography, *Oral Surg Oral Med Oral Pathol Oral Radiol Endod* 83:41–48, 1997.
Scarfe W, Farman A: What is cone-beam CT and how does it work? *Dental Clin N Am* 52:707–730, 2008.
Schering AG: *MRI made easy*, 35: 219–26. 2006.
Schulze D, Heiland M, Thurmann H, et al.: Radiation exposure during midfacial imaging using 4- and 16-slice computed tomography, cone beam computed tomography systems and conventional radiography, *Dentomaxillofac Radiol* 33:83–86, 2004.
Som PM, Brandwein M: Salivary glands. In Som PM, Curtin HD, editors: *Head and neck imaging*, vol. 2. St Louis, 1996, Mosby.
Ericson S: Conventional and oral computerized imaging of maxillary sinus pathology related to dental problems, *Oral Maxillofac Surg Clin North Am* 4:153–182, 1992.
Tyndall D, Rathore S: Cone-beam CT diagnostic applications: caries, periodontal bone assessment and endodontic applications, *Dental Clin N Am* 52:825–841, 2008. http://www.dentalcrest.com/dental-panoramic-anatomy/.
U.S. Nuclear Regulatory Commission, http://www.nrc.gov/reading-rm/doc-collections/cfr/part020/part020-1004.html.
van Rensburg LJ, Nortje CJ: Magnetic resonance imaging and computed tomography of malignant disease of the jaws, *Oral Maxillofac Surg Clin North Am* 4:75–112, 1992.
Wandtke JC: Chest imaging for the oral and maxillofacial surgeon, *Oral Maxillofac Surg Clin North Am* 4:241–252, 1992.
Weber AL: Imaging of cysts and benign odontogenic tumors of the jaw, *Oral Maxillofac Surg Clin North Am* 4:61–74, 1992.
WebMD: http://www.webmd.com/hw/health_guide_atoz/hw200283.asp.
Westesson P: Magnetic resonance imaging of the temporomandibular joint, *Oral Maxillofac Surg Clin North Am* 4:183–206, 1992.
White SC: Computer-assisted radiographic differential diagnosis of jaw lesions, *Oral Maxillofac Surg Clin North Am* 4:261–272, 1992.
White S, Pharoah M: *Oral radiology: principles and interpretation*, ed 7, 2014.

II

ANESTHESIA

CHAPTER 6

LOCAL ANESTHETICS

Ravi Agarwal, George Obeid, A. Omar Abubaker, Kenneth J. Benson

1. **What is the resting membrane potential for a neuron and how does that relate to transmission of neural impulses?**

   Like most cells, neurons have a resting membrane potential mostly created by the sodium-potassium pump in which sodium is pumped extracellularly and potassium pumped intracellularly. This concentration gradient, along with other factors, leads to a relative excess of anions inside the cell leading to a negative resting membrane potential (about −70 mV).

   Neural impulses are transmitted via changes in the electrical gradient along the nerve axon known as action potentials. To generate an action potential, there must be enough stimulation to the voltage-gated sodium channels to depolarize the cell to exceed the threshold potential (about −55 mV). Once reached, this allows depolarization of the cells through an influx of sodium intracellularly and propagation of the impulse along the nerve. Repolarization occurs with closure of these sodium channels and opening of the voltage-gated potassium channels to allow more potassium to exit the cell. The cell then returns to baseline gradient via the sodium-potassium pump (Fig. 6-1).

2. **What is the mechanism of action for local anesthetics?**

   Local anesthetics reversibly block conduction along the nerve distal to the site of application. Once injected into the tissue, the local anesthetic is a weak base and equilibrates into two forms: ionized and non-ionized. The non-ionized form is able to freely cross the cell membrane. Once inside the cell, re-equilibration occurs to the ionized form, which binds to specific sites on the voltage-gated sodium channels, impairing depolarization (Fig. 6-2). As concentration of the anesthetic increases and more receptors are occupied, action potentials are progressively slowed and then abolished. Although the resting membrane potential remains unchanged, the impulses never exceed the raised threshold to allow for an action potential.

3. **How does the onset and recovery of anesthesia proceed in a peripheral nerve block?**

   The onset and recovery of nerve blocks is determined by the organization of the nerve trunk itself. Generally, the outer (mantle) layers innervate proximal structures, whereas the inner (core) layers innervate distal structures. Since the local anesthetic diffuses through the nerve bundle from the outer (mantle) layer to the center (core) layers, the effects of anesthesia are noted on proximal structures faster than distal structures. For example, after inferior alveolar nerve block, anesthesia is noticed first at the site of injection, then from the molars to the incisors, and finally in the lower lip. Recovery also occurs from proximal to distal, with the lower lip being the last to recover.

4. **What is differential blockage and how does that relate to the order of sensation loss after an injection of local anesthesia?**

   Differential blockade refers to the ability of the local anesthetic to block noxious stimuli but still retain motor impulses. Classically, small nerve fibers (such as pain/proprioception fibers) are blocked faster than larger motor nerves. It is important to note, not all nerve fibers are equally affected, and the sensitivity to local anesthetics are determined by factors such as axonal diameter, frequency of impulses, length of nerve exposed to the drug, degree of myelination, and the type of local anesthetic. The classical order of sensation loss during local anesthesia is:
   - Pain
   - Cold
   - Warm
   - Touch
   - Deep pressure
   - Motor

5. **How are local anesthetics classified?**

   Local anesthetics can be classified based on their chemical structures, rate of onset, potency, or duration of action. Most commonly, the chemical structure determines if the anesthetic is an amide or an ester. All local anesthetics contain an aromatic, lipophilic ring linked to a hydrophilic amide group

Local anesthetics

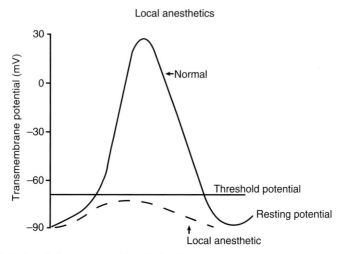

Figure 6-1. Local anesthetics slow the rate of depolarization of the nerve action potential such that the threshold potential is not reached. *(Modified from Stoelting RK, Miller RD: Local anesthetics. In Stoelting RK, Miller RD, editors:* Basics of anesthesia, *ed 3, New York, 1994, Churchill Livingstone.)*

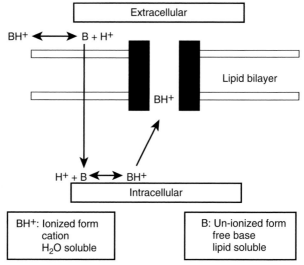

Figure 6-2. Mechanism of action of local anesthetics. *(Modified from Kumar S: Local anesthetics. In Duke J, editor:* Anesthesia secrets, *ed 3, Philadelphia, 2006, Mosby.)*

by an intermediate chain. The intermediate chain determines the chemical classification, either as an amide or an ester (Fig. 6-3).

In dentistry, ester local anesthetics are not available in dental cartridges due to lack of efficacy, potential for allergic reactions, and advantages of the amides.

An easy way to identify amide local anesthetics is to remember that the drug name contains an *i* plus -caine (lidocaine, mepivacaine, and bupivacaine). Esters such as Novocain, procaine, benzocaine, and tetracaine contain no *i*.

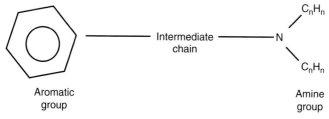

Figure 6-3. Structure of esters and amides. *(Modified from Kumar S: Local anesthetics. In Duke J, editor: Anesthesia secrets, ed 3, Philadelphia, 2006, Mosby.)*

Table 6-1. Properties of Local Anesthetics

AGENT	LIPID SOLUBILITY	PROTEIN BINDING	DURATION	PKa	ONSET TIME
Mepivacaine	1	75	Medium	7.6	Fast
Lidocaine	4	65	Medium	7.7	Fast
Bupivacaine	28	95	Long	8.1	Moderate
Tetracaine	80	85	Long	8.6	Slow

Articaine was approved for use in the United States in April 2000, although it has been used in other countries for some time. This local anesthetic contains both an amide and an ester link, although it is classified as an amide.

6. **How are local anesthetics metabolized?**
Amide local anesthetics are metabolized mainly by the microsomal P-450 enzymes in the liver. The rate of metabolism can be affected by decreases in liver function (e.g., cirrhosis) or liver blood flow (e.g., congestive heart failure), potentially leading to systemic toxicity. Articaine is considered an amide drug; however its ester side-chain does undergoes partial hydrolysis by nonspecific plasma esterases, leading to a short half-life and lower risk for toxicity.
   Ester local anesthetics are very rapidly metabolized by the plasma pseudocholinesterases. Benzocaine, a popular topical anesthetic, is metabolized to p-aminobenzoic acid (PABA), a known allergen.
   The elimination half-life for agents like lidocaine is about 90 minutes, whereas longer acting agents like bupivacaine is over 200 minutes. Articaine, because of its degradation in plasma, has a half-life ranging from 20 to 40 minutes.

7. **What determines the rate of onset of a local anesthetic?**
The pKa of a local anesthetic determines its speed of action. The pKa of a local anesthetic is the pH at which equal concentrations of ionized and un-ionized forms exist. It is the un-ionized form that must cross the axonal membrane to initiate neural blockade.
   Thus, the closer the pKa of a local anesthetic is to the pH of tissue (7.4), the more rapid the onset due to the greater amount of un-ionized agent available for diffusion (Table 6-1).

8. **Why are local anesthetics often ineffective when injected into an area of infection or inflammation?**
Local anesthetics exist in both an ionized (cation) and un-ionized (base) form. Keep in mind that infected tissue has a more acidic pH due to inflammatory mediators, neutralizing the un-ionized (base) form. Since there is less concentration of an un-ionized agent to diffuse across the nerve membrane, the onset time can be delayed significantly. Inflammatory exudates also enhance nerve conduction, making the blockage of nerve impulses more difficult.

9. **What determines the potency of a local anesthetic?**
The lipid solubility determines the potency of a local anesthetic. A greater lipid solubility produces a more potent local anesthetic due to the fact that nerve membranes are mostly lipid (see Table 6-1).

Bupivacaine is a more potent local anesthetic than lidocaine, for example. Therefore only a 0.5% solution is required to obtain comparable local anesthesia, instead of a 2% solution.

10. **What determines the duration of a local anesthetic?**
The degree of protein binding of a local anesthetic agent determines the duration of the anesthetic. Sodium channels and receptor sites for the local anesthetic are mostly protein, thus an agent with a greater degree of protein binding will have a longer duration of action (see Table 6-1). Also, protein binding creates a "reservoir" of local anesthetic availability to bind to receptors as they become unoccupied.
Because bupivacaine, tetracaine, and etidocaine are all highly protein bound, they are long-acting local anesthetics. Vasoconstrictors will also determine the duration of a local anesthetic, but for different reasons.

11. **Why are vasoconstrictors added to local anesthetics?**
Vasoconstrictors are added to prolong the duration of the anesthetic effect. Vasoconstrictors decrease the rate of absorption of the local anesthetic by vasculature, limit systemic toxic side effects, and decrease bleeding at the surgical sites. Because of the vasoconstriction, there is reduced blood flow and decreased vascular absorption of the local anesthetic. This decreases the blood concentrations of the local anesthetic and reduces the risk for toxicity.
The two vasoconstrictors available in dental cartridges are epinephrine and levonordefrin. Epinephrine can be found in concentrations of 1:50,000, 1:100,000, and 1:200,000. Levonordefrin is only found mixed with 3% mepivacaine in a concentration of 1:20,000.
Although the most commonly used formulation is 1:100,000, there is little added benefit from 1:200,000 epinephrine. The 1:50,000 may aid in surgical hemostasis but no effects with regard to the local anesthetic.

12. **What are the cardiovascular influences associated with vasoconstrictors?**
Vasoconstrictors have an impact on the cardiovascular system even with small amounts injected in the submucosal tissues. Epinephrine acts on alpha, beta-1, and beta-2 receptors, thus increasing the heart rate and myocardial contractility. The alpha effects cause vasoconstriction, but larger vessels in the body have beta-2 receptors leading to vasodilation. Thus, the mean arterial pressure has minimal change, although the systolic blood pressure increases and the diastolic pressure decreases.
Levonordefrin is a synthetic drug, closely resembling norepinephrine in action, hence the lack of beta-2 activity. Effects on blood pressure include increased systolic, diastolic, and mean arterial pressure leading to a reflex-induced slowing of the heart rate.
Generally, the hemodynamic effects of vasoconstrictors are seen within a few minutes and subside after 10 to 15 minutes. Peak influences are usually between 5 and 10 minutes.

13. **What is the mechanism of degradation of epinephrine?**
Epinephrine is rapidly metabolized and inactivated in the blood primarily by the enzyme catechol-O-methyltransferase (COMT) and monoamine oxidase (MAO). There is also rapid neuronal reuptake of epinephrine by adrenergic nerves.
One of the end breakdown products is vanillylmandelic acid (VMA). Only a small percentage (1%) of epinephrine is excreted unchanged in the urine.
The elimination half-life of epinephrine is rapid, typically in 1 to 3 minutes.

14. **What are potential drug interactions associated with vasoconstrictor use?**
Drug interactions associated with vasoconstrictors include tricyclic antidepressants (TCAs), monoamine oxidase inhibitors (MAOIs), digoxin, nonselective beta blockers, thyroid hormone, and any of the sympathomimetics such as drugs for weight control, attention deficit disorders, and/or cocaine. Vasopressors are not contraindicated in these patients, but they should be administered with caution.
TCAs (e.g., amitriptyline) increase the availability of endogenous norepinephrine, which could create an exaggerated heart rate or blood pressure response with the use of levonordefrin and to a lesser effect with epinephrine. Patients on TCAs or MAOIs can have some degree of cardiac excitement from the medications. Caution is advised when using vasoconstrictors, especially levonordefrin.
Nonselective beta blockers block both beta-1 and beta-2 receptors, influencing vasopressors to have a more pronounced alpha agonist response leading to elevated diastolic and mean arterial pressures. The elevated blood pressures can be significant, creating a reflex slowing of the heart rate. It is therefore prudent to limit the amount of vasoconstrictors used in these patients and to aspirate to prevent any intravascular injections.

Cocaine potentiates the effects of adrenergic vasoconstrictors. The dysrhythmic results of this interaction can be life threatening. Unfortunately, obtaining a factual health history from a cocaine user may be difficult. All suspected drug users should be made aware of these lethal side effects, especially if cocaine has been used recently.

15. **What is the maximum amount of 2% lidocaine with 1:100,000 epinephrine (in milligrams) that can be administered to a healthy 150-lb man?**

477 mg. The maximum dose of 2% lidocaine with 1:100,000 epinephrine for the adult patient is 7 mg/kg (Table 6-2). You first must convert pounds to kilograms by dividing the weight (in lbs) by 2.2.

$$150\,lb \div 2.2\,lb/kg = 68\,kg$$
$$68\,kg \times 7\,mg/kg = 477\,mg$$

16. **How do you calculate the amount, in milligrams, of any anesthetic and vasoconstrictor in a given solution?**

For local anesthetics, for every 1% solution there is 10 mg/mL. Therefore:

$$\text{Total milligrams} = \% \text{ of the solution} \times 10 \times \text{total milliliters}$$

For vasoconstriction, for every 1:100,000 there is 0.01 mg/mL. Therefore:

$$\text{Total milligrams} = \text{ratio} \times \text{total milliliters}$$

For example, a 1.8-mL dental cartridge of 2% lidocaine with 1:100,000 epinephrine has 20 mg/mL of lidocaine and 0.01 mg/mL of epinephrine. This totals to 36 mg of lidocaine and 0.018 mg of epinephrine.

17. **What is the maximum number of dental cartridges of 2% lidocaine with 1:100,000 that can be given to this 150-lb individual?**

13 cartridges. A standard dental cartridge (1.8 mL) contains 36 mg of lidocaine.

$$477\,mg \div 36\,mg/cartridge = 13.25\,cartridges.$$

18. **How many dental cartridges of lidocaine or mepivacaine can be administered to a 30-lb child?**

Maximum drug dosages are often unknown for the pediatric population. In addition, pharmaceutical manufacturers are reluctant to recommend maximum pediatric dosages of a drug because of variations in age and weight.

Table 6-2. Commonly Used Local Anesthetics in Dentistry

AGENT	CARTRIDGE SIZE (MG)	Maximum Dose		MAXIMUM DOSE
		(MG/KG)	(MG/LB)	
2% Lidocaine with 1:100,000 epinephrine	36	7	3.2	500
3% Mepivacaine	54	6.6	3.0	400
2% Mepivacaine with 1:20,000 levonordefrin	36	6.6	3.0	400
4% Prilocaine	72	8	3.6	600
4% Prilocaine with 1:200,000 epinephrine	72	8	3.6	600
0.5% Bupivacaine with 1:200,000 epinephrine	9	2.0	0.9	90
4% Articaine* with 1:100,000 epinephrine	72	7	3.2	500 (suggested)

*Articaine (Septocaine) dosages are based on a cartridge volume of 1.7 mL/cartridge.
*Maximum recommended dosages are based on an adult weight of 150lb or 70 Kg following manufacturers recommendation.
Table is adapted from Malamed S: Handbook of local anesthesia, ed 6.

Previously, Clark's rule was used to calculate the pediatric drug dose. The formula is:

Maximum pediatric dose = (weight of child in lb ÷ 150) × (maximum adult dose in mg).

It is now recommended to administer the local anesthetic based on the weight-dependent maximum recommended dose multiplied by the child's weight (Table 6-2). This calculated amount should never be exceeded.

The maximum number of cartridges for the 30-lb child for the following anesthetics is:

2% Lidocaine with 1:100,000 epinephrine	2.6 cartridges
3% Mepivacaine	1.6 cartridges

19. **What should be considered when selecting a local anesthetic for children?**

It is easy to exceed the maximum dose of local anesthetics with the pediatric patient.

Oftentimes, pediatric patients are treatment planned for multiple quadrant treatment such as extractions of four primary molars. If all four teeth are to be extracted in one appointment, the practitioner has to be very careful with the amount of local anesthetic administered in each quadrant.

It is often habitual to administer a full cartridge (1.8 mL) for each injection site in the pediatric patient. Remember, using large volumes of anesthetic in a child is not necessary! Children typically have a decreased bone density compared to adults, thus smaller volumes of anesthetics can achieve adequate pain control.

An anesthetic containing vasoconstrictors should be considered to limit the uptake of local anesthetic by the vasculature and thereby decrease systemic effects. With vasoconstrictors, a larger volume of anesthetic can be used. When working in one quadrant and the procedure is short (less then 30 minutes), "plain" local anesthetics are recommended. Always select a local anesthetic with duration of action appropriate for the planned procedure as prolonged anesthesia in children can lead to biting of the lip and tongue.

Generally, the safest local anesthetic to use in the pediatric patient is 2% lidocaine with 1:100,000 epinephrine. A conservative and easy method for remembering the pediatric dose of 2% lidocaine with vasoconstrictor is to use one cartridge for every 20 lbs of the child's weight. The maximum dose should be based on the child's weight.

Note:
- Articaine is not recommended for children younger than 4 years old.
- Bupivacaine is not recommended for children younger than 12 years old.

20. **What effect does narcotic sedation have on the maximum pediatric dose of local anesthetic?**

Amide local anesthetics and narcotics have a similar mechanism of action as both depress the central nervous system. These drugs when used at the same time can have an additive effect, thereby increasing the possibility of a toxic reaction. Narcotics can decrease the protein binding of local anesthetics, increasing the concentration of the local anesthetic in the bloodstream. Narcotics also cause respiratory depression, hence elevating arterial carbon dioxide. Both of these effects will increase central nervous system (CNS) sensitivity to convulsions.

It is advisable to use more conservative pediatric dosages of local anesthetics in pediatric patients undergoing sedation with narcotics.

21. **What is the maximum amount of epinephrine or levonordefrin that can be administered to a 70-kg patient with a history of cardiovascular disease?**

The general recommendation for a patient with a history of cardiovascular disease is no more than 0.04 mg (40 ug) of epinephrine or 0.20 mg (200 ug) of levonordefrin should be administered. Each dental cartridge of 1:100,000 epinephrine contains 0.01 mg/mL of epinephrine; therefore no more than two cartridges (3.6 mL) should be administered (total of 0.036 mg of epinephrine). Each dental cartridge of 1:20,000 levonordefrin contains 0.5 mg/mL of levonordefrin; therefore no more than two cartridges (3.6 mL) should be administered (Table 6-3).

When treating a patient with coronary artery disease, the objective is to prevent increases in heart rate. Increases in heart rate can decrease stroke volume and thereby decrease cardiac output. A decreased cardiac output will diminish the amount of oxygenated blood flowing to poorly perfused areas of the damaged pericardium.

Remember, this is a recommendation as maximal doses have not been established, and these guidelines should be used for stable patients. In any case, each patient should have full vital signs checked preoperatively to confirm a stable heart rate and blood pressure.

Table 6-3. Maximum Allowable Vasoconstrictor for the Cardiac Patient

VASOCONSTRICTOR CONCENTRATION AND TYPE	VASOCONSTRICTOR (MG/ML)	STANDARD DENTAL CARTRIDGE (MG/1.8 ML)	MAXIMUM ALLOWED CARTRIDGES
1:20,000 Levonordefrin	0.5	0.09	2
1:50,000 Epinephrine	0.02	0.036	1
1:100,000 Epinephrine	0.01	0.018	2
1:200,000 Epinephrine	0.005	0.009	4

Given that vasoconstrictors have a short elimination half-life and peak effects occur within 10 minutes, it is feasible to consider re-dosing another dental cartridge after 30 minutes if needed. Remember to re-assess the vital signs before administration.

Vasoconstrictors should not be used in patients with uncontrolled blood pressure (>200/115), uncontrolled hyperthyroidism, recent myocardial infarction, recent stroke, unstable angina, and cardiac dysrhythmias.

22. **Are there patients in whom vasoconstrictors should be avoided?**
Generally, vasoconstrictors should be avoided in patients with active or recent (within 3 to 6 months) cardiac abnormalities. These include recent myocardial infarction, unstable angina, and recent cerebrovascular accident. Patients with active dysrhythmias, especially ventricular arrhythmias, are sensitive to epinephrine, and the use of vasoconstrictors should be avoided. Other groups include uncontrolled hyperthyroidism and patients with uncontrolled blood pressures.

Consultation with the patient's physician is recommended if the history of cardiovascular disease is unclear. Make sure to specify the type and amount of local anesthetic/vasoconstrictor you plan to utilize when asking for the consultation. Remember, there is a balance between the risk in using vasoconstrictors versus obtaining adequate pain control and hemostasis.

23. **What are the clinical manifestations of local anesthetic toxicity?**
Systemic toxicity is the result of elevated plasma levels of local anesthetics. It is usually a manifestation of overdose or inadvertent intravascular injection. Toxicity from local anesthetics involves mostly the CNS and the cardiovascular system. Classic early symptoms are perioral numbness, metallic taste, or tinnitus.

Because the CNS is generally more sensitive to the toxic effects of local anesthetics, it is usually affected first. The manifestations are presented below, starting with early symptoms and progressing to late symptoms for each system.
CNS:
- Light-headedness, tinnitus, perioral numbness, confusion
- Muscle twitching, auditory and visual hallucinations
- Tonic-clonic seizure, unconsciousness, respiratory arrest
Cardiac:
- Hypertension, tachycardia
- Decreased contractility and cardiac output, hypotension
- Sinus bradycardia, ventricular dysrhythmias, circulatory arrest

24. **Which group of patients may accentuate the risk for local anesthetic toxicity?**
The potential for local anesthetic toxicity is greatest in geriatric and pediatric patients. Older individuals generally metabolize drugs at a slower rate. A geriatric patient who takes multiple medications may experience adverse drug reactions when lidocaine is administered. Cimetidine (Tagamet), a histamine H2-receptor antagonist, inhibits the hepatic oxidative enzymes needed for metabolism, thereby allowing lidocaine to accumulate in the circulating blood. This adverse reaction is seen only with cimetidine and not with other H2-receptor antagonists. Propranolol (Inderal), a beta-adrenergic blocker, can reduce both hepatic blood flow and lidocaine clearance. Therefore, a local anesthetic toxic reaction would not be expected with a routine injection of lidocaine in a patient who takes cimetidine or propranolol, but it may result if high doses of lidocaine are given.

In addition, a possible additive adverse drug reaction exists with the combined administration of local anesthetics and opioids in the geriatric and pediatric populations.

25. **What is methemoglobinemia, what are its causes and clinical manifestations, and how can it be treated?**

    A hemoglobin deficiency occurring when hemoglobin has been oxidized to methemoglobin. Oxidized hemoglobin cannot bind or carry oxygen. Excessive doses of prilocaine (above 600 mg) or articaine (above 500 mg) may result in the accumulation of an oxidized metabolite, *ortho*-toluidine, that is capable of allowing this conversion. Clinical manifestations include a decreased pulse oximeter reading, cyanosis, and chocolate-colored blood in the surgical field. This condition can be reversed with intravenous administration of 1 to 2 mg/kg of methylene blue over a 5-minute period.

    Benzocaine also has the potential to cause methemoglobinemia. It can be found in certain topical liquids, gels, ointments, and sprays (e.g., Hurricaine, Cetacaine). Benzocaine preparations should not be used in patients with a history of methemoglobinemia and in children <2 years of age. Methemoglobinemia formation can occur with benzocaine doses of 15 to 20 mg/kg. Benzocaine gels typically contain 18% to 20% benzocaine. Sprays containing 14% to 20% benzocaine can deliver 45 to 60 mg of benzocaine in 1 second. The signs and symptoms may occur within minutes or up to 2 hours after the use of benzocaine topical.

    Prilocaine is marketed as a 4% solution. A 4% solution contains 72 mg of prilocaine, with eight cartridges needed to obtain 600 mg. The use of a benzocaine topical along with prilocaine will reduce the maximum amount of injectable local anesthetic that can be used. In some countries other than the United States and Canada, prilocaine is marketed as a 3% solution, which is less likely to cause an excessive delivery of this local anesthetic.

    EMLA (eutectic mixture of local anesthetic) cream, used preoperatively before venous access, contains both lidocaine and prilocaine. EMLA cream should be used with caution in children, and it is not recommended for use in children younger than age 12 months because of potential methemoglobinemia development.

26. **A patient tells you he had an adverse reaction to local anesthetics in the past. What are common adverse reactions, and how do you rule out allergic reactions?**

    Patients often present to the dental office claiming they are allergic to local anesthetics. Common reactions to rule out are vasovagal syncope (loss of consciousness/brief seizure) during administration/injection and or symptoms related to vasoconstrictors such as heart palpitations or nervousness/excitability. True allergic reactions often can range from mild (rash or pruritus) to moderate (urticaria or wheezing) or to critical (anaphylaxis or airway compromise).

    Allergic reactions to local anesthetics have been reported. However, the reaction is most likely attributed to preservatives (methylparaben) or antioxidants (sulfites) contained in the solutions. Although the incidence is <1%, a thorough investigation is prudent. Allergies to the amides and ester local anesthetics have been reported. Cross-reactivity is theoretically possible, thus a referral to an allergist is recommended if a true allergy is suspected.

    In the past, procaine (Novocaine) was a commonly used ester local anesthetic in dentistry but now is no longer available in cartridges. Currently, benzocaine is a commonly used topical anesthetic found in sprays and gels. Both procaine and benzocaine are metabolized to compounds resembling PABA, which is a known allergen.

27. **What types of local anesthetics can be used in the pregnant and lactating patient?**

    Category B local anesthetics (see the following list) are recommended for the pregnant and lactating patient. Local anesthetics can cross the placental barrier but are generally not harmful unless excessive amounts are administered. A mother's normal tissue pH is 7.4, whereas the fetus has a pH of approximately 7.2. An excessive amount of local anesthetic could dangerously lower the fetus's pH (ion trapping).

Category B	*Category C*
Lidocaine	Articaine
Prilocaine	Bupivacaine
Etidocaine	Mepivacaine

Note: Category C medications are not recommended unless the potential benefits warrant their use.

28. **To what components of a local anesthetic are patients most likely to be allergic?**
Methylparaben, a bacteriostatic preservative, is found in multidose vials of local anesthetics. Oral and maxillofacial surgeons that use multidose vials need to be cautious of potential allergic reactions. Multidose vials are mostly encountered in the emergency room and the operating room. Since 1984, methylparaben is no longer added to dental cartridges. Because the cartridge is intended to be used as a single-dose vial, a preservative is not required.

    Bisulfites are commonly used as preservatives at salad bars and in wines. Any local anesthetic cartridge containing a vasoconstrictor will have metabisulfite added as a preservative for the vasoconstrictor. Patients with known bisulfite allergies need to be given local anesthetics without vasoconstrictors.

    Latex allergies should also be considered with the use of local anesthetics. The local anesthetic itself contains no latex, but its container may. The needle-puncture diaphragm of dental cartridges and multidose vials contains latex. The dental plunger of a dental cartridge may also contain latex. A disposable, latex-free syringe is recommended for the latex-allergic patient. The anesthetic solution may be drawn using a filtered needle or by removing the rubber diaphragm.

29. **Why is your knowledge of local anesthetics so important?**
With the possible exception of anesthesiologists, dental practitioners, especially oral and maxillofacial surgeons, use local anesthetics most frequently. Therefore, a thorough understanding of the pharmacokinetics and pharmacodynamics of local anesthetics is essential.

30. **Is there a method to reverse the clinical effects of local anesthetics?**
Traditionally, the effects of local anesthetics would wear off over time. However, an alpha receptor blocker, phentolamine mesylate (OraVerse, Septodont) has been approved in dental cartridges to accelerate the reversal of soft tissue anesthesia. Although not fully understood, it is thought to cause vasodilation in the identical site of the previous local anesthetic injection to increase absorption of the anesthetic agents.

    Although unlikely to be useful in the surgical setting, this drug may have a role in the dental office for routine procedures and patients wishing to have a faster return of function. OraVerse is approved for use in patients 6 years of age and older and weighing more than 15 kg.

31. **What are general concepts in the treatment of toxicity from local anesthesia?**
If you suspect local anesthetic toxicity, the initial steps should be to stop the injection, ensure oxygenation, stabilize the patient, and consider activating your emergency response team. Attention should be paid to airway compromise, hypotension, dysrhythmias, and seizures.

    Benzodiazepines are the drugs of choice for seizure control. Propofol can be used to control seizures but has the risk of potentiating cardiovascular collapse. Cardiovascular support should include fluid administration and vasopressors if needed.

    Also available are lipid emulsions (Intralipid), which can reverse the cardiac and neurologic effects of local anesthetic toxicity by extracting lipid soluble molecules from the plasma. These lipid emulsions have been successful in treating toxicity, especially with bupivacaine, that is part of the Advanced Cardiac Life Support (ACLS) support guidelines.

32. **What are the common reasons for failure to obtain adequate local anesthesia during the removal of a mandibular molar?**
The inferior alveolar block has a high failure rate in dentistry. Here are some considerations to improve the success rate when anesthetizing mandibular molars.
Technical considerations:
- Allow adequate time for the anesthetic to take effect. Sit the patient in an upright position after delivering the inferior alveolar block and wait an additional 5 to 10 minutes. This is difficult for the oral and maxillofacial surgeon who is inherently impatient.
- Often the needle is inserted too low and too anterior on the ramus. Consider re-administering the local anesthetic at a higher level and deeper on the ramus.
- Adjust your entry position and angle of entry for the block. There is a significant difference in success rates between the right and left inferior alveolar block, which is operator dependent.
Anatomic considerations:
- Consider innervations from the mylohyoid nerve and anesthetize accordingly (lingual to the mandibular second molar).

- Administer another cartridge of anesthetic at the highest level possible by using the Gow-Gates technique (intraoral condylar injection) to anesthetize all branches of cranial nerve V3.
  Physiologic considerations:
- Consider using a higher pH anesthetic solution (one without a vasoconstrictor) to help overcome the acidity created by possible infection/inflammation.
- Alkalinize (buffer) your anesthetic by adding sodium bicarbonate to your local anesthetic just before injecting.
- Use a larger amount (but do not exceed the maximum recommended dose) of local anesthetic to overcome the acidity created by the infection.

33. **Is there an easy way to remember important data about lidocaine?**
    Yes. Because lidocaine is one of the safest and most commonly used local anesthetics, it is useful to commit to memory certain information about this drug. Its molecular weight is 234, its protein binding is 56%, and its pKa is 7.8, so just remember 2, 3, 4, 5, 6, 7, 8.

BIBLIOGRAPHY

American Academy of Pediatric Dentistry (AAPD): *Guideline on use of local anesthesia for pediatric dental patients*, Chicago 2009, American Academy of Pediatric Dentistry (AAPD).
Becker DE: Drug allergies and implications for dental practice, *Anesth Prog* 60(4):188–197, 2013.
Becker DE, Reed XL: Local anesthetics: review of pharmacological considerations, *Anesth Prog* 59(2):90–101, 2012.
Cummings DR, Yamashita DD, McAndrews JP: Complications of local anesthesia used in oral and maxillofacial surgery, *Oral Maxillofac Surg Clin North Am* 23:369–377, 2011.
Giovannittis JA, Rosenberg MB, Phero JC: Pharmacology of local anesthetics used in oral surgery, *Oral Maxillofac Surg Clin N Am* 25:453–465, 2013.
Kumar S: Local anesthetics. In Duke J, editor: *Anesthesia secrets*, ed 4, Philadelphia, 2010, Mosby.
Malamed SF: *Handbook of local anesthesia*, ed 6, St Louis, 2012, Mosby.
Mastrello CL, Abubaker AO, Benson KI: Local anesthetics. In Abubaker AO, Benson KI, editors: *Secrets of oral and maxillofacial surgery*, ed 2, Philadelphia, 2007, Elsevier.
Moore PA: Adverse drug interactions in dental practice: interactions associated with local anesthetics, sedatives and anxiolytics, *J Am Dental Assoc* 130:541–554, 1999.
Morgan GE, Mikhail MS, Murray MJ: Local anesthetics. In Morgan GE, Mikhail MS, Murray MJ, editors: *Clinical anesthesiology*, ed 4, New York, 2005, McGraw-Hill.
Ogle OE, Majhoubi G: Local anesthesia: agents, techniques, and complications, *Dent Clin North Am* 56:133–148, 2012.
Reed KL, Malamed SF, Fonner AM: Local anesthesia part 2: technical considerations, *Anesth Prog* 59(3):127–136, 2012.
Stoelting RK, Miller RD: Local anesthetics. In Stoelting RK, Miller RD, editors: *Basics of anesthesia*, ed 4, New York, 2000, Churchill Livingstone.
Wilburn-Goo D, Lloyd LM: When patients become cyanotic: acquired methemoglobinemia, *J Am Dental Assoc* 130: 826–831, 1999.
Yagiela JA: Adverse drug interactions in dental practice: interactions associated with vasoconstrictors, *J Am Dent Assoc* 130:701–709, 1999.

CHAPTER 7

INTRAVENOUS SEDATION

Jason A. Jamali, A. Omar Abubaker

1. **What are the different levels of sedations?**
   See Table 7-1.

2. **How is an intravenous (IV) anesthetic agent used in anesthesia?**
   An IV anesthetic is a drug that is intravenously injected to induce unconsciousness at the beginning of general anesthesia. At the same time, it allows rapid recovery after termination of its effect.

3. **What are the properties of an ideal induction agent?**
   - Water soluble, compatible with IV solutions, and stable in aqueous solution
   - Rapid onset and recovery of anesthesia (within 1 arm-brain circulation time)
   - Absence of unwanted cardiovascular or neurologic side effects
   - Anticonvulsant, antiemetic, analgesic, and amnestic properties
   - It should not impair renal or hepatic function or steroid synthesis.

4. **What are the commonly used intravenous anesthetic agents?**
   See Table 7-2.

5. **What effect does age have on dosing of induction agents?**
   With increasing age, elimination time and renal clearance time increase, resulting in longer lasting drug effects. Elderly patients are more sensitive to intravenous anesthetics; therefore dose reductions are necessary in this group of patients.

6. **What are the cardiovascular effects of commonly used induction agents?**
   See Table 7-3.

7. **What are barbiturates?**
   As derivatives of barbituric acid, they exhibit a dose-dependent central nervous system (CNS) depression with hypnosis and amnesia. They are very lipid soluble, which results in a rapid onset of action. When used for induction, they produce unconsciousness in less than 30 seconds.

8. **What are the pharmacologic effects of barbiturates?**
   Barbiturates modulate the interaction of gamma-aminobutyric acid (GABA) with its receptors. GABA, an inhibitory neurotransmitter, causes an increase in chloride concentration within the membranes of postsynaptic neurons resulting in hyperpolarization. Barbiturates are capable of depressing the reticular activating system, which is important in maintaining wakefulness and medullary ventilatory centers to decrease responsiveness to ventilatory stimulant effects of carbon dioxide. In addition, barbiturates induce depression of the medullary vasomotor center, causing decreased sympathetic nervous system impulses from autonomic ganglia. This results in decreases in blood pressure (10 to 20 mm Hg) secondary to peripheral vasodilation. Finally, barbiturates are potent cerebral vasoconstrictors resulting in decreases in cerebral blood flow, cerebral blood volume, and intracranial pressure (ICP).

9. **What are the pharmacokinetics of barbiturates?**
   Maximal uptake of barbiturates by the brain occurs within 30 seconds after IV administration. This accounts for the rapid (1 arm-brain circulation) induction of anesthesia. The redistribution of these drugs from the brain to inactive tissues, especially skeletal muscle and fat, results in prompt awakening. The elimination of barbiturates is dependent on hepatic function because less than 1% of the administered dose is cleared unchanged by the kidneys.

10. **What are the most commonly used barbiturates for induction of anesthesia?**
    Thiopental sodium (Pentothal) is a thiobarbiturate usually prepared as a 2.5% solution. The pH of thiopental is 10.5. When injected intravenously, it can be irritating. An induction dose of 3 to 5 mg/kg produces a loss of consciousness within 30 seconds and recovery in 5 to 10 minutes. Because the

Table 7-1. Continuum of Sedation

	MINIMAL SEDATION	MODERATE SEDATION	DEEP SEDATION	GENERAL ANESTHESIA
Comment	Anxiolysis	Conscious sedation Drug-induced depression of consciousness	Drug-induced depression of consciousness	Drug-induced loss of conscious-ness
Cognitive/ physical coordination		Impaired		
Responsiveness	Responds normally to verbal com-mands	Purposeful response to verbal or tactile stimulation	Purposeful response follow-ing repeated or painful stimulation	Unarousable even with painful stimulus
Airway	Unaffected	No intervention	Intervention may be required	Required
Spontaneous ventilation	Unaffected	Adequate	Inadequate	Inadequate
Cardiovascular function	Unaffected	Maintained	Maintained	Impaired

Table 7-2. Commonly Used Intravenous Anesthetic Agents

AGENT	COMMENTS
Etomidate	Anesthetic agent that provides hemodynamic stability. Excellent for compro-mised cardiac patient. Major side effect is adrenal suppression.
Propofol	Most popular anesthetic agent used in office anesthesia due to fast onset, short duration, and antiemetic property. Major disadvantage is its association with myocardial depression and vasodilation.
Ketamine	NMDA receptor antagonism. It causes dissociative anesthetic state. Its usage has gained popularity due to its uniqueness in providing anesthesia, amnesia, and analgesia as a single agent. Major side effect is associated with its sympathomimetic properties.
Midazolam	Short-acting water-soluble benzodiazepam. Benzodiazepam carries anxiolysis, sedation, and amnesia properties. It also has minimal effect on cardiovascu-lar system.
Fentanyl	Short-acting opioid that is used commonly with other anesthetic agents to provide synergistic effect. Opioid (except meperidine) carries vagolytic effect in high dose.
Dexmedetomidine	It is a centrally acting alpha-2 agonist. It has a short half-life and good safety profile. When given as an intravenous bolus, significant hypotension can be observed due to activation of peripheral alpha-1 antagonist effect.

elimination half-life is 6 to 12 hours, patients may experience a slow recovery. After 24 hours, approxi-mately 28% to 30% may be detectable in the body. Thiopental is not used to maintain anesthesia because of accumulation in inactive tissues with repeated doses.

Methohexital (Brevital) is somewhat less lipid soluble and less ionized at physiologic pH than thiopental. The pH is 10.5. An induction dose of 1 to 2 mg/kg produces loss of

Table 7-3. Cardiovascular Effects of Induction Agents

AGENT	MAP	HR	SVR	CO
Ketamine	++	++	+	+
Midazolam	0	0	0	0
Propofol	−	+	−	0
Etomidate	0	0	0	0
Fentanyl	0	0	0	0

CO, Cardiac output; *HR*, heart rate; *MAP*, mean arterial pressure; *SVR*, systemic vascular resistance.
Modified from Duke J: Anesthesia secrets, ed 4.

consciousness in less than 20 seconds and recovery in 4 to 5 minutes. The elimination half-life of methohexital is 3 hours, which allows a clearance rate that is three to four times faster than that of thiopental.

11. **Why is propofol the best agent for outpatient anesthesia?**
   - Rapid induction and recovery
   - Lower incidence of nausea and vomiting
   - Patients regain cognitive function quickly, which leads to a shorter recovery period.

12. **What are the properties of propofol?**
   Propofol is a sedative-hypnotic that works via GABA pathways to produce anesthesia (without analgesia) with a relatively rapid recovery time. It may be used as a sedative as well as an induction and maintenance agent for general anesthesia. It has mostly supplanted the use of barbiturates given the faster emergence during recovery.
   The systemic effects include:
   - Decreased cerebral blood flow and ICP
   - Myocardial depression, decreased systemic vascular resistance (SVR), and hypotension (20% to 30% reduction)
   - Respiratory depression
   - Antiemetic properties
   Propofol should be avoided in patients with soy and egg allergies as well as lipid disorders.

13. **What are the pros and cons of using dexmedetomidine (Percedex) over traditional anesthetic agents?**
   Dexmedetomidine is a centrally acting alpha-2 agonist. Its short half-life, fast onset, and limited effects on the respiratory system make it a great anesthetic alternative. Studies have also suggested a better emergence profile (i.e., delirium) than propofol. The major disadvantages with dexmedetomidine are the relative high cost compared with generic propofol and midazolam and its association with hypotension when given in bolus dose intravenously. Its sedation dose is 0.2 to 0.7 mcg/kg/hr.

14. **What are the pharmacologic properties and side effects of etomidate?**
   Etomidate (Amidate) is a carboxylated imidazole derivative. An induction dose of 0.2 to 0.5 mg/kg IV produces rapid induction of anesthesia that lasts 3 to 12 minutes. The CNS effects are dose dependent, and recovery of psychomotor skills is equal to that of thiopental. Rapid awakening results from redistribution and nearly complete hydrolysis to inactive metabolites. Because etomidate produces no noticeable cardiovascular changes, it is used in patients with limited cardiac reserve. In addition, etomidate decreases cerebral blood flow and ICP. Like methohexital, it activates seizure foci.
   Side effects include venoirritation with rapid infusion, involuntary skeletal muscle movements, and a high incidence of nausea and vomiting. Also, etomidate suppresses adrenocortical function for up to 8 hours after administration. During this time, the adrenal cortex is unresponsive to adrenocorticotropic hormone (ACTH).

15. **What is ketamine, and how does it exert its physiologic action?**
   Ketamine, a phencyclidine (PCP) derivative, is 10 times more lipid soluble than thiopental, enabling it to cross the blood-brain barrier (BBB) quickly. It produces dissociative anesthesia, which can be seen on electroencephalogram (EEG) as dissociation between the thalamus and limbic system.

Rapid CNS depression with hypnosis, sedation, amnesia, and intense analgesia occurs in 30 to 60 seconds after IV administration. The anesthetic induction doses are 1 to 2 mg/kg IV, with effects lasting 5 to 10 minutes, or 10 mg/kg intramuscular (IM), which acts in 2 to 4 minutes. A ketamine dart contains 4 mg/kg.

IM can be administered to uncooperative patients to facilitate completion of short procedures.

16. **What are the pharmacologic effects and side effects of ketamine?**
Ketamine is highly lipid soluble, is rapidly redistributed to muscle and fat, and undergoes extensive hepatic metabolism to a weakly active metabolite, norketamine. Ketamine stimulates the cardiovascular system, increasing the heart rate, blood pressure, and cardiac output. In patients with ischemic heart disease, ketamine may adversely increase myocardial oxygen requirements. In addition, ketamine produces bronchial smooth muscle relaxation because of sympathetic stimulation, which may be beneficial in patients with bronchospasm or asthma. Airway secretions are increased by ketamine, creating the need for anticholinergics such as glycopyrrolate in the preoperative period. Ketamine is a potent cerebral vasodilator and will increase ICP in patients with intracranial lesions. Finally, emergence from ketamine anesthesia may be associated with unpleasant auditory, visual, and out-of-body illusions that can progress to delirium. It is recommended that benzodiazepines or droperidol be administered either preoperatively or after induction to decrease the incidence of emergence delirium.

17. **What are the dosages for ketamine?**

Route/Anesthetic Type	Dosage
IV induction	1-2 mg/kg
IV sedation	0.25-0.75 mg/kg
IM ketamine dart	4 mg/kg

18. **What are the onset and duration of ketamine when administered via IV versus IM route?**

	IV	IM
Onset	30-60 seconds	2-4 minutes
Duration	10-15 minutes	30-60 minutes

19. **What are the clinical uses for benzodiazepines?**
- Preoperative medication
- Intravenous sedation
- Induction of anesthesia
- Maintenance of anesthesia
- Suppression of seizure activity

Anterograde amnesia, minimal depression of ventilation and the cardiovascular system, and sedative properties make benzodiazepines favorable preoperative medications.

20. **Where in the CNS do benzodiazepines exert their amnestic effects?**
These effects occur at benzodiazepine receptors, which are found on postsynaptic nerve endings in the CNS. Benzodiazepine receptors are part of the GABA receptor complex. The GABA receptor complex consists of two alpha subunits, to which benzodiazepines bind, and two beta subunits, to which GABA binds. A chloride ion channel exists in the middle of the receptor complex. Benzodiazepines enhance the binding of GABA to beta subunits, which opens the chloride ion channel. Chloride ions flow into the neuron, hyperpolarizing it and inhibiting action potentials.

21. **What clinical properties make benzodiazepines good preoperative medications?**
At lower doses, only anxiolysis is obtained. Anterograde amnesia, sedation, and anxiolysis are produced at higher concentrations. At this concentration, patients are conscious and can maintain their own airway but will not remember events during surgery. Finally, at even higher concentrations, benzodiazepines will produce unconsciousness, although they are not complete anesthetics. A complete general anesthetic produces the effects already mentioned plus analgesia, control of the autonomic nervous systems, and occasionally muscle relaxation. Benzodiazepines do not provide analgesia, and they should not be used alone to produce general anesthesia. They are best used in low doses to supplement inhaled or intravenous anesthetics to provide amnesia.

22. **What benzodiazepines are most commonly used as amnestics in anesthesiology?**
    - Induction of anesthesia: Midazolam (most common)
    - Induction of anesthesia: Lorazepam
    - Induction of anesthesia: Diazepam

23. **What are the properties and pharmacokinetics of midazolam?**
    Midazolam is prepared as a water-soluble compound that is transformed into a lipid-soluble compound by exposure to the pH of blood upon injection. This unique property of midazolam improves patient comfort during administration. This also prevents the need for an organic solvent such as propylene glycol (venoirritation), which is required for diazepam and lorazepam. Midazolam is the most lipid soluble of the three and, as a result, has a rapid onset and a relatively short duration of action. (See Table 7-4.)

24. **What is the antagonist for benzodiazepines?**
    Flumazenil, a competitive antagonist, given in increments of 0.2 mg IV every 60 seconds, will reverse unconsciousness, sedation, respiratory depression, and anxiolysis. Flumazenil has a rapid onset with the peak effect occurring in about 1 to 3 minutes. The effect of flumazenil lasts for about 20 minutes, and resedation may occur.

25. **What is the concept of context-sensitive half-time and its relevance to opioids?**
    Context-sensitive half-time is the time required for 50% reduction in the plasma concentration of a drug on termination of a constant infusion. This time is determined by both elimination and redistribution, and it varies considerably as a function of infusion duration for commonly used opioids.

26. **What is the mechanism of action of opioids?**
    Opioids act as agonists through complex interactions with mu, delta, and kappa receptors in the CNS. Supraspinally, mu receptors are responsible for analgesia, euphoria, miosis, nausea and vomiting, urinary retention, depression of ventilation, and bradycardia. Delta and kappa receptors are active at the spinal level, mediating spinal analgesia, sedation, and miosis. In addition, opioids may act presynaptically to interfere with the release of neurotransmitters such as acetylcholine, dopamine, norepinephrine, and substance P.

27. **How are opioids used clinically?**
    Uses include provision of analgesia before or after surgery, synergistic effects with inhaled anesthetics being used for maintenance of anesthesia, induction and maintenance of anesthesia (particularly in patients with severe cardiac dysfunction), and inhibition of reflex sympathetic nervous system activity. Usually, opioids are administered intermittently in lower doses during maintenance of anesthesia or as continuous infusions to augment inhaled anesthetics. Often, small doses of fentanyl, sufentanil, or alfentanil are administered just before direct laryngoscopy and tracheal intubation to attenuate blood pressure and heart rate responses evoked by these stimuli.

28. **What are the pharmacologic effects of opioids?**
    Opioids are cardiac-stable drugs. In many settings, opioids are used as the principal anesthetic agent for cardiac anesthesia because of their hemodynamic stability; however, they do lack an amnestic effect. At the same time, opioids can cause a dose-dependent bradycardia resulting from vagal stimulation in the medulla. In contrast, meperidine will cause tachycardia because it is structurally similar to atropine and elicits atropine-like effects. Opioids act on the medullary ventilatory centers to produce rapid and sustained dose-dependent depression of ventilation. This is characterized by increases in the resting $PaCO_2$ and decreased responsiveness to the ventilatory stimulant effects of carbon dioxide. In the CNS, opioids do not produce unconsciousness reliably. They do, however, stimulate dopamine receptors in the

Table 7-4. The Properties and Pharmacokinetics of Midazolam

DRUG	DOSAGE	ONSET	ELIMINATION HALF-LIFE
Midazolam (IV-sedation)	0.01-0.1 mg/kg	0.5-2 minutes	2 hours
Midazolam (IV-induction)	0.1-0.3 mg/kg		
Diazepam IV	2-10 mg prn	1-3 minutes	20-90 hours
Lorazepam IV	2-4 mg prn	1-5 minutes	10-20 hours

chemoreceptor trigger zone of the medulla, causing nausea and vomiting. Finally, rapidly administered high doses can cause spasm of the thoracoabdominal muscles, resulting in hypoventilation.

29. **What is remifentanil, and how does it differ from other opioids?**
Remifentanil is an ultrashort-acting opioid with a duration of 5 to 10 minutes. It has a context-sensitive half-time of 3 minutes. It is metabolized by nonspecific plasma esterases. It is commonly used as a continuous infusion. Intravenous bolus administration has been associated with increased incidence of bradycardia and chest-wall rigidity. It also has been shown to induce hyperalgesia and acute opioid tolerance.

30. **What are the pharmacokinetics among the commonly used opioids?**
See Table 7-5.

31. **Which opioids stimulate the release of histamine?**
Morphine, codeine, and meperidine (Demerol) cause histamine release, resulting in vasodilation and possible hypotension. Fentanyl, sufentanil, and alfentanil do not stimulate histamine release.

32. **What opioid antagonist is most commonly used in clinical anesthesia?**
Naloxone is the pure mu-receptor antagonist that is used to reverse the effects of opioids. Naloxone will reverse overdoses and respiratory depressant effects; however, at the same time, it reverses the analgesic effects. Normal dosages may cause abrupt reversal, which can result in tachycardia, hypertension, pulmonary edema, and cardiac dysrhythmias. To avoid these adverse effects, naloxone should be given in doses of 40 mg (0.1 mL), repeated every few minutes.

33. **Which intravenous induction agents are recommended for use in major trauma or other hypovolemic states?**
Etomidate is an agent commonly used because of its cardiac stability in patients with limited cardiac reserve. Ketamine is recommended for patients who are hypovolemic because of the direct stimulation of sympathetic outflow from the CNS. However, patients with depleted endogenous catecholamines may not be able to respond to the stimulation, resulting in more hypotension. The induction dose of etomidate is 2 to 3 mg/kg and that of ketamine is 1 to 2 mg/kg.

34. **Which induction agents alter ICP?**
Thiopental, propofol, etomidate, and fentanyl reduce ICP because they cause decreases in cerebral blood flow and cerebral metabolic consumption of oxygen. Ketamine increases cerebral blood flow, cerebral metabolism, and ICP.

35. **What are the roles of anticholinergic medicines in sedation and the differences among the options?**
Anticholinergic medications can be used as antisialagogues as well as in the management of bradycardia. Variability of the CNS effects relates to the differential ability to cross the BBB. Scopolamine crosses the BBB without difficulty, causing CNS depression and amnesia. Atropine has less pronounced CNS effects than scopolamine but produces greater tachycardia, whereas glycopyrrolate

Table 7-5. Pharmacokinetics among the Commonly Used Opioids

	MORPHINE	FENTANYL	REMIFENTANYL	MEPERIDINE
Potency (compared with IV morphine)	1	100	250	0.1
Dosage (sedation/analgesic)	2-10 mg IV	Sedation: 0.5 mcg/kg (load); 0.01-0.04 mcg/kg/min (maint)	0.5-1 mcg/kg load (infused over 30-60 seconds); 0.025-0.2 mcg/kg/min (maint)	50-150 mg IV q3-4 hours
Onset (minutes)	5-15	1-3	1.5-2	15
Peak (minutes)	20-30	3-5	2	5-7
Duration (hours)	3-4	0.5-1	0.1-0.2	2-3
Clearance	Renal	Liver	Esterases	Liver

does not readily cross the BBB. As a result, only scopolamine and atropine have a risk of central anticholinergic syndrome (CAS), and emergence delirium can be treated with physostigmine 0.01 to 0.03 mg/kg, which may be repeated.

36. **What is the management of an inadvertent intraarterial injection?**
    - Induction of anesthesia. Leave the catheter in place.
    - Induction of anesthesia. Administer 2 to 10 cc of 1% procaine (vasodilation may attenuate the arteriospasm).
    - Induction of anesthesia. Assess the pulse/color of the extremity.
    - Induction of anesthesia. Consider a vascular consult.

BIBLIOGRAPHY

Allen DM: Intravenous anesthetics and benzodiazepines. In Duke J, editor: *Anesthesia secrets*, ed 3, Philadelphia, 2006, Mosby.

American Society of Anesthesiologists: Task force on sedation and analgesia by nonanesthesiologists: practice guidelines for sedation and analgesia by non-anesthesiologists, *Anesthesiology* 96:1004–1017, 2002.

Hatheway J: Opioids. In Duke J, editor: *Anesthesia secrets*, ed 2, Philadelphia, 2000, Hanley & Belfus.

Hudson RJ, Stanski DR, Burch PG: Pharmacokinetics of methohexital and thiopental in surgical patients, *Anesthesiology* 59:215–219, 1983.

Malamed S: *Sedation: a guide to patient management*, ed 5, Mosby, 2009.

McDowell G: Intravenous induction agents. In Duke J, editor: *Anesthesia secrets*, ed 2, Philadelphia, 2000, Hanley & Belfus.

Nabonsal J: Preoperative medications. In Duke J, editor: *Anesthesia secrets*, ed 2, Philadelphia, 2000, Hanley & Belfus.

Nutt DJ: New insights into the role of the $GABA_A$—benzodiazepine receptor in psychiatric disorder, *Br J Psychiatry* 179:390–396, 2001.

Reves JG, Fragen RJ, Vinik HR, et al.: Midazolam: pharmacology and uses, *Anesthesiology* 62:310–324, 1985.

Stoelting RK, Miller RD: Intravenous anesthetics. In Stoelting RD, Miller RD, editors: *Basics of anesthesia*, New York, 1999, Churchill Livingstone.

Swank KM: Preoperative evaluation. In Duke J, editor: *Anesthesia secrets*, ed 3, Philadelphia, 2006, Mosby.

Winkelmann G: Benzodiazepines. In Duke J, editor: *Anesthesia secrets*, ed 2, Philadelphia, 2000, Hanley & Belfus.

CHAPTER 8

INHALATION ANESTHESIA AND NEUROMUSCULAR BLOCKING AGENTS

Matthew Cooke

1. **What inhalational anesthetics are currently available, and how are they delivered in clinical use?**
   Three volatile liquids (desflurane, isoflurane, and sevoflurane) and one gas (nitrous oxide) are used clinically. The volatile liquids require a vaporizer for inhalational administration. Additionally, the desflurane vaporizer has a heating component to allow delivery at room temperature.
   Inhalational anesthetic delivery systems exist for the delivery of one or multiple agents. These delivery systems have mandatory scavenging and fail-safe mechanisms to optimize safety. Inhalation agents are administered in hospital operating rooms and outpatient environments, such as surgery centers and dental offices.

2. **What is the mechanism of action of inhalational anesthetics?**
   The mechanism of action of volatile anesthetics, along with their molecular and cellular actions, remains elusive. Volatile anesthetics act on synaptic transmission in the central nervous system but proof remains a matter of debate.
   Inhalational anesthetics act in the central nervous system. They disrupt synaptic transmission, interfere with the release of neurotransmitters from presynaptic nerve terminals, alter reuptake of neurotransmitters, change binding of neurotransmitters to the postsynaptic receptor sites, and influence the ionic conductance.
   The Meyer-Overton theory postulates that anesthesia occurs when a sufficient number of inhalation anesthetic molecules dissolve in the lipid cell membrane. However, the Meyer-Overton theory does not describe why anesthesia occurs. The Critical Volume Hypothesis believes that the absorption of anesthetic molecules could expand the volume of a hydrophobic region within the cell membrane and subsequently distort channels necessary for sodium ion flux and the development of action potentials necessary for synaptic transmission.
   The protein interaction theory hypothesizes that anesthetics bind to specific proteins that affect ion flux during membrane excitation, resulting in either potentiation of inhibitory neurotransmitters (e.g., GABA, glycine) or inhibition of excitatory neurotransmitters (e.g., glutamate NMDA receptors). This is supported by a steep dose response curve.

3. **How long can oxygen at 2L/min be delivered from an E cylinder with a reading of 500psi?**
   A full E cylinder of oxygen (O_2) contains approximately 600L at a pressure of 2000psi. At 2L/min, a full E cylinder will deliver O_2 for approximately 300minutes, or 5hours. A reading of 500psi will therefore give you approximately 1 hour and 15minutes of O_2.

4. **How long can nitrous oxide (N_2O) at 2L/min be delivered from an E cylinder that reads 750psi?**
   N_2O has a pressure of 750psi, and approximately 1600L of N_2O is contained in an E cylinder. N_2O is a compressed liquid and not a compressed gas like O_2. A compressed liquid does not show a linear correlation between volume and pressure as does a compressed gas. N_2O pressure will remain at 750psi until all the liquid has been vaporized. Therefore an estimated time cannot be determined.

5. **Why is N_2O use contraindicated in patients with conditions involving closed gas spaces?**
   N_2O has a low blood-to-gas partition coefficient (0.46) and therefore low solubility. It can leave the blood and enter air-filled cavities 34 times more quickly than nitrogen can leave the cavity to enter

the blood. The use of N_2O can increase the expansion of compliant cavities, such as a pneumothorax, bowel gas in a bowel obstruction, and an air embolism. An increase in pressure will occur when N_2O is used with noncompliant cavities, such as the middle ear or sinuses.

The oral and maxillofacial surgeon needs to be cautious when treating the recent trauma patient (e.g., motor vehicle accident victim). An asymptomatic, undiagnosed closed pneumothorax can double in size in 10 minutes after the administration of 70% N_2O. Nitrous oxide-oxygen sedation should be postponed in patients with gastrointestinal obstructions, middle ear disturbances, and, possibly, sinus infections.

6. Should a patient with an upper respiratory infection (URI) be given N_2O via a nasal hood?

Because a patient with a URI has nasal blockage, the delivery of the N_2O is limited and the potential for leakage of N_2O around the hood is more likely. In addition, patients with a URI are also more likely to have associated middle ear and sinus infections. Therefore the use of N_2O with patients with URI is unwise.

7. Can inhalational anesthetics be administered to patients with chronic obstructive pulmonary disease (COPD)?

Administration of volatile anesthetics (desflurane, isoflurane, and sevoflurane) is safe for patients with COPD (asthmatic bronchitis, emphysema, and chronic bronchitis). Volatile anesthetics are potent bronchodilators and, therefore, beneficial to patients with COPD.

N_2O, however, should be used cautiously. Carbon dioxide (CO_2) is a respiratory stimulus for patients with normal respiratory physiology. Patients with COPD retain larger amounts of CO_2 in their lungs and, over time, lose their respiratory drive. COPD patients thus develop a hypoxic drive. The potential for the hypoxic drive to cease with the severe chronic patient exists when O_2 is >21% room air (i.e., N_2O-O_2 at 70/30%).

Patients with COPD have increased incidence of pulmonary bullae or blebs (combined alveoli). Because of N_2O's low blood solubility, it can increase the volume and pressure of these lung defects, which could create an increased risk of barotrauma and pneumothorax. Duration of exposure and concentration of N_2O must be considered.

During sedation with an open airway, keep patients breathing spontaneously, and do not take away their respiratory drive. O_2 supplementation should be used with caution in patients with severe COPD. Supplemental O_2 via nasal cannula delivers low FiO_2, which should not affect hypoxic drive. It is recommended that oxygen concentrations not exceed an FiO_2 of 40. Remember, 4 L through a nasal cannula equals 36% O_2.

$$\text{Nasal cannula (3 to 6 L/min): } FiO_2 = 20 + 4 \times L/\text{min}$$
$$\text{Face mask with reservoir (6 to 10 L/min): } FiO_2 = 10 \times L/\text{min}$$

Asthma or reactive airways may occur at any age and could easily be encountered in the office. Patients with debilitating emphysema and chronic bronchitis are often chronically ill and are not seen commonly in an office setting. They may, however, be encountered in nursing homes and hospitals.

8. When is administration of N_2O sedation contraindicated in an asthmatic patient?

There are no absolute contraindications for the use of N_2O sedation in asthmatic patients. Because anxiety is a stimulus for an asthmatic attack, N_2O sedation is actually beneficial for these patients.

9. What is the second gas effect?

This occurs when one gas speeds the rate of increase of the alveolar partial pressure of a second gas. This effect is normally associated with an inhalational induction involving a large volume of N_2O and a volatile anesthetic. N_2O's low blood solubility allows it to be absorbed quickly by the alveoli, thus causing an increase in the alveolar concentration of the concomitantly administered volatile anesthetic. In theory, a high concentration of one gas (e.g., 70% N_2O) could speed the induction of a second gas (e.g., sevoflurane).

Inhalational inductions are normally used in energetic pediatric patients. Obtaining intravenous access in children who cannot sit still is difficult, and a quick induction is desirable. The speed of induction with sevoflurane should be increased when it is used concurrently with 70% N_2O.

10. What is minimal alveolar concentration (MAC)?

MAC is the concentration of an inhaled anesthetic at 1 atm that prevents skeletal muscle movement response to a painful stimulus (e.g., surgical skin incision) in 50% of patients (Table 8-1). A MAC of 1.3 prevents skeletal movement in approximately 95% of individuals undergoing surgery. The potency of anesthetic gases can be compared using MAC.

Table 8-1. Minimal Alveolar Concentration (MAC) of Commonly Used Agents

AGENT	MAC
Nitrous oxide	104
Isoflurane	1.15
Halothane	0.77
Desflurane	6.0
Sevoflurane	1.71

11. What factors affect MAC?

Factors that **decrease** *MAC:*	*Factors that* **increase** *MAC:*
Higher altitudes (Ø barometric pressure)	Increased central neurotransmitter levels (MAOIs,
Pregnancy	Cocaine, ephedrine, levodopa)
Hypothermia	Hyperthermia
Hyponatremia	Alcohol (chronic use)
Alcohol (acute use)	Hypernatremia
Barbiturates	
Calcium channel blockers	
Opioids	

12. How can MAC values be used to gauge awareness during surgery?
    Intraoperative patient awareness is a concern with all patients undergoing a deep sedation or general anesthesia. Volatile anesthetics have amnestic properties at an adequate MAC. Intravenous medications are often used in conjunction with volatile anesthetics, which often cause a decrease in MAC. This decreased MAC may prevent an amnestic state. Although specific concentrations of volatile agents have not been established for the elimination of intraoperative recall, clinical studies show that awareness is eliminated between 0.4 and 0.6 MAC for isoflurane. Attaining a MAC of 0.8 has been recommended to guarantee unconsciousness and, therefore, lack of awareness.
    Awareness precautions need to be taken with certain anesthetic techniques. An anesthetist may be tempted to decrease the concentration of a volatile anesthetic when a paralytic has been used because surgical stimulation has been eliminated. The addition of midazolam, an amnestic benzodiazepine, can be used in situations where MAC has been reduced below 0.8. MAC is often reduced in patients who develop intraoperative hypotension because of volatile inhalational vasodilating properties. Vasopressors, such as ephedrine and phenylephrine, may be necessary to maintain a MAC of 0.8 when additional amnestic medications are not being used.

13. Why are additive values of MAC for inhalational anesthetics beneficial?
    Additive values are beneficial when a decrease in volatile anesthetics is desired. MAC values are additive; therefore the simultaneous administration of N_2O with a volatile anesthetic will decrease the MAC of both agents. For example, using 0.5 MAC N_2O (approximately 50%) with 0.5 MAC isoflurane (approximately 0.6%) results in a MAC of 1.0.
    The only inhalational anesthetics that would be administered simultaneously would be a volatile anesthetic (desflurane, halothane, isoflurane, and sevoflurane) and N_2O. Fail-safe mechanisms exist on anesthetic machines to prevent the simultaneous administration of two volatile agents.
    N_2O has a MAC >100% and therefore is not used as a sole anesthetic agent, because a minimum of 21% O_2 is required at 1 atm. Typically, N_2O concentrations of 20% to 70% are used.

14. What are the hemodynamic effects of volatile anesthetics?
    Volatile anesthetics depress the cardiovascular system, which results in a reduced mean arterial pressure. Desflurane, isoflurane, and sevoflurane cause primarily a decrease in systemic vascular resistance, which is reflected by a reduced blood pressure.

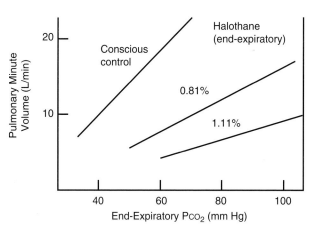

Figure 8-1. The CO_2 response curve. Note the effects of inhalational anesthetics on the pulmonary minute volume.

15. **What are the hemodynamic considerations of the combined use of a volatile anesthetic and the intravenous anesthetic propofol?**
    The inhalational anesthetics desflurane, isoflurane, and sevoflurane and the intravenous agent propofol are potent vasodilators. Additive effects causing hypotension from a decrease in systemic vascular resistance occur with simultaneous administration of these two anesthetic groups. Combining these agents should be done cautiously in elderly patients and patients taking hypertensive medications. Preoperative blood pressures are extremely important. Selection of an alternative intravenous anesthetic agent may be indicated. If propofol is used along with a volatile anesthetic, then vasopressors (e.g., ephedrine, phenylephrine) should be prepared and made readily available.

16. **What are the respiratory effects of volatile anesthetics?**
    Volatile anesthetics will cause a dose-dependent decrease in ventilation. Volatile anesthetics cause a decrease in tidal volume (TV) with a compensatory increase in respiratory rate (RR) but a net decrease in minute ventilation (mV).

    $$\text{Volatile anesthetics: net } \downarrow mV = \uparrow RR \times \downarrow TV$$

    This decreased minute ventilation causes an increase in CO_2. An increase in CO_2 stimulates the respiratory drive in the unanesthetized patient. Inhalational anesthetics, however, shift the CO_2 response curve to the right and lessen the ventilatory response to hypercarbia and hypoxia (Fig. 8-1).

17. **What is partition coefficient? How can it influence the speed of induction?**
    A partition coefficient is defined as a distribution ratio of a volatile anesthetic as it distributes itself between two phases at equilibrium when the temperature, pressure, and volume are the same (Table 8-2). A blood-to-gas coefficient therefore describes the distribution of anesthetic between blood and gas. High blood solubility requires a greater concentration of inhaled anesthetic to be dissolved in the blood before equilibrium can occur. The blood acts as an inactive reservoir that prevents the anesthetic from reaching the site of action, thereby slowing induction.
    Gases with low solubility in blood and adipose equilibrate more rapidly. Nitrous oxide has very low solubility and therefore achieves equilibration most rapidly. This explains why nitrous oxide has the fastest onset among inhalation agents (Fig. 8-2). Relative onset of effect is directly proportional to solubility, when all other factors are equal (e.g., alveolar concentration, cardiac output). The lower solubility of sevoflurane compared with isoflurane explains why sevoflurane is a more rapid induction agent.

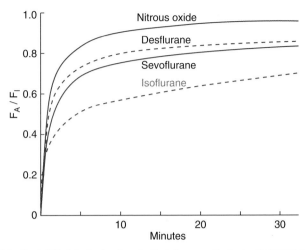

Figure 8-2. Relative Onset of Effect. Gas tensions throughout body tissues equilibrate when the inspired gas tension (FI) equals that in the alveoli (FA). *(Becker D, Rosenberg M: Nitrous oxide and the inhalation anesthetics,* Anesth Prog *55(4): 124–131, 2008 Winter.)*

Table 8-2. Partition Coefficients for Inhaled Anesthetics

	DESFLURANE	ISOFLURANE	N$_2$O	SEVOFLURANE
Blood:gas	0.42	1.4	0.46	0.68
Brain:blood	1.3	1.6	1.1	1.7
Muscle:blood	2.0	2.9	1.2	3.1
Fat:blood	27	45	2.3	48
Oil:blood	18.7	90.8	1.4	47.2

18. **Which volatile anesthetic has the quickest wake-up potential after a long (>5 hours) surgical procedure?**
Anesthetics take time to be distributed from the blood to the tissues (e.g., muscle, fat). As the length of time of a surgery increases and tissues become increasingly saturated with an anesthetic, wake-up times increase. The fat-to-blood partition coefficient for desflurane is the lowest for all volatile anesthetics, and it provides the quickest wake-up. A common misconception is that sevoflurane has a quick wake-up time because it has a quick onset. For short surgeries this is true, because tissue saturation has not had time to occur. For long surgeries, however, sevoflurane does not provide a quick wake-up. (See sevoflurane's tissue:blood coefficients in Table 8-2.)

19. **What is diffusion hypoxia?**
Although its existence has been questioned, diffusion hypoxia is postulated to occur when the administration of N$_2$O has been discontinued with the spontaneous breathing of room air. The theory holds that N$_2$O's low blood solubility allows it to leave the blood rapidly and enter the alveoli. Excessive N$_2$O in the alveoli dilutes the O$_2$ and makes the patient hypoxic. This phenomenon has been refuted by many studies. Nonetheless, because of side effects such as headaches, nausea, vomiting, and lethargy, administering O$_2$ for 3 to 5 minutes following N$_2$O use is recommended.

20. **What are the concerns to administration of N$_2$O sedation to an obstetric patient?**
N$_2$O crosses the placenta and therefore has the potential to cause teratogenic effects to the fetus. The greatest potential for problems exists during the first trimester when organs are forming. Significant exposure during the first 6 weeks can inhibit DNA synthesis. Consequently, female surgeons and staff who are not aware that they are pregnant may be at greater risk than patients.

Recent research has refuted the claim that N_2O is dangerous to the fetus. Although N_2O has been used safely for years in obstetrics, it would be wise to obtain a medical consult before its administration in pregnant women who are in their second or third trimesters. Even if N_2O sedation is approved by the patient's obstetrician, it should be used only for short procedures, and no more than 50% N_2O should be administered.

21. **What are neuromuscular blocking agents (NMBs)?***

NMBs, commonly called muscle relaxants, are drugs that interrupt transmission at the neuromuscular junction. These drugs provide skeletal muscle relaxation and, consequently, can be used to facilitate tracheal intubation, assist with mechanical ventilation, and optimize surgical conditions. Occasionally, they may be used to reduce the metabolic demands of breathing; in the management of status epilepticus (although they do not diminish central nervous system activity), status asthmaticus, or tetanus; and to facilitate the treatment of raised intracranial pressure.

These drugs inhibit the function of all skeletal muscle, including the diaphragm, and must be administered only by personnel skilled in airway management. NMBs should never be given without preparation to maintain the airway and ventilation. The concomitant use of sedative-hypnotic or amnestic drugs is indicated, because NMBs alone achieve complete paralysis while allowing the patient complete awareness.

22. **How are NMBs classified?***

These drugs are classified into two groups according to their actions at the neuromuscular junction:
1. Depolarizing NMB (succinylcholine [SCh]): SCh mimics the action of acetylcholine by depolarizing the postsynaptic membrane at the neuromuscular junction. The postsynaptic receptor is occupied/depolarized and remains refractory to further stimulation.
2. Nondepolarizing NMBs: These agents act by competitive blockade of the postsynaptic membrane, so that acetylcholine is blocked from the receptors and cannot have a depolarizing effect.

23. **What is the mechanism of action of SCh?***

SCh is the only depolarizing agent to be used widely in clinical anesthetic practice. The depolarizing agent mimics the action of acetylcholine. However, because SCh is hydrolyzed by plasma cholinesterase (pseudocholinesterase), which is present only in the plasma and not at the neuromuscular junction, the length of blockade is directly related to the rate of diffusion of SCh away from the neuromuscular junction. Consequently, the resultant depolarization is prolonged when compared with acetylcholine. Depolarization gradually diminishes, but relaxation persists as long as SCh is present at the postsynaptic receptor.

24. **What are the indications for using SCh?***

In clinical situations in which the patient has a full stomach and is at risk for regurgitation and aspiration when anesthetized, rapid paralysis and airway control are priorities. Such situations include diabetes mellitus, hiatal hernia, obesity, pregnancy, severe pain, and trauma.

SCh provides the most rapid onset of any NMB currently available. In addition, the duration of blockade induced by SCh is only 5 to 10 minutes. Respiratory muscle function returns quickly should the patient prove difficult to intubate. SCh is indicated for the treatment of laryngospasm unresponsive to positive pressure ventilation.

25. **What is the breakdown and elimination process of nondepolarizing NMBs?***

Atracurium and cisatracurium are unique in that they undergo spontaneous breakdown at physiologic temperatures and pH (Hoffmann elimination), as well as ester hydrolysis. These properties allow safe delivery in patients with compromised hepatic or renal function.

Aminosteroid relaxants (pancuronium, vecuronium, pipecuronium, and rocuronium) are deacetylated in the liver, and their action may be prolonged in the presence of hepatic dysfunction. Vecuronium and rocuronium also have significant biliary excretion, and their action may be prolonged with extrahepatic biliary obstruction.

Relaxants with significant renal excretion include tubocurarine, metocurine, doxacurium, pancuronium, and pipecuronium.

---

*Reprinted from Warnecke DE: Neuromuscular blocking agents. In Duke J, editor: *Anesthesia secrets*, ed 2, Philadelphia, 2000, Hanley & Belfus.

Table 8-3. Neuromuscular Blocking Reversal Agents

DRUG	DOSE (MG/KG)	ONSET (MIN)	DURATION (MIN)
Edrophonium	0.5-1.0	2	45-60
Neostigmine	0.035-0.07	7	60-90
Pyridostigmine	0.15-0.25	11	60-120

26. **Is it possible to reverse the effects of the nondepolarizing NMBs?***

Just as competition at the receptor sites of the neuromuscular junction allows the relaxant to overcome the effects of acetylcholine, medications that increase the amount of acetylcholine at the neuromuscular junction facilitate reversal of relaxation. Reversal agents are **acetylcholinesterase inhibitors** and include neostigmine, pyridostigmine, and edrophonium (Table 8-3). These drugs inhibit the enzyme that breaks down acetylcholine, making more of this neurotransmitter available at each receptor. Physostigmine, another acetylcholinesterase inhibitor, crosses the blood-brain barrier and is not used for reversal of muscle relaxants. Pyridostigmine is used in the management of patients with myasthenia gravis. The acetylcholinesterase inhibitors possess positively charged quaternary ammonium groups, are water-soluble, and are renally excreted.

27. **NMB reversal agents cause an increase in available acetylcholine. Is this a problem?***

It is important to remember that the muscarinic effects of these drugs at cholinergic receptors in the heart must be blocked by atropine or glycopyrrolate to prevent bradycardia. The degree of bradycardia may be significant. Even asystole has been noted. The most common doses used for this purpose are 0.01 mg/kg of atropine and 0.005 to 0.015 mg/kg of glycopyrrolate.

To prevent bradycardias associated with the anticholinesterases, it is important to administer an anticholinergic with a similar onset of action. Atropine is administered with edrophonium and glycopyrrolate with neostigmine.

28. **The heart is a muscle. Do muscle relaxants decrease contraction of the myocardium?***

The NMBs have their primary effect at nicotinic cholinergic receptor sites. The myocardium is a muscle with nerve transmission accomplished via adrenergic receptors using norepinephrine as the transmitter. Consequently, muscle relaxants have no effect on cardiac contractility. NMBs also have no effect on smooth muscle.

29. **How do we make muscle relaxants work faster if we need to secure the airway sooner?***

By overwhelming the sites of action (receptors in the neuromuscular junction), one can provide a competitive advantage for the blocking drug over acetylcholine. This is exactly what is done with the standard intubating dose of a nondepolarizing relaxant. The usual intubating dose is approximately three times the ED95 (the dose expected to show 95% reduction in twitch height on electrical stimulation). For relaxants with cardiovascular stability, further increases in initial dose can provide some decrease in onset time without producing side effects. However, with the exception of the nondepolarizing NMB rocuronium, it is very difficult to decrease the onset time to that of SCh. For drugs with side effects such as histamine release, increases in dose usually increase side effects as well.

Another method of decreasing onset time is the priming technique. By giving one-third of the ED95 at 3 minutes before the intubating dose, one can decrease onset time by as much as 1 minute. However, sensitivity to the paralyzing effects of these agents varies greatly among patients, and some patients may become totally paralyzed with a priming dose. Other patients may experience distressing diplopia, dysphagia, or the sensation of not being able to take a deep breath. For this reason, the practice of administering "priming" doses of relaxants is discouraged by many anesthesiologists. Once relaxants are administered at any dose, the anesthetist should be in the position to assist ventilation.

---

*Reprinted from Warnecke DE: Neuromuscular blocking agents. In Duke J, editor: *Anesthesia secrets*, ed 2, Philadelphia, 2000, Hanley & Belfus.

30. **What is plasma cholinesterase (pseudocholinesterase)?***

    Plasma cholinesterase is produced in the liver and metabolizes SCh as well as ester local anesthetics. A reduced quantity of plasma cholinesterase may be the result of liver disease, pregnancy, malignancies, malnutrition, collagen vascular disease, and hypothyroidism. This reduction could result in a prolonged duration of blockade with SCh.

31. **What is the importance of a dibucaine number?***

    The dibucaine number is used to identify individuals at risk for prolonged paralysis following administration of SCh. Dibucaine number is the percent of pseudocholinesterase (PChE) enzyme activity that is inhibited by dibucaine. Dibucaine inhibits normal plasma cholinesterase by 80%, whereas atypical plasma cholinesterase is inhibited by only 20%. A patient with normal SCh metabolism will have a dibucaine number of 80. If a patient has a dibucaine number of 40 to 60, then that patient is heterozygous for this atypical plasma cholinesterase and will have a moderately prolonged block with SCh. If a patient has a dibucaine number of 20, the patient is homozygous for atypical plasma cholinesterase and will have a very prolonged block with SCh.

    It is important to remember that a dibucaine number is a qualitative, and not quantitative, measurement. Consequently, a patient may have a dibucaine number of 80 but have prolonged blockade with SCh related to decreased levels of normal plasma cholinesterase.

32. **Are clinicians accurate in determining arterial desaturation by "visual oximetry" (how red is the blood)?[†]**

    No. Pulse oximetry should be regarded as the fifth vital sign.

33. **Can any other environmental or clinical conditions result in inaccurate pulse oximetry values?[†]**

    Reliability depends on a strong arterial pulse plus good light transmission. Inaccuracy results with hypotension (mean arterial pressure $<50\,mm\,Hg$), hypothermia ($<35°\,C$), vascular disease (poor peripheral perfusion), and vasopressor therapy (vasoconstriction). Bright lights, intravenous dyes, nail polish, and excessive motion each may produce bad information.

34. **What is the relationship between oxyhemoglobin saturation (SaO_2) and partial pressure of oxygen (PaO_2)?[†]**

    Proper interpretation of pulse oximetry requires recall of the oxyhemoglobin dissociation curve (Fig. 8-3). A rightward shift (decreased hemoglobin affinity for oxygen) facilitates oxygen unloading at the tissue level. Increasing temperature, increasing $PaCO_2$, increasing 2,3-diphosphoglycerate, and increasing hydrogen ion concentration—all "increases"—shift the curve to the right. When the PaO_2 is $>100\,mm\,Hg$, however, the curve is virtually flat. Consequently, a large drop in PaO_2 (e.g., from 200 to $100\,mm\,Hg$) may occur with no discernible change in SaO_2.

35. **How should a hypoxic event be managed?[†]**

    Before you even start trying to make the diagnosis, give oxygen. The first maneuver for intubated patients is to hand-ventilate with an Ambu bag. A ruptured endotracheal tube cuff is self-evident, whereas difficult bagging implies airway obstruction, bronchospasm, or tension pneumothorax. Inability to pass a suction catheter confirms endotracheal tube obstruction. If the obstruction is not reversible by changing head position or by cuff deflation, the endotracheal tube must be replaced immediately. If there is difficulty with bagging and no evidence of airway obstruction, listen to the chest for breath sounds to exclude a tension pneumothorax. The mechanical ventilator and breathing circuit must be examined for malfunction. Send arterial blood gases to confirm hypoxia (low PO_2) and rule out hypoventilation (high PCO_2).

    Next, get a chest X-ray (to rule out a pneumothorax and to confirm the correct position of the endotracheal tube) and review recent medications, interventions (e.g., suctioning, position changes, nursing care), and changes in clinical status. Most acute hypoxic events in the intensive care unit are the result of easily identified and reversible mechanical problems, such as disconnects from oxygen delivery systems or mucus plugging that requires suctioning.

*Reprinted from Warnecke DE: Neuromuscular blocking agents. In Duke J, editor: *Anesthesia secrets*, ed 2, Philadelphia, 2000, Hanley & Belfus.

[†]Reprinted from Haenel J, Johnson JL: Oxygen monitoring and assessment. In Harken AH, Moore EE, editors: *Abernathy's surgical secrets*, ed 5, Philadelphia, 2005, Mosby.

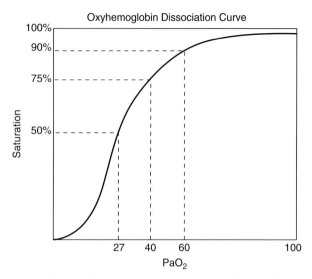

Figure 8-3. The oxyhemoglobin dissociation curve describes the nonlinear relationship between PaO_2 and percentage saturation of hemoglobin with oxygen (SaO_2). In the steep part of the curve (50% region), small changes in PaO_2 result in large changes in SaO_2. The converse is true when PaO_2 rises above 60 mm Hg. Three regions of the curve have been marked. *(From Edwards RK: Pulse oximetry. In Duke J, editor:* Anesthesia secrets, *ed 3, Philadelphia, 2006, Mosby.)*

36. How long does it take before changes in oxygen saturation are reflected in pulse oximeter readings?

    Approximately 20 seconds. It takes time for O_2 delivered to the lung to influence oxygenation at the fingertip. Pulse oximeter signals are also averaged over different periods. This is mainly to reduce spurious pulse oximeter readings, such as those caused by patient movement. The trade-off is that true reductions in pulse oximeter readings are delayed (a patient desaturating faster than the pulse oximeter indicates). Similarly, once adequate delivery of oxygen is restored, there will be a delay in recovery of the pulse oximeter readings. The period of signal averaging can often be changed in commonly used pulse oximeters.

BIBLIOGRAPHY

Adamson DT: Oxygenation and ventilation. In Duke J, editor: *Anesthesia secrets*, ed 2, Philadelphia, 2000, Hanley & Belfus.
Becker D, Rosenberg M: Nitrous oxide and the inhalation anesthetics, *Anesth Prog* 55(4):124–131, 2008.
Browne MD: Volatile anesthetics. In Duke J, editor: *Anesthesia secrets*, ed 3, Philadelphia, 2006, Mosby.
Cahalan MK, Lurz FW, Eger 2nd EI, et al.: Narcotics decrease heart rate during inhalation anesthesia, *Anesth Analg* 66:166–170, 1987.
Christensen LQ, Bonde J, Kampmann JP: Drug interactions with inhalational anaesthetics, *Acta Anesthesiol Scand* 37:231–244, 1993.
Clark MS, Brunick AL: *Handbook of nitrous oxide and oxygen sedation*, ed 2, St Louis, 2003, Mosby.
Duke J: Airway management. In Duke J, editor: *Anesthesia secrets*, ed 3, Philadelphia, 2006, Mosby.
Eger 2nd EI, Saidman LJ: Hazards of nitrous oxide anesthesia in bowel obstruction and pneumothorax, *Anesthesiol* 26:61–66, 1965.
Gomez R, Guatimosim C: Mechanism of action of volatile anesthetics: involvement of intracellular calcium signaling, *Curr Drug Targets CNS Neurol Disord* 2:123–129, April 2003.
Foltz B, Benumof J: Mechanisms of hypoxia and hypercarbia in the perioperative period, *Crit Care Clin* 3:269–286, 1987.
Haenel JB, Johnson JL: Oxygen monitoring and assessment. In Duke J, editor: *Anesthesia secrets*, ed 2, Philadelphia, 2000, Hanley & Belfus.
Hayashi Y, Kamibayashi T, Sumikawa K, et al.: Adrenoreceptor mechanism involved in thiopental-epinephrine-induced arrhythmias in dogs, *Am J Physiol* 265:H1380–H1385, 1993.
Johnston RR, Eger 2nd EI, Wilson C: A comparative interaction of epinephrine with enflurane, isoflurane, and halothane in man, *Anesth Analg* 55:709–712, 1976.
Kamibayashi T, Hayashi Y, Takada K, et al.: Adrenoreceptor mechanism involved in thiopental-induced potentiation of halothane-epinephrine arrhythmias in dogs, *Res Comm Mol Pathol Pharmacol* 93:225–234, 1996.

Katz RL, Matteo RS, Papper EM: The injection of epinephrine during general anesthesia with halogenated hydrocarbons and cyclopropane in man. 2. Halothane, *Anesthesiol* 23:597–600, 1962.

Leichliter C: Awareness during anesthesia. In Duke J, editor: *Anesthesia secrets*, ed 3, Philadelphia, 2006, Mosby.

Malamed SF: *Sedation: a guide to patient management*, ed 4, St Louis, 2003, Mosby.

Miller HJ: Chronic obstructive pulmonary disease. In Duke J, editor: *Anesthesia secrets*, ed 3, Philadelphia, 2006, Mosby.

Rosen MA: Management of anesthesia for the pregnant surgical patient, *Anesthesiol* 91:1159–1163, 1999.

Stoelting RK, Miller RD: Effects of inhaled anesthetics on ventilation and circulation. In Stoelting RK, Miller RD, editors: *Basics of anesthesia*, ed 3, New York, 1994, Churchill Livingstone.

Warnecke DE: Neuromuscular blocking agents. In Duke J, editor: *Anesthesia secrets*, ed 2, Philadelphia, 2000, Hanley & Belfus.

Wenker O: Review of currently used inhalation anesthetics: part I, *Internet J Anesthesiol* 3(2), 1998.

CHAPTER 9

ANESTHESIA FOR DIFFICULT PATIENTS

Stuart Lieblich

1. **What important physiological changes occur during pregnancy?**
   - Cardiovascular: An increase in cardiac output of up to +40% is seen by the second trimester. This is a result of both an increase in heart rate and stroke volume. Blood pressure is normally decreased due to effects of progesterone on peripheral vascular resistance. During the third trimester, the uterus can cause compression of both the vena cava and the abdominal aorta, resulting in postural decrease in venous return and a drop in cardiac output and blood pressure. Patients during their third trimester should be positioned on the left side with the right hip elevated with the use of a pillow.
   - Pulmonary: There is a decrease in functional residual capacity due to decrease in both expiratory reserve volume and residual volume that results in lowering of oxygen reserve. Resting minute ventilation and tidal volume increase by 40% to 50%, which results in hyperventilation and lower mean arterial CO_2 levels.
   - Hematological: Hematocrit and hemoglobin levels decrease during pregnancy. By the third trimester, the hematocrit averages 31% to 33% and hemoglobin 11 g/dl. Several coagulation factors such as factors VII, VIII, X, and fibrinogen increase during pregnancy. In addition the fibrinolytic activity is decreased, causing an overall hypercoagulable state during pregnancy.
   - GI: There is a decrease in GI motility and delayed gastric emptying as well as compromised gastro-esophageal sphincter. These changes predispose pregnant patients to reflux and increased risk of aspiration during deep sedation and general anesthesia.
   - Renal: There is an increase in renal blood flow and glomerular filtration rate resulting in faster clearance of drugs that are cleared by kidneys.

2. **When is the fetus most sensitive to teratogenic influences of anesthetic drugs?**
   Teratogens have either a lethal effect or no effect on the embryo in the first two weeks of intrauterine life. Organogenesis takes place between the third and eighth week; drug exposure during this period can produce major developmental abnormalities. After completion of organogenesis teratogen exposure results in only minor morphological abnormalities but can also produce significant physiological abnormalities and growth retardation.

3. **What are the categories in evaluating the severity of obesity?**
   Body mass index (BMI) has been used to categorize severity of obesity. BMI greater than 25 kg/m² is considered overweight, 30 to 39 kg/m² is considered obese, and anyone with BMI greater than 40 kg/m² is considered morbidly obese.

4. **What is Pickwickian syndrome?**
   Pickwickian syndrome is also known as obesity hypoventilation syndrome. It is a condition in which obese patients fail to breathe rapidly enough or deeply enough, resulting in low blood oxygen levels and high blood carbon dioxide levels.

5. **What are the pharmacokinetic differences in the obese population compared to that in healthy adults?**
   Obese patients will have reduced total body water volume, increased body fat, and increased renal clearance because of increased GFR. A hypophilic drug has an increased volume of distribution, which translates into longer time for drug elimination.

6. **What factors make office-based anesthesia more difficult for patients with Obstructive Sleep Apnea (OSA)?**
   OSA patients are very sensitive to central nervous system (CNS) depressant drugs, especially opioids that are routinely used in office-based anesthesia. Peripherally, CNS depressant drugs can

alter normal phasic negative pressure reflex, which is important in protecting the upper airway from collapse during inspiration. Centrally, opioids act on the medulla respiratory center to blunt the response to a hypercapnia challenge. Several studies have also shown that moderate-severe OSA results in both difficult mask ventilation and difficult tracheal intubation. In addition, OSA is associated with several metabolic and cardiovascular comorbidities such as HTN, MI, strokes, insulin resistance, and GERD.

For the reasons outlined above, OSA patients are at increased risk of developing respiratory events, which emphasizes the importance of screening all patients for OSA and identifying suitable candidates for office-based anesthesia.

7. **What screening tool can you use to detect patients with high risk of OSA?**
The STOP-BANG questionnaire should be used to screen for patients that are considered to be at risk for OSA before anesthesia. This includes all middle-aged obese men and postmenopausal women. The total score received on the questionnaire is related directly to the severity of OSA. A score of 4 or more answered "yes" questions indicates a high risk for OSA. A score of 5 to 8 is predictive of moderate-severe OSA. A score of 3 or less predicts a low risk for OSA.
S = Snoring
T = Tiredness
O = Observed apnea
P = Pressure (HTN)
B = BMI >35 kg/m^2
A = Age >50 years
N = Neck circumference >40 cm
G = Male gender

8. **What physical findings are consistent with obstructive sleep apnea?**
   1. BMI greater than 35 (95th percentile for age and gender)
   2. Neck circumference greater than 17 inches (men) or 16 inches (women)
   3. Craniofacial abnormalities affecting airway
   4. Anatomic nasal obstruction
   5. Tonsils nearly touching or touching in the midline

9. **What general considerations should be taken into account in sedating patients with obstructive sleep apnea?**
For most dentoalveolar surgeries, local anesthesia, with or without minimal sedation, should be considered. If minimal sedation is used, ventilation should be continuously monitored by capnography due to increased risk of undetected airway obstruction in these patients. Patients should be placed in a sitting position and an independent head holder should maintain neck extension. Reversal agents should be immediately available to rescue from deeper levels of anesthesia. A nasopharyngeal airway can be helpful in maintaining a patient's SpO$_2$ above 90%. Lastly, one should strongly consider general anesthesia with a secure airway in an operating room over office-based anesthesia without a secure airway for patients with moderate-severe OSA.

10. **What general consideration should be taken into account in postoperative management of patients with obstructive sleep apnea?**
The supine position should be avoided and patients should sleep upright while taking opioids. Nonopioid medications such as NSAIDs should be considered for pain management. Nasal CPAP should be used strictly, especially while taking opioids. Patients should be kept in close contact during the first postoperative week to monitor pain levels and opioid use.

11. **List some of the important anatomical abnormalities seen in Trisomy 21 syndrome patients. What anesthetic consideration should be taken into account in managing these patients?**
Some of the concerning abnormalities seen in Down syndrome patients include a short neck, irregular dentition, mental retardation, hypotonia, and a large tongue. Additionally, congenital heart disease (particularly ventricular septal defect) is seen in 40% of these patients. Due to the mentioned anatomical differences, these patients often have difficult airways. Neck flexion during laryngoscopy and intubation may result in atlantooccipital dislocation due to congenital laxity of these ligaments. Special consideration must be taken to avoid air bubbles in the intravenous line because of possible right-to-left shunts (paradoxical air embolus).

12. **What is cerebral palsy?**
    Cerebral palsy (CP) is a nonprogressive motor and posture disorder of cerebral or cerebellar origin. The primary impairment involves significant deficits in motor planning and control (patient can be spastic, dyskinetic, or ataxic). Although the disorder is nonprogressive, clinical manifestations often change over time as the functional expression of the underlying brain is modified by normal brain development and maturation.

13. **What are the anesthetic concerns for cerebral palsy patients?**
    Muscle spasticity and limb contractures can make airway management, intravenous access, and surgical positioning difficult. Medical findings, such as seizure disorder, GI reflux, scoliosis, and multiple history of pulmonary infections are commonly found in this population. CP patients may also have impaired pharyngeal function, which leads to pooling of oral secretions and increasing risk of aspiration. If muscle relaxant is needed, a nondepolarizing skeletal muscle relaxant is preferred to prevent hyperkalemic episodes; however, a higher dose of depolarizing agent may be needed due to drug resistance.

14. **What are the special considerations in the perioperative assessment of alcohol-abusing patients?**
    Chronic alcohol-abusing patients can have multiorgan diseases. Alcohol-induced cardiac disease should be evaluated with preoperative 12-lead ECG. These patients are also less sensitive to endogenous or parenteral catecholamine. Electrolyte imbalance (hypokalemia), hypoglycemia, anemia, and coagulopathy should also be evaluated. Hypervolemia is also a major concern for a long operating procedure, but less so in the outpatient setting.

15. **What is the mechanism of action for marijuana and its physiological effects?**
    The active substances in marijuana are tetrahydrocannabinol and cannabinoids, which stimulate cannabinoid receptors to produce euphoric, analgesic, anxiolytic, and sedative effects. Low-dose marijuana can stimulate the sympathetic nervous system, which leads to hypertension and tachycardia. High-dose marijuana inhibits the sympathetic system, which results in bradycardia and hypotension. Marijuana smokers also have similar pulmonary effects to tobacco users (airway irritation and increased CO-Hb level).

16. **What are the withdrawal signs and symptoms of chronic opioid users?**
    Agitation, hypotension, tachycardia, lacrimation, and diarrhea are the typical withdrawal signs and symptoms found in chronic opioid users. Naloxone and mixed agonist-antagonist agents (buprenorphine) are relatively contraindicated in this patient population as they can precipitate withdrawal symptoms.

17. **What is the management strategy of the chronic opioid user, who is currently on mixed agonist-antagonist agents (buprenorphine), when required to undergo surgery?**
    Buprenorphine is a mixed agonist-antagonist opioid receptor modulator that is used to treat opioid addiction in high dosage. A patient who is on this medication and undergoes major surgery should discontinue the medication one to three days preoperatively to prevent its antagonist effect against postoperative opioid medication. Low-dose opioid may be needed to prevent withdrawal symptoms during this time. Postoperatively, buprenorphine can be resumed once acute pain is no longer an issue. For a minor procedure, patients should continue buprenorphine until the morning of surgery to prevent withdrawal symptoms.

18. **What are the anatomical differences between a pediatric and adult airway?**
    A pediatric patient has a larger tongue size, floppier omega-shaped epiglottis, and funnel-shaped larynx. The narrowest point of the airway is lower in the subglottic region. Patients in this group also have decreased compliance in the upper airway, which makes them more prone to collapse. They also have decreased total lung capacity and faster respiratory and metabolic rates.

19. **How is an endotracheal tube (ET) of appropriate size chosen?**
    Age/4 + 4 = mm of diameter for ET tube. Patient variation does exist; a half size above and a half size below the estimated size should be available. The leak around the tube should be <30 cc, H_2O, and the ET should be placed to a depth of approximately three times its internal diameter.

20. **What is the appropriate size laryngeal mask airway for pediatric patient?**
    The laryngeal mask airway should be based on the patient's age and weight (Table 9-1).

21. **What is malignant hyperthermia (MH)?**
    A hypermetabolic state involving skeletal muscle that is precipitated by certain anesthetic agents in genetically susceptible individuals.

Table 9-1. Laryngeal Mask Airways for Children

SIZE OF CHILD	LARYNGEAL MASK SIZE
Neonates up to 5 kg	1
Infants 5-10 kg	1.5
Children 10-20 kg	2
Children 20-30 kg	2.5
Children/small adults >30 kg	3
Children/adults >70 kg	4
Children/adults >80 kg	5

22. **Which patients are at risk of developing MH?**
    Patients at risk of developing MH include those with:
    - A diagnosis of MH (see question 6)
    - A first-degree relative with a diagnosis of MH
    - An elevated resting creatine kinase (CK) and family with suspected MH tendency
    - Central core disease
    - Musculoskeletal disease associated with MH (see question 23)

23. **With which muscle diseases has MH been associated?**
    - Dystrophinopathy
    - Myotonia
    - Phosphorylase deficiency
    - King-Denborough and Barnes myopathies
    - Minicore disease

24. **How are susceptible patients diagnosed?**
    The diagnosis of MH in susceptible patients is made by the muscle contracture test. Muscle fibers from MH-positive patients produce an exaggerated response to electrical stimulation when exposed to halothane and caffeine. When a muscle contracture test is not possible, muscle biopsy may be performed. Characteristic findings on muscle biopsy include variable muscle fiber size, increased number of internalized nuclei, and the presence of "moth-eaten" fibers. These findings are nonspecific and cannot be used alone to establish diagnosis. Patients with MH also may have elevated baseline CK levels.

25. **Which anesthetic drugs are known to trigger MH?**
    Inhalation anesthetics:
    - Halothane
    - Desflurane
    - Enflurane
    - Sevoflurane
    - Isoflurane
    Depolarizing neuromuscular blockade agents:
    - Succinylcholine
    - Decamethonium
    - Suxamethonium

26. **What are the three early presenting signs and symptoms of MH during an anesthetic procedure?**
    1. Early masseter contracture following administration of succinylcholine
    2. An unexplained rise in end-tidal CO_2 following induction of anesthesia
    3. An unexplained tachycardia following induction of anesthesia

27. **What is the initial management of an acute attack of MH in the adult patient?**
    1. Discontinue the anesthetic agent.
    2. Hyperventilate with 100% oxygen.
    3. Administer dantrolene sodium intravenously until heart rate and end-tidal CO_2 decrease.

4. Begin infusion of iced intravenous (IV) fluids (avoid lactated Ringer's).
5. Cool patient with iced saline lavage of stomach, bladder, and rectum; cooling blankets; and ice packs.
6. Draw blood for serum electrolytes, arterial blood gases, prothrombin time (PT), partial thromboplastin time (PTT), and myoglobin studies.
7. Monitor vital signs, electrocardiogram (ECG), end-tidal CO_2, blood gases, temperature, and urine output.
8. Treat metabolic acidosis with sodium bicarbonate.
9. Treat arrhythmias with antiarrhythmic drugs (avoid calcium channel blockers).
10. Treat hyperkalemia with glucose and insulin.
11. Maintain urinary output of greater than 2 mL/kg/hr with hydration and diuretics (furosemide or mannitol).

28. What is dantrolene sodium, and how does it work?

Dantrolene sodium is a hydantoin-derivative muscle relaxant that exerts its muscle relaxant effect by interfering with excitation-contraction coupling in the muscle fiber. Dantrolene sodium is used in the treatment of MH because it blocks calcium release from the sarcoplasmic reticulum calcium channels.

29. What is the recommended dose of dantrolene sodium for treatment of MH?

- 2 to 3 mg/kg IV every 5 minutes up to a total dose of 10 mg/kg.
- 1 mg/kg IV every 6 hours for 24 to 48 hours in recovery.
- Then oral dantrolene for an additional 24 hours.

III

PERIOPERATIVE CARE

1. **What is the distribution of water in the human body?**
   Total body water (TWB) in men is 60% of body weight and in women comprises 50% of body weight. The water is then split between intracellular fluid (ICF) and extracellular fluid (ECF). ICF is two-thirds of TWB, and ECF is one-third of TBW. The ECF is then further divided with one-third resting in the intravascular space and two-thirds in the interstitial fluid.

2. **What is the TBW, ECF volume (ECFV), and blood volume in a 70-kg man?**
   TBW: $6 \times 70 = 42\,L$
   ECFV: $42\,L \times 1/3 = 14\,L$
   Intravascular fluid (blood volume): $14\,L \times 1/3 = 4.66\,L$

3. **What are the major extracellular and intracellular cations?**
   The major extracellular cation is sodium, and it is responsible for most of the osmotic force that maintains the size of the ECFV. The concentration is usually kept within a narrow range (135 to 145 mEq/L). Potassium is the major intracellular cation. The intracellular concentration is about 130 to 140 mEq/L, and the extracellular concentration is 3.5 to 5.0 mEq/L. A stable plasma concentration is essential for normal cellular function, cardiac rhythm, and a proper neuromuscular transmission.

4. **How is TBW maintained?**
   Total body water is maintained through numerous systemic systems including the hypothalamic center, antidiuretic hormone (ADH), and the renin-angiotensin-aldosterone system. The hypothalamic thirst center is stimulated when the plasma becomes hypertonic. The hypothalamus secretes vasopressin (ADH), stimulating more water reabsorption. ADH is also secreted in the renin system. Low perfusion of the kidney stimulates renin secretion, which stimulates production of angiotensin 1. Angiotensin 1 is converted to angiotensin 2 in the lungs. Angiotensin 2 stimulates ADH release from the pituitary, leading to an increase in sodium and water reabsorption.

5. **What is the water exchange process in a normal person?**
   An average adult takes in approximately 2.5 L of water in one day, with approximately 1.5 L from drinking. The remaining 1 L is extracted from food. Water is excreted through the kidneys (500 to 1500 cc/day), stool (250 cc/day), and insensible losses (600 cc/day).

6. **What is normal urine output in an adult patient?**
   One cc/kg/hr is considered normal urine output. However, the patient's systemic issues may play a role in volume status and may affect urine output. For example, patients with sepsis will have higher insensible losses; patients with liver failure will have more third spacing of fluid.

7. **How is maintenance fluid calculated?**
   The 4/2/1 rule is used with 4 cc/kg for the first 10 kg, 2 cc/kg for the next 10 kg, and 1 cc/kg for every kg over 20 kg. As mentioned before, the patient's total health needs to be considered and additional fluid is necessary in those patients with fevers, sepsis, or burns. Decreased fluid infusion should be considered in those patients with edematous states, hypothyroidism, and renal failure.

8. **What is body osmolality?**
   Osmolality is the ratio of solutes to water in body compartments. The main solutes include sodium, glucose, and urea.
   Calculated osmolality $= 2[Na+] + [glucose]/18 + [BUN]/2.8$
   When the measured osmolality is greater than the calculated osmolality, an osmolar gap is calculated. When the gap is greater than 10, extra solutes such as ethylene glycol, methanol, and ethanol may be found.

9. **What is tonicity (effective osmolality)?**
   Tonicity is the ability of solutes to generate an increase in osmotic pressure, when they are restricted to a compartment, causing water to move from an intracellular compartment to an extracellular one to establish osmotic equilibrium. These solutes are termed effective osmoles. Sodium, glucose, mannitol, and sorbitol are effective osmoles. An increase in tonicity is the main stimulus for thirst and the release of ADH to help water regulation.

10. **What are some causes of hypovolemia?**
    Volume depletion can be secondary to renal losses because of diuretic use, adrenal insufficiency, osmotic diuresis, and Diabetes Inspidus (DI). Third spacing is common in soft tissue injuries, infections, pancreatitis, and intestinal obstruction. Fluid can also be lost through the skin and lungs in cases of high fever, sweating, increased respiratory rate, and hyperventilation.

11. **What are signs of a hypovolemic fluid status?**
    Patients will typically develop oliguria with acute renal failure secondary to prerenal azotemia, orthostatic hypotension, tachycardia, decreased Central Venous Pressure (CVP), and pulmonary capillary wedge pressure. Central nervous system findings can include mental status changes and sleepiness. These patients may also develop weakness, dry mucous membranes and hypothermia, and will exhibit poor skin turgor.

12. **How is hypovolemia diagnosed?**
    Urine output will decrease, serum sodium will be elevated, BUN/Cr ratio will be greater than 20:1, and hematocrit will increase 3% for each liter of deficit.

13. **How is hypovolemia treated?**
    Crystalloid therapy is the gold standard except in cases of severe blood loss; 2 L of isotonic crystalloid fluid should initially be bolused. It is important to note that in these patients, close monitoring of vitals is imperative. Urine output should be maintained at 1 cc/kg/hr. Colloid therapy is more expensive and has not shown any benefit over crystalloid therapy. In cases of severe hemorrhagic hypovolemia or shock, blood transfusion should be used. Patients with cardiac history should be cautioned in replenishing their fluid deficiency.

14. **What are clinical signs of hypervolemia, and when does volume excess occur?**
    Peripheral edema, pulmonary rales secondary to edema, low albumin, elevated CVP, and jugular venous distention are all signs of volume excess. These patients will often exhibit weight gain. Typically volume excess occurs when water and sodium intake/retention are greater than renal and extrarenal losses. The etiology of hypervolemia includes liver disease, congestive heart failure, acute renal failure, and nephrotic syndrome.

15. **What is edema?**
    Edema is a condition of volume excess that occurs in the interstitial or extracellular space and is not evident until 3 to 4 L of fluid have accumulated.

16. **Which commonly used parenteral fluid most closely resembles ECF? How does its composition differ from 5% dextrose in half-normal saline (D5-1/2 NS) (Table 10-1)?**

Table 10-1. Commonly Used Parenteral Fluids

	Electrolyte Content (mEq/L)						OSMO-LARITY (IN OSM)
	SODIUM	POTASSIUM	CALCIUM	MAGNESIUM	CHLORIDE	HCO$_3$	
Lactated Ringer's	130	4	3	–	109	28 (as lactate)	273
ECF	142	4	5	3	103	27	280-310
D$_5$-1/2 NS	77	–	–	–	77	–	407

17. **What is the most common electrolyte disorder in hospitalized patients? What are general considerations?**

Hyponatremia is the most common electrolyte disorder in hospitalized patients. It is defined as having a serum sodium concentration <130 mEq/L. It is usually caused by a water imbalance because of increased water intake or a decrease in excretion by the kidney. The most common type is a hypoosmolar form in which the serum osmolarity is reduced to <280 mOsm/kg. Two other types must be ruled out. One is an isotonic form, in which the serum osmolality is normal (280 to 295 mOsm/kg) and is caused by hyperproteinemia, hyperlipemia, and posttransurethral resection (TUR) prostatectomy. The other is a hyperosmolar form with a serum osmolality >295 mOsm/kg caused by hyperglycemia, mannitol, and radiocontrast agents.

18. **How is the concentration of sodium maintained?**

Sodium is restricted to the extracellular space and is the main osmotic cation in the extracellular fluid. When sodium intake is increased, there is a concurrent increase in the extracellular fluid volume. This will then increase sodium excretion through the renal system.

19. **What is hypoosmolar hyponatremia?**

Hypoosmolar hyponatremia can occur with normal TBW (euvolemic hyponatremia), excess TBW (hypervolemic hyponatremia), and low TBW (hypovolemic hyponatremia). The most common cause of hyponatremia with euvolemia is SIADH. Other causes of this can be drugs (nonsteroidal antiinflammatory drugs, Diabinese, Tegretol, cytotoxin), diuretics, pulmonary infection, meningitis, and oat cell carcinoma. Hypervolemic hyponatremia is a depletion of the effective circulating volume with no restriction of water intake [Congestive Heart Failure (CHF), hepatic cirrhosis, nephritic syndrome]. Hypovolemic hyponatremia can be nonrenal in origin (vomiting, diarrhea, sweating) when the urine sodium concentration is <10 mEq/L, or renal (diuretics, a salt-losing renal disease or adrenal insufficiency) when the urine sodium concentration is >20 mEq/L. Rapid correction can lead to irreversible central nervous system (CNS) damage.

20. **How is hyponatremia diagnosed?**

Hyponatremia is caused by too much water; however, the etiology and diagnosis is found when serum osmolality is calculated. A normal serum osmolality is isotonic hyponatremia and is typically caused by hyperlipidemia and hyperproteinemia. A high serum osmolality is hypertonic hyponatremia and is caused by hyperglycemia. When serum osmolality is low, hypotonic hyponatremia is the diagnosis; however, it needs to be further classified based on volume status. In the hypotonic hyponatremic setting, the patients who are hypovolemic are losing salt, the euvolemic patients can have SIADH, hypothyroidism, or psychogenic polydipsia, and the hypervolemic patients are typically in renal failure, congestive heart failure, or liver failure.

21. **What are symptoms of hyponatremia?**

The most common are neurologic symptoms that are caused by an increase in ICF volume leading to headaches, hyperactive deep tendon reflexes, weakness, and irritability. Other symptoms include hypertension, nausea, vomiting, ileus, and oliguria.

22. **What are the critical levels of hyponatremia, and how can this condition be corrected?**

Symptoms usually occur during an acute, sudden decrease of sodium levels to <130 mEq/L or during a chronic, gradual decrease to <120 mEq/L. Treat the underlying cause or restrict free water intake first. Treat only acutely hyponatremic and profoundly symptomatic patients, and raise serum sodium levels by 2 mEq/L/hr but no higher than 125 mEq/L, with 3% NaCl.

$$\frac{2 \text{ mEq/L} \times 0.6 \times (\text{body weight in kg}) \times 1000}{513 \text{ mEq/L}} = \text{mL/hr of 3\% NaCl}$$

For example, for a 70-kg patient:

$$\frac{2 \times 0.6 \times (70) \times 1000}{513} = 160 \text{ mL/hr of 3\% NaCl}$$

23. **What is hypernatremia?**

A sodium greater than 145 and diagnosed based on volume status. A hypovolemic hypernatremia is from renal failure and renal losses; an isovolemic hypernatremia is related to diabetes insipidus; and hypervolemic hypernatremia is secondary to Cushing's syndrome, exogenous glucocorticoids, and can be iatrogenic.

24. Discuss the symptoms of hypernatremia.

Again, neurologic symptoms are the most common with altered mental status, restlessness, focal neurologic deficits, and seizures all possible.

25. How is hypernatremia treated?

The hypovolemic patients should be given isotonic fluid gradually by calculating their water deficit:

Water deficit $= 0.6 \times$ (body weight in kg) $\times [(Na/140)-1]$

In addition, underlying disorders should be addressed such as diabetes insipidus in isovolemic patients, and hypervolemic patients can be treated with diuretics.

26. When can D5W be used, and why?

One liter of D5W contains 1 L of free water and 50 g of glucose. Because it contains no sodium, it is used in patients with hypernatremia. Free water will distribute evenly between the ICFV and the ECFV, and the glucose will move into the cell. Pure water is not given because it can cause hemolysis. It is not used in diabetics because it can cause hyperglycemia; so in nondiabetics, it is used to give medications. It should not be used in patients with depletion of ECFV because it is a hypotonic solution and its use could cause hyponatremia. It can be used in patients with ECFV overload as a KVO (keep vein open) solution.

27. When is a hypotonic saline solution used?

A hypotonic saline solution such as 0.45% saline is used to expand the ECFV in someone who is volume depleted and to correct hypertonicity in someone who is hyperglycemic or hypernatremic.

28. What are the risks of rapid correction of hyponatremia or hypernatremia?

Rapid correction of hyponatremia with hypertonic solution may lead to permanent brain damage, seizures, and pontine myelinolysis. Rapid expansion of the ECF compartment can also worsen preexisting conditions, such as CHF. Rapid correction of hypernatremia and a severe decrease in serum osmolarity can cause convulsions, coma, and death.

29. What is the difference between SIADH and DI?

SIADH has an increase in ADH secretion, which causes water retention and hyponatremia. In DI, ADH secretion is decreased, leading to a large volume of dilute urine. Central DI has no ADH release leading to the kidneys being unable to concentrate urine. Nephrogenic DI has a normal amount of circulating ADH, but water is unable to be absorbed by the collecting tubules. Hypernatremia arises in both central and nephrogenic DI.

30. What is central DI?

In the absence or lack of ADH, the kidney is unable to concentrate urine. This can lead to excessive loss of water from the kidney and hypernatremia. This is manifested by polyuria and polydipsia.

31. What is nephrogenic DI?

In this syndrome, there are adequate levels of circulating ADH; however, water is not absorbed because the permeability of collecting tubules is not increased. This results in hypernatremia because of excessive water loss.

32. What are normal levels of potassium?

Levels between 3.5 and 5 are considered normal, with most of the potassium being found intracellularly.

33. What causes hypokalemia?

GI losses including vomiting, diarrhea, laxatives, and renal losses from diuretics, renal disease, magnesium deficiency, and excess of glucocorticoids. Other causes of hypokalemia are secondary to redistribution, such as with insulin excess or a metabolic alkalosis.

34. Discuss symptoms of hypokalemia.

Arrhythmias secondary to hypokalemia as the cardiac cycle will be prolonged. Polyuria, polydipsia, and nausea/vomiting or altered mental status, as well. On ECG, the T wave will flatten and a U wave may be present.

35. How is hypokalemia treated?

Any underlying cause should immediately be addressed. Oral potassium replacement is the safest method for replacement. For every dose of 10 mEq of KCl, the potassium should increase by 0.1 mEq/L. IV forms are available, but serum potassium needs very close monitoring in these patients.

36. **What causes hyperkalemia?**
    A redistribution of potassium from intracellular to extracellular in cases of insulin deficiency, hemolysis, GI bleeding, and acidosis. Renal failure, blood transfusion, spironolactone, and ACE inhibitors can all increase potassium levels. Renal failure with oliguria is the most common cause of true hyperkalemia.

37. **What ECG changes are noted in hyperkalemic patients?**
    Peaked T waves, prolonged PR interval, and QRS widening are seen on ECG. The patient may enter ventricular fibrillation when potassium levels are high enough.

38. **How is hyperkalemia treated?**
    The goal is to shift the potassium back from extracellular to intracellular sources. In severe cases of hyperkalemia, IV calcium is given to stabilize the myocardium and decrease the excitability. Sodium bicarbonate will shift potassium intracellularly and insulin will also push potassium intracellularly. When giving insulin, it is important to also provide the patient with glucose to prevent hypoglycemia. Removing potassium is possible with Kayexalate and dialysis.

39. **How is calcium maintained by the body?**
    Maintenance is hormonal and based on Parathyroid Hormone (PTH), calcitonin, and vitamin D. All of these hormones act on the gut, kidney, and bones. PTH increases plasma calcium and decreases plasma phosphate, calcitonin decreases plasma calcium and decreases plasma phosphate, and vitamin D increases plasma calcium and increases plasma phosphate.

40. **How is calcium found in plasma?**
    There is a protein-bound form that is bound to albumin, and a free, ionized form. An increase in pH will increase calcium-albumin binding. Hypoalbuminemia is the most common cause of hypocalcemia. For every 1 g/dL decrease in albumin below 4 g/dL, the total serum calcium is corrected by adding 0.8 mg/dL. The free ionized form is the physiologically active calcium and is independent of albumin levels.

41. **What are the causes and symptoms of hypocalcemia?**
    Hypocalcemia is defined by an ionized calcium level below 2 or a serum calcium lower than 9. Hypocalcemia is commonly caused by renal failure and hypoalbuminemia (most common). Other causes include a vitamin D deficiency, hypoparathyroidism, pancreatitis, and rhabdomyolysis. Increased neuromuscular irritability is common with perioral numbness, hyperactive deep tendon reflexes, grand mal seizures, and cardiac arrhythmias. Chvostek's sign and Trousseau's sign are both seen in hypocalcemia. Chvostek's sign is twitching of the facial muscles when the facial nerve is tapped. Trousseau's sign causes carpal spasm after occluding forearm blood flow for 3 minutes. Patients with a chronic hypocalcemia may exhibit no symptoms.

42. **What are clinical features of hypercalcemia?**
    Stones, bones, groans, and psychiatric overtones is a mnemonic for this problem. Patients have kidney stones, bone aches with brown tumors, muscle pain, gout, constipation, and can have signs of depression, anxiety, and lethargy. A shortened QT interval is seen on ECG.

43. **What are some of the signs that should alert you to a patient having an acid–base disorder?**
    A patient who has a change in mental status; tachypnea; Kussmaul breathing; cyanosis; respiratory failure; severe fluid loss from vomiting, diarrhea, or shock; and a history of an endocrine disorder, renal problems, or drug ingestion should be suspected of having an acid–base problem.

44. **What is metabolic acidosis?**
    Decreased blood pH with a decreased bicarbonate; there are two types: an anion gap metabolic acidosis (gap >12) and a nonanion gap acidosis.

45. **What is the significance of an anion gap?**
    A normal anion gap typically ranges from 8 to 12 mmol/L. It is significant in the presence of metabolic acidosis. A normal anion gap acidosis is due to a drop in bicarbonate, whereas an anion gap acidosis is due to an increase in anions.
    $Anion\ Gap = [Na+] + [K+] - [Cl-] - [HCO_3-]$

46. **What is the etiology of metabolic acidosis?**
    MUDPILES is a common mnemonic for the etiology of anion gap metabolic acidosis.
    Methanol ingestion
    Uremia

Diabetic ketoacidosis
Paraldehyde ingestion
Isoniazid ingestion
Lactic acidosis
Ethylene glycol ingestion
Salicylate ingestion
Nonanion gap acidosis occurs secondary to GI and renal losses.

47. **What are signs of metabolic acidosis, and how is it treated?**
Decreased tissue perfusion, decreased cardiac output, altered mental status, arrhythmias, hyperkalemia, and a compensatory hyperventilation. Treatment relies on determining the underlying cause of the acidosis and treating the etiology. Sodium bicarbonate has been shown to be ineffective and is only used in cases of rapid deterioration.

48. **What is metabolic alkalosis?**
The pH levels increased secondary to an increase in bicarbonate. The etiology is based on extracellular fluid volumes. An expansion of the ECF with a metabolic alkalosis is common in adrenal disorders. ECF contraction in the face of a metabolic alkalosis points the etiology toward renal and GI losses. Again, the treatment of metabolic alkalosis relies on treating the underlying disorder.

49. **What are the signs, symptoms, and treatment of respiratory acidosis?**
Respiratory acidosis is a decreased blood pH with $PaCO_2 > 40$. Signs and symptoms include confusion, headaches, CNS depression, and fatigue. Commonly this is secondary to COPD and hypoventilation. Acute respiratory acidosis will have no renal compensation; however, chronic respiratory acidosis will show renal compensation with an increase in plasma bicarbonate. These patients are treated with supplemental oxygen and possible mechanical ventilation in severe cases.

50. **What is respiratory alkalosis?**
This is an increased blood pH with a decrease in $PaCO_2$ secondary to hyperventilation. The etiology of this phenomenon includes pregnancy, sepsis, anxiety, asthma, and pulmonary embolism.

51. **What are signs, symptoms, and treatment of respiratory alkalosis?**
Signs include perioral numbness, anxiety, arrhythmias, and decreased cerebral blood flow. Severe cases can cause tetany. The treatment includes inhaling carbon dioxide and treatment of the underlying disorder.

52. **What is a desirable parenteral fluid level in a sickle cell crisis patient who weighs 150 lb?**
1/2 NS will create an osmotic gradient to distribute water intracellularly.
    This is thought to cause cellular swelling and reduce sickling of red blood cells.
kg = lb − 10/2 = 150 − 10/2 = 70 kg
    "4, 2, 1 method": 40 mL first 10 kg/hr + 20 mL second 10 kg/hr + 10 mL for each additional 10 kg/hr. Therefore the 70-kg patient will receive 110 mL/hr of 1/2 NS.

53. **What is the maintenance fluid requirement of a healthy 72-kg adult who is restricted from oral intake (NPO) while awaiting surgery?**
Maintenance fluid should be replaced with lactated Ringer's solution or D5-1/2 NS with 20 mEq KCl/L in the following amount:
40 mL/hr for the first 10 kg of body weight + 20 mL/hr for second 10 kg + 10 mL/hr for each additional 10 kg
Therefore for a 72-kg patient, the fluid requirement is:
40 mL/hr + 20 mL/hr + 52 mL/hr = 112 mL/hr (for practical purposes, 115 mL/hr)

54. **How will the same situation be managed in a patient with end-stage renal disease?**
Intravenous (IV) fluids will be restricted to minimal level, usually 30 mL/hr of D5-1/2 NS regardless of weight. Potassium usually will be avoided.

55. **What is the drug therapy for an unconscious patient who develops DI after extensive panfacial and cranial fractures? How does therapy differ for a patient who is conscious and alert?**
Unconscious patients may receive 5 U of the ADH analogue desmopressin (1-deamino-8-D-arginine vasopressin; DDAVP) subcutaneously every 4 hours along with slow replacement of free water.

Patients who are alert and have sufficient oral intake of water may receive 2 to 4 mg of intranasal DDAVP twice a day.

56. **How is the true serum calcium level calculated in a patient with a lab calcium concentration of 7.5 mg/dL and an albumin level of 2.0 g/dL? What other lab value might be helpful?**
Most serum calcium is bound to albumin, and therefore hypoalbuminemia will give a false reading of hypocalcemia. The minimal normal albumin level is 3.5 g/L, and the corrected calcium level is calculated as:

(3.5 g/dL – albumin level) × 0.8 + calcium level (mg/dL)
(3.5 – 2.0) × 0.8 + 7.5 = 8.7 mg/dL of corrected calcium level

The measurement of ionized calcium (iCa) in serum will give a true level of available calcium in serum.

57. **An 11-month-old infant who underwent palatoplasty had minimal blood loss but is refusing any type of feeding and will be temporarily started on parenteral fluids. She weighs 22 lb. What is her TBW? What is her minimal acceptable urine output? What maintenance parenteral fluids should be prescribed?**
TBW in infants represents 75% to 80% of the kilogram body mass (in comparison to 50% to 60% in adults). Adequate urinary output in children younger than age one is 2.0 mL/kg/hr (in comparison to 0.5 to 1.0 mL/kg/hr in adults).
   Maintenance IV fluids would be D5-1/4 NS + 20 mEq KCl/L in the amount of 40 mL/hr. The amount of fluids is calculated the same way as in adults. The sodium and potassium intake requirements for infants are 3 mEq/kg/day and 2 mEq/kg/day, respectively.

58. **A young, healthy woman who was hospitalized and treated for Ludwig's angina is unable to have any oral intake and is currently running a fever of 39.4° C. She weighs 60 kg, and her electrolytes are within normal limits. How should her parenteral fluids be managed?**
Add 2 to 2.5 mL/kg/day per each degree above 37.0° C to the appropriate maintenance fluid requirement to compensate for insensible losses due to fever. This patient's baseline would be 100 mL/hr of lactated Ringer's solution, and 12 mL/hr would be added according to the formula:

$$\frac{2 \times 6 \,(\text{kg})}{24 \text{ hours}} \times 2.4 \,(^\circ C) = 12 \text{ mL/hr}$$

59. **A patient has hyposmolar, hypervolemic hyponatremia 24 hours after surgery. What is the initial treatment?**
Restrict oral fluid intake (usually to about 1000 mL/24 hours). This patient most likely has been over-hydrated with hypotonic IV fluid. If the sodium level is not in the range that needs emergent correction, the patient will mobilize the fluid, and the sodium level will be corrected slowly on its own.

60. **A trauma patient who has undergone repair of maxillofacial fractures develops oliguria with a serum osmolarity of 1000 mOsm/dL. What is the most likely diagnosis?**
SIADH, probably due to trauma.

61. **A patient who has been on IV antibiotics for 7 days develops diarrhea. The patient is hemodynamically stable. What is the most appropriate fluid to administer initially?**
This patient is suffering from insult to normal intestinal function. Thus the patient is losing sodium, potassium, and, to a lesser extent, other ions (e.g., calcium, magnesium). Lactated Ringer's solution is the best fluid for this situation because it contains sodium, potassium, calcium, lactic acid, and sodium bicarbonate, which resemble the fluid lost from the small intestine.

62. **A patient with a history of CHF is on loop diuretics and digoxin. He is admitted for maxillofacial surgery. Perioperatively, what is the most important electrolyte to check and adjust?**
Potassium. Loop diuretics (e.g., furosemide) are potassium-wasting drugs. Digoxin is an inotrope, which blocks Na/K channels. The serum potassium level of patients who take digoxin and loop diuretics should be safely above 4.0 mEq/L to prevent arrhythmia. This patient has the potential to develop

hypokalemia because of the loop diuretic. Thus paying close attention to the serum potassium level is critical for prevention of cardiac dysfunction.

63. A patient manifests signs and symptoms of muscle twitching and prolonged QT on ECG. What electrolyte should be checked?

Calcium. Hypocalcemia increases excitation of the neuromuscular system, causing cramps and tetany. Chvostek's sign and Trousseau's sign (carpopedal spasm following occlusion of arterial blood supply to the arm for 3 minutes) are clinically important indications of hypocalcemia. Prolonged QT may lead to arrhythmias and subsequent heart failure if not treated.

64. A trauma patient develops polyuria with low osmolarity on day 1 of hospital admission. What is the most likely diagnosis, and what is the initial management?

DI is the most likely diagnosis. The initial management would be IV 1/2 NS and DDAVP. In DI, ADH is not adequately released from the posterior pituitary. In this patient, trauma to the stalk in the pituitary gland is probably the cause. Therefore the patient is losing free water. The patient requires IV fluid to keep him hemodynamically stable and prevent hyperosmolar hypovolemic hypernatremia. This is best accomplished with a hypotonic solution, such as 1/2 or 1/4 NS. The patient also needs exogenous replacement of ADH. Thus DDAVP needs to be administered intravenously to prevent free water loss.

65. After a motor vehicle accident, a patient is on a ventilator, receives appropriate fluid, has a Foley catheter, and has no oral intake. What is the source of his insensible fluid loss?

Perspiration. Sensible losses are through the kidneys and feces. Insensible losses are through the skin and lungs. When a patient is on a closed-system ventilator, there is really no insensible loss through the lungs. Thus the only insensible loss that needs to be replaced is the evaporated sweat.

66. A patient who has a past medical history significant for chronic renal failure is put on a regular diet. The next day, the patient develops flaccid muscles and decreased urine output. His magnesium is normal. Which electrolyte is the most likely cause?

Potassium. Hyperkalemia is characterized by flaccid muscles, fatigue, and ECG abnormalities in severe cases. Considering the patient's history, he might have hypermagnesemia or hyperkalemia, but the magnesium is reported as normal. Therefore the potassium level must be checked and treated accordingly.

67. Twenty-four hours after an elderly patient underwent oral maxillofacial surgery, she develops tonic-clonic seizures. Her lab results indicate that her serum sodium is 119 mEq/L and her serum osmolarity is 250 Osm. The patient is euvolemic with stable vital signs. What is the appropriate fluid management of the patient?

Fluid restriction and very slow replacement with hypertonic saline solution (usually 3% NaCl). Many conditions can cause hypotonic, euvolemic hyponatremia. This patient is symptomatic (seizure), which should be treated first (e.g., with Valium). Sodium must be replaced very slowly to prevent CNS damage.

CHAPTER 11

NUTRITIONAL SUPPORT

Hani F. Braidy, Vincent B. Ziccardi

1. **When is enteral feeding/nutrition indicated?**
   - Inability to ingest food normally because of maxillofacial trauma
   - Protein-energy malnutrition
   - Normal functioning bowel

2. **What are the indications for nutritional support?**
   - Inadequate intake for more than 5 days
   - Malnourished patients undergoing surgery
   - Major trauma (burn victims, blunt or penetrating injury, etc.)

3. **What are the causes of malnutrition?**
   - Neglect (e.g., severe alcoholics, extreme of ages)
   - Digestive problems
   - Inadequate food intake
   - Chronic illness
   - Dysphagia
   - Stress and trauma
   - Vomiting

4. **What is the definition of malnutrition according to the World Health Organization (WHO)?**
   According to the WHO, malnutrition is "the cellular imbalance between supply of nutrients and energy and the body's demand for them to ensure growth, maintenance, and specific functions."

5. **What are the two forms of protein-energy malnutrition?**
   Marasmus and kwashiorkor.

6. **What is marasmus?**
   Marasmus is a form of protein malnutrition in the presence of inadequate total calorie intake. It is endemic in third-world countries and characterized by decreased weight, decreased body fat, loss of muscle mass, hypothermia, apathy, and dehydration.

7. **What is kwashiorkor?**
   Kwashiorkor is a form of protein malnutrition in the presence of near-normal total calorie intake. It is endemic in third-world countries and characterized by hypoalbuminemia, edema, muscle wasting, immunosuppression, fatty liver, and distension of the abdomen. Patients with marasmus undergoing major surgery or stress may suffer subsequently from kwashiorkor.

8. **What vitamin deficiency is commonly found in chronic alcoholics, and what are the common symptoms associated with it?**
   Thiamin (vitamin B1) deficiency is commonly found in severe alcoholics. The following symptoms and clinical pictures are classically described:
   - Beriberi: fatigue, weakness, depression, right- or left-sided congestive heart failure, peripheral vasodilation, neuropathy
   - Wernicke-Korsakoff's syndrome: symptoms of beriberi in addition to ophthalmoplegia, gait disturbance, nystagmus, confusion, amnesia, dementia

9. **If a patient is at risk for aspiration, which short-term feeding route is indicated?**
   If a patient is at risk for aspiration, the nasoduodenal and nasojejunal (postpyloric) routes are best. The technique of nasoduodenal feeding can overcome problems of gastric retention. There are fewer problems with gastroesophageal reflux and subsequent risk of tracheobronchial aspiration. The technique of nasojejunal feeding bypasses an obstructive lesion or motor abnormalities involving the gastrointestinal (GI) tract proximal to the jejunum.

10. **What route of administration is indicated for long-term enteral feeding?**
For long-term enteral feeding, enterostomies are the preferred access route. Percutaneous endoscopic gastrostomy (PEG) involves placement of a 16- to 18-gauge latex or silicone catheter through the abdominal wall and directly into the stomach.

11. **Which feeding route is preferred when a patient is at risk for aspiration?**
If a patient is at risk for aspiration, the feeding tube should be placed in the small intestine either surgically via a jejunostomy or nonsurgically via a percutaneous jejunostomy tube.

12. **Where does a nasogastric tube (NGT) extend, and what are some advantages to its use?**
The NGT extends from the nose into the stomach. NGTs are advantageous because:
    - The NGT tolerates high osmotic loads without cramping, distention, vomiting, diarrhea, or fluid and electrolyte shifts.
    - It allows intermittent or bolus feedings because the stomach has a large reservoir capacity.
    - It is easier to position a tube into the stomach than into the jejunum.
    - The presence of hydrochloric acid in the stomach may help prevent infection.

13. **Where does a nasoduodenal tube (NDT) extend, and when is it indicated?**
The NDT extends from the nose through the pylorus and into the duodenum. NDT feedings are indicated in:
    - Patients at risk for aspiration.
    - Patients who are debilitated, demented, stuporous, or unconscious.
    - Patients with gastroparesis or delayed gastric emptying.

14. **What is meant by continuous feeding, and what are its advantages and disadvantages?**
Continuous feeding allows a patient to receive a constant infusion of enteral feedings. The advantages of continuous feeding are decreased risk of aspiration, bloating, distention, and osmotic diarrhea with improved patient tolerance. The disadvantages of continuous feeding are that it requires the patient to be physically connected to the apparatus during infusion and the expense associated with the purchase of volumetric infusion pumps.

15. **What three macronutrients are required when infusing total parenteral nutrition (TPN)?**
    1. Glucose
    2. Protein
    3. Lipids

16. **What parameters should be monitored in patients receiving TPN?**
    - Metabolic parameters: sodium, potassium, chloride, CO_2, blood urea nitrogen (BUN), creatinine, glucose, hematocrit, hemoglobin, white blood cell (WBC) count, calcium, magnesium, phosphorus, and platelets
    - Nutrition: daily weight evaluations, albumin, and prealbumin
    - Fluid status
    - Infection: If WBC count is increasing or the patient is febrile, a blood culture should be obtained and consideration given to changing the central line.

17. **What are some of the physical findings clinically seen in malnutrition?**
    - Temporal wasting, decreased skinfold (pinch test)
    - Glossitis, cheilosis, decreased taste
    - Hair loss, dry skin, edema
    - Confusion, gait abnormalities, loss of tactile sense, peripheral neuropathies

18. **What are the lab values typically assessed when evaluating a patient for malnutrition?**
    - Albumin (20 days half-life, 3.5 to 5.0 g/dL)
    - Transferrin (7 to 10 days half-life, 200 to 400 mg/dL)
    - Prealbumin (2 days half-life, 16.0 to 35.0 mg/dL)
    - Vitamin and mineral levels

19. **What is the Harris-Benedict equation?**
This equation is an estimation of the daily calorie requirement at rest (expenditure) in relation to a patient's weight, height, and age. It usually overestimates by 20% to 60%.
Males: $66.5 + 13.8 \times weight(kg) + 5 \times height(cm) - 6.8 \times age$.
Females: $655.1 + 9.5 \times weight(kg) + 1.8 \times height(cm) - 4.7 \times age$.
This estimation can be adjusted to various levels of stress. For instance, in a patient who sustained severe trauma, this equation can be multiplied by 1.6.

20. **Other than the Harris-Benedict equation, what other method can be used to esti-mate the daily total calorie requirement?**
30 cal/kg is a gross estimation of the total daily calorie requirement in a nonstressed patient.

21. **How many calories are provided by different organic fuels (glucose, protein, fat)?**
Glucose   3.7 cal/g
Protein   4.0 cal/g
Fat   9.1 cal/g

22. **How much carbohydrates, fat, and protein are required in the diet of the surgical patient?**
The bulk of the energy requirement should be provided by carbohydrates (70%) and lipids (30%). Proteins are calculated in relation to a patient's catabolic state. Normally, 0.8 to 1.0 g/kg of proteins are necessary, whereas 1.2 to 1.6 g/kg are required in the stressed patient.

23. **Which amino acid is critical for bowel mucosa function?**
Glutamine.

24. **What is enteral nutrition?**
Enteral nutrition is a technique to provide nutrition to a patient through the gut using a tube placed in the GI tract. An orogastric tube (OGT) or NGT can be used to deliver special liquid formulas. These formulations are especially useful in patients who have undergone oral and maxillofacial surgical procedures and in malnourished patients. Long-term enteral feedings are best achieved through a percutaneous gastrostomy tube inserted endoscopically (PEG).

25. **What are the contraindications for enteral nutrition?**
Enteral nutrition is possible only if the gut is functioning. In patients with intestinal ischemia, ileus, or bowel obstruction, enteral nutrition is contraindicated. It is also contraindicated in patients in shock and those with severe pancreatitis.

26. **What are some of the problems associated with enteral nutrition?**
Insertion of the tube into the trachea is possible and potentially fatal due to aspiration pneumonia. Sometimes, tube occlusion can occur. Pulmonary aspiration (80% occurrence), nausea, and vomiting can ensue if the infusion rate is too high. Diarrhea is a common side effect. When the carbohydrate intake is too high, a hyperosmolar state or diabetes can complicate the feedings. Most of the issues associated with enteral nutrition can be rectified by changing the rate or the osmotic content of the enteral solution.

27. **What are the main components of enteral feeding formulas?**
Protein   Usually 35 to 40 g/L
Calories   Between 1 and 2 cal/mL
Osmolality   Usually between 280 and 1100 mOsm/L, a value that is directly related to the amount of carbohydrates

28. **What is the best way to confirm nasogastric tube (NGT) placement?**
Reviewing an abdominal radiograph showing the NGT tip in the stomach.

29. **In patients undergoing enteral tube feedings, what is the minimal gastric residual volume that may require the use of promotility agents?**
250 cc. Promotility agents (such as metoclopramide) will increase gastrointestinal transit and may decrease tube feed complications such as aspiration, gastric distension, bloating, nausea, and vomiting.

30. **At which gastric residual volume may you elect to hold tube feedings?**
500 cc. High residuals can increase risks outlined in question 29.

31. What is parenteral nutrition?

Parenteral nutrition is a way to feed the patient intravenously. It can be delivered centrally through a central venous catheter, most commonly in the superior vena cava or peripherally (PPN) via a peripheral vein.

32. What is total parenteral nutrition (TPN)?

TPN is the delivery of all the required nutrients parenterally. It is a solution containing proteins, carbohydrates, fat, vitamins, and minerals. Because of the high osmolarity of the solution and the risk of phlebitis, it is usually given centrally rather than peripherally. Consequently, solutions delivered peripherally need to be diluted and may not meet the complete nutritional requirements of the patients.

33. When are TPN and PPN indicated?

TPN is indicated when patients need long-term nutritional support but are not able to receive enteral feedings (nonworking GI tract, shock, pancreatitis, bone marrow transplant, etc.). PPN is indicated in patients requiring short-term nutritional support (<10 days) to restrict protein breakdown.

34. What are the complications of parenteral nutrition?

Hyperglycemia, fatty liver, hypercapnia, acute respiratory distress syndrome, GI mucosal atrophy (predisposing the gut for bacterial translocation and septicemia). Catheter-related complications include infections and pneumothorax.

BIBLIOGRAPHY

Braidy HF, Ziccardi VB: Oral surgery, diet and nutrition. In Touger-Decker R, editor: *Nutrition and oral medicine*, ed 2, New York, 2014, Humana Press, pp 333–347.

Kasper DL, Braunwald E, Fauci A, et al.: *Harrison's principles of internal medicine*, ed 16, New York, 2004, McGraw-Hill.

Marino PL: *The ICU book*, ed 3, Philadelphia, 1998, Lippincott Williams & Wilkins.

Rolandelli RH, Bankhead R, Boullata J, et al.: *Clinical nutrition: enteral and tube feeding*, ed 4, Philadelphia, 2005, Saunders.

Souba WW: Nutritional support, *N Engl J Med* 336:41–48, 1997.

Thomson AD: Mechanism of vitamin deficiency in chronic alcohol misusers and the development of the Wenicke-Korsakoff syndrome, *Alcohol & Alcoholism* 35(Suppl. 1):2–7, 2000.

POSTOPERATIVE COMPLICATIONS

Amber Johnson, Dean M. DeLuke

CHAPTER 12

1. **What is a fever?**
   A fever (also known as pyrexia) is a reaction to a systemic inflammatory process that raises the core body temperature to >38°C. It is a physiologic response to infection or inflammation.

2. **What causes fever?**
   Pyrogenic cytokines (interleukin-1, tumor necrosis factor, and interferon) are released by macrophages that are activated during inflammation and infection. These cytokines act on the hypothalamic thermoregulatory center and cause release of prostaglandins, resulting in fever.

3. **What are the most common causes of fever in the first 24 hours after surgery?**
   - Aspiration pneumonia
   - An ill-defined response to the surgery itself (a response to the systemic inflammatory process associated with the surgical trauma)

   Many surgical textbooks state that atelectasis is the usual cause of postoperative fever in the first 48 hours, but this theory is not evidence based. Experimental studies have been performed in animals in which induced atelectasis did not produce fever unless there was a coexisting pulmonary infection.

4. **What are the most common causes of postoperative fever in the first 24 to 72 hours?**
   - Bacterial pneumonia
   - Thrombophlebitis
   - An ill-defined response to the surgery itself

   In a low-risk patient, a fever within the first 72 hours of surgery is usually a clinically benign process and does not typically warrant a further work-up (cultures, chest X-rays, etc.) unless dictated by clinical findings.

5. **What are the most common causes of fever 72 hours after surgery?**
   - Pneumonia
   - Wound infection
   - Pulmonary emboli
   - Urinary tract infection
   - Intravenous (IV) catheter infection

6. **What are the five Ws of postoperative fever?**
   The five *W*s are a summary of the possible causes of any postoperative fever: wind (atelectasis-controversial, pneumonia), water (UTI), wound (surgical site infection), walking (thrombophlebitis, deep venous thrombosis [DVT]/PE), and wonder drugs (reaction to medications).

7. **When can the surgical site be considered the source of postoperative fever?**
   Typically, the surgical site should not be considered the primary source of postoperative fever until at least 48 to 72 hours after surgery. However, surgical wound infection may develop between 12 hours and 7 days postoperatively.

8. **How are the development of fever and the patient's heart rate interrelated?**
   For every 1°C rise in body temperature, there is a corresponding 9 to 10 beats/minute increase in the patient's heart rate.

9. **Can fever be treated?***
   Yes. Aspirin, acetaminophen, and ibuprofen are cyclooxygenase (COX) inhibitors that block the formation of prostaglandin E2 in the hypothalamus and effectively control fever.

10. Should fever be treated?*
    This is controversial. No evidence suggests that suppression of fever improves patient outcome. Patients are more comfortable, however, and the surgeon receives fewer calls from the nurses.

11. Should fever be investigated?*
    Yes. Fever indicates that something (frequently treatable) is going on. The threshold for inquiry depends on the patient. A transplant patient with a temperature of 38° C requires scrutiny, whereas a healthy young person with an identical temperature of 38° C 24 hours after an appendectomy can be ignored.

12. Summarize a fever work-up.*
    • Order blood cultures, urine Gram stain and culture, and sputum Gram's stain and culture.
    • Look at the surgical incisions.
    • Look at old and current IV sites for evidence of septic thrombophlebitis.
    • If breath sounds are worrisome, obtain a chest X-ray.

13. What are the most common late causes of postoperative fever?*
    Septic thrombophlebitis (from an IV line) and occult (usually intraabdominal) abscesses tend to present 2 weeks after surgery.

14. How often should IV catheter sites be changed to avoid infection?
    In general, IV access sites should be changed no more frequently than every 72 to 96 hours, but the sites should be examined daily for signs of infection or phlebitis.

15. What are the common signs and symptoms of phlebitis?
    • Pain
    • Erythema
    • Tenderness
    • Streaking of the limb
    • Edema

16. What is the treatment for phlebitis?
    • Remove the IV catheter.
    • Elevate the affected limb.
    • Apply warm, moist packs to the infected site.
    • If infection is suspected, initiate IV antibiotics for appropriate staphylococcus coverage.

17. What are the most frequent respiratory complications following oral and maxillofacial surgery?
    • Pulmonary atelectasis
    • Aspiration pneumonia
    • Pulmonary embolus

18. Which group of patients is predisposed to the development of postoperative atelectasis?
    Postoperative atelectasis occurs more often in smokers than in any other subset of patients.

19. How can a patient improve atelectasis?
    Deep breathing exercises, especially with incentive spirometry.

20. Where is the most common site for aspiration pneumonia to develop?
    If aspiration pneumonia occurs, it is most likely to manifest itself initially in the patient's right lung.

21. What are the risk factors for aspiration pneumonia?
    • Reduced consciousness (trauma patients with low Glasgow Coma Scale, patients under sedation or general anesthesia)
    • Disorders of the upper GI tract (GERD, gastroparesis)
    • Dysphagia
    • Tracheostomy
    • NPO status

---

*Reprinted from Harken AH: What does postoperative fever mean? In Harken AH, Moore EE, editors: *Abernathy's surgical secrets*, ed 6, Philadelphia, 2009, Mosby.

22. How can aspiration be prevented?
Aspiration can be prevented by avoiding general anesthesia in patients who have recently eaten, positioning the patient correctly before endotracheal intubation, and using high-volume, low-pressure cuffs on the endotracheal tube. If the risk of aspiration is high, metoclopramide or ondansetron should be administered before surgery to minimize the incidence of aspiration pneumonia.

23. Which surgical patients are predisposed to aspiration?
Tracheostomy patients. Incidence as high as 80% has been reported.

24. Why does postoperative pneumonia develop?
After surgery, a patient's host defense against pneumonia is compromised. This impairment is likely caused by several factors: The cough mechanism may be impaired and may not effectively clear the bronchial tree, the mucociliary transport mechanism may be damaged by endotracheal intubation, and the alveolar macrophage may be compromised by a number of factors that may be present during and after surgery (e.g., hypoxia, pulmonary edema, aspiration, or corticosteroid therapy). All these factors may decrease the patient's immune response to infection with pneumonia and increase the incidence of postoperative pneumonia.

25. What is the primary pathogen in postoperative pneumonia?
Approximately half the pulmonary infections that follow surgery are caused by gram-negative bacilli, which are usually acquired by aspiration of oropharyngeal secretions.

26. What is the treatment for postoperative pneumonia?
Appropriate antibiotic therapy, which can be determined through sputum culture and sensitivity, and clearing of secretions through aggressive suctioning and chest physical therapy.

27. Where do most postoperative pulmonary emboli originate?
In the deep venous systems of the lower extremities, especially in non-ambulatory patients.

28. What is Virchow's triad?
Virchow's triad is the name given to the three chief causes of DVT: (1) damage to the endothelial lining of the vessel, (2) venous stasis, and (3) hypercoagulability (a change in blood constituents attributable to postoperative increase in the number and adhesiveness of the patient's platelets).

29. What are the classical clinical features of DVT?
- Calf swelling and tenderness
- Sudden dyspnea
- Fever
- Tachypnea
- Chest pain

30. What is Homans' sign?
Homans' sign is pain in the calf that is elicited by forced dorsiflexion of the foot. It was once considered pathognomonic for the presence of DVT, but this test is no longer taught because performing this maneuver can increase the risk of movement of an existing thrombus.

31. What is the immediate treatment of DVT?
A patient who has developed DVT should be started immediately on systemic anticoagulation with elevation of the affected limb. Subcutaneous heparin and low molecular weight heparin are choices to consider. Thrombolytics are not indicated.

32. What are some common causes of postoperative bleeding?
- Incompletely ligated or cauterized vessels
- Wound infection
- Coagulopathy
- Rebound effect of hypotensive anesthesia

33. What are some common causes of postoperative hypotension?
A good differential diagnosis for the development of hypotension should include intravascular hypovolemia, rewarming vasodilation, myocardial depression, and hypothyroidism.

34. What are the most common causes of postoperative hypertension?
- Pain and anxiety
- Hypoxia

- Over-distention of the bladder
- Hypercapnia

35. What are some possible treatment options for postoperative hypotension?
- Elevation of the lower extremities
- Administration of carefully monitored fluid boluses
- Administration of vasopressors (e.g., ephedrine)

36. What is the most common cardiac arrhythmia observed in the postoperative period? Why?
The most common postoperative arrhythmia is the development of ventricular complexes or premature ventricular contractions (PVCs). Hypoxia, pain, or fluid overload, all of which are common in the postoperative period, can precipitate PVCs.

37. What are the common causes of postoperative cardiac arrhythmias?
Postoperative arrhythmias are generally related to reversible factors such as hypokalemia, hypoxemia, alkalosis, and digitalis toxicity, but they could be the first sign of postoperative myocardial infarction. Postoperative myocardial infarction is rare, with an incidence of 0.7% for patients without preexisting cardiac disease. However, incidence increases to 6% for patients with preexisting cardiac disease.

38. Why is postoperative myocardial infarction difficult to diagnose?
More than one third of postoperative myocardial infarctions are asymptomatic as a result of the residual effects of anesthesia and analgesics administered postoperatively.

39. What is the most common cause of dysuria in the immediate postoperative period?
The agents incorporated in the administration of general anesthesia can inhibit the micturitic reflex, and the patient can suffer bladder distention, which itself may inhibit the ability to micturate.

40. What are some other causes of dysuria in the postoperative period?
- Positional inhibition (many patients find it difficult to pass urine while supine)
- Preexisting prostatism
- Inadequate fluid replacement during surgery, which creates a hypovolemic state

41. What are the treatment options for postoperative dysuria in a patient with suprapubic pain and an obviously distended bladder elicited by palpation in the first 4 to 6 hours after surgery?
Treatment of postoperative dysuria should begin simply by having the patient stand by or sit on the toilet while running water in the sink. If this does not help and there is no evidence of a hypovolemic state, then the patient should be catheterized. If the residual measures >300 mL, then the catheter should be left in overnight.

42. What are some risk factors for postoperative nausea and vomiting (PONV)?
Female gender, childhood history of PONV or motion sickness, non-smokers, intra and postoperative opioid use, increased duration of surgery, gastric distention (e.g., swallowed blood), type of anesthetic (volatile agents), and type of surgery (e.g., ear and eye surgery).

43. What is a seroma, and how can it be prevented?
A seroma is fluid (other than pus or blood) that has collected in the wound. Seromas often appear after surgical procedures that involve elevation of skin flaps and transection of numerous lymphatic channels. The incidence of seromas can be decreased if proper pressure dressing is applied to the wound after surgery.

44. What is the treatment for seroma?
Seromas should be evacuated either by needle aspiration or by incision and drainage because they can delay healing and provide an excellent medium for bacterial growth. A pressure dressing should be placed immediately after drainage to help seal lymphatic leaks and prevent additional accumulation of fluids.

45. What is a surgical wound infection?
Surgical wound infections or surgical site infections (SSIs) usually occur within 30 days of surgery. In cases where a foreign body is left in situ, the onset of postoperative infection may be delayed much longer, even occurring a year or more after surgery.

46. **What are the types of surgical wound infection?**
Depending on the depth of tissue involvement, SSIs can be subdivided into three categories:
- **Superficial incisional SSIs**, involving only the skin and subcutaneous tissue
- **Deep incisional SSIs**, involving deep soft tissue layers, such as fascial or muscle layers of the incision
- **Organ space SSIs**, involving any anatomic structure opened or manipulated during the operative procedure.

47. **What are the classic signs of superficial incisional SSI?**
Signs of superficial incisional infection are calor (heat), rubor (redness), tumor (swelling), dolor (pain), and purulent drainage.

48. **What are the signs of deep-space SSIs?**
Deep-space infection should be suspected in the presence of systemic signs and symptoms: fever, ileus, and shock. Definitive diagnosis of deep-space SSIs may require imaging studies.

49. **What are patient risk factors for SSIs?**
Smoking, obesity, poor nutritional status, and advanced age.

50. **What can surgeons do to decrease the risk of SSIs?**
Perform proper hand washing, administer prophylactic antibiotics (given within 1 hour of surgical incision), eliminate dead space, minimize placement of foreign material (implants, suture material, etc.), appropriately wash out wounds, and control hemorrhage.

51. **Are certain wounds prone to infection?***
Each milliliter of human saliva contains 10^8 aerobic and anaerobic, gram-positive and gram-negative bacteria. Therefore, all human bite wounds must be considered contaminated. Animal bite wounds typically are less contaminated.

52. **Do incisions become infected early after surgery?***
The incision must be examined in a patient with a fever ($39°$C) <12 hours after surgery. Look for a foul-smelling, serous discharge in a particularly painful wound (all incisions hurt) with or without crepitus. Gram's stain of the serous discharge for gram-positive rods confirms or excludes the diagnosis of clostridial infection.

53. **When do urinary tract infections (UTIs) occur?***
The longer the urethral (Foley) catheter is in place, the more likely a urinary tract infection (UTI) will develop. Urologic instrumentation at the time of surgery may accelerate the process considerably. Pathogens migrate along the outside of the urethral catheter, and by 5 to 7 days after surgery, most patients harbor infected urine.

54. **How is a UTI diagnosed?***
Urine culture with >105 bacteria/mL defines a UTI. White blood cells on urinalysis are highly suggestive of UTI.

BIBLIOGRAPHY

Barie PS: Modern surgical antibiotic prophylaxis and therapy: less is more, *Surg Infect* 1:23–29, 2000.

Harken AH: What does postoperative fever mean? In Harken AH, Moore EE, editors: *Abernathy's surgical secrets*, ed 6, Philadelphia, 2009, Mosby.

Hollingsworth JW, Govert JA: Fever in the critical care patient. In Jafek BW, Murrow BW, editors: *ENT secrets*, ed 3, Philadelphia, 2005, Hanley & Belfus.

Kluytmans J, Voss A: Prevention of postsurgical infections: some like it hot, *Curr Opin Infect Dis* 15:427–432, 2002.

Leigh JM: Postoperative care. In Rowe NL, Williams IL, editors: *Maxillofacial injuries*, vol II. New York, 1985, Churchill Livingstone.

Lesperance R, Lehman R, et al.: Early postoperative fever and the "routine" fever work-up: results of a prospective study, *J Surg Res* 171(1):245–250, 2011.

Nicholau D: Postanesthesia recovery. In Miller R, editor: *Basics of anesthesia*, ed 6, Philadelphia, 2011, Elsevier.

Meyer LE: Postoperative problems. In Kwan PH, Laskin DM, editors: *Clinical manual of oral and maxillofacial surgery*, ed 2, Carol Stream, IL, 1997, Quintessence.

---

*Reprinted from Harken AH: What does postoperative fever mean? In Harken AH, Moore EE, editors: *Abernathy's surgical secrets*, ed 6, Philadelphia, 2009, Mosby.

Myles PS, Iacono GA, Hunt JO, et al.: Risk of respiratory complications and wound infection in patients undergoing ambulatory surgery, *Anesthesiology* 97:842–847, 2002.

Narayan M, Medinilla S: Fever in the postoperative patient, *Emergency Med Clin N Am* 31:1045–1058, 2013.

O'Grady N, et al.: *Guidelines for the prevention of intravascular catheter-related infections*, CDC, 2011. www.cdc.gov/hicpac/BSI/BSI-gudelines-2011.html.

Pellegrini CA: Postoperative complications. In Way L, editor: *Current surgical diagnosis and treatment*, ed 6, Los Altos, CA, 1983, Lange.

Peterson SL: Surgical wound infection. In Harken AH, Moore EE, editors: *Abernathy's surgical secrets*, ed 6, Philadelphia, 2009, Mosby.

Singer AJ, Quinn JV, Thode Jr HC, et al.: Trauma Seal Study Group: determinants of poor outcome after laceration and surgical incision repair, *Plast Reconstr Surg* 110:429–435, 2002.

INTRODUCTION TO MECHANICAL VENTILATION AND ICU CARE

Alia Koch

1. **When is it appropriate to mechanically ventilate a patient?**
   Mechanical ventilation is a clinically based decision. Patients who should be mechanically ventilated are those with significant respiratory muscle fatigue, patients in respiratory distress, patients who are unable to protect their own airway either secondary to swelling or those who have depressed levels of consciousness, and patients with a metabolic acidosis, respiratory acidosis, or significant hypoxemia.

2. **What are the goals of mechanical ventilation?**
   To correct hypoxemia and to maintain alveolar ventilation.

3. **What are the different ventilator settings?**
   - Assist-control ventilation (AC): This is an initial setting used for most patients. It is a safe mode that ensures the patient receives a breath at a certain preset rate. Every time the patient initiates a breath, the ventilator will deliver a breath to the patient. If the patient does not initiate a breath, the ventilator will still deliver a breath of preset tidal volume at the predetermined rate.
   - Synchronous intermittent mandatory ventilation (SIMV): This setting allows the patient to breathe on his/her own and is used for weaning patients off the ventilator. It does not have a preset tidal volume, only a preset breathing rate. If the patient takes a spontaneous breath, the mandatory breath is given in synchrony by the ventilator. If the patient does not take a spontaneous breath, the ventilator does provide a breath to the patient.
   - Continuous positive airway pressure (CPAP): This setting only has predetermined positive end expiratory pressure and pressure support. In other words, positive pressure is continuously given by the ventilator. The patient otherwise breathes on his/her own. This setting is also used when weaning patients from a ventilator.

4. **How is correct intubation determined when a patient is on a ventilator?**
   Postintubation chest X-ray is used to determine location of the tip of the tube. The endotracheal tube should sit approximately 3 to 5 cm above the carina. It is also important to hear bilateral breath sounds on exam.

5. **What criteria is used to determine if a patient is ready for extubation?**
   - Tidal volumes of more than 5 cc/kg
   - Oxygen saturation of at least 90% with less than 5 cm H_2O PEEP and FiO_2 less than 40%
   - Respiratory rate of less than 30 breaths/min
   - Vital capacity of greater than 10 cc/kg
   - Intact cough

6. **What is PEEP?**
   PEEP is positive pressure maintained at the end of passive exhalation. It is used to keep alveoli open and improve gas exchange. Usually, PEEP is used to prevent alveolar collapse and atelectasis; it is most commonly used in patients with Acute Respiratory Distress Syndrome (ARDS). PEEP also allows for a decrease in inspired oxygen concentration, which decreases the risk of oxygen toxicity. If PEEP is too high, complications include barotrauma, pneumothorax, and low cardiac output secondary to decreased venous return.

7. **What is an appropriate tidal volume in most patients on a mechanical ventilator?**
   Initially, patients can be set at 8 to 10 cc/kg; however, smaller tidal volumes are used in those patients with ARDS.

8. **What inspiratory:expiratory ratio on a mechanical ventilator is most similar to a normal respiratory pattern?**
   A ratio of 1:2.

9. **What is used to prevent tracheal stenosis in intubated patients?**
   Cuffs on endotracheal tubes, which are large volume and low pressure.

10. **What are the different types of shock?**
    - Cardiogenic, typically caused by myocardial infarction causing a decreased cardiac output and increased systemic vascular resistance
    - Hypovolemic, secondary to trauma and bleeding with decreased cardiac output and increased systemic vascular resistance
    - Distributive, typically secondary to neurogenic changes, sepsis, or anaphylaxis. This type of shock will show increased cardiac output and decreased systemic vascular resistance

11. **What are the stages of shock?**
    Initially, shock is reversible, and no signs are seen on exam. The compensatory stage is when the body uses mechanisms to try to reverse the symptoms. Next is the progressive stage, when the shock is no longer reversible. Compensatory mechanisms are not working, and worsening acidosis with decreased organ perfusion is seen. Finally, the last stage is refractory, with organ failure and death.

12. **How is shock treated?**
    Shock requires an ICU admission. Cardiogenic shock is treated with decreased afterload, increasing cardiac output, and decreasing myocardial oxygen demand. Other forms of shock are treated with aggressive fluid hydration and treatment of the underlying cause.

13. **What are the indications of placing an arterial line?**
    - Inability to obtain noninvasive blood pressures
    - Hemodynamic instability
    - Rigorous blood pressure control is needed.
    - Frequent arterial blood sampling is needed.

14. **What are the indications for central line placement?**
    - Monitoring the central venous pressure
    - Infusing concentrated vasopressors
    - Delivering total parenteral nutrition
    - Inability to gain peripheral venous access

15. **What are the most common causes of postoperative fever in the intensive care unit?**
    In the ICU, the most common are ventilator-associated pneumonia, vascular catheter-related infections, wound infections, and catheter-related urinary tract infections.

16. **Which patients should be prophylaxed for stress ulcers?**
    Patients who have been mechanically ventilated for more than 48 hours, patients with a history of GI ulcers or bleeding within the past year, patients with a coagulopathy, patients with traumatic brain injury, patients with burn injuries, and patients with two or more minor criteria: sepsis, steroid therapy, an ICU stay of more than a week, and occult GI bleeding for more than 5 days.

17. **What are the contraindications to enteral feeding in the critically ill patient population?**
    Contraindications include patients who are hemodynamically unstable or who are not fully resuscitated, bowel obstruction, ileus, vomiting and diarrhea, major GI bleeding, and GI ischemia.

CHAPTER 14

BASIC LIFE SUPPORT, ADVANCED CARDIAC LIFE SUPPORT, AND ADVANCED TRAUMA LIFE SUPPORT

Robert A. Strauss, Amber Johnson, Robert C. Lampert, Shahid R. Aziz, John Wessel

BASIC LIFE SUPPORT*

1. What are the four steps of basic life support (BLS)?
   1. Check responsiveness (also check for absent or abnormal breathing by scanning the chest for movement).
   2. Activate the emergency response system/get automated external defibrillator (AED).
   3. Circulation (check the carotid pulse): if no pulse within 10 seconds, start CPR.
   4. Defibrillate.

2. What is the new sequence of CPR?
   CABD: Chest compressions, airway, breathing, defibrillation.
      The 2010 guidelines emphasize chest compressions for both trained and untrained rescuers. Chest compressions should be initiated prior to ventilation. If a person is not CPR trained, he or she should provide Hands-Only (compression-only) CPR. This change of sequence allows for chest compressions to be initiated sooner, increasing the patient's chance of survival.

3. What is the American Heart Association (AHA) Emergency Cardiovascular Care Adult Chain of Survival?
   1. Immediate recognition of cardiac arrest and initiation of the emergency response system
   2. Early CPR (emphasizing chest compressions)
   3. Rapid defibrillation
   4. Effective advanced life support
   5. Integrated post-cardiac arrest care

4. At what point should EMS be activated with an adult victim?
   Immediately upon finding an unresponsive adult. The victim should be checked for responsiveness and breathing, and then the emergency response system should be activated and an AED should be retrieved, if available. Return to the victim to check a pulse and begin CPR. Most adults in cardiac arrest are in ventricular fibrillation (V-fib); therefore the time from collapse until defibrillation is the single greatest factor in survival.

5. At what point should EMS be activated with an infant or child victim?
   If the arrest was not witnessed, call EMS after five cycles (approx. 2 minutes) of CPR. It is believed that many children develop respiratory arrest and bradycardia prior to cardiac arrest. During this time (prior to progression to cardiac arrest), these younger victims have a higher survival rate if CPR is started. Once a child progresses to cardiac arrest, his or her chance of survival is much lower. If the arrest is sudden and witnessed, call EMS first.

6. What length of time is used when assessing for a pulse?
   <10 seconds. If a pulse is not felt within 10 seconds, begin CPR. Assess the carotid pulse in children and adult. Assess the brachial pulse in infants.

---

*Written by Robert Strauss and Amber Johnson.

7. When an adult victim has a pulse but is breathless, what is the recommended rate of rescue breathing?
Once every 5 to 6 seconds (10 to 12 breaths/min).

8. When a child or infant has a pulse but is breathless, what is the recommended rate of rescue breathing?
Once every 3 seconds (20 breaths/min). Add compressions if the pulse remains <60 with signs of poor perfusion.

9. What is the best indicator of effective ventilation?
Seeing the chest rise when delivering breaths.

10. What are the effects of excessive ventilation?
Excessive ventilation (giving breaths too rapidly or with too much force) may decrease cardiac output and increase the risk of regurgitation and aspiration.
    Excessive ventilation increases intrathoracic pressure, decreasing venous return to the heart and in turn diminishing cardiac output. It increases the risk of regurgitation and aspiration by forcing air into the stomach, causing gastric inflation once the esophageal opening pressure is exceeded. To reduce the risk of aspiration, you should deliver air until you make the victim's chest rise and take 1 second to deliver the breath. You should also watch the victim's chest fall as you allow time for the lungs to empty.

11. In a victim with a pulse, how often should the pulse be checked during rescue breathing?
Once every 2 minutes.

12. What happens if chest compressions are interrupted?
There will be a decreased organ perfusion. During CPR, blood flow is completely dependent on chest compressions. Any interruption in CPR results in a lack of blood flow during that time.

13. In a pulseless victim, how often should the pulse/rhythm be checked during CPR?
Every 2 minutes. The goal is to minimize interruption during compressions. Do not take longer than 10 seconds to assess the pulse.

14. What are the indicators of effective CPR?
   • Seeing the chest rise when rescue breathing is delivered
   • Presence of a pulse during chest compressions (Intra-arterial relaxation pressures of less than 20 mm Hg will not achieve return of spontaneous circulation [ROSC].)
   • Capnography (end-tidal CO_2) >10 to 15 mm Hg (End-tidal CO_2 of less than 10 mm Hg will not achieve ROSC.)
       The team leader should also monitor the quality of the compressions and instruct another provider to switch if unable to provide high-quality compressions.

15. What are the signs of mild versus severe airway obstruction?
   • Mild: good air exchange, forceful cough, possible wheezing
   • Severe: poor to no air exchange, weak or absent cough, high-pitched noises during inhalation, no noises, respiratory difficulty, unable to speak, cyanosis (turning blue), universal choking sign

16. In the initial assessment, when is breathing assessed?
When assessing the patient for responsiveness, also check for normal breathing. Scan the chest for movement (for 5 to 10 seconds). If the patient is not breathing or is not breathing normally, begin chest compressions. After 30 chest compressions, open the airway and deliver two breaths. Abnormal breathing includes gasping for air or agonal breathing. "Look, listen, and feel" was removed from the 2010 AHA guidelines as a way to assess breathing due to excess delay and confusion when patients exhibited agonal gasping.

17. What is the most frequent cause of airway obstruction in an unconscious person?
The tongue.

18. Where is the correct location for applying pressure for external chest compressions in adult and children victims?
The center of the chest, between the nipples (lower half of the sternum). In adults, use the heels of both hands, with one stacked on the other to perform the compressions. In children ages 1 to 8 years, use the heel of one hand.

19. **Where is the ideal location for applying pressure for external chest compressions in infants?**
One finger width below the nipple line, with care being taken to stay off the xiphoid process. Use two fingers to perform the compressions or use the two thumb encircling hand technique if two rescuers are available.

20. **What is the depth of external chest compressions in adults?**
At least 2 inches.

21. **What is the depth of external chest compressions in children?**
At least one-third the depth of the child's chest (about 2 inches).

22. **What is the depth of external chest compressions in infants?**
At least one-third the depth of the infant's chest (about 1.5 inches).

23. **What is the rate of external chest compressions for adults, children, and infants?**
>100/min. The number of chest compressions delivered per minute is determined not only by the rate of compressions, but also by the frequency and duration of interruptions. You must provide an adequate compression rate and minimize interruptions to provide for adequate compressions.

24. **What is the ratio of external chest compressions to breaths for one or two rescuers with an adult victim?**
30 compressions for every two breaths (30:2) for both one- and two-rescuer CPR.

25. **What is the rate of external chest compressions to breaths for one or two rescuers with a child or infant?**
   - One rescuer: 30:2 (30 compressions for every two breaths).
   - Two rescuer: 15:2 (15 compressions for every two breaths).

26. **What is the rate of ventilation in a patient with an advanced airway?**
One breath every 6 to 8 seconds (8 to 10 breaths/min). These breaths are not synchronous with chest compressions.

27. **What is the length of time recommended to deliver each breath to an adult victim?**
About 1 second/breath. You should see visible chest rise. Allow for full exhalation between breaths.

28. **Why is it important to allow for full chest recoil?**
When the chest recoils (re-expands) after each compression, it allows blood to flow into the heart. This allows for the next chest compression to create blood flow because compressions pump the blood in the heart into the rest of the body. If the chest does not completely recoil, it decreases the blood flow created by each chest compression.

29. **What is the recommended method of clearing foreign body airway obstructions in infants?**
A combination of back slaps and chest thrusts: five back slaps followed by five chest thrusts, repeated until the object is dislodged. Do not use the Heimlich maneuver because an infant's liver is not well protected by the ribs and is at risk for injury with this technique. If the infant becomes unresponsive, begin CPR.

30. **What is the recommended method of clearing foreign body airway obstructions in responsive children and adults? What do you do if the victim is unresponsive?**
The Heimlich maneuver (abdominal thrusts) is used in responsive victims. If the victim is pregnant or obese, perform chest thrusts instead of abdominal thrusts. If the victim becomes unresponsive, activate EMS and begin CPR, starting with compressions.

31. **Why should blind finger sweeps not be used in children and infants?**
The object may be pushed deeper in the airway. Only attempt to remove the object if you can see it and it can be easily removed with your fingers.

32. **After successful resuscitation (ROSC), what is done with the patient?**
If signs of circulation and breathing return, place the patient in the recovery position. Continue to monitor pulse and blood pressure. Leave the AED in place and turned on while monitoring the patient. The patient should be transported to the appropriate hospital or critical care unit. Multidisciplinary care is vital.

33. **What are four conditions that require you to change how you use an AED?**
    1. Victim is in water (remove to dry area and dry off chest)
    2. Victim has implanted pacemaker or defibrillator (place electrodes away from device)
    3. Victim has transdermal patch (remove and clean area)
    4. Victim has a hairy chest (quickly pull pads to remove hair and replace pads)

34. **Can you use an AED in children and infants?**
    Yes. Ideally, in children from 1 to 8 years of age an AED should be used with a dose attenuator if available. If not available, a standard AED may be used. For infants (<1 year old), a manual defibrillator is preferred. If not available, then an AED with a pediatric dose attenuator would be the next choice, but if neither is available a standard AED may be used.

35. **What does an AED/defibrillator do?**
    An AED/defibrillator delivers an electric shock to the heart that stops the movement of the heart muscle fibers and allows the electrical system to reset itself. It does not restart the heart, but it resets it, hopefully allowing an organized rhythm to take over. If an organized rhythm occurs and the heart starts contracting effectively, a pulse will be generated, indicating ROSC.

36. **What are the major differences between initial resuscitation efforts for pediatric patients vs. adult patients?**
    With a child or infant victim, CPR should be started promptly prior to EMS activation if the arrest is not witnessed. EMS should be called after five cycles (approx. 2 minutes) of CPR have been performed. In adults, EMS should be activated immediately. Another major difference is, when two rescuers are available, the compression to breath ratio for children and infants should be 15:2 (compared to adults, for whom the ratio stays at 30:2).

37. **Where should you check for a pulse in an infant? In a child?**
    The brachial pulse in an infant and the carotid or femoral pulse in a child.

38. **What age ranges delineate infants and children?**
    An infant is younger than age 1, and a child is age 1 year old to puberty.

39. **What are the four universal steps of AED operation?**
    1. Power on AED.
    2. Attach AED pads to victim's chest (use adult pads for victims >8 years old).
    3. Clear victim and analyze heart rhythm.
    4. Clear victim and deliver shock if indicated.
       Directly after the shock is delivered (or if no shock is needed), immediately resume chest compressions.

40. **What is the goal for when a shock should be delivered after a victim collapses?**
    Less than 3 minutes. Early defibrillation results in better outcomes, and the goal is shock delivery within 3 minutes from the time of collapse.

41. **What is the predominant determinant of successful CPR?**
    Time to restoration of spontaneous circulation, which itself is a function of the time to effective chest compression and time to defibrillation in ventricular fibrillation. Early CPR, minimizing interruptions, and reducing the time from collapse to defibrillation can result in quicker restoration of spontaneous circulation, which improves survival in hospital and nonhospital settings.

42. **How do you open an airway? What do you do differently if the victim is an infant?**
    The two basic maneuvers to open an airway are head tilt with chin lift and jaw thrust. If the victim is an infant, do not extend the head beyond the neutral position because it may block the airway.

43. **What maneuver should the rescuer first use to open the airway in an otherwise uninjured patient? What if the patient has a suspected neck injury?**
    In an uninjured patient, perform the head tilt with chin lift maneuver to open the airway. In an unconscious patient with a suspected neck injury, the jaw thrust should be performed. The jaw thrust pulls the mandible forward, which pulls the tongue and epiglottis anteriorly off the upper airway (with minimal cervical hyperextension). This is only possible with two rescuers.

44. How much oxygen does mouth-to-mouth deliver compared to other techniques?
    - Mouth-to-mouth ventilation delivers approximately 17% inspired oxygen and 4% carbon dioxide.
    - Bag-mask ventilation delivers 21% oxygen.
    - Bag-mask ventilation with an oxygen supply can deliver close to 100% oxygen.

45. What are some of the complications of external chest compression?
    Rib and sternal fractures are the most common iatrogenic injuries. Other complications include cardiac or pericardial injuries (hematomas, lacerations, ruptures) and damage to other adjacent structures (e.g., pneumothorax, GI laceration), but these injuries are rare. The number of iatrogenic injuries increases when the compression depths exceed 6 cm (2.3 inches), but these injuries are rarely fatal. Do not let fear of complications interfere with effective chest compression.

46. What are the components of high-quality CPR?
    According to the advanced cardiac life support (ACLS) guidelines, the following are components of high-quality CPR:
    1. Rate ≥100/min
    2. Compression depth of ≥2 inches in adults
    3. Complete chest recoil after each compression
    4. Minimize interruptions in compressions.
    5. Switch providers every 2 minutes to prevent fatigue.
    6. Avoid excessive ventilations; one should only provide 500 to 600 ml of tidal volume per breath, which correlates to half a bag squeeze on the AMBU bag.

47. Why do we need to avoid excessive ventilation during CPR?
    Over-ventilation during CPR means too much volume is forcefully delivered into the patient. This causes multiple problems including gastric distention, which is caused when pressure overcomes the esophageal sphincters. This may lead to increased risk of aspiration. Over-ventilation also increases intrathoracic pressure, which decreases venous return and decreases chances of survival.

48. How can one monitor the quality of CPR?
    - End-tidal CO_2 of less than 10 mm Hg will not achieve ROSC.
    - Intra-arterial relaxation pressures of less than 20 mm Hg will not achieve ROSC.
    - The team leader should also monitor the quality of the compressions and instruct another provider to switch if unable to provide high-quality compressions.

ADVANCED CARDIAC LIFE SUPPORT†

49. Why the change from ABC to CAB?
    When an adult suffers from cardiac arrest, it is most often caused by ventricular fibrillation or ventricular tachycardia. The heart is quivering but fails to effectively deliver blood to the heart and other organs. By initiating chest compressions, the responder serves to pump blood and deliver oxygen to organs. By bypassing the "Airway and Breathing" part of the algorithm, one can deliver oxygen without additional delays and increase the chance of survival. Chest compressions will generate negative pressure upon recoil that will allow ambient air to be entrained into the pulmonary system.

50. When should a responder alter the CAB and utilize the ABC algorithm for resuscitation?
    Airway and Breathing algorithm components should be emphasized when the clinical scenario justifies their use, such as a patient in cardiac arrest secondary to drowning or asphyxiation. For a drowned patient, clearing the airway and providing rescue breaths will allow increased oxygen delivery. Patients with airway obstruction and the resulting hypoxia benefit from efficient maneuvers to clear the airway. To put it another way, if the patient's heart started beating again, but he had a collapsed airway, no oxygen would be delivered and resuscitation would be futile.

51. What is agonal breathing?
    Absent breathing or nonfunctional breathing. This includes gasping, which does not move oxygen. Agonal gasps are not effective breathing. One should not be fooled into a false sense of security with agonal breathing; respiratory arrest is occurring and treatment should commence.

---

†Written by Robert C. Lampert and Shahid R. Aziz.

52. **What are the major updates for ACLS based on the 2010 AHA guidelines?**
    1. For the cardiac arrest algorithm, emphasis is centered on a 2-minute cycle of chest compressions.
    2. Continued emphasis for vasopressors to be used every 3 to 5 minutes. This may be either epinephrine or vasopressin.
    3. Administer amiodarone for refractory ventricular fibrillation or ventricular tachycardia.
    4. Atropine is no longer recommended for use in pulseless electrical activity or asystole.

53. **When should hypothermia be considered in the ACLS protocol?**
    The goal of controlled hypothermia is to optimize survival and neurologic function when brain injury is suspected. Hypothermia is the only intervention shown to improve neurologic recovery. This intervention should be considered for any patient who is comatose after ROSC and V-fib was the presenting rhythm. Multiple studies have demonstrated improved outcomes for patients whose temperature was decreased to 32-34° C for 12 to 24 hours.

54. **What is the function and significance of waveform capnography?**
    Waveform capnography is a measure of CO_2 with respiration. The waveform rises with expiration and returns to zero upon inhalation. It serves as the most reliable indicator of endotracheal tube position after intubation. It also serves as a monitor for effectiveness of chest compressions.

55. **What are the current guidelines for cricoid pressure?**
    Per the 2010 guidelines, the AHA states one should not routinely use cricoid pressure during cardiac arrest. Cricoid pressure is a maneuver that is difficult to master, may not prevent aspiration as once thought, and may delay or prevent placement of advanced airway.

56. **Where are the sites that intraosseous access can be achieved?**
    In general, the anatomic sites that are common include sternum, humeral head, anterior superior iliac spine, medial malleolus, distal radius, distal femur, and proximal tibia. Certain devices are site specific, so one should be familiar with the specific device at one's institution. Similar to with all ACLS medications, one should flush the meds with normal saline to propel the medication into the central circulation.

57. **How is the diagnosis of cardiac arrest established?**
    By definition, the patient is in full cardiac arrest if he or she:
    - Is not responsive
    - Is not breathing
    - Has no pulse

58. **What are the three mechanisms of cardiac arrest?**
    1. V-fib/pulseless VT
    2. Pulseless electrical activity
    3. Asystole
    V-fib is most commonly present during the first minute following the onset of cardiac arrest.

59. **Which types of chest pain suggest cardiac ischemia?**
    - Uncomfortable squeezing pressure, fullness, or pain in the center of the chest lasting longer than 15 minutes
    - Pain that radiates to the shoulder, neck, arm, and jaws
    - Pain between the shoulder blades
    - Chest discomfort with light-headedness, fainting, sweating, and nausea
    - A feeling of distress, anxiety, or impending doom

60. **What is the recommended initial management for a stable adult patient with chest pain that is suggestive of ischemia?**
    1. Call for help.
    2. Perform immediate assessment including:
       - Vital signs and SaO_2 monitoring
       - IV access and electrocardiogram (ECG)
       - Targeted history and physical exam
       - Initial serum cardiac marker levels, electrolytes, and coagulation studies
       - Portable chest X-ray

3. Immediate general treatment:
   - Oxygen at 4 L/min
   - Aspirin (160 to 325 mg)
   - Nitroglycerin (sublingual or spray)
   - Morphine (IV) if pain is not relieved by nitroglycerin
   - Memory aid: "MONA greets all patients" (morphine, oxygen, nitroglycerin, and aspirin).

61. **What is the initial assessment of a 12-lead ECG in patients with cardiac ischemia?**
    - ST-segment elevation or new-onset left bundle branch block (LBBB) strongly suggests a myocardial injury. New LBBB is caused by occlusion of the left anterior descending (LAD) branch of the left coronary artery. LAD occlusion causes a loss of a large amount of myocardium.
    - ST-segment depression or T-wave inversion (ischemia)
    - Non-diagnostic or normal ECG

62. **What is the relationship between 12-lead EGC findings and coronary artery disease?**
    ECG relationship:
    - Anterior myocardium injury or infarct: leads V3 and V4
    - Septal myocardium injury or infarct: leads V1 and V2
    - Lateral myocardium injury or infarct: leads I, aVL, V5, and V6
    - Inferior myocardium injury or infarct: leads II, III, and aVF
    Coronary artery branches relationship:
    - LAD artery occlusion: leads V1 through V6
    - Circumflex artery occlusion: leads I, aVL, possibly V5, and V6
    - Right coronary artery occlusion: leads II, III, aVF

63. **What is the most common arrhythmia following electrical shock?**
    The most common arrhythmia caused by electrocution is V-fib; hence cardiac arrest is the primary cause of death from electrical shock. Other rhythms that may occur following electrical shock are VT progressing to V-fib and asystole.
    Electrical shock is the cause of more than 1000 deaths/year in the United States. It results in injuries ranging from unpleasant sensation to instant cardiac death. Exposure to high-tension current (>1000 V) is more likely to produce serious injury. However, death can result from exposure to relatively low voltage (100 V) household currents. Alternating current (AC) is more dangerous than direct current (DC). AC produces muscle tetany, which may prevent the victim from releasing the electrical source and thus prolong the contact.

64. **What is V-fib?**
    V-fib is a cardiac dysrhythmia that occurs when multiple areas within the ventricles display unsynchronized depolarization and repolarization. As a result, the ventricles do not contract as a unit. Instead, the ventricles appear to quiver, or fibrillate, as multiple areas of the ventricle are contracting and relaxing in a disorganized fashion. The net result is no cardiac output and no pulse.

65. **How is V-fib/pulseless VT treated initially according to the AHA recommendations?**
    1. The initial treatment for V-fib is always defibrillation.
    2. Begin with the universal algorithm:
       - Assess the airway, breathing, and circulation (ABCs).
       - Ascertain that the patient is in cardiac arrest.
       - Begin CPR with cycles of 30 compressions and two breaths until defibrillator is attached, and confirm V-fib.
    3. Give one shock:
       - Manual biphasic: device specific (120 to 200 J)
       - AED: device specific
       - Monophasic: 360 J
    4. If V-fib persists:
       - Resume CPR immediately, intubate, and establish IV access.
       - Administer epinephrine 1 mg IV/IO (intraosseous) and repeat every 3 to 5 minutes, or you may administer one dose of vasopressin 40 U IV/IO to replace the first or second dose of epinephrine.

5. Give five cycles of CPR.
6. Give one shock if the rhythm is shockable.
7. Resume CPR immediately after the shock.
8. Consider antiarrhythmic medications.

66. **What is tachycardia?**
Tachycardia means that there is a rapid heart rate. The normal adult heart rate is considered by most to be between 60 and 100 beats/min. Thus a heart rate of >100 beats/min can be classified as tachycardia. Not all patients with a heart rate of 100 beats/min or more will require treatment. The following cardiac rhythms are considered tachyarrhythmias:
1. Atrial flutter (A-flutter)/atrial fibrillation (A-fib)
2. Narrow-complex tachycardia:
   - Junctional tachycardia
   - Paroxysmal supraventricular tachycardia (PSVT)
   - Multifocal or ectopic atrial tachycardia
3. Wide-complex tachycardia:
   - SVT with aberrant conduction
   - Stable monomorphic VT
   - Stable polymorphic VT (with and without normal baseline QT interval)
   - Torsades de pointes
   A patient with tachycardia or tachyarrhythmia needs treatment when there are signs and symptoms associated with the rapid heart rate. The following signs and symptoms indicate that the patient is already or is becoming hemodynamically unstable:
   - Symptoms: shortness of breath, chest pain, dyspnea on exertion, and altered mental status
   - Signs: pulmonary edema, rales, rhonchi, hypotension, orthostasis, jugular vein distention, peripheral edema, ischemic ECG changes, ventricular rate >150 beats/min

67. **Which tachyarrhythmias are supraventricular?**
If the QRS complex is narrow, then the tachyarrhythmia is **supraventricular**. This means the arrhythmia is originating at or above the level of the atrioventricular (AV) node:
- Sinus tachycardia
- A-flutter
- A-fib
- PSVT
   If the QRS complex is wide, then the tachycardia is of **ventricular** origin:
- Wide-complex tachycardia of uncertain type
- VT

68. **What is the pathophysiology of PSVT?**
PSVT is a distinct clinical syndrome characterized by repeated episodes of tachycardia with abrupt onset lasting a few seconds to many hours. PSVT is due to a reentry mechanism involving the AV node alone or automatic focus.

69. **What are the types of narrow-complex tachycardia?**
- PSVT: caused by a reentry circuit mechanism
- Ectopic or multifocal atrial tachycardia: caused by an automatic focus
- Junctional tachycardia: caused by automatic focus that originates within or near the AV node
   Reentry tachycardia responds well to antiarrhythmic medications and electrical cardioversion. Automatic focus tachycardias do not respond to electrical cardioversion and should be treated with medications that suppress the ectopic foci.

70. **What are the signs and symptoms of A-fib and A-flutter?**
A-fib may result from multiple areas of reentry within the atria or from multiple ectopic foci. A-fib may be associated with sick sinus syndrome, hypoxia, increased atrial pressure, and pericarditis. Because there is no uniform atrial depolarization, no P-wave will be seen on ECG. Hypotension may result from A-fib.
   A-flutter is the result of a reentry circuit within the atria. A-flutter rarely occurs in the absence of organic disease. It is seen in association with mitral or tricuspid valvular disease, acute cor pulmonale, and coronary artery disease. Signs and symptoms include hypotension, ischemic pain, and severe congestive heart failure.

71. **How are A-fib and A-flutter treated?**

    According to the AHA, the protocol for treatment of A-fib and A-flutter is:

    1. Rule out precipitating causes for A-fib and A-flutter:
       - Heart failure
       - Pulmonary embolism
       - Acute MI/substance abuse
       - Hyperthyroidism
       - Hypokalemia
       - Hypoxia
       - Hypomagnesemia
    2. Control the rate:
       - Preserved heart function: diltiazem (or another calcium channel blocker) or metoprolol (or another beta blocker), flecainide, propafenone, procainamide, amiodarone, or digoxin
       - Impaired heart function: diltiazem, digoxin, or amiodarone
       - Patients with Wolff-Parkinson-White (WPW) syndrome: Avoid adenosine, calcium channel blockers, beta blockers, and digoxin to control the rate. Convert the rhythm (electrical cardioversion if drug therapy is unsuccessful) if the duration is 48 hours or less.
       - Preserved heart function: DC cardioversion, amiodarone, ibutilide, flecainide, propafenone, procainamide
       - Impaired heart function: DC cardioversion, amiodarone
    3. Convert the rhythm if the duration is >48 hours.
    4. Urgent cardioversion: begins with IV heparin, followed by transesophageal echocardiogram to exclude atrial clot. Then cardiovert within 24 hours and give anticoagulation for 4 weeks.
    5. Delayed cardioversion: anticoagulation for 3 weeks; then cardiovert and anticoagulate for 4 more weeks.

72. **What are the types of wide-complex tachycardias and their AHA treatment recommendations?**

    1. Unknown type:
       - Attempt to identify and distinguish between VT and SVT with aberrant conduction due to the different treatment options for SVT that might compromise a patient with VT.
       - Always assume that any wide-complex tachycardia is VT until proven otherwise, because there is little danger in treating a wide-complex SVT as if it were VT.
       - **Treatment:** DC cardioversion, procainamide, or amiodarone for preserved cardiac function. Treat with DC cardioversion or amiodarone for impaired cardiac function.
    2. Monomorphic VT:
       - QRS complexes appear identical in shape.
       - **Treatment:** procainamide, amiodarone, lidocaine, or sotalol with normal cardiac function. Lidocaine or amiodarone should be given to patients with impaired cardiac function.
    3. Polymorphic VT:
       - QRS complexes are subdivided into normal baseline QT and prolonged baseline QT interval.
       - Associated with metabolic derangement such as electrolyte abnormalities or drug toxicities.
       - **Treatment:** search for the metabolic derangement. Use DC cardioversion, procainamide, amiodarone, or beta blockers.
       - Torsades de pointes is an example of this VT with a unique rhythm strip. The drug of choice for torsades associated with hypomagnesemia is magnesium sulfate.

73. **What is WPW syndrome? Which drugs can be harmful in the treatment of A-fib or A-flutter associated with WPW syndrome?**

    If there is an extra conduction pathway, the electrical signal may arrive at the ventricles too soon. This condition is called Wolff-Parkinson-White (WPW) syndrome. It is in a category of electrical abnormalities called pre-excitation syndromes.

    It is recognized by certain changes on the ECG, which is a graphical record of the heart's electrical activity. The ECG will show that an extra pathway or shortcut exists from the atria to the ventricles.

    Many people with WPW syndrome who have symptoms or episodes of tachycardia (rapid heart rhythm) may have dizziness, chest palpitations, fainting, or, rarely, cardiac arrest. Other people with WPW syndrome never have tachycardia or other symptoms. About 80% of people with symptoms first have them between the ages of 11 and 50.

Drugs that selectively block the AV node without also blocking coexisting accessory conduction pathways (e.g., adenosine, calcium channel blockers, beta blockers, and digoxin) are contraindicated when pre-excitation syndromes are present. These medications can increase conduction through the accessory pathway and paradoxically increase the heart rate. For patients with A-fib or A-flutter, this poses severe risks and is associated with a very high incidence of clinical deterioration.

74. **What is bradycardia?**

The term *bradycardia* simply means that the heart rate is slow. Normal adult heart rate is considered by most to be 60 to 100 beats/min. According to this definition, every patient with a heart rate <60 beats/min is bradycardic. Not all patients with a heart rate <60 beats/min will need treatment. Autonomic influence or intrinsic disease affecting the cardiac conduction system most often causes bradycardia.

A patient may have a relative bradycardia. An example is the patient with severe hypotension but with a heart rate of 70 beats/min; the heart rate of 70 in a hypotensive patient may not sustain the cardiac output.

75. **What are the principal types of bradyarrhythmias?**

- Sinus bradycardia
- A-fib with slow ventricular response
- AV block:
  - First-degree heart block
  - Second-degree heart block, types I and II
  - Third-degree heart block
- Relative bradycardia

Other rhythms that may also be considered bradyarrhythmias are:

- Pulseless electrical activity
- Asystole

76. **When does sinus bradycardia need treatment?**

A patient with a slow heart rate needs treatment only if there are serious signs or symptoms associated with the slow heart rate that indicate the patient is already or is becoming hemodynamically unstable. These signs and symptoms include:

- **Signs:** hypotension, congestive heart failure, pulmonary congestion, and acute MI
- **Symptoms:** chest pain, shortness of breath, and decreased level of consciousness

77. **How is a patient with a bradyarrhythmia initially managed according to AHA protocol?**

1. Supportive actions:
   - Assess ABCs
   - Chest X-ray
   - Oxygen, IV, monitors, and pulse oximetry
   - Brief history and targeted physical exam
   - 12-lead ECG
2. Determine if bradycardia is hemodynamically significant.
   - Monitor patient.
   - Be prepared to begin transcutaneous pacing (TCP) on standby.
   If the patient is hemodynamically unstable:
   - Atropine, 0.5 to 1.0 mg IV
   - Epinephrine infusion, 2 to 10 mg/min
   - TCP
   - Isoproterenol infusion, 2 to 10 mg/min
   - Dopamine infusion, 5 to 20 mg/kg/min

78. **What is meant by the term *heart block*?**

Heart block is used interchangeably with the correct term, *atrioventricular (AV) block*. AV block describes a delay or interruption in conduction between the atria and the ventricles, which may be caused by one or more of the following:

- Lesion in the conduction pathway
- Prolonged refractory period along the conduction pathway
- Supraventricular heart rates that surpass the refractory period of the AV node

79. **What is first-degree heart block?**
First-degree heart block is the prolonged delay in conduction at the AV node or the bundle of His. The diagnosis of first-degree heart block is based on the PR interval. First-degree heart block exists when the PR interval is longer than 0.2 seconds.

80. **According to AHA protocol, how is first-degree heart block treated?**
First-degree heart block requires no treatment unless there are associated symptoms.

81. **What is second-degree heart block?**
In second-degree heart block, not every atrial impulse is able to pass through the AV node into the ventricles. The atrial impulses that are conducted to the ventricle will stimulate ventricular contraction. Therefore the ratio of P to QRS will be >1:1.
   Type I second-degree heart block (Wenckebach):
- Occurs at the level of the AV node
- Is usually due to increased parasympathetic tone or drug effects
- Is characterized by progressive elongation of the PR interval
- Conduction velocity through the AV node gradually decreases until the impulse is blocked, resulting in a skipped ventricular beat.
   Type II second-degree heart block:
- Occurs below the level of the AV node, uncommonly at the bundle of His
- Is usually due to a lesion along the pathway
- Has a PR interval that does not lengthen before a skipped ventricular beat
- May have more than one skipped ventricular beat in a row
- Has a poorer prognosis than type I second-degree heart block
- Is more likely to progress to complete heart block than type I

82. **According to AHA protocol, how is type I second-degree heart block treated?**
Type I second-degree heart block rarely requires treatment unless symptoms associated with bradycardia develop. Treatment should be directed at addressing the underlying cause of the block, such as:
- Decreased parasympathetic tone
- Propranolol toxicity/overdose
- Digitalis toxicity
- Verapamil toxicity/overdose
   If serious symptoms occur, then the following treatment is recommended:
- Atropine, 0.5 to 1.0 mg
- Epinephrine infusion, 1 to 2 µg/min
- TCP
- Fluid challenge if appropriate
- Dopamine infusion, beginning with 5 µg/kg/min

83. **According to AHA protocol, how is type II second-degree heart block treated?**
Type II second-degree heart block requires no treatment unless symptoms associated with bradycardia develop.
   If serious symptoms develop, then the following treatment is recommended:
- Atropine, 0.5 to 1.0 mg
- Epinephrine infusion, 1 to 2 µg/min
- TCP
- Fluid challenge if appropriate
- Dopamine beginning with 5 µg/kg/min

84. **What is third-degree heart block?**
Third-degree heart block occurs when no atrial impulses are transmitted to the ventricles. The atrial rate will be equal to or greater than the ventricular rate. If block occurs at the AV node, a junctional pacemaker may initiate ventricular depolarizations at a regular rate of 40 to 60 beats/min. If the block is infranodal, usually both bundle branches are blocked and there is significant disease of the conduction pathway.

85. **According to AHA protocol, how is third-degree heart block treated?**
Third-degree heart block is treated only if there are signs and symptoms that the patient is or is becoming hemodynamically unstable. Recommended treatment for third-degree heart block is:
- Atropine, 0.5 to 1.0 mg
- Epinephrine infusion, 1 to 2 mg/min

- TCP
- Fluid challenge if appropriate
- Dopamine infusion beginning with 5 µg/kg/min

86. **What is pulseless electrical activity (PEA)?**
This term is used to describe a group of diverse ECG rhythms that manifest electrical activity but are similar in that the patient will be without a pulse. Therefore the PEA is a nonperfusing rhythm. The types of rhythms included in the PEA group are:
- **EMD:** organized ECG rhythm present, no pulse
- **Pseudo-EMD:** as above, but with some meaningful cardiac contraction
- **Idioventricular, ventricular escape:** wide-QRS, no atrial activity, and no pulse
- **Bradyasystolic:** profound bradycardia with periods of asystole, no pulse
PEA is almost always a secondary disorder resulting from some underlying condition.

87. **What are the causes of PEA?**
The underlying causes of PEA can be remembered easily using the mnemonic 5 H's and 5 T's.
Five causes that start with **H**:
Hypovolemia
Hypoxia
Hydrogen ion (acidosis)
Hyperkalemia/hypokalemia
Hypothermia
Five causes that start with **T**:
Table (ABCDs): antidepressants, beta blockers, calcium channel blocker, and digitalis
Tamponade (cardiac)
Tension pneumothorax
Thrombosis (coronary)
Thrombosis (pulmonary)
Alternatively, the causes of PEA can be divided into three basic categories:
1. Inadequate ventilation:
   - Intubation of right main stem bronchus
   - Tension pneumothorax
   - Bilateral pneumothorax
2. Inadequate circulation:
   - Pericardial effusion with tamponade
   - Myocardial rupture
   - Ruptured aortic aneurysm
   - Massive pulmonary embolus
   - Hypovolemia
3. Metabolic disorder:
   - Electrolyte disturbances (hyperkalemia or hypokalemia, hypomagnesemia)
   - Persistent severe acidosis (diabetic ketoacidosis or lactic acidosis)
   - Tricyclic overdose
   - Hypothermia

88. **According to AHA protocol, how is PEA treated?**
1. Continue CPR.
2. Intubate/establish IV access.
3. Assess blood flow using Doppler.
4. Consider and treat underlying causes.
5. Epinephrine, 1 mg IV/IO. Repeat every 3 to 5 minutes, or you may give one dose of vasopressin 40 U IV/IO to replace the first or second dose of epinephrine.
6. Atropine, 1 mg IV push if pulse is present and absolute bradycardia is <60 beats/min. Repeat every 3 to 5 minutes (up to three doses).

89. **What is asystole?**
The term *asystole* indicates the absence of ventricular activity. The patient will be without a pulse. ECG will show characteristic flat-line tracing without P-waves and QRS complexes. The underlying causes of asystole can be remembered using the mnemonic PHD:
Preexisting acidosis

Hypoxia, hyperkalemia, hypokalemia, hypothermia
Drug overdose

90. **How is a flat-line rhythm verified to be asystole?**
    - The patient is pulseless.
    - The patient is unresponsive.
    - The monitoring leads are correctly hooked up.
    - There is a flat-line recording in more than one lead.

91. **What four conditions other than asystole can lead to a flat-line tracing on ECG?**
    1. Fine V-fib
    2. No power
    3. Loose electrode leads
    4. Signal gain is turned down.

92. **What four conditions are pulseless?**
    There are four conditions in which the patient will present without a pulse and which are therefore considered nonperfusing conditions:
    1. V-fib
    2. Pulseless VT
    3. PEA:
       - Electromechanical dissociation
       - Pseudo-EMD (pulse will be very faint and evident only by Doppler)
       - Ventricular escape rhythms
       - Postdefibrillation idioventricular rhythms
    4. Asystole

93. **According to AHA protocol, what is the treatment for asystole?**
    The treatment sequence for asystole is virtually the same algorithm for PEA:
    1. Continue CPR.
    2. Intubate/establish IV access.
    3. Confirm asystole.
    4. Consider and treat underlying causes.
    5. TCP only if started early.
    6. Epinephrine, 1 mg IV/IO. Repeat every 3 to 5 minutes, or you may give one dose of vasopressin 40 U IV/IO to replace the first or second dose of epinephrine.
    7. Atropine, 1 mg IV/IO. Repeat every 3 to 5 minutes (up to three doses).

94. **What is shock?**
    The term *shock* denotes a clinical syndrome in which there is inadequate cellular perfusion and inadequate oxygen delivery for the metabolic demands of the tissues. Types of shock include:
    - Cardiogenic shock
    - Neurogenic shock
    - Hypovolemic shock
    - Flow disruption shock
    - Septic shock
    - Anaphylactic shock
        In general, shock is characterized by:
    - Increased vascular resistance
    - Anxiety
    - Cool mottled skin
    - Vomiting
    - Oliguria
    - Diarrhea
    - Tachycardia
    - Myocardial ischemia
    - Adrenergic response
    - Mental status changes
    - Diaphoresis

95. When is synchronized cardioversion used?
    - Tachycardia
    - A-fib
    - PSVT
    - A-flutter

96. What are the signs and symptoms of cardiac tamponade?
    - Persistent tachycardia with falling blood pressure
    - Pulsus paradoxus
    - Pulsatile neck veins
    - Enlarging heart shadow on chest X-ray

97. What are the signs and symptoms of hypovolemic shock?
    - Cardiac output will be low due to inadequate left ventricular filling.
    - Hypotension may lead to changes in the ECG.

98. How is hypovolemic shock treated?
    - Volume loss can be diagnosed through history and clinical evaluation.
    - Replace volume with crystalloid or colloid solution when the hematocrit is normal.
    - With active bleeding, hemostasis must be achieved first. If the hematocrit is dangerously low, transfusion of whole blood or packed red blood cells is indicated.

99. What are the four life-threatening conditions that may mimic acute MI and lead to cardiovascular collapse?
    1. Massive pulmonary embolism
    2. Cardiac tamponade
    3. Hypovolemic and septic shock
    4. Aortic dissection

100. What drugs can be administered through the endotracheal tube?
    L-E-A-N (**L**idocaine, **A**tropine, **E**pinephrine, **N**arcan). Administer all tracheal medications at 2 to 2.5 times the recommended IV dosage, diluted in 10 mL of normal saline or distilled water. Tracheal absorption is greater with the distilled water as the diluent than with normal saline, but distilled water has a greater adverse effect on PaO_2.

101. How is sudden cardiac death defined?*
    Sudden V-fib or PEA. Acute coronary ischemia and preexisting cardiac disease are the most common causes. V-fib is becoming less common.

102. Is there an immediate need for an airway?*
    No. Defibrillation and chest compression should be initiated first. Waiting for intubation to be completed before initiation of these interventions is one of the most common mistakes in advanced life support. Children, in whom primary respiratory arrest is more common, are an exception. Restoration of ventilation in children often reveals that pulselessness was severe shock, not cardiac arrest.

103. Is the central line the best access to the circulation?*
    Yes. Large volumes of fluid can be delivered to the venous system more quickly, however, via large-bore peripheral venous catheters. A 14-gauge, 5-cm catheter (peripheral) can deliver twice the flow of a 16-gauge, 20-cm catheter (central). Central line placement may be associated with significant complications, including pneumothorax, air embolus, and arterial puncture. In hypovolemic patients, in whom central veins are collapsed and peripheral veins are constricted, venous cannulation can be difficult.

104. Does a central line offer therapeutic and diagnostic advantages?*
    Yes. A central line permits bolus administration of drugs to the right side of the heart. Identification of a high central venous pressure may indicate the need to treat reversible causes of PEA, such as cardiac tamponade or tension pneumothorax.

105. Which is preferred: colloid or crystalloid resuscitation fluid?*
    Colloid advocates claim that the big molecules remain in the intravascular space and are more effective in elevating blood volume. Crystalloid advocates state that capillaries leak albumin, especially in the shock state. Resuscitation with crystalloid is clearly safe. Given its availability, low cost,

and safety, crystalloid (lactated Ringer's solution) is the choice for initial fluid resuscitation. When true cardiac arrest has occurred, however, volume is of little importance.

106. **In a patient exhibiting asystole, bradycardia, PEA, or fine fibrillation, what is your primary goal?***

Adequate vital organ perfusion, especially to the coronary arteries. Done properly, CPR may cause PEA to progress to stable hemodynamics or V-fib to become coarse enough for successful countershock.

107. **When should adenosine be used?**

Adenosine is the first line drug of choice for managing stable narrow-complex tachycardia. Adenosine is effective in terminating arrhythmias due to reentry at the AV or SA node. It is often used as a agent, to decrease the heart rate for better appreciation of the underlying rhythm. Adenosine will NOT convert atrial fibrillation, atrial flutter, or ventricular tachycardia. During rapid IV push, adenosine will often cause short-lived side effects including asystole or significant bradycardia, chest pain, and flushing. Adenosine is also safe to be used during pregnancy.

108. **When should Amiodarone be used?**

Amiodarone is a drug that affects sodium, potassium, and calcium channels in addition to having alpha- and beta-adrenergic blocking components. The AHA recommends that amiodarone be prescribed by physicians well versed in the treatment of arrhythmias and fully aware of its risks and benefits. Beyond its warning, amiodarone is indicated for patients with V-fib, pulseless VT unresponsive to defibrillation, CPR and vasopressors, and recurrent, unstable VT. The first dose is 300 mg IV push, followed by a second dose of 150 mg as necessary. Avoid using amiodarone with other drugs that increase the QT interval (e.g., procainamide).

109. **When should aspirin be used in the ACLS protocol?**

Administer to all patients with suspected acute coronary syndrome; this includes patients with crushing chest pain, chest pressure, or other symptoms consistent with cardiac ischemia. The dose is 160 to 325 mg non-enteric coated tablet and should be chewed. A rectal suppository may be substituted in those who cannot take PO medications. The rectal dose is 300 mg. One must weigh the benefits and risks of giving aspirin (ASA) to someone with a history of active ulcer disease or asthma. The only true contraindication is someone with a known allergy to ASA.

110. **When should atropine be used?**

Atropine is the first line drug in symptomatic sinus bradycardia. The 2010 AHA guidelines have eliminated atropine from the PEA or systole algorithm. The dose for bradycardia is 0.5 mg IV q 3 to 5 min, and not to exceed 3 mg. Doses less than 0.5 mg may cause paradoxical slowing of the heart rate. Judicious use should be performed in the patient with myocardial ischemia and hypoxia, as atropine will increase the myocardial oxygen demand. The other indication for atropine use outside of the ACLS algorithm is for organophosphate poisoning.

111. **When should diltiazem be used?**

Use to control ventricular rates in the atrial fibrillation and atrial flutter. It is also used to rate control refractory reentry SVT. For acute rate control one should use 15 to 20 mg IV over 2 minutes. A second dose of 20 to 25 mg IV may be given 15 minutes later over 2 minutes. Do NOT use calcium channel blockers in patients with Wolff-Parkinson-White Syndrome. Calcium channel blockers will cause a drop in blood pressure from peripheral vasodilation. Avoid calcium channel blockers in patients already receiving IV beta blockers, as this combination may cause severe hypotension.

112. **When should epinephrine be used?**

There are several indications for epinephrine:
- Cardiac arrest: which includes V-fib, pulseless VT, asystole, and PEA. The dose is 1 mg administered q 3 to 5 min (10 mL of 1:10k solution). As with all medications in cardiac arrest, they should be flushed with 20 mL saline and elevation of the limb.
- Symptomatic bradycardia
- Severe hypotension: a dose of 2 to 10 mcg/min is used as a vasopressor.
- Anaphylaxis

---

*Reprinted from Paradis NA, Harken AH: Cardiopulmonary resuscitation. In Harken AH, Moore EE, editors: *Abernathy's surgical secrets*, ed 5, Philadelphia, 2005, Mosby.

Epinephrine will raise blood pressure and increase heart rate causing increased myocardial oxygen consumption. Epinephrine is a medication that may be given through the endotracheal tube.

113. **When should magnesium sulfate be used?**

There are two major indications for magnesium sulfate: the first is in situations of torsades de pointes with suspected hypomagnesemia; the second is in ventricular arrhythmias secondary to digitalis toxicity. In the setting of cardiac arrest with torsades de pointes, the dose is 1 to 2 g diluted in 10 ml D5W IV.

114. **When should morphine be used?**

Morphine is a powerful opiate that provides profound analgesia and euphoria. It is to be used in cases of chest pain with acute coronary syndrome that does not respond to nitrates. Two well-known side effects of opiates are respiratory depression and hypotension. For ST-elevation myocardial infarction (STEMI) patients, the dose is 2 to 4 mg IV, and it may be increased depending on patient tolerance and response. Morphine should be used judiciously in patients with right ventricular infarction, as these patients are preload dependent and decreases in blood pressure will worsen coronary perfusion.

115. **When should oxygen be delivered to the patient?**

Oxygen should be used when there is any suspicion of cardiac or pulmonary emergencies. All patients with shortness of breath and/or chest pain should receive supplemental oxygen. ACLS guidelines recommend administering oxygen to patients once oxygen saturation levels fall to <94%. Oxygen may be delivered via a variety of devices ranging from a nasal cannula to an endotracheal tube. Oxygen toxicity is a concern for intubated patients. FiO_2 higher than 60% may cause free radical damage resulting in atelectasis and lung consolidation. In general, one should titrate FiO_2 to achieve 100% saturation at the lowest possible FiO_2. In addition, any patient on supplemental oxygen should have continuous pulse oximetry.

116. **Can you summarize the Acute Coronary Syndrome Algorithm?**

The ACS Algorithm should be activated when there is suspicion that a heart attack may be occurring. Suspicion should be heightened on patients with multiple risk factors (e.g., chest pain radiating to left arm, age >70, male sex, diabetes mellitus, and history of ischemic heart disease). Once initiated, the patient should be connected to cardiac monitors, given supplemental oxygen, and IV access should be initiated. Aspirin should be given and chewed. Nitroglycerin and morphine may be given depending on the patient's blood pressure and symptoms. A 12-lead ECG should be obtained to determine STEMI versus non-STEMI. Labs should be drawn that include electrolytes, coagulation studies, and cardiac markers. A portable CXR should be taken. A checklist for reperfusion should be initiated. If the patient is not in a hospital setting, then EMS should notify a hospital equipped for Percutaneous Cardiac Intervention (PCI).

The ECG result will dictate the next step in treatment. If the patient has STEMI, then a focus on reperfusion therapy should be priority. The AHA recommends door-to-balloon (PCI) time of 90 minutes, or door-to-needle (fibrinolysis) goal of 30 minutes. Other adjunctive therapy should be initiated such as nitroglycerin, heparin, antiplatelet agents, and rate control with beta blockers. All patients with STEMI should be admitted to monitored beds and frequently monitored.

If the patient has ST-segment depression or dynamic T-wave inversion, there is a high likelihood of ischemia. Adjunctive treatment as listed above should be started. Serial troponin markers should be measured and the patient should be monitored for signs of heart failure, persistent ECG changes, or arrhythmias. If these occur, the patient should be considered for invasive therapy (PCI).

Last, if the patient has a normal ECG, then one should evaluate serial cardiac markers and perform noninvasive imaging. If these tests are positive for pathology, then the patient should be treated with adjunctive therapy and be considered for more invasive imaging and intervention. Most patients with ACS will benefit from an HMG CoA reductase inhibitor, ASA, and blood pressure control.

117. **When should nitroglycerin be avoided in the ACLS patient?**

Nitrates cause veno-dilation and are used for the treatment of ischemic chest pain. They should be avoided when the patient cannot tolerate an additional drop in blood pressure caused by the veno-dilation. The AHA recommends caution with nitrates when SBP <90 mm Hg or >30 mm Hg below baseline. Avoid nitrates in patients with inferior wall MI and suspected right ventricular involvement, as these patients are preload dependent. Last, avoid nitrates in someone who has used phosphodiesterase inhibitors in the past 24 to 48 hours.

118. **What are the time limit goals for reperfusion therapy?**

Percutaneous coronary intervention within 90 minutes of arrival at the emergency department. Alternatively, fibrinolytic therapy within 30 minutes of arrival at the emergency department. To facilitate this rapid intervention, the chain of response must be tightened. Obtaining a 12-lead ECG in the field by EMS and forwarding to the emergency department of a PCI-equipped facility, helps to eliminate unnecessary delay. This will minimize delays and maximize optimum outcomes.

119. **Describe the algorithm for managing a patient with cardiac arrest.**

Once a cardiac arrest is suspected, the first action is to activate the emergency response by calling for help, or calling for a Code Team. In a hospital setting, cardiac arrest triggers a Code Blue. Depending on the number of rescuers, clear roles should be assigned; the code leader should be clear. The next step is immediately starting CPR. With the heart no longer pumping oxygen to the tissues, the rescuer must preserve the function of these organs by artificially pumping oxygen via chest compressions. While one person maintains chest compressions at a rate of 30:2 with respirations, another should be preparing the defibrillator. Emphasis should be placed on activating the defibrillator as soon as possible, as delay in defibrillation is associated with worse outcomes. The defibrillator will search for a shockable or nonshockable rhythm. If nonshockable (asystole or PEA), immediately return to performing CPR. If shockable, rescuers must stand clear until shock is delivered. The shock is 120 to 200 J on biphasic units, and 360 J on monophasic units. During CPR, attempts should be made to obtain IV access. Consideration for advanced airways must be made (either LMA, endotracheal intubation, or an emergency surgical airway). If an advanced airway is placed, then respirations change to 8 to 10/min and chest compressions continue without interruption for 2 minutes. Waveform capnography should be used to confirm proper placement of advanced airway. Every 2-minute cycle of CPR triggers a rhythm check by the defibrillator, a drug therapy check, and reevaluation of the treatment so far. Drug therapy consists of giving a vasopressor (epinephrine or vasopressin) or antiarrhythmic such as amiodarone. A search for "H's and T's" must be performed to identify and ultimately treat a potential source for cardiac arrest. One should not deviate from the ACLS algorithm, as deviations are associated with worse outcomes.

120. **What are the steps to be taken after return of spontaneous circulation (ROSC)?**

The goal after ROSC is to minimize damage from ischemia. Therefore, oxygenation saturation must be maintained at a level of ≥94%. Consider placing an advanced airway if oxygenation is tenuous. Avoid hyperventilation as this may prevent venous return and cause gastric insufflation. Start at a rate of 10 to 12 breaths/min and titrate to target end tidal CO_2 of 35 to 40 mm Hg. Along with oxygenation, perfusion must be maintained. Perfusion may be estimated from blood pressure. The goal is to maintain systolic BP ≥90 mm Hg. To achieve this goal, IVF bolus and vasopressors may be used. A search for reversible causes must continue (H's and T's). Evaluation of mental status will determine if induced hypothermia is necessary. If the patient cannot follow commands, then induced hypothermia is recommended. If the initial cardiac arrest was suspected to be STEMI or acute myocardial infarction, then coronary reperfusion should be initiated as quickly as possible. Induced hypothermia and coronary reperfusion can be initiated simultaneously when indicated.

121. **What is the algorithm for bradycardia?**

The first step is identifying the appropriateness of the heart rate for a given clinical scenario (e.g., marathon runners may have heart rates in the 40s and be normal). In general, a heart rate <50/min is considered a bradyarrhythmia. Once determined to be pathologic, a search for the underlying cause should begin. One should obtain IV access, cardiac monitoring, and supplemental oxygen if hypoxemic. 12-lead ECG should be obtained with all arrhythmias. The next step is determining the severity of the bradyarrhythmia. If the patient has signs of hypotension, altered mental status, ischemic chest pain, acute heart failure, or shock, then treatment to raise the heart must begin. Without these signs of symptoms the patient may be monitored and observed. If symptomatic, atropine is the first line agent to be used. A dose of 0.5 mg bolus may be repeated q 3 to 5 min until a maximum of 3 mg is reached. If atropine is ineffective in raising the heart rate, TCP or dopamine infusion or epinephrine infusion may be started. Transvenous pacing may be required but should be performed by an expert.

122. **Can you explain the algorithm for tachycardia?**

The first steps are similar to evaluating the patient with bradycardia. First, one must identify the appropriateness of the heart rate for a given clinical scenario (e.g., strenuous activity will raise HR in a physiologic manner). In general, heart rate ≥150/min is considered a tachyarrhythmia. Once determined to be pathologic, a search for underlying causes should begin. One should obtain IV access, cardiac monitoring, and supplemental oxygen if hypoxemic. Monitoring blood pressure frequently is crucial in determining the severity of tachyarrhythmias. There are two significant checkpoints in the evaluation of tachyarrhythmias: (1) is the tachyarrhythmia causing hypotension, altered mental status, ischemic chest pain, acute heart failure, or signs of shock? These are signs of hemodynamic instability. (2) Is the QRS complex wide or narrow (defined by ≥0.12 s)? The former must be evaluated first. If the patient has signs of hemodynamic instability, proceed to immediate synchronized cardioversion. The energy for cardioversion is dictated by the arrhythmia: narrow regular = 50 to 100 J; narrow irregular = 120 to 200; wide regular = 100 J. Sedation may be considered if the clinical course permits. If the patient has no signs of instability, then evaluate the QRS complex; if wide, consider adenosine only if regular and monomorphic, consider antiarrhythmic infusion, and obtain expert consultation. Antiarrhythmic infusions for stable wide-QRS tachycardia consist of procainamide, amiodarone, and sotalol. If the QRS complex is narrow, perform vagal maneuvers, administer adenosine (if regular), beta blockers, or calcium channel blockers, and obtain expert consultation.

123. **When is it appropriate to give adenosine for wide-complex tachycardia?**
Adenosine may be given in cases of regular, monomorphic wide-complex tachycardia. However, one should avoid adenosine in cases of irregular, wide-complex tachycardia as it may cause degeneration into ventricular fibrillation.

124. **What are the reversible causes of the ACLS protocol?**
Commonly known as the H's and T's. These are factors that may be causing or may be contributing to cardiac arrest, bradycardia, or tachycardia. They include:
- H's: Hypovolemia, Hypoxia, Hydrogen ion (acidosis), Hypo/Hyperkalemia, Hypothermia
- T's: Tension pneumothorax, Tamponade (cardiac), Toxins, Thrombosis (pulmonary or coronary)

125. **For maternal cardiac arrest, what are the unique reversible causes specific for this demographic?**
The causes form the acronym BEAU–CHOPS: Bleeding/DIC, Embolism (coronary/pulmonary/amniotic fluid), Anesthetic complications, Uterine atony, Cardiac disease, Hypertension (preeclampsia/eclampsia), Other, Placenta aburptio/previa, Sepsis.

126. **What is the Cincinnati Prehospital Stroke Scale?**
A system developed to predict if a stroke occurred. The test centers around three observations: facial droop, arm drift, and speech. If any one of these three is abnormal, the probability of stroke is 72%.

127. **What is the Suspected Stroke Algorithm?**
This is a time-sensitive protocol designed to preserve vital brain tissue in a patient suspected of having a stroke. The first step is identifying the signs and symptoms of a stroke. The EMS team should perform a prehospital stroke assessment and determine time of symptom onset. The patient should be transported to a stroke center; the center should be notified that the patient is en route. Once the patient enters the emergency department (ED), ABC's, vitals, IV access, glucose levels, neurologic screening, 12-lead ECG, CT scan, and activation of the stroke team should be performed within 10 minutes. Within 45 minutes the CT scan should be reviewed and a determination must be made: is there hemorrhage or no hemorrhage? If hemorrhage is found, a neurosurgeon should be notified for possible surgical intervention. If no hemorrhage is found, acute ischemic stroke is likely and fibrinolytic therapy should be considered. The checklist for fibrinolytic exclusion criteria must be completed. If no contraindications to fibrinolytic therapy, it should be administered within 60 minutes of arrival at the ED. If not a candidate for fibrinolytic therapy, then administer ASA. Regardless of pathway, BP monitoring must be performed frequently. Serial neurologic exams must be performed. All patients who sustain a stroke must be admitted to a stroke unit or ICU.

128. **What are the time limit goals for acute ischemic stroke?**
Three hours from the onset of symptoms to fibrinolytic therapy. For a select group of patients the fibrinolytic treatment goal limit may be extended to 3 to 4.5 hours. Similar to PCI for ACS patients, fibrinolytic therapy response for acute ischemic stroke patients should be initiated as soon as possible to minimize the damage to brain parenchyma. Patients with suspected strokes should be transported to a comprehensive stroke center for optimal outcomes.

129. **According to the AHA, what are the absolute contraindications to fibrinolytic therapy?**
Prior intracranial bleeding, known cerebral vascular lesion, known malignant intracranial mass, suspected aortic dissection, active bleeding, significant facial/head trauma within 3 months, and ischemic stroke within 3 months, with the exception of an acute ischemic stroke within 3 hours.

130. For unstable atrial fibrillation, what is the recommended voltage for synchronized cardioversion?
Initial biphasic energy dose is between 120 and 200 J.

131. For unstable supraventricular tachycardia or unstable atrial flutter, what is the recommended energy dose for synchronized cardioversion?
50 to 100 J.

132. For monophasic waveforms, what is the recommended energy dose for synchronized cardioversion?
An initial dose of 200 J. One should increase the energy in regular intervals if no response is seen.

133. For unstable monomorphic ventricular tachycardia, what is the recommended energy dose for synchronized cardioversion?
An initial dose of 100 J. One should increase the energy in regular intervals if no response is seen.

ADVANCED TRAUMA LIFE SUPPORT†

134. In treating the seriously injured patient, what are the components of the appropriate systematic approach essential in instituting life preserving therapy?
Primary and secondary surveys are used for rapid, systematic, and thorough evaluation of the seriously injured patient.

135. What are the components of the primary survey?
The primary survey includes the ABCDE's: **A**irway maintenance with cervical spine protection, **B**reathing and Ventilation, **C**irculation with hemorrhage control, **D**isability (neurological status), **E**xposure/Environmental control (undressing patient completely while preventing hypothermia).

136. What are the components of the secondary survey, and when does it begin?
The secondary survey only begins once the primary survey is completed, resuscitative efforts are underway, and normalization of vital functions has been demonstrated. The secondary survey is a complete head-to-toe history and physical examination of the trauma patient. This includes a thorough exam of the skull, head, maxillofacial, neck, chest, abdomen, perineum/rectum/vagina, musculoskeletal system, and neurological system.

137. What is the useful mnemonic in aiding the complete medical assessment with the history of the mechanism of the injury?
The AMPLE history can be used for complete medical assessment as well as history of mechanism of the injury: **A**llergies, **M**edications currently used, **P**ast illnesses or **P**regnancy, **L**ast meal, **E**vents/**E**nvironment related to injury.

138. What assumption should be made regarding patients with maxillofacial or head trauma?
Patients with maxillofacial or head trauma should be presumed to have an unstable cervical spine injury. Therefore, these patients should have an immobilized neck until all aspects of the cervical spine are carefully and adequately studied.

139. When should a definitive airway be placed in the trauma patient?
If there is any doubt in the patient's ability to maintain airway integrity. Examples include an altered level of consciousness or a Glasgow Coma Scale (GCS) score of eight or less, severe maxillofacial trauma, risk for aspiration (bleeding/vomiting), and risk for obstruction (neck hematoma, laryngeal/tracheal injury, or stridor).

140. What are the initial radiographic studies obtained for the blunt trauma patient?
Anteroposterior (AP) chest, AP pelvic, and cervical spine films should be obtained and can guide resuscitation efforts in patients with blunt trauma.

---

†Written by John Wessel and Shahid R. Aziz.

141. **What are the signs of laryngeal fracture?**
Although fracture of the larynx is a rare injury, it can present with acute airway obstruction. The triad of clinical signs is hoarseness, subcutaneous emphysema, and palpable fracture.

142. **How is proper endotracheal tube placement confirmed?**
Proper position of the tube is best confirmed by chest X-ray once the possibility of esophageal intubation is excluded. A carbon dioxide detector is indicated to help confirm proper intubation of the airway. Proper placement of the tube is suggested but not confirmed by hearing equal and bilateral breath sounds.

143. **How many intravenous (IV) catheters should be introduced in the trauma patient?**
A minimum of two large caliber IV catheters should be introduced in the trauma patient.

144. **What determines the maximum rate of fluid administration through a catheter?**
The maximum rate of fluid administration is determined by the internal diameter of the catheter and inversely by its length. The size of the vessel into which the catheter is placed has no effect on flow rate.

145. **What is the optimal urinary output for adult and pediatric trauma patients?**
In an adult patient, urinary output should be at least 0.5 mL per kilogram per hour. In the pediatric patient older than age 1, it should be 1 mL per kilogram per hour.

146. **What is the definition of shock?**
Shock is an abnormality of the circulatory system that results in inadequate organ perfusion and tissue oxygenation.

147. **What are the most common forms of shock encountered in trauma patients?**
Most patients in shock are hypovolemic, but they may also suffer from neurogenic, obstructive, cardiogenic, or septic shock.

148. **What is the earliest measurable circulatory sign of shock?**
Tachycardia is the earliest measurable circulatory sign of shock. The release of endogenous catecholamines increases peripheral vascular resistance. This increases diastolic blood pressure and reduces pulse pressure but does not increase organ and tissue perfusion.

149. **Why do pediatric patients with hemorrhagic injuries deteriorate rapidly?**
The ability for a pediatric patient to compensate in the beginning phases of blood loss due to their abundant physiologic reserve may create an illusion of hemodynamic stability, resulting in inadequate fluid or blood product resuscitation and rapid deterioration.

150. **What is cardiogenic shock?**
Cardiogenic shock occurs when the blood flow decreases due to an intrinsic defect in cardiac function in either the heart muscle or the heart valves. A classic example is an acute myocardial infarction resulting in ischemic damages to the heart muscle impeding cardiac contractility. The decreased contractility causes a decrease in stroke volume, resulting in decreased cardiac output and blood pressure; high left ventricular filling pressures (backward failure); increased systemic vascular resistance (from vasoconstriction, which is a sympathetic compensatory response to the low blood pressure); and increased heart rate (sympathetic compensatory response to the low blood pressure). Other features of cardiogenic shock, such as cool extremities, decreased urine output, and sweating, may also be explained by the sympathetic compensatory response.

151. **How is hemorrhage classified?**
There are four classes of hemorrhage: **Class I** hemorrhage is where the patient has up to 15% blood volume loss (up to 750 mL). The clinical symptoms are minimal and crystalloid is the initial fluid replacement. **Class II** hemorrhage is where the patient has between 15% and 30% blood volume loss (750 to 1500 mL). Clinically, the patient has a slightly increased pulse rate (100 to 120) and respiratory rate (20 to 30 beats/min). Crystalloid is the initial fluid replacement therapy. **Class III** hemorrhage is a complicated hemorrhagic state where the patient has between 30% and 40% (1500 to 2000 mL). Clinically, the patient has an even increased pulse rate (between 120 and 140), as well as an increased respiratory rate (30 to 40 bpm). This patient will require both crystalloid infusion and blood product replacement. In **Class IV** hemorrhage where the patient lost

greater than 40% total blood volume (greater than 2000 mL), the patient will deteriorate very quickly unless aggressive measures are taken. This patient is considered preterminal and may die within minutes. Clinically, the pulse rate is >140 and respirations are >35 beats/min.

152. **What are the urinary outputs expected in each stage of hemorrhagic shock in mL/hr?**
Class I is 30 mL; Class II is 20 to 30 mL; Class III is 5 to 15 mL; Class IV is negligible.

153. **What are the steps in a Rapid Sequence Intubation?**
    1. Prepare for the need for a possible surgical airway.
    2. Prepare section and the ability to deliver positive pressure ventilation.
    3. Preoxygenate the patient with 100% oxygen.
    4. Apply cricoid pressure.
    5. Administer an induction agent or sedation, according to local practice.
    6. Administer IV succinylcholine (1 to 2 mg per kilogram).
    7. Direct laryngoscopy and intubation of the patient.
    8. The endotracheal tube cuff is inflated and tube placement is confirmed by equal and bilateral breath sounds on auscultation. An end-tidal CO_2 detector is used at this point if available.
    9. Cricoid pressure is released.
    10. The patient is ventilated.

154. **Why is etomidate (Amidate) the drug of choice for sedation for intubation of the trauma patient?**
Etomidate is more cardio-stable, not having a significant effect on blood pressure or intracranial pressure. Etomidate inhibits adrenal steroidogenesis; repeated doses should not be used because of the risk of adrenal suppression.

155. **In which patient is a surgical cricothyroidotomy contraindicated?**
Children (under age 11), crush injury to larynx, and known preexisting laryngeal or tracheal pathology are generally contraindications to surgical cricothyroidotomy.

156. **What is a tension pneumothorax?**
A tension pneumothorax is a true surgical emergency that requires immediate diagnosis and treatment. A tension pneumothorax develops when there is a violation of the visceral space and the visceral pleura acts as a one-way valve, allowing air to escape into the pleural space. As the pneumothorax expands, the diaphragm is pushed downward and the mediastinum is shifted to the contralateral hemithorax. This causes impaired venous return and a decline in cardiac output.

157. **How is a tension pneumothorax diagnosed?**
Diagnosis of a tension pneumothorax should be made based on clinical evaluation.

158. **What are some signs or symptoms of a tension pneumothorax?**
Acute respiratory distress, subcutaneous emphysema, absent breath sounds, hyperresonance to percussion, and tracheal deviation support the diagnosis of a tension pneumothorax.

159. **What is the treatment of a tension pneumothorax?**
A tension pneumothorax requires immediate thoracic decompression and is managed initially by rapidly inserting a needle into the second intercostal space along the mid-clavicular line of the affected hemithorax.

160. **What are epidural and subdural hematomas and how do they differ?**
These hematomas are focal brain lesions. **Epidural** hematomas are neurosurgical emergencies and occur in 0.5% of all brain-injured patients. They are located outside the dura but within the skull and are typically biconvex or lenticular in shape. They are typically caused by laceration of an anterior or posterior division of the middle meningeal artery and are most often located in the temporal or temporoparietal region; less commonly they can be caused by laceration over a large intracranial venous sinus with resultant accumulation of blood in the epidural space. **Subdural** hematomas occur in approximately 30% of severe brain injuries. These brain injuries result from hemorrhage into the subdural space from laceration of the bridging veins, laceration of a cortical vessel, or laceration of the cortex itself and commonly cover the entire surface of the hemisphere. An acute subdural hematoma usually results in much more severe brain damage than an epidural hematoma.

161. What are the clinical characteristics and presentations of an epidural hematoma?
    - Loss of conscious state followed by an intervening lucid interval
    - Secondary depression of consciousness
    - Development of hemiparesis on the contralateral side
    - A fixed and dilated pupil on the ipsilateral side of the impact area

162. What is the Glasgow Coma Scale (GCS)?
    The Glasgow Coma Scale provides a quantitative measure of the patient's level of consciousness. The GCS is scored between 3 and 15, with 3 being the worst and 15 the best. This scale is composed of three parameters: eye response, verbal response, and motor response.
    Best Eye Response:
    No eye opening: one point
    Eye opening to pain: two points
    Eye opening to verbal command: three points
    Eyes open spontaneously: four points
    Best Verbal Response:
    No verbal response: one point
    Incomprehensible sounds: two points
    Inappropriate words: three points
    Confused, but able to answer questions: four points
    Orientated: five points
    Best Motor Response:
    No motor response: one point
    Extension to pain: two points
    Flexion to pain: three points
    Withdrawal from pain: four points
    Localizing pain: five points
    Obeys commands: six points

163. How is GCS used to classify the severity of the brain-injured patient?
    - Mild head injury: GCS of 14 to 15
    - Moderate head injury: GCS of 9 to 13
    - Severe head injury: GCS score of eight or less

164. What is focused assessment sonography (FAST) and its indications?
    FAST is a rapid bedside ultrasound exam performed to identify intraperitoneal hemorrhage or pericardial tamponade. FAST examines four areas for free fluid: perihepatic and hepatorenal space, perisplenic, pelvis, and pericardium. FAST assessment is indicated in trauma patients who have a history of abdominal trauma, are hypotensive, or are unable to provide a reliable history because of impaired consciousness resulting from head injury or drugs. FAST is an adjunct to the ATLS primary survey and therefore follows the performance of the ABCs.

165. What is diagnostic peritoneal lavage (DPL) and its indications?
    DPL involves passing a small catheter into the peritoneal cavity, usually at the umbilicus just inferior to it (3 to 4 cm). If blood can be aspirated through this catheter, this is referred to as a diagnostic positive aspiration (DPA). If no blood can be aspirated, a liter of warm crystalloid solution is run into the peritoneal cavity and then allowed to drain out by gravity after sitting for 5 to 10 min. This lavage fluid is then sent to the lab for analysis of red blood cell count, white blood cell count, and any bowel contents. A rule of thumb for a positive DPL is the inability to read newsprint through the lavage fluid. Further surgical intervention is required if lab results of the submitted specimen indicate that the presence of 100,000 RBCs/mm^3 or more, and > WBCs/mm^3. DPL is used as an alternative to the FAST scan to identify intraperitoneal hemorrhage in blunt abdominal trauma. The role of DPL in the hemodynamically normal patient with penetrating abdominal injury is to identify hollow viscus injury (stomach, small bowel, or colon) or diaphragmatic injury. The primary disadvantages of the DPL are that it is invasive, does not evaluate the retroperitoneum, and has a significant false positive rate.

166. What is spinal shock?
    Loss of reflexes and flaccidity, seen after spinal cord injury. Owing to shock, the injured cord may appear completely functionless, although all areas are not necessarily destroyed.

167. What are the classifications of spinal cord injuries?
    1. Level
    2. Severity of neurologic deficit
    3. Spinal cord syndrome
    4. Morphology

168. What are the most common spinal cord syndromes?
    - **Central cord syndrome:** identified by greater loss of motor function in the upper extremities than the lower extremities, with varying sensory loss
    - **Anterior cord syndrome:** identified by paraplegia with loss of temperature and pain sensation

169. What are three proper ways for assessment of the trauma patient's extremities?
    1. **Primary survey:** identification of life-threatening injury
    2. **Secondary survey:** identification of limb-threatening injuries
    3. **Continuous reevaluation:** systematic review to decrease the chances of missing any other musculoskeletal injury

170. What is the most common cause of cardiac arrest in the pediatric patient?
    Hypoxia is the most common cause of cardiac arrest in the pediatric patient. Before cardiac arrest, hypoventilation causes a respiratory acidosis, which is the most common acid–base abnormality during resuscitation of the pediatric trauma patient.

171. What are the different degrees of thermal burns?
    - **First-degree burn:** It is identified by erythema with absence of blisters.
    - **Second-degree burn (partial-thickness burn):** It is identified by a mottled or erythematous appearance with swelling and blister formation. The surface may be wet and weeping; it is painful and hypersensitive.
    - **Third-degree burn (full-thickness burn):** It is identified by skin that appears dark, translucent, leathery, and mottled. The surface does not blanch with pressure. The skin is dry, painless, and red.
    It is important to ascertain the depth of a burn to properly plan for wound care and predict cosmetic and functional outcome.

BIBLIOGRAPHY

Basic Life Support

Berg RA, Hemphill R, et al.: Part 5: Adult Basic Life Support: 2010 American Heart Association Guidelines for Cardiopulmonary Resuscitation and Emergency Cardiovascular Care, *Circulation* 122:S685–S705, 2010.

Hazinki MF, Hunter-Wilson SL, editors: *BLS for healthcare providers manual*, Dallas, TX. American Heart Association, 2011.

Hellevo H: Deeper chest compression: more complications for cardiac arrest patients? *Resuscitation* 84:760–765, 2013.

Highlights of the 2010 American Heart Association Guidelines for Cardiopulmonary Resuscitation and Emergency Cardiovascular Care, Dallas, TX, American Heart Association, 2010.

Ohgali MA: Basic Life Support. In Abubaker O, Benson K, editors: *Oral and maxillofacial surgery secrets*, ed 2, Philadelphia, 2007.

Advanced Cardiac Life Support

Arrich J, Holzer M, Havel C, et al.: Hypothermia for neuroprotection in adults after cardiopulmonary resuscitation, *Cochrane Database Syst Rev* 9:CD004128, 2012.

Brindley PG, Markland DM, Mayers I, et al.: Predictors of survival following in-hospital adult cardiopulmonary resuscitation, *Can Med Assoc J* 167:343–348, 2002.

Chan PS, Krumholz HM, Nichol G, et al.: Delayed time to defibrillation after in-hospital cardiac arrest, *N Engl J Med* 358:9–17, 2008.

Danciu SC, Klein L, Hosseini MM, et al.: A predictive model for survival after in-hospital cardiopulmonary arrest, *Resuscitation* 62:35–42, 2004.

Dager WE, Sanoski CA, Wiggins BS, et al.: Pharmacotherapy considerations in advanced cardiac life support, *Pharmacotherapy* 12:1703–1729, 2006.

Girotra S, Nallamothu DK, Spertus JA, et al.: Trends in survival after in-hospital cardiac arrest, *N Engl J Med* 367:1912–1920, 2012.

McEvoy MD, Field LC, Moore HE, et al.: The effect of adherence to ACLS protocols on survival of event in the setting of in-hospital cardiac arrest, *Resuscitation* 85:82–87, 2013.

Paradis NA, Harken AH: Cardiopulmonary resuscitation. In Harken AH, Moore EE, editors: *Abernathy's surgical secrets*, ed 5, Philadelphia, 2005, Mosby.

Rajab BM, Banks KA: Advanced cardiac life support. In Abubaker O, Benson KJ, editors: *Oral and maxillofacial surgery secrets*, Philadelphia, 2007, Mosby/Elsevier.

Sinz E, Navarro K, Soderberg E, et al.: *Advanced cardiovascular life support provider manual*, Dallas, American Heart Association, 2011.

Advanced Trauma Life Support

Advanced Trauma Life Support Student Course Manual, ed 9, American College of Surgeons, 2012.

Kozlovsky E, Aziz SR: Advanced trauma life support. In Abubaker O, Benson KJ, editors: *Oral and maxillofacial surgery secrets*, Philadelphia, 2007, Mosby/Elsevier.

Kress TD, et al.: Cricothyroidotomy, *Ann Emerg Med* 11:197, 1982.

Mattox KL, Feliciano DV, Moore EE: *Trauma*, ed 7, McGraw-Hill, 2012.

CHAPTER 15

TRACHEOSTOMY AND CRICOTHYROTOMY

Andrew Yampolsky, Shahid R. Aziz, A. Omar Abubaker

1. **What are the different methods of achieving and securing an airway in an emergency?**
   Securing the airway is of paramount importance in both emergencies and critically ill patients. A simple chin lift and jaw thrust will relieve airway obstruction in most patients. If a patient is unable to generate adequate respiratory effort on his or her own, bag mask ventilation is attempted first. Oral and nasal airways may be used in conjunction with these techniques to assist in providing adequate ventilation. To definitively secure an airway, endotracheal intubation is performed. In certain situations, oral intubation is unsuccessful or contraindicated, such as in severe panfacial trauma, massive upper airway bleeding, spasm of facial muscles, and laryngeal stenosis or deformities of the oronasopharynx. A surgical airway (whether by needle or surgical technique) must be performed, thus bypassing any possible area of obstruction.

2. **What are the advantages of cricothyrotomy?**
   Cricothyrotomy should be viewed as the method of choice in procuring a patent airway in patients with acute airway obstruction that fail traditional intubation. It is faster and is technically easier to perform with minimal instrumentation in an emergency setting and with low incidence of operative and postoperative complications.

3. **What anatomy is pertinent to cricothyrotomy?**
   The thyroid cartilage consists of two quadrilateral laminae of hyaline cartilage that fuse anteriorly. The anterosuperior edge of the thyroid cartilage, the laryngeal prominence, is known as the Adam's apple. The angle at which these laminae converge is more acute in men than women and therefore is more easily located in men. The thyroid prominence is the most important landmark in the neck when performing a cricothyrotomy. The next cartilaginous ring below the larynx (and the only complete ring) is the cricoid cartilage. It helps to maintain the laryngeal lumen and forms the inferior border of the cricothyroid membrane. This membrane, another important landmark, is a dense fibroelastic membrane located between the thyroid cartilage superiorly and the cricoid cartilage inferiorly and bounded laterally by the cricothyroid muscles. It is approximately 22 to 30 mm wide, 9 to 10 mm high, and 13 mm inferior to the vocal cords. This membrane can be identified by palpating a notch (a slight indentation or dip) in the skin inferior to the laryngeal prominence in an adult. Although the right and left cricothyroid arteries (branches of the right and left superior thyroid arteries, respectively) traverse the superior part of the cricothyroid membrane, these vessels are not of clinical significance or the cause of problems when performing a cricothyrotomy.

   The tissue layers involved in cricothyrotomy include the subcutaneous tissue, cervical fascia, cricothyroid membrane, and tracheal mucosa. The distance from skin to tracheal lumen is only 10 mm in most adult patients. In contrast to the main body of the trachea, the posterior wall at this level of the upper airway is rigidly separated from the esophagus by the tall posterior cricoid cartilage shield, making esophageal perforation unlikely during cricothyrotomy. The highly vascular thyroid gland lies over the trachea at the level of the second and third tracheal rings. If the tracheal rings or the thyroid gland is encountered when performing a cricothyrotomy, the incision is too low in the neck and must be redirected more superiorly.

4. **What is the cricothyrotomy technique?**
   If there are no known or suspected cervical spine injuries, the patient's head may be hyperextended. Identify and palpate the notch or dip in the neck below the laryngeal prominence. Once the pertinent landmarks are identified, the right-handed surgeon then stabilizes the thyroid cartilage between the thumb and middle finger of his left hand and identifies the cricothyroid space with his left index finger. If local anesthetic is used, it should also be injected into the tracheal lumen to diminish the cough

reflex during tube placement. A 3- to 4-cm transverse or vertical skin incision is made. A vertical incision is preferred in an emergency situation because if the skin incision is too high or too low, it may be extended easily, saving time and avoiding a second incision. A short, horizontal stab incision (about 1 cm long) is made with a No. 11 blade in the lower part of the cricothyroid membrane (nearer the cricoid ring) to avoid the cricothyroid arteries. Mayo scissors are spread horizontally in the incision to widen the space. Alternatively, the handle of the scalpel may be inserted and twisted 90 degrees. Next, the opening is enlarged with Trousseau dilators or a curved hemostat. After stabilization of the larynx, the tracheostomy tube is inserted, the dilator or hemostat is removed, and the cuff of the tracheostomy tube is inflated (Fig. 15-1).

5. **What is percutaneous transtracheal jet ventilation (PTJV)?**
   PTJV is an option to provide temporary ventilation for a patient in situations when the equipment for a formal airway or skilled personnel are not available. A needle cricothyrotomy must first be performed. A large bore needle with an IV catheter (14 gauge) is attached to a small syringe with sterile saline and advanced through skin, subcutaneous tissues, and the cricothyroid membrane at a 45-degree

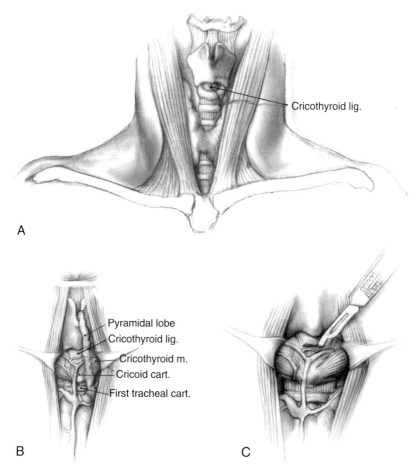

Cricothyroid lig.

A

Pyramidal lobe
Cricothyroid lig.
Cricothyroid m.
Cricoid cart.
First tracheal cart.

B   C

Figure 15-1. A and **B,** Surface anatomy and landmarks for cricothyroidotomy. **C,** A horizontal stab incision is made through the ligament. *(From Morris WM: Cricothyroidotomy. In Loré JM, Medina JE, editors:* An atlas of head and neck surgery, *ed 4, Philadelphia, 2005, Saunders.)*

angle until air is aspirated. The syringe and needle are then removed, and the IV catheter is left in place. A manual jet ventilator device is then attached and 100% oxygen is administered intermittently. This technique does not allow for adequate exhalation, as such CO_2 and airway pressure eventually builds up. Therefore, this should only be used as a temporizing measure until a definitive airway is established.

6. **When is a tracheostomy the preferred emergency surgical airway?**
In pediatric patients younger than ages 10 to 12. The pediatric airway is described as funnel shaped with the narrowest part below the cords as such entrance through the cricothyroid membrane may not bypass the airway obstruction. Furthermore, the small 3-mm-wide cricothyroid membrane and poorly defined anatomic landmarks make cricothyrotomy all but impossible in children.

7. **What are the surface anatomy landmarks for a tracheostomy?**
The most important anatomic landmarks for the tracheostomy procedure are the thyroid notch, cricoid ring, sternal notch, and innominate artery, which is above the sternal notch in approximately 25% of patients. The location for skin incision (approximately 4 to 6 cm long) for tracheostomy should be about 2 cm below the cricoid ring or midway between this ring and the sternal notch.

8. **From the skin to the trachea, what are the layers encountered during dissection for tracheostomy?**
   - Skin
   - Subcutaneous connective tissue
   - Platysma
   - Investing fascia
   - Line alba of the infrahyoid muscles
   - Thyroid isthmus
   - Pretracheal fascia
   - Tracheal rings

9. **What is the technique for performing a tracheostomy?**
A 4- to 6-cm incision is carried through skin, subcutaneous tissue, and platysma. Flaps are retracted superiorly, and a vertical incision is made in the fascia overlying the strap muscles. After the cricoid cartilage is identified, the thyroid isthmus may be retracted superiorly or divided and tied off. This exposes the second, third, and fourth tracheal rings. Using a hypodermic needle and a syringe, aspirate air from the trachea and inject 1 to 2 mL of local anesthetic to minimize coughing when entering the trachea. Make a 1-cm horizontal incision into the trachea above and below the ring of choice. This ring is cut so that a small rectangular window into the trachea is made. Place sutures in each side of the trachea to facilitate locating the tracheal stoma should the tube become dislodged. Insert the tracheostomy tube into the opening, taking care not to tear the cuff and not to insert the tube in the space anterior or lateral to the trachea. Once the tube is in place, inflate the cuff and check the chest for breath sounds. Leave the skin edges around the tube open or only partially closed with nonresorbable sutures, leaving a small space to minimize the danger of air escape into the subcutaneous tissue. Suture the tube to the skin, and secure it with a tape tied in a square knot around the neck (Fig. 15-2).

10. **What major vessels may be encountered during tracheostomy?**
The anterior jugular vein and the jugular venous arch are found in the suprasternal space of Burns. The infrahyoid vein and artery and thyroid artery all lie in the space between the pretracheal and infrahyoid fascia.

11. **Which tracheal rings are covered by the thyroid isthmus? What do you do if the thyroid is encountered during your dissection?**
The second through fourth rings. If the thyroid isthmus is encountered during dissection, it can be managed depending on surgeon preference. Some surgeons prefer to gently mobilize it and retract it caudally or cranially. Others ligate and divide it to prevent postoperative bleeding.

12. **What are the possible intraoperative complications associated with tracheostomy?**
    - **Hemorrhage:** The anterior jugular system and its anastomoses, thyroid isthmus, high aortic arch (elevated into the surgical field by hyperextension of the neck in children and elderly patients), thyroid veins and arteries, left innominate or brachiocephalic veins.

- **Subcutaneous emphysema:** This can result from a wound that has been closed too tightly around the tracheostomy tube, sutures that are placed after decannulation, or the tracheostomy tube being placed in a false passage.
- **Recurrent laryngeal nerve injury:** The laryngeal nerve innervates the trachea, esophagus, and all the intrinsic muscles of the larynx except the cricothyroid. Damage to this nerve produces vocal cord paralysis.

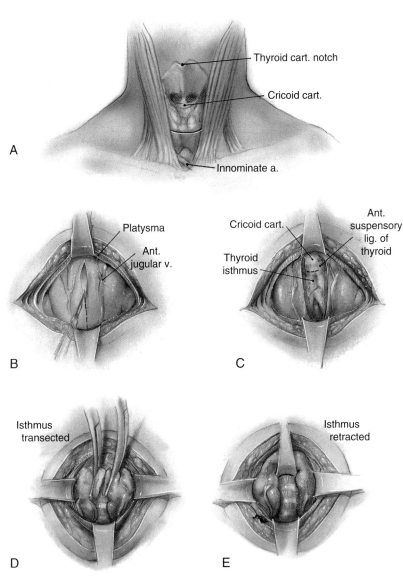

Figure 15-2. A, Surface anatomy landmarks for tracheostomy. **B,** After skin and platysma incisions are completed, a vertical incision is made in the fascia at midline between the strap muscles. **C,** The cricoid cartilage and thyroid isthmus exposed. **D-F,** The thyroid isthmus transected, retracted, and secured with ligature.

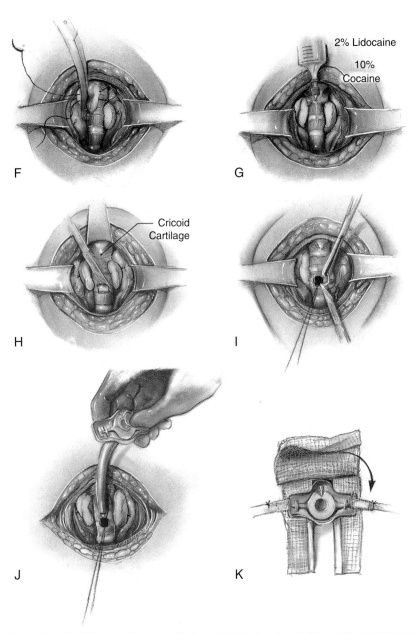

Figure 15-2, cont'd. G, Using a smaller gauge needle, air is aspirated into the syringe, 2% lidocaine (Xylocaine) is injected into the lumen of the trachea. **H** and **I,** A window is cut into the second, third, or fourth ring of the trachea. Alternatively, the ring is left pedicle inferiorly and sutured to the skin. **J** and **K,** The tracheostomy tube is inserted into the trachea and secured in place. *(From Loré JM: The trachea and mediastinum. In Loré JM, Medina JE, editors: An atlas of head and neck surgery, ed 4 Philadelphia, 2005, Saunders.)*

- **Pneumothorax or pneumomediastinum:** These are more common in pediatrics, in which the lung apex extends farther into the lower neck. They can also result from false passage of a tracheostomy tube between the anterior tracheal surface and the mediastinal tissues.
- **Other complications include:** insertion into a false passage, airway fire, laceration of the posterior tracheal wall, esophageal injury, loss of airway, aspiration, and even death

13. What are the possible postoperative complications associated with tracheostomy?
    - **Atelectasis.** This is caused if blood or foreign material is aspirated into the tube or if the tracheostomy tube is directed into one mainstem bronchus, resulting in collapse of the opposite lung.
    - **Tracheoesophageal fistula.** This rarely occurs in an orderly tracheostomy. It may accompany an emergency stab type of tracheotomy, or it may occur if an ill-fitting tracheostomy tube rubs against the posterior tracheal wall.
    - **Subglottic edema and tracheal stenosis.** These are preventable by entering the trachea below the second tracheal ring. The most common symptom is increasing stridor.
    - **Persistent fistula after decannulation.** Vertical incisions heal more rapidly than horizontal ones. This may require operative closure with resection of the tracheotomy tract.
    - **Tracheo-innominate fistula** resulting in devastating hemorrhage
    - **Other complications include:** vocal chord paralysis, dysphagia, tracheal stenosis, pneumonia, and difficult decannulation

14. What is the postoperative care for a tracheostomy?
    Once the tracheostomy procedure is completed, diligent postoperative care and observation are essential to prevent postoperative complications associated with this procedure. Both the surgeons and the nursing staff should supply this care, including:
    - Obtaining a chest X-ray within the immediate postoperative period to check the position of the tube and for presence of a pneumothorax
    - Using humidified air to keep the tracheal mucosa moist
    - Frequently suctioning the tracheostomy tube, because the tracheotomy reduces the efficiency of coughing, and initially there are more secretions from the trachea and mucous that may plug the tracheostomy tube and result in respiratory distress
    - Performing routine wound care and changing/cleaning the inner cannula or the tube itself
    - Removing the sutures once a tract is formed
    - Ensuring that the tube is appropriately secured and that the ventilator tubing is not abnormally pulling on the tube
    - Downsizing the tracheostomy and weaning the patient

15. What are the components of a typical tracheostomy tube? What kinds of tracheostomy tubes exist? How do you select a proper tracheostomy tube?
    See Figure 15-3 and Table 15-1.
    Tracheostomy tubes exist in a variety of styles and materials and are made by multiple manufacturers. Traditionally made from stainless steel, the so-called Jackson tracheostomy tubes are infrequently used currently. Modern tracheostomy tubes are typically made from polyvinyl chloride or silicone, which provide some degree of compliance and flexibility, allowing the tube to conform to the patient's anatomy.
    Tracheostomy tubes have a variety of variables in their construction that must be considered when selecting the proper tube, including outer diameter (OD), inner diameter (ID), curvature, proximal and distal length, presence of an inner cannula, presence of a cuff, type of cuff, and fenestration of the tube.
    Depending on the manufacturer, the tracheostomy tubes come in a variety of sizes. Table 15-1 is based off the traditional Jackson tubes and can be used as a rough guide, with the understanding that there is variation depending on the specific manufacturer.
    Proximal and distal length is an important consideration when selecting an appropriate tube. Longer proximal length "XLT" tubes are used in patients with a large neck circumference (i.e., obese patients). Longer distal length is used in patients with tracheal anomalies such as tracheomalacia. The internal diameter is a consideration in terms of facilitating airway clearance and minimizing resistance through the tube. Outer diameter is determined by the overall diameter of the patient's airway, taking into account the importance of being able to pass laryngeal air around the tube as is required for phonation. Fenestrated tubes are also often used by some clinicians in situations when the patient will need to phonate with a tracheostomy tube in place. The use of a tube with a cuff is determined

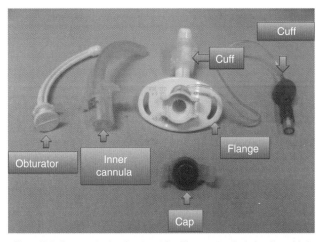

Figure 15-3. Components of tracheostomy tube. *(Photo courtesy Dr. Andrew Yampolsky.)*

Table 15-1. Jackson Tracheostomy Tube Size

JACKSON	ID WITH IC	ID WITHOUT IC	OUTER DIAMETER
Size	(mm)	(mm)	(mm)
4	5	6.7	9.4
6	6.4	8.1	10.8
8	7.6	9.1	12.2
10	8.9	10.7	13.8

by the patient's age, requirement of mechanical ventilation, and possible affects on aspiration. The general consensus is that cuffed tubes are contraindicated in the pediatric population because of a risk of affecting the development of the immature trachea and potential for long-term squalae such as tracheal stenosis. Cuffed tubes are often used during periods of mechanical ventilation. Generally speaking, it is easier to maintain proper hygiene of the airway when an interchangeable inner cannula is used; the inner cannula can be easily replaced when it becomes soiled with airway secretions or if an obstructive mucus plug develops.

16. **What are the indications for a tracheostomy? What are the benefits of an early tracheostomy?**

Commonly cited indications for the placement of a tracheostomy include: facilitating weaning from positive pressure ventilation in acute respiratory failure or prolonged ventilation, securing the airway in the upper respiratory tract where obstruction is a risk, facilitating removal of respiratory secretions, improved pulmonary toilet, decreased sedation requirements, improved patient comfort and mobility, to allow a patient to be weaned off mechanical ventilation quicker and in a less monitored setting, and to obtain an airway for patients with head and neck pathology or those undergoing head and neck surgery.

It was generally accepted that patients who were expected to require mechanical ventilation for 21 days or more have tracheostomies performed.

More recently, however, it is suggested that early tracheostomy (tracheostomy performed before day 10 of ICU admission) can be beneficial. Such benefits include reduced time of ventilation, hospitalization, and thus hospitalization cost This is likely due to decreased dead space of a tracheostomy, improved pulmonary toilet, decreased airway resistance, improved patient comfort, and ability to wean patients outside the critical care setting.

Generally speaking, early tracheostomies are recommended for patients who have anatomical anomalies that make emergent intubation difficult or impossible. These include many head and neck surgery patients and patients with head and neck infections causing trismus or airway obstruction.

17. **What is the purpose of downsizing a tracheostomy? How do you downsize a tracheostomy?**
The indications for downsizing a tracheostomy include improving patient comfort, reducing pressure on the tracheal mucosa, and facilitating the passage of air around the tracheostomy tube for speech. Typically, as a prerequisite, the patient should have had the tracheostomy in place for at least 7 to 10 days to ensure a proper track has formed, thus making tube exchange less risky. The patient must be hemodynamically stable, and off mechanical ventilation.

    It is prudent to have the patient in a monitored environment with pulse oximetry during the decannulation process. The patient should be preoxygenated and the tracheostomy tube and oropharynx suctioned to remove any secretions that may become dislodged when the cuff is deflated. The patient should be placed in a supine position with the neck extended. Any sutures or ties securing the tracheostomy tube are removed, the cuff, if present, is deflated, the old tube is removed at the peak of inspiration, and the new, smaller tracheostomy tube is inserted with the obturator in place. The new tracheostomy tube is secured, and the patient is monitored to ensure no respiratory distress is present. This procedure may also be performed over a tube exchanger to ensure that the tube is not placed in a false passage.

18. **What are the most common life-threatening postoperative complications of a tracheostomy?**
Hemorrhage, tube dislodgment, and tube obstruction.

19. **What are the possible causes of postoperative bleeding in tracheostomy patients?**
A small amount of bleeding from the tissues surrounding a recent tracheostomy is common and can usually be controlled with local measures such as pressure dressings around the tracheostomy tube. Continued bleeding that does not resolve may be an indication for surgical exploration. Tracheo-innominate fistula is a rare complication that may result in catastrophic hemorrhage.

20. **What do you do if a tracheostomy tube becomes dislodged?**
Management of accidental decannulation depends on an initial, rapid evaluation of the patient's oxygenation and ventilation status. If the patient is not in apparent respiratory distress, then one should carefully attempt reinserting a well-lubricated tube with the obturator in place; consideration should be given to inserting a smaller tube if available.

    In situations when the tracheostomy was placed recently and the tract is not yet fully formed, rapid replacement of the tube is paramount as the tract may collapse, making simple replacement of the tube impossible. If stay sutures are present, apply traction to bring the trachea anteriorly, facilitating insertion.

    If the patient is in respiratory distress, then one should administer supplemental oxygen and consider oral bag mask ventilation and orotracheal intubation.

    Ultimately, the most important factor is preventing dislodgment in the first place. This involves ensuring that an appropriately sized tube is selected, there is no excessive coughing or agitation, the tube is properly secured, and the patient is appropriately monitored.

21. **What do you do if a tracheostomy tube is obstructed?**
A possible cause of respiratory distress in a tracheostomy patient is tube obstruction. One must initially inspect the inner cannula; if any mucus plugging is noted, it can be readily replaced with a clean one. Continued respiratory distress may indicate that the tube has been displaced into a false passage or that there is an obstruction in the distal tube or trachea itself. A bedside maneuver that can be performed to further elucidate the nature of the distress is passing a soft suction catheter. If it passes easily and secretions are readily suctioned, that suggests that the tube was partially obstructed by secretions. If one is unable to pass the soft suction catheter more than a few centimeters, the tube may be lodged in a false passage or the tube itself may be clogged. In patients with immature stomas, the best course of action is to then secure the airway via an orotracheal tube, thus providing an opportunity to revise the tracheostomy.

22. **How do you identify and manage a tracheo-innominate (TI) fistula?**

    A TI fistula is one of the most life-threatening tracheostomy complications. Associated risk factors include overinflated cuff, high-pressure cuff, excessive movement of the tracheostomy, and caudal tracheostomy placement. The pathophysiology involves pressure of the cuff or tube on the tracheal mucosa, eventually eroding through the trachea and into the innominate (brachiocephalic) artery, which typically is located at the ninth tracheal ring. The complication most commonly occurs at the third to fourth postoperative week, and mortality approaches 100%.

    This complication is avoided by preventing prolonged hyperextension of the patient's neck, using lightweight tubing to avoid traction of the tracheostomy tube, and deflating the cuff when mechanical ventilation is no longer necessary.

    Early diagnosis is said to be the key to successful management. Many patients have sentinel hemorrhages that precede the devastating hemorrhage. These should be evaluated appropriately. A ridged bronchoscopy may be performed in a setting where potential intervention is possible. If inconclusive, angiography should be performed to further elucidate the vascular anatomy.

    In the event of an acute hemorrhage, an attempt must be made to control the hemorrhage at bedside. The cuff is overinflated, and the tube withdrawn with pressure directed at the anterior tracheal wall, in an attempt to occlude the innominate artery. If this fails, the patient should be orally intubated, the tracheostomy tube should be removed, and a finger can be used to bluntly dissect through the pretracheal fascia, attempting to occlude the artery against the anterior chest wall. If successful, the maneuvers can be used to help stabilize the patient during transport to the operating room for definitive management.

23. **What are the advantages of a percutaneous tracheostomy (PCT)?**

    The advantages of percutaneous techniques are that they use smaller incisions, cause potentially less tissue trauma, are potentially less invasive, are more readily performed at bedside in a critical care setting, and, according to some studies, have lower complication rates. There are multiple techniques described in the literature for performing a PCT, as well as several commercially available kits.

24. **What is the surgical technique for a percutaneous tracheostomy?**

    The patient is positioned, prepped, and draped in the same manner as for a standard tracheostomy, with the neck extended. Anatomical landmarks are identified, including the cricothyroid membrane and the sternal notch; ideally the entrance point into the trachea is to be at the second and third rings. A bronchoscope is then passed into the airway, and the tracheal anatomy is visualized. The bronchoscope is then used to monitor the placement of the introducer needle as well as subsequent dilation and eventual insertion of the tracheostomy tube.

    Local anesthesia with epinephrine is administered into the planned surgical site, and a 1-cm incision is made in the midline, through the skin and subcutaneous tissue. The introducer needle is then inserted at a 45-degree angle to the skin until air is aspirated. Care is taken to not advance the needle through the posterior wall of the trachea, and the needle introduction is simultaneously observed through the bronchoscope to ensure correct positioning.

    In what is referred to as the Seldinger technique, a guide wire is then passed through the introducer needle into the trachea. The needle is then removed, and a lubricated dilator is passed over the wire. Depending on the set used, there are variations in the dilator sequence and specific dilating instruments. The basic concept, however, remains unchanged. Once dilated to the appropriate diameter, the tracheostomy tube is inserted. Once in place, the ET tube is withdrawn, end-tidal CO_2 is confirmed, peak pressures and tidal volumes are confirmed, and the tracheostomy tube is secured. It is important to note that when performing a percutaneous tracheostomy, one must always be prepared to convert to a standard open tracheostomy in the event that complications occur.

25. **What is the purpose of the inner cannula, and how should it be cared for?**

    Inner cannulas should be regularly examined and cleaned both for hygiene as well as to prevent mucus plugging. Many clinicians recommend that they be checked several times daily. Mucus plugging is one possible cause of an airway emergency in a tracheostomy-dependent patient that can be easily mitigated by regular inner cannula changes.

26. **Do tracheostomy patients require speech and swallow evaluations prior to feeding? Does the inflated cuff prevent aspiration?**

    Currently, there is no evidence that placement of a tracheostomy results in increased rates of dysphagia and aspiration. Instead it appears that aspiration postoperatively is more dependent on the patient's preoperative status, prolonged mechanical ventilation, and associated comorbid conditions that may affect the swallowing mechanisms. As such, patients who do not have associated physical or cognitive deficits that might result in aspiration do not require a speech and swallow evaluation prior to resuming oral intake.

The inflated cuff does not provide much protection against aspiration, as secretions will eventually leak around the cuff unless frequently suctioned.

27. **What is the process of decannulation?**

Decannulation is the final step in weaning a patient from a tracheostomy and may occur when a patient no longer requires mechanical ventilation or airway protection. Typically a patient's tracheostomy tube is gradually downsized until translaryngeal air is able to pass around the tube to the point that it is possible to "cap" the tube without any evidence of respiratory distress. In situations when it is not expected that the patient will undergo further operations, it acceptable to remove the tracheostomy tube if the patient has been able to tolerate a "capped" tube for 48 hours. Immediately following removal of the tube, a dressing is placed on the stoma. One option is to use petroleum gauze secured with silk tape. The patient is instructed to apply pressure to the dressing when speaking or coughing, thus preventing the dressing from becoming dislodged. The dressing should be changed daily until the stoma closes over the next several days to weeks.

BIBLIOGRAPHY

Abubaker AO, Benson KJ: Tracheostomy and cricothyrotomy. In *Oral and maxillofacial surgery secrets*, ed 2, St Louis, 2007, Mosby Elsevier.

Allan JS, Wright CD: Tracheoinnominate fistula: diagnosis and management, *Chest Surg Clin N Am* 13:331, 2003.

Bradley PJ: Management of airway and tracheostomy. In Hibbert J, editor: *Otolaryngology: laryngology and head and neck surgery*, ed 6, Bath, England, 1997, Butterworth–Heinernann.

Braun RF, Cutilli BJ: Cricothyrotomy. In Braun RF, Cutilli BJ, editors: *Manual of emergency medical treatment for the dental team*, Baltimore, 1999, Williams & Wilkins.

Demas PN, Sotereanos GC: The use of tracheotomy in oral and maxillofacial surgery, *J Oral Maxillofac Surg* 46:483–486, 1988.

Engels PT, Bagshaw SM, Meier M, Brindley PG: Tracheostomy: from insertion to decannulation, *Can J Surg* 52:427, 2009.

Epstein SK: Late complications of tracheostomy, *Respir Care* 50:542, 2005.

Feinberg SE, Peterson LJ: Use of cricothyrotomy in oral and maxillofacial surgery, *J Oral Maxillofac Surg* 45:873–878, 1987.

Groves DS, Durbin Jr. CG: Tracheostomy in the critically ill: indications, timing and techniques, *Curr Opin Crit Care* 13:90, 2007.

Jones JW, Reynolds M, Hewitt RL, Drapanas T: Tracheo-innominate artery erosion: successful surgical management of a devastating complication, *Ann Surg* 184:194, 1976.

Koch T, Hecker B, Hecker A, et al.: Early tracheostomy decreases ventilation time but has no impact on mortality of intensive care patients: a randomized study, *Langenbecks Arch Surg* 397:1001, 2012.

Leder SB, Ross DA: Confirmation of no causal relationship between tracheotomy and aspiration status: a direct replication study, *Dysphagia* 25:35, 2010.

Lewis RJ: Tracheostomy. Indications, timing, and complications, *Clinic Chest Med* 13:137–149, 1992.

Lore JM: Emergency procedures. In Lore JM, Medina JE, editors: *An atlas of head and neck surgery*, ed 4, Philadelphia, 2005, Saunders.

Montgomery WW: *Surgery of the upper respiratory system*, ed 2, Philadelphia, 1989, Lea & Febiger.

Morris LL, Whitmer A, McIntosh E: Tracheostomy care and complications in the intensive care unit, *Crit Care Nurse* 33:18, 2013.

Parsons DS, Smith WC: Difficult tracheostomy decannulation. In Gates GA, editor: *Current therapy in otolaryngology head and neck surgery*, ed 6, St Louis, 1998, Mosby.

Patel RG: Percutaneous transtracheal jet ventilation: a safe, quick, and temporary way to provide oxygenation and ventilation when conventional methods are unsuccessful, *Chest* 116:1689, 1999.

Paul A, Marelli D, Chiu RC, Vestweber KH, Mulder DS: Percutaneous endoscopic tracheostomy, *Ann Thorac Surg* 47:314, 1989.

Plummer AL, Gracey DR: Consensus conference on artificial airways in patients receiving mechanical ventilation, *Chest* 96:178, 1989.

Stothert Jr JC, Stout MJ, Lewis LM, Keltner Jr RM: High pressure percutaneous transtracheal ventilation: the use of large gauge intravenous-type catheters in the totally obstructed airway, *Am J Emerg Med* 8:184, 1990.

Terk AR, Leder SB, Burrell MI: Hyoid bone and laryngeal movement dependent upon presence of a tracheotomy tube, *Dysphagia* 22:89, 2007.

Weissler MC: Tracheostomy and intubation. In Bailey BJ, editor: *Head and neck surgery–otolaryngology*, Philadelphia, 1993, J.B. Lippincott.

White AC, Kher S, O'Connor HH: When to change a tracheostomy tube, *Respir Care* 55:1069, 2010.

IV

MANAGEMENT CONSIDERATIONS FOR THE MEDICALLY-COMPROMISED PATIENTS

CARDIOVASCULAR DISEASES: ISCHEMIC HEART DISEASE, MYOCARDIAL INFARCTION, AND VALVULAR HEART DISEASE

David W. Lui, A. Omar Abubaker

1. **What are the known risk factors for the development of ischemic heart disease (IHD)?**
   Age, male gender, positive family history, hypertension, smoking, hypercholesterolemia, and diabetes mellitus. Sedentary lifestyle and obesity are often associated factors.

2. **What are the determinants of myocardial oxygen supply and demand?**
   Oxygen (O_2) supply to the myocardium is determined by oxygen content and coronary blood flow. Oxygen content can be calculated by the following equation:

$$O_2 \text{ content} = [1.39 \text{ mL } O_2/g \text{ of hemoglobin} \times \text{hemoglobin } (g/dL) \times \% \text{ saturation}] + [0.003 \times PaO2]$$

   Coronary blood flow occurs mainly during diastole, especially to the ventricular endocardium. Coronary perfusion pressure is determined by the difference between diastolic blood pressure and left ventricular end-diastolic pressure (LVEDP). Anemia, hypoxemia, tachycardia, diastolic hypotension, hypocapnia (coronary vasoconstriction), coronary occlusion (IHD), vasospasm, increased LVEDP, and hypertrophied myocardium all may adversely affect myocardial O_2 supply.

   Myocardial O_2 demand is determined by heart rate, contractility, and wall tension. Increases in heart rate increase myocardial work and decrease the relative time spent in diastole (decreased supply). Contractility increases in response to sympathetic stimulation, which increases O_2 demand. Wall tension is the product of intraventricular pressure and radius. Increased ventricular volume (preload) and increased blood pressure (BP) (afterload) both increase wall tension and O_2 demand.

3. **What is the pathophysiology of myocardial ischemia?**
   Ischemia occurs when coronary blood flow is inadequate to meet the needs of the myocardium. Atherosclerotic lesions that occlude 50% to 75% of the vessel lumen are considered hemodynamically significant. Non-stenotic causes of ischemia include aortic valve disease, left ventricular hypertrophy, ostial occlusion, coronary embolism, coronary arteritis, and vasospasm.

   The right coronary artery system is dominant in 80% to 90% of people and supplies the sino-atrial node, atrioventricular node, and right ventricle. Right-sided coronary artery disease often manifests as heart block and dysrhythmias. The left main coronary artery gives rise to the circumflex artery and left anterior descending artery, which supply the majority of the interventricular septum and left ventricular wall. Significant stenosis of the left main coronary artery (left main disease) or the proximal circumflex and left anterior descending arteries (left main equivalent) may cause severely depressed myocardial function during ischemia.

4. **What is the pathogenesis of a perioperative myocardial infarction?**
   A myocardial infarction (MI) is usually caused by platelet aggregation, vasoconstriction, and thrombus formation at the site of an atheromatous plaque in a coronary artery. Sudden increases in myocardial O_2 demand (tachycardia, hypertension) or decreases in O_2 supply (hypotension, hypoxemia, or anemia) can precipitate MI in patients with IHD. Complications of MI include dysrhythmias, hypotension, congestive heart failure (CHF), acute mitral regurgitation, pericarditis, ventricular thrombus formation, ventricular rupture, and death.

5. What clinical factors increase the risk of a perioperative MI following non-cardiac surgery?

IHD (prior MI or angina) and CHF are historically the strongest predictors of an increased risk for perioperative MI. Other risk factors include valvular heart disease (particularly aortic stenosis), arrhythmias caused by underlying heart disease, advanced age, type of surgical procedure, and poor general medical status. Hypertension alone does not place a patient at increased risk for perioperative MI, but these patients are at increased risk for IHD, CHF, and stroke.

6. How can cardiac function be evaluated on history and physical exam?

If a patient's exercise capacity is excellent even in the presence of IHD, then chances are good that the patient will be able to tolerate the stresses of surgery. Poor exercise tolerance in the absence of pulmonary or other systemic disease indicates an inadequate cardiac reserve. All patients should be questioned about their ability to perform daily activities, such as cleaning, yard work, shopping, and golfing, for example. The ability to climb two to three flights of stairs without significant symptoms (angina, dyspnea, syncope) is usually an indication of adequate cardiac reserve. Signs and symptoms of CHF including dyspnea, orthopnea, paroxysmal nocturnal dyspnea, peripheral edema, jugular venous distention, a third heart sound, rales, and hepatomegaly must be recognized preoperatively.

7. What is the significance of a history of angina pectoris?

Angina is a symptom of myocardial ischemia, and nearly all patients with angina have coronary artery disease. Stable angina is defined as no change in the onset, severity, and duration of chest pain for at least 60 days. Syncope, shortness of breath, or dizziness that accompanies angina may indicate severe myocardial dysfunction resulting from ischemia. Patients with unstable angina are at high risk for developing an MI and should be referred for medical evaluation immediately. Patients with diabetes mellitus and hypertension have a much higher incidence of silent ischemia. Perioperatively, most ischemic episodes are silent (as determined by ambulatory and postoperative electrocardiogram [ECG]) but probably significant in the final outcome of surgery.

8. Should all cardiac medications be continued throughout the perioperative period?

Patients with a history of IHD are usually taking medications intended to decrease myocardial oxygen demand by decreasing the heart rate, preload, or contractile state (beta blockers, calcium channel antagonists, nitrates) and to increase the oxygen supply by causing coronary vasodilation (nitrates). These drugs are generally continued throughout the perioperative period. Abrupt withdrawal of beta blockers can cause rebound increases in heart rate and BP. Calcium channel blockers can exaggerate the myocardial depressant effects of inhaled anesthetics but should be continued perioperatively.

9. What ECG findings support the diagnosis of IHD?

The resting 12-lead ECG remains a low-cost, effective screening tool in the detection of IHD. It should be evaluated for the presence of ST-segment depression or elevation, T-wave inversion, old MI as demonstrated by Q waves, disturbances in conduction and rhythm, and left ventricular hypertrophy. Ischemic changes in leads II, III, and aVF suggest right coronary artery disease, leads I and aVL monitor circumflex artery distribution, and leads V3-V5 look at the distribution of the left anterior descending artery. Poor progression of anterior forces suggests significant left ventricular dysfunction, possibly related to IHD.

10. What tests performed by medical consultants can help further evaluate patients with known or suspected IHD?

Exercise ECG is a noninvasive test that attempts to produce ischemic changes on ECG (ST depression = 1 mm from baseline) or symptoms by having the patient exercise to maximum capacity. Information obtained relates to the thresholds of heart rate and BP that can be tolerated. Maximal heart rates and BP response, as well as symptoms, guide interpretation of results.

Exercise thallium scintigraphy increases the sensitivity and specificity of the exercise ECG. The isotope thallium is almost completely taken up from the coronary circulation by the myocardium and can then be visualized radiographically. Poorly perfused areas that later refill with contrast delineate areas of myocardium at risk for ischemia. Fixed perfusion defects indicate infarcted myocardium.

Dipyridamole thallium imaging is useful in patients who are unable to exercise. This testing is frequently required in patients with peripheral vascular disease who are at high risk for IHD and limited by claudication. Dipyridamole is a potent coronary vasodilator that causes differential flow between normal and diseased coronary arteries detectable by thallium imaging.

Echocardiography can be used to evaluate left ventricular and valvular function and to measure ejection fraction. Stress echocardiography (dobutamine echo) can be used to evaluate new or worsened regional wall motion abnormalities in the pharmacologically stressed heart. Areas of wall motion abnormality are considered at risk for ischemia.

Coronary angiography is the gold standard for defining the coronary anatomy. Valvular and ventricular function can be evaluated and measurements of hemodynamic indices taken. Because angiography is invasive, it is reserved for patients who require further evaluation based on previous tests or who have a high probability of severe coronary disease.

11. **Based on the initial evaluation, which patients should be referred for further testing?**
Patients at risk for IHD but with good exercise tolerance may not require further work-up, especially if they are undergoing procedures with a low to moderate risk of perioperative MI. Patients with decreased exercise tolerance for unclear reasons or with unreliable histories should be evaluated with dipyridamole thallium testing.

Patients with documented IHD (prior MI or chronic, stable angina) with good exercise tolerance can sometimes proceed with low-risk surgery without further evaluation. Patients with known IHD and poor exercise tolerance should be referred for dipyridamole thallium testing or coronary angiography before all but the most minor surgical procedures.

12. **Which surgical procedures carry the highest risk of perioperative MI?**
In general, major abdominal, thoracic, and emergency surgeries carry the highest risk of perioperative MI. The highest risk non-cardiac procedure is aortic aneurysm repair. These patients have a high incidence of IHD, and cross-clamping of the aorta during surgery and postoperative complications can place great stress on the heart.

13. **How long should a patient with a recent MI wait before undergoing elective non-cardiac surgery?**
The risk of re-infarction during surgery after a prior MI has traditionally depended on the time interval between the MI and the procedure. The highest risk of re-infarction is between 0 and 3 months post-MI; lower risk is from 3 to 6 months; and a baseline risk level is reached after 6 months (approximately 5% in most studies). A study using discharge summaries demonstrated that the postoperative MI rate decreased substantially as the length of time from MI to operation increased (0 to 30 days = 32.8%; 31 to 60 days = 18.7%; 61 to 90 days = 8.4%; and 91 to 180 days = 5.9%), as did the 30-day mortality rate (0 to 30 days = 14.2%; 31 to 60 days = 11.5%; 61 to 90 days = 10.5%; and 91 to 180 days = 9.9%).

14. **What if surgery cannot safely be delayed for 6 months?**
The patient's functional status after rehabilitation from an MI is probably more important than the absolute time interval. Patients with ongoing symptoms may be candidates for coronary revascularization before their non-cardiac procedure. Patients who quickly return to good functional status after an MI can be considered for necessary non-cardiac surgery between 6 weeks and 3 months without undue added risk, due to the advance of percutaneous coronary intervention. According to 2014 American College of Cardiology/American Heart Association perioperative guidelines, ≥ 60 days should elapse after an MI before non-cardiac surgery in the absence of a coronary intervention.

15. **How is premedication useful in the setting of IHD and surgery?**
Patient anxiety can lead to catecholamine secretion and increased oxygen demand. In this regard, the goal of premedication is to produce sedation and amnesia without causing deleterious myocardial depression, hypotension, or hypoxemia. Morphine, scopolamine, and benzodiazepines, alone or in combination, are popular choices to achieve these goals. All premedicated patients should receive supplemental oxygen. Patients who use sublingual nitroglycerin should have access to their medication. Transdermal nitroglycerin can be applied in the perioperative period as well.

16. **What are the hemodynamic goals of induction and maintenance of general anesthesia in patients with IHD?**
The anesthesiologist's goal must be to maintain the balance between myocardial O_2 supply and demand throughout the perioperative period. During induction, wide swings in heart rate and BP should be avoided. Ketamine should be avoided because of the resultant tachycardia and hypertension. Prolonged laryngoscopy should be avoided, and the anesthesiologist may wish to blunt the

stimulation of laryngoscopy and intubation by the addition of opiates, beta blockers, or laryngotracheal or intravenous lidocaine.

Maintenance drugs are chosen with knowledge of the patient's ventricular function. In patients with good left ventricular function, the cardiac depressant and vasodilatory effects of inhaled anesthetics may reduce myocardial O_2 demand. A narcotic-based technique may be chosen to avoid undue myocardial depression in patients with poor left ventricular function. Muscle relaxants with minimal cardiovascular effects are usually preferred.

BP and heart rate should be maintained near baseline values. This can be accomplished by blunting sympathetic stimulation with adequate analgesia and aggressively treating hypertension (anesthetics, nitroglycerin, nitroprusside, beta blockers), hypotension (fluids, sympathomimetics, inotropic drugs), and tachycardia (fluids, anesthetics, beta blockers).

17. What monitors are useful for detecting ischemia intraoperatively?

The V5 precordial lead is the most sensitive single ECG lead for detecting ischemia and should be monitored routinely in patients at risk for IHD. Lead II can detect ischemia of the right coronary artery distribution and is the most useful lead for monitoring P waves and cardiac rhythm.

Transesophageal echocardiography can provide continuous intraoperative monitoring of left ventricular function. Detection of regional wall motion abnormalities with this technique is the most sensitive for myocardial ischemia.

The pulmonary artery occlusion (wedge) pressure gives an indirect measurement of left ventricular volume and is a useful guide for optimizing intravascular fluid therapy. Sudden increases in the wedge pressure may indicate acute left ventricular dysfunction resulting from ischemia. The routine use of pulmonary artery catheters in patients with IHD has not been shown to improve outcome. However, close hemodynamic monitoring (including pulmonary artery catheter data) may be beneficial, depending on the patient's condition and the nature of the surgical procedure.

18. What is the basic pathophysiology of valvular heart disease?

Mitral and aortic stenosis cause pressure overload of the left ventricle, which produces hypertrophy with a cardiac chamber of normal size. Mitral and aortic regurgitation causes volume overload, which leads to hypertrophy with a dilated chamber. The net effect of left-sided valvular lesions is an impedance to forward flow of blood into the systemic circulation. Although right-sided valvular lesions occur, left-sided lesions are more common and usually more hemodynamically significant. This chapter deals only with left-sided lesions.

19. What are common findings of the history and physical exam in patients with valvular heart disease?

A history of rheumatic fever, intravenous drug abuse, or heart murmur should alert the examiner to the possibility of valvular heart disease. Exercise tolerance is frequently decreased. Patients may exhibit signs and symptoms of CHF, including dyspnea, orthopnea, fatigue, pulmonary rales, jugular venous congestion, hepatic congestion, and dependent edema. Compensatory increases in sympathetic nervous system tone manifest as resting tachycardia, anxiety, and diaphoresis. Angina may occur in patients with a hypertrophied left ventricle, even in the absence of coronary artery disease. Atrial fibrillation frequently accompanies diseases of the mitral valve.

20. Which tests are useful in the evaluation of valvular heart disease?

The **EGC** should be examined for evidence of ischemia, arrhythmias, atrial enlargement, and ventricular hypertrophy. The **chest radiograph** may show enlargement of cardiac chambers, suggest pulmonary hypertension, or reveal pulmonary edema and pleural effusions. **Cardiac catheterization** is the gold standard in the evaluation of such patients and determines pressures in various heart chambers, as well as pressure gradients across valves. **Cardiac angiography** allows visualization of the coronary arteries and heart chambers.

21. How is echocardiography helpful?

Doppler echocardiography characterizes ventricular function and valve function. It can be used to measure the valve orifice area and transvalvular pressure gradients, which are measures of the severity of valvular dysfunction. The function of prosthetic valves is also measured echocardiographically.

22. Which invasive monitors aid the anesthesiologist in the perioperative period?

An arterial catheter provides beat-to-beat BP measurement and continuous access to the bloodstream for sampling. Pulmonary artery catheters enable the anesthetist to measure cardiac output and provide central access for the infusion of vasoactive drugs. The pulmonary capillary wedge pressure is an index of left ventricular filling and is useful for guiding intravenous fluid therapy. Transesophageal echocardiography can be used intraoperatively to evaluate left ventricular volume and function, to detect ischemia (segmental wall motion abnormalities) and intracardiac air, and to examine valve function before and after repair.

23. **What is a pressure–volume loop?**

A pressure–volume loop plots left ventricular pressure against volume through one complete cardiac cycle. Each valvular lesion has a unique profile that suggests compensatory physiologic changes by the left ventricle.

24. **What is the pathophysiology of aortic stenosis?**

Aortic stenosis is a fixed outlet obstruction to left ventricular ejection. Concentric hypertrophy (thickened ventricular wall with normal chamber size) develops in response to the increased intraventricular systolic pressure and increased wall tension necessary to maintain forward flow. Ventricular compliance decreases, and end-diastolic pressures increase. Contractility and ejection fraction are usually maintained until late in the disease process. Atrial contraction may account for up to 40% of ventricular filling (normally 20%). Aortic stenosis is usually secondary to calcification of a congenital bicuspid valve or rheumatic heart disease. Patients often present with angina, dyspnea, syncope, or sudden death. Angina occurs in the absence of coronary artery disease because the thickened myocardium is susceptible to ischemia (increased oxygen demand) and elevated end-diastolic pressure reduces coronary perfusion pressure (decreased oxygen supply).

25. **What is the pathophysiology of aortic insufficiency?**

Chronic aortic insufficiency is usually rheumatic in origin. Acute aortic insufficiency may be secondary to trauma, endocarditis, or dissection of a thoracic aortic aneurysm. The left ventricle experiences volume overload, because part of the stroke volume regurgitates across the incompetent aortic valve in diastole. Eccentric hypertrophy (dilated and thickened chamber) develops. A dilated orifice, slower heart rate (relatively more time spent in diastole), and increased systemic vascular resistance increase the amount of regurgitant flow. Compliance and stroke volume may be significantly increased in chronic aortic insufficiency, whereas contractility gradually diminishes. Ideally, such patients should have valve replacement surgery before the onset of irreversible myocardial damage. In acute aortic insufficiency, the left ventricle is subjected to rapid, massive volume overload with elevated end-diastolic pressures and displays poor contractility. Hypotension and pulmonary edema may necessitate emergent valvular replacement.

26. **What is the pathophysiology of mitral stenosis?**

Mitral stenosis is usually secondary to rheumatic disease. Critical stenosis of the valve occurs 10 to 20 years after the initial infection. As the orifice of the valve narrows, the left atrium experiences pressure overload. In contrast to other valvular lesions, the left ventricle shows relative volume underload resulting from the obstruction of forward blood flow from the atrium. The elevated atrial pressure may be transmitted to the pulmonary circuit and thus may lead to pulmonary hypertension and right-sided heart failure. The overdistended atrium is susceptible to fibrillation with resultant loss of atrial systole, leading to reduced ventricular filling and cardiac output. Symptoms (fatigue, dyspnea on exertion, hemoptysis) may be worsened when increased cardiac output is needed, as with pregnancy, illness, anemia, and exercise. Blood stasis in the left atrium is a risk for thrombus formation and systemic embolization.

27. **What is the pathophysiology of mitral regurgitation?**

Chronic mitral regurgitation is usually due to rheumatic heart disease, ischemia, or mitral valve prolapse. Acute mitral regurgitation may occur in the setting of myocardial ischemia and infarction with papillary muscle dysfunction or chordae tendineae rupture. In chronic mitral regurgitation, the left ventricle and atrium show volume overload, which leads to eccentric hypertrophy. Left ventricular systolic pressures decrease as part of the stroke volume escapes through the incompetent valve into the left atrium, leading to elevated left atrial pressure, pulmonary hypertension, and eventually right-sided heart failure. As in aortic insufficiency, regurgitant flow depends on valve orifice size, time available for regurgitant flow, and transvalvular pressure gradient. The valve orifice increases in size as the left ventricle increases in size. In acute mitral regurgitation, the pulmonary circuit and right side of the heart are subjected to sudden increases in pressure and volume in the absence of compensatory ventricular dilatation, which may precipitate acute pulmonary hypertension, pulmonary edema, and right-sided heart failure.

PERIOPERATIVE CONSIDERATIONS IN VALVULAR HEART DISEASE

28. What are the surgical risks for patients with valvular heart disease?

Patients with valvular heart disease present varying degrees of surgical risk, depending on the nature and severity of the valvular disease. The risk is generally one of three types:
1. Hemodynamic risk
2. Risk associated with medications taken for this disease
3. Risk of bacterial endocarditis

29. Is the following statement true or false? Patients with valvular stenosis are at greater surgical risk than those with valvular regurgitation.

True. Among patients with valvular heart disease, valvular stenosis poses higher risks intraoperatively than valvular regurgitation, although careful fluid management is important in both entities. Such management prevents increases in afterload and possibly pulmonary edema. In addition, patients with valvular stenosis are poorly tolerant of tachyarrhythmias, and care should be taken to avoid them.

30. What is the perioperative management of medications for valvular heart disease?

Patients with valvular heart disease, especially with mechanical valves, often receive anticoagulation therapy to render the prothrombin time at 1.3 to 1.5 times control, or an international normalized ratio (INR) of 2 to 3. When oral surgical procedures are to be performed on these patients, the risk of thromboembolism has to be weighed against the risks of postoperative hemorrhage. A decision should be made, in consultation with the patient's cardiologist, on stopping such medications.

In general, if the risk of thromboembolism is moderate, Coumadin can be stopped for 72 hours preoperatively and resumed the same or following day postoperatively. If the patient is at high risk for thromboembolic phenomena, then heparin can be started intravenously after Coumadin has been discontinued; heparin is discontinued 6 hours before surgery. Once hemostasis of the surgical site is assured, heparin and Coumadin can be resumed postoperatively, but close monitoring for evidence of hemorrhage is continued.

31. Which cardiac conditions require preoperative antibiotic prophylaxis for prevention of bacterial endocarditis?

1. Prosthetic cardiac valve or prosthetic material used for cardiac valve repair
2. Previous infective endocarditis
3. Congenital heart disease (CHD)
   a. Unrepaired cyanotic CHD, including palliative shunts and conduits
   b. Completely repaired congenital heart defect with prosthetic material or device, whether placed by surgery or by catheter intervention, during the first 6 months after the procedure
   c. Repaired CHD with residual defects at the site or adjacent to the site of a prosthetic patch or prosthetic device (which inhibit endothelialization)
4. Cardiac transplantation recipients who develop cardiac valvulopathy

32. Which dental and oral surgical procedures require preoperative antibiotic prophylaxis for prevention of bacterial endocarditis?

All dental procedures that involve manipulation of gingival tissue or the periapical region of teeth or perforation of the oral mucosa. The following procedures and events do not need prophylaxis: routine anesthetic injections through noninfected tissue, taking dental radiographs, placement of removable prosthodontic or orthodontic appliances, adjustment of orthodontic appliances, placement of orthodontic brackets, shedding of deciduous teeth, and bleeding from trauma to the lips or oral mucosa.

33. What are the different antibiotic prophylactic regimens for dental and oral surgical procedures?

See Table 16-1.

HYPERTENSION

34. What is hypertension?

Hypertension is a sustained elevated arterial blood pressure resulting from increased peripheral vascular resistance. An adult patient with a BP reading above 140/90 mm Hg is generally considered to be hypertensive.

Table 16-1. Antibiotic Prophylactic Regimens for Dental and Oral Surgical Procedures

SITUATION	AGENT	Regimen: Single Dose 30-60 Minutes Before Procedure	
		ADULTS	**CHILDREN**
Oral	Amoxicillin	2 g PO	50 mg/kg PO
Unable to take oral medication	Amoxicillin	2 g IM or IV	50 mg/kg IM or IV
	Cefazolin or Ceftriaxone	1 g IM or IV	50 mg/kg IM or IV
Allergic to penicillins or ampicillin (oral)	Cephalexin*	2 g PO	50 mg/kg PO
	Clindamycin	600 mg PO	20 mg/kg PO
	Azithromycin or Clarithromycin	500 mg PO	15 mg/kg PO
Allergic to penicillins or ampicillin and unable to take oral medication	Cefazolin or Ceftriaxone	1 g IM or IV	50 mg/kg IM or IV
	Clindamycin phosphate	600 mg IM or IV	20 mg/kg IM or IV

*Or other first- or second-generation oral cephalosporin in equivalent adult or pediatric dosage. Cephalosporins should not be used in an individual with a history of anaphylaxis, angioedema, or urticaria with penicillins or ampicillin.
IM, Intramuscularly; IV, intravenously; PO, orally.
Total children's dose should not exceed adult dose.
Adapted from Wilson W, Taubert KA, Gewitz M, et al.: Prevention of infective endocarditis: guidelines from the American Heart Association: a guideline from the American Heart Association Rheumatic Fever, Endocarditis, and Kawasaki Disease Committee, Council on Cardiovascular Disease in the Young, and the Council on Clinical Cardiology, Council on Cardiovascular Surgery and Anesthesia, and the Quality of Care and Outcomes Research Interdisciplinary Working Group, *Circulation* 116:1736–1754, 2007.

35. **What are the general categories of hypertension, based on the presentation and level of need for treatment?**
Hypertension clinically presents in one of four generally recognized settings: hypertensive emergencies, hypertensive urgencies, mild uncomplicated hypertension, and transient hypertensive episodes.

36. **What is the difference between hypertensive emergency and hypertensive urgency? How are these conditions managed?**
A hypertensive *emergency* is an increased BP with **end-organ damage or dysfunction**. The brain, heart, or kidneys may be affected. BP can be as high as systolic >210 mm Hg and diastolic >120 mm Hg. Treatments for a hypertensive emergency should be rapid and aggressive, attempting to lower the BP within 60 minutes in a controlled fashion.
   Hypertensive *urgency* is an elevation of BP to a potentially harmful level **without end-organ dysfunction**. Hypertensive urgency should be treated over a longer period (1 to 2 days).

37. **What is the difference between primary and secondary hypertension?**
Primary or essential hypertension is a sustained elevated BP of unknown etiology. Secondary hypertension is an elevated BP that results from an identifiable cause, such as renal artery stenosis; chronic renal parenchymal disease; aldosteronism/Cushing's syndrome; acromegaly; hypercalcemia; coarctation of the aorta; pheochromocytoma; or oral contraceptives.

38. **During the perioperative period, when are the highest mean arterial pressure (MAP) readings typically recorded?**
The highest MAP readings are typically observed in response to laryngoscopy and intubation. A single dose of a beta-adrenergic blocker 90 minutes before induction in a patient with hypertension has been shown to reduce intraoperative BP, myocardial ischemia, and postoperative morbidity.

39. **How is hypertension classified?**
There are different systems for classifying hypertension. For example, hypertension can be classified as high normal, mild, moderate, or severe based on the diastolic pressure alone (85-89, 90-104, 105-114, and >115, respectively). However, hypertension typically is classified based on both the

systolic and diastolic pressures into four stages. BP readings below these stages are considered either normal (<130 for systolic and <85 for diastolic) or high normal (130-139 for systolic and 85-89 for diastolic). The four stages of hypertension are:

Stage I (mild): 140-159 systolic and 90-99 diastolic
Stage II (moderate): 160-179 systolic and 100-119 diastolic
Stage III (severe): 180-209 systolic and 110-119 diastolic
Stage IV (very severe): >210 systolic and >120 diastolic

40. **What behavior modifications can help treat hypertension?**
Patients with hypertension are encouraged to modify their lifestyle. Weight loss (10 pounds or more in overweight people), limitation of alcohol intake to <1 oz/day for men and 0.5 oz for women, and aerobic physical activity for 30 to 45 minutes three to five times/week are recommended. Patients are also encouraged to maintain adequate intake of potassium, calcium, and magnesium; reduce sodium, fat, and cholesterol; and quit smoking. All these measures have been shown to lower BP (Table 16-2).

41. **What pharmacologic therapy exists for hypertension?**
Drug therapy for hypertension is based on the individual's needs and condition. For example, initial drug therapy for uncomplicated hypertension consists of diuretics and beta blockers. Beta blockers also may be prescribed for patients with hypertension after experiencing an MI. **Diuretics** can be used when there is concomitant CHF. **Calcium channel blockers** are recommended for older patients with IHD. **Angiotensin-converting enzyme (ACE) inhibitors** benefit hypertensive patients who have diabetes and proteinuria.
   Note: Nonsteroidal antiinflammatory drugs (NSAIDs) may reduce the efficacy of ACE inhibitors, diuretics, and beta blockers. However, the reduction appears to be more likely in the NSAID class, dose, and duration not commonly prescribed for oral and maxillofacial surgery procedures. In addition, calcium channel blockers may cause gingival hyperplasia similar to the hyperplasia associated with Dilantin used to treat epilepsy.

42. **Is it safe to administer local anesthesia with epinephrine to a hypertensive patient?**
Cartridges of local anesthetic as used in dentistry contain epinephrine concentrations of 1:50,000 (0.02 mg/mL), 1:100,000 (0.01 mg/mL), or 1:200,000 (0.005 mg/mL). One cartridge contains 1.8 mL solution of local anesthetic and epinephrine; therefore one cartridge with an epinephrine concentration of 1:100,000 contains 1.8 mL × 0.01 mg/mL or 0.018 mg of epinephrine. According to American Dental Association/American Heart Association guidelines, a patient with cardiovascular disease can receive up to 0.04 mg of epinephrine, or up to two cartridges of this epinephrine-containing lidocaine preparation.
   If, however, the patient has poorly controlled hypertension or an otherwise significant medical risk, then the use of epinephrine becomes a clinical judgment of risk vs. benefit and is performed on a case-by-case basis. These patients are medical risks, not only concerning epinephrine, but also because of their overall poor medical status.

43. **What is the Goldman Cardiac Risk Index? Which factors are most important in assigning risk?**
The Goldman Cardiac Risk Index was established based on the study of more than 1000 patients undergoing non-cardiac surgery who were evaluated preoperatively. The evaluation examined certain variables obtained from the history, physical exam, ECG, and general status (pulmonary, kidney, or liver disease) and factored in the type of operation to determine the risk factors that predispose a patient to a cardiac event.
   The cardiac risk index is based on a point system, and patients are assigned to four different cardiac risk index classes (Tables 16-3 and 16-4). According to this study, the presence of an S_3 heart sound, indicating heart failure or MI within the last 6 months, poses the greatest risk for a significant perioperative event.

44. **What are the different sympathetic nervous system receptors relative to hypertension and antihypertensive agents?**
These receptors are classified into two major categories: alpha and beta receptors. Each of these is further divided into two subdivisions: alpha-1 and alpha-2 receptors, and beta-1 and beta-2 receptors.
   • Alpha-1 site stimulation causes constriction of vascular smooth muscles and thus increases peripheral vascular resistance.

Table 16-2. Classification of Adult Blood Pressure and Treatment Modifications

CATEGORY	SYSTOLIC (mm Hg)	DIASTOLIC (mm Hg)	TREATMENT
Normal	<130	<85	No modification
High normal	130-139	85-89	No modification
Hypertension			
Stage I	140-159	90-99	No modification, medical referral, inform patient
Stage II	160-179	100-109	Selective care,* medical referral
Stage III	180-209	110-119	Emergent non-stressful procedures†
			Immediate medical referral or consultation
Stage IV	≥210	≥120	Emergent non-stressful procedures†
			Immediate medical referral

*Selective care may include but is not limited to atraumatic removal of teeth, biopsies, etc.
†Emergent non-stressful procedures may include but are not limited to procedures that alleviate pain, infection, or masticatory dysfunction. These procedures should have limited physiologic and psychological effects (e.g., incision and drainage of an abscess). In all cases, the medical benefit of the procedure should outweigh the risk of complications secondary to the patient's hypertensive state.

Table 16-3. Points Awarded for Cardiac Risk Factors

RISK FACTOR	POINTS
Third heart sound or jugular venous distention	11
Recent myocardial infarction	10
Rhythm other than sinus or premature atrial contractions on last ECG	7
>5 premature ventricular contractions/min at any time	7
Intraperitoneal, intrathoracic, or aortic operation	3
Age >70 years	5
Important aortic stenosis	3
Emergent operation	4
Poor general medical condition	3
PO_2 <60 or PCO_2 >50 mm Hg K^+ <30 mEq/L HCO_3^- <20 mEq/L Creatinine >3 mg/dL or BUN >50 mg/dL Chronic liver disease	

BUN, Blood urea nitrogen; ECG, electrocardiogram.
Adapted from Goldman L: Multifactorial index of cardiac risk in noncardiac procedures, N Engl J Med 297:945–950, 1977.

- Alpha-2 stimulation inhibits the release of norepinephrine (the negative feedback to sympathetic neurons).
- Beta-1 stimulation increases heart rate and the strength of cardiac contraction.
- Beta-2 stimulation causes dilatation of smooth muscles of the blood vessels and airway, relaxation of uterine smooth muscle, and a variety of endocrine effects, including secretion of renin.

45. Is the following statement true or false? There are six different categories of oral antihypertensive agents.

     False. Antihypertensive agents are generally classified into three major categories based on their mechanisms of action: diuretics, sympatholytics, and vasodilators (Table 16-5).

Table 16-4. Goldman Cardiac Risk Index

Class	Point total	NO OR ONLY MINOR COMPLICATION ($n=943$) (%)	LIFE-THREATENING COMPLICATIONS* ($n=39$) (%)	CARDIAC DEATHS ($n=19$) (%)
I ($n=537$)	0-5	532 (99)	4 (0.7)	1 (0.2)
II ($n=316$)	6-12	295 (93)	16 (5)	5 (2)
III ($n=130$)	13-25	112 (86)	15 (11)	3 (2)
IV ($n=18$)	>26	4 (22)	4 (22)	10 (56)

*Documented intraoperative or postoperative myocardial infarction, pulmonary edema, or ventricular tachycardia.
Adapted from Goldman L: Multifactorial index of cardiac risk in noncardiac procedures, *N Engl J Med* 297: 945–950, 1977.

Table 16-5. Categories and Classes of Oral Antihypertensive Agents

CATEGORY	CLASS	SUBCLASS	AGENT
Diuretics	Thiazide type		Chlorothiazide, chlorthalidone, hydrochlorothiazide, indapamide, metolazone
	Potassium-sparing		Spironolactone, triamterene, amiloride
	Loop		Bumetanide, ethacrynic acid, furosemide, torsemide
Sympatholytics	Adrenergic-receptor blockers	Beta	Acebutolol, atenolol, betaxolol, bisoprolol, carteolol, metoprolol, nadolol, penbutolol, pindolol, propranolol, timolol
		Alpha: alpha-1	Doxazosin, prazosin, terazosin
		alpha-1+ alpha-2	Phenoxybenzamine
		Alpha and beta	Labetalol
	Central alpha-2 agonists Postganglionic blockers		Clonidine, guanabenz, guanfacine, methyldopa Bethanidine, guanadrel, guanethidine, reserpine
Vasodilators	Calcium channel blockers	Benzothiazepines, Phenylalkylamines Dihydropyridines	Diltiazem, verapamil, amlodipine, felodipine, isradipine, nicardipine, nifedipine
	ACE inhibitors		Benazepril, captopril, enalapril, fosinopril, lisinopril, quinapril, ramipril
	Direct vasodilators		Hydralazine, minoxidil

Adapted from Dym H: The hypertensive patient. Therapeutic modalities, *Oral Maxillofac Clin North Am* 10:349–362, 1998.

46. What are the doses, mechanisms of action, and possible complications of commonly used antihypertensive agents?
    See Table 16-6.

47. What are the commonly used parenteral agents for treatment of hypertensive emergencies?
    See Table 16-7.

Table 16-6. Doses, Mechanisms of Action, and Possible Complications of Antihypertensive Drugs

AGENT AND DOSE	MECHANISM OF ACTION	POSSIBLE COMPLICATIONS
Diuretics		
Thiazide 25-50 mg/day	Increases urinary excretion of Na and water by inhibiting Na reabsorption in cortical diluting tubule in nephron; exact mechanism of antihypertension is unknown; may be partially from direct arteriolar vasodilation	Hypokalemia, dehydration, hyperglycemia, hyperuricemia, decreased lithium clearance
Loop diuretics 40-240 mg/day	Inhibits Na and chloride reabsorption in proximal ascending loop of Henle; also has renal and peripheral vasodilatory effects	Hypokalemia, dehydration, hypochloremic alkalosis
Spironolactone 50-100 mg/day	Potassium-sparing; competitively inhibits aldosterone effects on distal renal tubules (increases Na and water excretion); also may block aldosterone effect on vascular smooth muscle	Hyperkalemia, gynecomastia, dehydration
Central Antiadrenergics		
Alpha-methyldopa PO 500-2000 mg/day IV 250-500 mg over 30-60 minutes q6h	Metabolite (alpha-methylnorepinephrine) stimulates inhibitory alpha-adrenergic receptors and inhibits sympathetic nervous system outflow, thus decreasing total peripheral resistance	Sedation, hepatic dysfunction, lupus-like symptoms, rebound hypertension, positive Coombs' test
Clonidine PO 0.1-2.4 mg/day topical transdermal patch q7d	Stimulates inhibitory alpha-2 receptors and inhibits sympathetic outflow	Sedation, xerostomia, rebound HTN, 50% decrease in minimal alveolar concentrations of volatile anesthetics
Peripheral Antiadrenergics		
Prazosin (Minipress) 220 mg/day	Selective and competitive postsynaptic alpha-receptor blockade leads to arterioles and vasodilation	Alters test results for pheochromocytoma, false-positive test results for ANA, increased liver function tests
Terazosin (Hytrin) 1-5 mg/PO/day	Selectively inhibits alpha receptors in vascular smooth muscles; dilates both arteriolar and venules	Decreases hematocrit, hemoglobin, albumin, leukocytes, and total protein
Guanethidine (Ismelin) 100-300 mg/day	Peripherally inhibits alpha receptors and release of NE; depletes stores of NE in adrenergic nerve endings	Peripherally inhibits alpha receptors and release of NE; depletes stores of NE in adrenergic nerve endings
Labetalol 100-400 mg PO twice daily 10-80 mg IV q10min	Competitive antagonist at beta- and alpha-adrenergic receptors	Contraindicated in asthmatic, second- or third-degree AV block, CHF, or "brittle" diabetes
Vasodilators		
Hydralazine 10-50 mg PO four times/day 5-10 mg IV q20min	Direct relaxing effect on vascular smooth muscle (arterioles) veins	Lupus-like syndrome in 1%-20% of patients on long-term therapy, decreases DBP, >SBP, increases heart rate
Minoxidil 5-10 mg/ day PO		Fluid retention, pericardial effusion, and hypertrichosis

Continued on following page

Table 16-6. Doses, Mechanisms of Action, and Possible Complications of Antihypertensive Drugs—*(continued)*

AGENT AND DOSE	MECHANISM OF ACTION	POSSIBLE COMPLICATIONS
ACE Inhibitors		
Benazepril (Lotensin) 10-40 mg/day PO Captopril (Capoten) 6.25-150 mg PO three times/day Enalapril (Vasotec) 5-40 mg/day PO 1.25 mg/IV q6h Lisinopril (Zestril) 10-40 mg/day PO	Competes with ACE, prevents pulmonary conversion of angiotensin I to angiotensin II (a potent vasoconstrictor); decreases peripheral arterial resistance; leads to decreased aldosterone secretion, thereby reducing Na and water retention	10% get rash with fever and joint pain, proteinuria, neutropenia, and cough
Calcium Channel Blockers		
Diltiazem (Cardizem) 30-90 mg PO four times/day 0.25 mg/kg IV over 2 min 5-15 mg/h IV drip Isradipine (DynaCirc) 2.5-5 mg PO twice daily Nifedipine (Procardia) 10-30 mg PO three times/day	Blocks calcium movement across cell membranes, causing arterial vasodilation; nifedipine is the most potent peripheral and coronary artery vasodilator of calcium channel blockers; diltiazem has less negative inotropic effects than verapamil and has some selective coronary vasodilatory effects	CHF, nodal changes, edema, headaches, hyperkalemia, flushing, tachycardia (with nifedipine only)
Verapamil (Calan, Isoptin) 0.075-0.3 mg/kg IV over 2 min 80-120 PO three times/day		

ACE, Angiotensin-converting enzyme; *ANA,* antinuclear antibody; *AV,* atrioventricular; *CHF,* congestive heart failure; *DBP,* diastolic blood pressure; *HTN,* hypertension; *IV,* intravenously; *Na,* sodium; *NE,* norepinephrine; *PO,* orally; *q6h,* every 6 hours; *q7d,* every 7 days; *q10min,* every 10 minutes; *q20min,* every 20 minutes; *SBP,* systolic blood pressure.

Adapted from Dym H: The hypertensive patient. Therapeutic modalities, *Oral Maxillofac Clin North Am* 10:349–362, 1998.

48. What are the commonly used oral drugs for treatment of hypertensive urgencies?
    See Table 16-8.

CONGESTIVE HEART FAILURE

49. What is congestive heart failure?
    CHF results from impaired pumping ability by the heart. A ventricular ejection fraction below 50% is indicative of CHF. Causes of CHF include MI, IHD, poorly controlled hypertension, structural heart defects, and cardiomyopathy.

50. What are the potential effects of long-term hypertension on end organs?
    Chronically elevated BP often leads to serious consequences for the heart, central nervous system, and kidneys. Persistent hypertension may lead to left ventricular hypertrophy; angina pectoris with the potential for MI; CHF; and cardiomyopathy. Neurologic complications of hypertension include retinal damage with focal spasm; narrowing of arterioles or papilledema, or both; cerebral infarction

Table 16–7. Parenteral Drugs Used for Treatment of Hypertensive Emergencies

DRUG	DOSAGE	ONSET OF ACTION	ADVERSE EFFECTS
Vasodilators			
Nitroprusside (Nipride, Nitropress)	0.25-10 mg/kg/min as IV infusion	Instantaneous	Nausea, vomiting, muscle twitching, sweating, thiocyanate, intoxication
Nitroglycerin	5-100 g/min as IV infusion	2-5 min	Tachycardia, flushing, headache, vomiting, methemoglobinemia
Diazoxide (Hyperstat)	50-100 mg IV bolus repeated or 15-30 mg/min by IV infusion	2-4 min	Nausea, hypotension, flushing, tachycardia, chest pain
Hydralazine (Apresoline)	10-20 mg IV bolus	10-20 min	Tachycardia, flushing, headache, vomiting, aggravation of angina
Enalapril (Vasotec IV)	1.25-5 mg IV bolus q6h	15 min	Precipitous fall in blood pressure in high renin states; response variable
Nicardipine	5-10 mg/h as IV infusion	10 min	Tachycardia, headache, flushing, local phlebitis
Adrenergic inhibitors			
Phentolamine (Regitine)	5-15 mg IV bolus	1-2 min	Tachycardia, flushing
Trimethaphan (Arfonad)	0.5-5 mg/min as IV infusion	1-5 min	Paresis of bowel and bladder, orthostatic hypotension, blurred vision, dry mouth
Esmolol (Brevibloc)	500 mg/kg/min for first 4 min, then 150-300 mg/kg/min as IV infusion	1-2 min	Hypotension
Propranolol (Inderal)	1-10 mg load; 3 mg/h	1-2 min	Beta blocker side effect, e.g., bronchospasm, decreased cardiac output
Labetalol (Normodyne, Trandate)	10-80 mg IV bolus q10min; 0.5-2 mg/min IV as infusion	5-10 min	Vomiting, scalp tingling, burning in throat, postural hypotension, dizziness, nausea

IV, Intravenous; *q6h*, every 6 hours; *q10min*, every 10 minutes.
Adapted from Dym H: The hypertensive patient. Therapeutic modalities, *Oral Maxillofac Clin North Am* 10:349–362, 1998.

or hemorrhage; cerebral vascular microaneurysms (Charcot-Bouchard aneurysms); hypertensive encephalopathy; and stroke. Renal complications include renal insufficiency and renal failure.

51. **What are the clinical signs and symptoms of CHF?**
Fatigue and dyspnea on exertion are often the primary symptoms of CHF. Patients may also report ankle edema and 2- to 3-pillow orthopnea. Palpitation, nocturia, cough, nausea, and vomiting are associated findings. Physical findings include gallop rhythm (S_3 or S_4), murmurs, and jugular venous distention. Pulmonary exam may reveal rales over the lung bases and decreased breath sounds. Cyanosis is often present in severe CHF.

52. **What are the different classifications of heart failure?**
There are different methods of classification of heart failure, such as left-sided versus right-sided, high output versus low output, backward versus forward, acute versus chronic, and compensated versus decompensated.

Table 16-8. Oral Drugs Used for Hypertensive Urgencies

DRUG	CLASS	DOSAGE	ONSET	DURATION
Nifedipine (Procardia)	Calcium entry blocker	5-10 mg sublingual	5-15 min	3-5 h
Clonidine (Catapres)	Central sympatho-lytic	0.2 mg initially, then 0.1 mg/h up to 0.7 mg total	0.5-2 h	6-8 h

Adapted from Dym H: The hypertensive patient. Therapeutic modalities, *Oral Maxillofac Clin North Am* 10:349–362, 1998.

53. What are the causes of heart failure?

Cardiac	**Non-cardiac**
Ischemia	Hypertension

Cardiac

Ischemia
- Cardiomyopathy   Pulmonary embolus
- Toxic   High-output states
- Metabolic   Thyrotoxicosis
- Infectious, inflammatory
- Infiltrative
- Genetic
- Idiopathic

Valvular heart diseases
- Aortic stenosis, regurgitation
- Mitral stenosis, regurgitation

Restrictive disease
- Pericardial
- Myocardial

Congenital disease

Electrical abnormalities
- Tachydysrhythmias
- Ventricular dyssynergy

Non-cardiac

Hypertension

54. What are the major physiologic alterations in patients with heart failure?
- Loss of artery compliance
- Arteriolar narrowing
- Vascular smooth muscle hypertrophy
- Enhanced vasoconstrictor activity secondary to elevated sympathetic nervous system activity
- Activation of the renin-angiotensin system resulting in sodium and water retention
- Increased levels of arginine, vasopressin and endothelin
- Possible decrease in the local release of endothelium-derived relaxing factor (nitric oxide)

55. Which lab studies are useful in evaluating the patient with CHF?
Chest X-ray, ECG, echocardiogram, and radionuclear ventriculography are all useful in the evaluation of patients with heart failure. **Chest X-ray** may show cardiomegaly or evidence of pulmonary vascular congestion, including perihilar engorgement of the pulmonary veins, cephalization of the pulmonary vascular markings, or pleural effusions. The **ECG** in these patients is often nonspecific, although 70% to 90% of patients demonstrate ventricular or supraventricular dysrhythmias. **Echocardiography** is used to demonstrate chamber size, wall motion, valvular function, and left ventricular wall thickness. **Radio-nuclear ventriculography** is helpful in providing an assessment of left ventricular ejection fraction.

56. How is the severity of heart failure classified?
The status of patients with CHF is typically classified on the basis of symptoms, impairment of lifestyle, or severity of cardiac dysfunction. The New York Heart Association uses four categories that describe the symptomatic limitations of the patient with heart failure. These classifications are:
Class I: Ordinary physical activity does not cause symptoms.
Class II: Ordinary physical activity causes symptoms.

Class III: Less than ordinary activity results in symptoms.
Class IV: Symptoms occur at rest.

57. **What are the principles of management for CHF?**
The mnemonic MOIST'N DAMP is helpful in listing the methods generally used in combination for the management of CHF:
- **M**orphine
- **O**xygen
- **I**notropes (digitalis)
- **S**it-'em-up
- **T**ourniquets
- **N**itrates
- **D**iuretics
- **A**CE inhibitors and afterload reduction (aminophylline)
- **M**echanical ventilator
- **P**hlebotomy

58. **What are the different classes of drugs used in the treatment of heart failure?**
Drugs used in the treatment of CHF typically fall into one of five categories: diuretics, ACE inhibitors, calcium channel blockers, digitalis, and beta blockers.
   Diuretics are used when patients with CHF exhibit signs or symptoms of circulatory congestion. *Thiazide* diuretics are often used for mild fluid retention. *Loop* diuretics, such as furosemide, may be substituted when thiazides fail to produce an adequate response. Addition of a second diuretic, such as metolazone, may induce an effective diuresis in patients resistant to loop diuretics alone.
   ACE inhibitors are effective therapy for patients who can tolerate them. They improve left ventricular function and exercise tolerance and may prolong life. Hypotension and azotemia are the major side effects. A dry cough is fairly common but rarely necessitates discontinuation of therapy. A combination of the vasodilators hydralazine and isosorbide dinitrate also has been shown to be effective in improving exercise tolerance and life span.
   Calcium channel blockers may produce favorable hemodynamic responses, but negative inotropic effects. These agents are used in patients with concurrent myocardial ischemia.
   Digitalis is effective in patients with underlying arterial fibrillation or a dilated left ventricle with poor systolic function.
   Beta blockers may produce favorable long-term effects in patients with IHD.

59. **What are the signs and symptoms of digitalis toxicity?**
Patients with digitalis toxicity may present with any of the following signs and symptoms: anorexia, nausea, vomiting, abdominal pain, confusion, paresthesias, amblyopia, and scotomata. ECG findings are usually nonspecific and include atrial or ventricular dysrhythmias, such as premature ventricular contractions, bigeminy, trigeminy, ventricular tachycardia, delayed atrioventricular node conduction, and complete heart block. Older patients and patients with hypothyroidism, decreased renal function, hypokalemia, hypercalcemia, and/or hypomagnesemia are more predisposed to digitalis toxicity.

60. **What are the important elements of postoperative care for patients with CHF?**
The peak evidence of postoperative MI occurs about 72 hours postoperatively; therefore closely monitor the patient's cardiac status during this period. Improve pulmonary function with incentive spirometry, pulmonary toilet, and bronchodilators when appropriate. Observation of renal function and urine output is also important in these patients, because postoperative renal failure has ominous implications. Pain must be well controlled to minimize physiologic stress.
   Other possible postoperative complications to avoid include gastrointestinal ischemia, bleeding, stroke, graft infection, distal arterial thrombosis, and pulmonary embolism.

BIBLIOGRAPHY

Dajani AS, Taubert KA, Wilson W, et al.: Prevention of bacterial endocarditis. Recommendations by the American Heart Association, *JAMA* 277:1794–1801, 1997.
Disease in the Young, and the Council on Clinical Cardiology, Council on Cardiovascular Surgery and Anesthesia, and the Quality of Care and Outcomes Research Interdisciplinary Working Group, *Circulation* 116: 1736–1754, 2007.
Dym H: The hypertensive patient. Therapeutic modalities, *Oral Maxillofac Surg Clin North Am* 10:349–362, 1998.
Eagle KA, Coley CM, Nussbaum SR, et al.: Combining clinical and thallium data optimizes preoperative assessment of cardiac risk before major vascular surgery, *Ann Intern Med* 110:859–866, 1989.

Fleisher LA, Fleischmann KE, Auerbach AD, et al.: 2014 ACC/AHA Guideline on perioperative cardiovascular evaluation and management of patients undergoing noncardiac surgery: executive summary, *Circulation*, August 1, 2014. [published online].

Glick M: New guidelines for prevention, detection, evaluation, and treatment of high blood pressure, *J Am Dent Assoc* 129:1588–1594, 1998.

Goldman L, Caldera DL, Nussbaum SR, et al.: Multifactorial index of cardiac risk in patients in noncardiac surgical procedures, *N Engl J Med* 297:945–950, 1977.

McCabe JC, Roser SM: Evaluation and management of the cardiac patient for surgery, *Oral Maxillofac Surg Clin North Am* 10:429–443, 1998.

Muzyka BC, Glick M: The hypertensive dental patient, *J Am Dent Assoc* 128:1109–1120, 1997.

Seres T: Congestive heart failure. In Duke J, editor: *Anesthesia secrets*, ed 3, Philadelphia, 2006, Mosby.

Wilson W, Taubert KA, Gewitz M, et al.: Prevention of infective endocarditis: guidelines from the American Heart Association: a guideline from the American Heart Association Rheumatic Fever, Endocarditis, and Kawasaki Disease Committee, Council on Cardiovascular.

CHAPTER 17

RESPIRATORY DISORDERS

Yedeh Ying, Zachary S. Peacock, Osama Soliman

1. **What is the normal adult oxyhemoglobin dissociation curve for blood at 37%, pH of 7.4, and PCO_2 of 40 mm Hg?**
   See Fig. 17-1.

2. **What are the general rules concerning the dissociation curve shifts?**
   - A low pH or a high PCO_2 shifts the curve to the right.
   - A high pH or a low PCO_2 shifts the curve to the left.
   - Elevated body temperature shifts the curve to the right.
   - Lower body temperature shifts the curve to the left.
   - Carbon monoxide in the blood increases the affinity of remaining oxygen for hemoglobin and shifts the curve to the left.

3. **How does the interpretation of the curve change when the curve shifts to the left?**
   The P50 is a conventional measure of the hemoglobin affinity for oxygen. If the curve is shifted to the left, there is less PO_2 (mm Hg) in the blood needed to achieve the P50. In other words, there is an increased hemoglobin affinity to O_2 with a left curve shift.

4. **What is 2,3-diphosphoglycerate (2,3-DPG)?**
   It is produced by erythrocytes and normally is present in fairly high concentrations in red blood cells (RBCs).

5. **When is 2,3-DPG produced?**
   It is produced mainly during chronic hypoxic conditions. An increase in 2,3-DPG shifts the curve to the right and allows more O_2 to be released from hemoglobin at a particular O_2 level. With a decrease in 2,3-DPG, the curve will shift to the left, indicating an increased affinity for O_2 by hemoglobin. Hemoglobin does not release O_2 in the tissues except at a very low PO_2.

6. **How does 2,3-DPG affect blood supply in blood banks?**
   Blood stored for as little as 1 week will have depleted 2,3-DPG unless steps are taken to restore normal levels of 2,3-DPG.

7. **How does the aging process affect $PaCO_2$?**
   $PaCO_2$ and alveolar ventilation are unchanged by the aging process.

8. **How does the aging process affect PaO_2?**
   PaO_2 decreases with age. This decrease can be calculated according to the following formula:

   $$PaO_2 = 100.1 - (0.323 \times \text{age in years})$$

   Thus the PaO_2 of a 30-year-old person would be calculated as $100.1 - (0.323 \times 30) = 90.41$.

9. **What are the anatomic volumes of the lungs?**
   TV: tidal volume, the amount of air moved with each breath (Fig. 17-2)
   IRV: inspiratory reserve volume, the maximum additional amount of air that can be inhaled after the end of inspiration
   IC: inspiratory capacity, the maximum volume of air that can be inspired (VT + IRV)
   RV: residual volume, the remaining volume of air after maximal expiration
   ERV: expiratory reserve volume, the maximum additional amount of air that can be exhaled after expiration
   FRC: functional residual capacity, the volume in the lungs after passive expiration (RV + ERV)
   VC: vital capacity, the maximum amount of air that can be exhaled after maximum inspiration (IC + ERV)
   TLC: total lung capacity, the volume in the lungs at maximal inspiration (RV + VC)

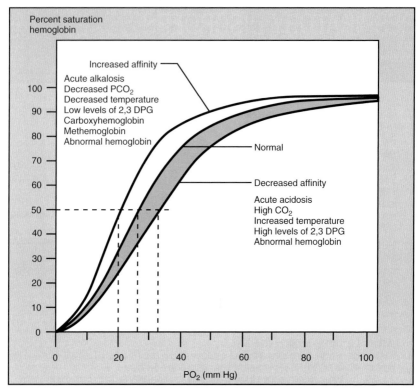

Figure 17-1. Normal oxyhemoglobin dissociation curve. *DPG*, Diphosphoglycerate; *COHb*, carboxyhemoglobin; *Hb*, hemoglobin. *(From Cairo JM, Pilbeam SP: Mosby's respiratory care equipment, ed 9, St Louis, 2009, Mosby.)*

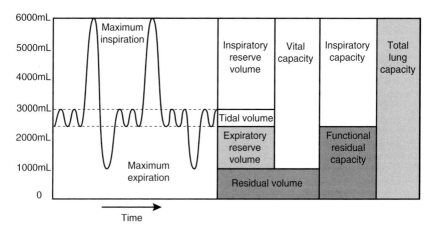

Figure 17-2. Lung volumes and capacities. *(From Nagelhout JJ, Plaus K: Nurse anesthesia, ed 4, St Louis, 2010, Saunders.)*

10. What are pulmonary function tests (PFTs), and why are they used?
    PFTs are an adjunct to history and physical examination and provide an overall assessment of the respiratory system. The tests include (1) measurements of airflow (spirometry), (2) lung volumes, and (3) diffusing capacity for inspired carbon monoxide (DLCO). The tests are reported as a percentage of predicted normal values based on age and height.

11. What useful measurements are used in spirometry?
    FVC: Forced vital capacity
    FEV_1: the volume of air that can forcibly be blown out in 1 second, after full inspiration
    FVC/FEV_1 ratio: known as the Tiffeneau-Pinell index

12. What is the normal FVC/FEV_1 ratio?
    The normal FVC/FEV_1 ratio is 70% to 80%.

13. What is the FVC/FEV_1 ratio in obstructive and restrictive disease?
    In obstructive pulmonary disease, expiratory resistance increases, resulting in an increase in the FEV_1. The FVC may also increase, but not to the same extent, resulting in a decreased ratio below 70%. In restrictive disease such as pulmonary fibrosis, the FVC and the FEV_1 are both reduced proportionally, resulting in a normal ratio or even increased as a result of decreased lung compliance.

14. How is the forced expiratory volume in 1 second (FEV_1) changed with age?
    FEV_1 declines linearly with age increase.

15. What are the most significant changes of pulmonary function associated with aging?
    • Loss of lung elasticity, which leads to increased mean alveolar diameter and volume and reduced FEV_1
    • Decreased power of the respiratory musculature
    • Increased rigidity of rib cage
    All these changes start becoming apparent in the third decade of life.

16. What is the normal rate of breathing?
    The normal respiratory rate (RR) is 10 to 20 breaths/min in adolescents and adults (>12 years old), 30 to 60 in infants (0 to 1 year), 24 to 40 in toddlers (1 to 3 years), 22 to 34 in those 3 to 6 years old, and 18 to 30 in those 6 to 12 years old. For adolescents and adults, an RR >20/min is considered tachypnea and <10/min is bradypnea.

17. Where is the respiratory center?
    The respiratory center is a widely dispersed group of neurons located bilaterally in the reticular substance of the medulla oblongata and pons.

18. What influences the respiratory center?
    Excess CO_2 and hydrogen ions (H+) affect respiration mainly by direct excitatory effects on the respiratory center itself. Oxygen does **not** have a significant direct effect on the respiratory center. O_2 acts almost entirely peripherally on the carotid and aortic bodies.

19. What does PEEP mean?
    Positive **E**nd-**E**xpiratory **P**ressure during mechanical ventilation. PEEP aids in preventing alveolar and small airway collapse and may help recruit lung units that were previously collapsed.

20. What are the beneficial effects of PEEP?
    • Increased functional residual capacity
    • Increased compliance
    • Increased PaO_2
    • Increased ventilation–perfusion (V/Q) ratio (when initially low)
    • Decreased pulmonary shunt

21. What is the effect of PEEP on cardiac output?
    Because of increased intrathoracic pressure and decreased venous return when using PEEP, cardiac output may be decreased.

22. What are the normal blood gas values?
    pH7.40 ± 0.05 units
    (H+) 40 ± 5 mEq/L

PCO_2 40 ± 5 mm Hg

A 0.1 decrease in pH corresponds to a 12 mm Hg of PCO_2 increase, which equals a base change of 6 mEq/L.

- Golden rule no. 1: A pH of 0.08 = $PaCO_2$ of 10 mm Hg.
- Golden rule no. 2: A pH of 0.15 = base change of 10 mEq/L.

23. **What are the common causes of acid–base disorders?**
    - Respiratory alkalosis: hyperventilation, sepsis, anxiety, pain
    - Respiratory acidosis: CNS depression, neuromuscular disorders, upper and lower airway abnormalities
    - Metabolic alkalosis: emesis, volume depletion, nasogastric tube (NGT) drainage, diuretic use, exogenous alkali, mineralocorticoid excess
    - Metabolic acidosis: ketoacidosis, lactic acidosis, renal failure, ingestion of toxins (e.g., methanol and propylene glycol)

24. **How is the diagnosis of respiratory acidosis made?**
    Respiratory acidosis is usually evident from the clinical exam, especially if respiration is obviously depressed. Analyses of arterial blood gases (ABGs) will confirm the diagnosis. Arterial pH will be <7.35, and PCO_2 will be >45 mm Hg.

25. **What are some causes of respiratory acidosis?**
    Any disease or condition that may affect the respiratory function can cause respiratory acidosis, including:
    - Chronic obstructive pulmonary disease (COPD)
    - Chest wall or airway injury
    - Drug effects
    - Pulmonary edema
    - Central nervous system (CNS) depression
    - Cardiac arrest
    - Extreme obesity (e.g., pickwickian syndrome)
    - Pneumonia

26. **How is the diagnosis of respiratory alkalosis made?**
    Clinically, respiratory alkalosis usually manifests as hyperventilation. However, depending on its severity and acuteness, hyperventilation may not be evident, but an analysis of ABGs will demonstrate an arterial pH of >7.45 and a PCO_2 of <35 mm Hg.

27. **What are some causes of respiratory alkalosis?**
    - Hyperventilation
    - Pulmonary embolus
    - CNS injury
    - Excessive mechanical ventilation
    - Fever

28. **What is Cheyne-Stokes breathing?**
    Periods of hyperpnea (deep breathing) alternating with periods of apnea. The crescendo–decrescendo pattern of breathing is associated with changes in PO_2 and PCO_2. Children and the elderly normally show this pattern in sleep. In normal adults, causes of this pattern of breathing include heart failure, uremia, drug-induced respiratory depression, and brain damage.

29. **What are the causes of hypoxemia?**
    - Low inspired oxygen concentration (low FiO_2): when inadequate oxygen level is supplied or available (e.g., asphyxiation)
    - Hypoventilation: inadequate minute ventilation (e.g., sedation or CNS depression, brainstem stroke)
    - Right to left shunt: perfusion without ventilation; when blood bypasses the pulmonary system by flowing from the right heart to the left without exposure to inhaled oxygen (e.g., atrial or ventricular septal defect, pulmonary edema, pneumonia)
    - Ventilation/perfusion mismatch: Ventilation (V) should ideally match perfusion (Q) at the alveolar-capillary level. Areas of ventilation without perfusion are termed dead space (e.g., pulmonary embolus).
    - Diffusion abnormality: abnormality of the alveolar-capillary membrane causing inefficient exchange of oxygen to the bloodstream (e.g., diseases of the lung parenchyma or interstitium)

30. **What causes stridor?**
Stridor, an airway emergency that demands immediate attention, is caused by partial obstruction of the airway at the level of the larynx or trachea. This high-pitched breath sound can be noted on inspiration or expiration or can even be biphasic.

31. **What is the definition of acute respiratory failure?**
Respiratory failure is an inadequate exchange of O_2 and CO_2 secondary to failure of the ventilatory apparatus or gas exchange system. It results in hypoventilation and, therefore, hypercapnia and hypoxemia.

32. **How is the diagnosis of respiratory failure made?**
Respiratory failure is primarily based on ABGs: hemoglobin saturation of <92% (which corresponds to a PaO_2 of <60 mm Hg, a $PaCO_2$ of >50 mm Hg, and a pH of <7.35 [respiratory acidosis]).

33. **How is respiratory failure treated?**
Secure and maintain a patent airway to deliver appropriate O_2 therapy using mechanical or supportive ventilation. The airway may be in the form of oral and nasal endotracheal intubation, tracheostomy, or cricothyrotomy.

34. **What are the indications for elective intubation and mechanical ventilation?**
The indications for intubation and mechanical ventilation are based on clinical and lab values. These include:
- Respiratory rate >30 to 40 breaths/min
- Negative inspiratory pressure <25 cm H_2O
- Vital capacity <10 to 15 mL/kg or a $PaCO_2$ >50 mm Hg with a pH < 7.3

35. **What are the guidelines for withdrawing mechanical ventilatory support (weaning parameters)?**
Mechanical ventilation can be withdrawn if one or more of the following parameters are met:
- PaO_2 >60 mm Hg with an FiO_2 < 0.4
- Minute ventilation <10 L/min
- $PaCO_2$ (35 to 45) acceptable with normal pH
- Respiratory rate <25 breaths/min
- Tidal volume >4 to 5 mL/kg
- Negative inspiratory pressure >20 cm H_2O
- Vital capacity >10 to 15 mL/kg

36. **What is pleural effusion?**
Pleural effusion occurs when fluid accumulates in the pleural space (i.e., volume overload, infection) and the air-filled lung separates from the chest wall.

37. **What is atelectasis?**
Atelectasis occurs when mucus or a foreign object obstructs airflow in a main stem bronchus causing collapse of the affected lung tissue into an airless state. It typically occurs 36 hours postoperatively and presents with mild dyspnea.

38. **What chest X-ray findings are noted in a patient with atelectasis?**
Radiologic signs of lobar atelectasis can be categorized as direct or indirect. Direct signs include increased opacification of the airless lobe and displacement of fissures. Indirect signs include displacement of hilar and cardiomediastinal structures toward the side of collapse, narrowing of the ipsilateral intercostal spaces, elevation of the ipsilateral hemidiaphragm, compensatory hyperinflation and hyperlucency of the remaining aerated lung, and obscuration of the structures adjacent to the collapsed lung.

39. **How is postoperative atelectasis managed?**
Treatment of postoperative atelectasis is aimed at expansion of the lung, and, for most patients, incentive spirometry is adequate. However, in patients with severe atelectasis, endotracheal suction and even bronchoscopy may be warranted.

40. **What are the signs of pneumothorax?**
Pneumothorax occurs when air leaks into the pleural space, causing the lung to recoil from the chest wall. The signs of intraoperative pneumothorax include unexplained hypotension, ventilatory hypoxia with

bulging diaphragm, jugular venous distention, tympanic thorax, and trachea deviated to one side. In an awake patient, a pneumothorax typically presents with dyspnea, chest pain, absence of breath sounds on the affected side, and evidence of pneumothorax on chest X-ray. Tracheal deviation may be present.

41. What is the appropriate treatment of pneumothorax?

Pneumothorax is definitively treated with placement of a thoracostomy tube connected to closed suction of 20 cm H_2O. However, if tension pneumothorax is suspected, immediate needle decompression through the second intercostal space in the midclavicular line using a 14-gauge needle should be performed.

42. What is the mechanism of bronchial asthma?

Asthma is a chronic disorder characterized by inflammation and increased responsiveness of the tracheobronchial tree to diverse stimuli resulting in a varying degree of airway obstruction.

43. What is the clinical presentation of bronchial acute asthma?

Patients present with dyspnea or tachypnea, wheezing, hypoxemia, and, occasionally, hypercapnia.

44. How is bronchial asthma classified?

One of the classifications of asthma is based on the severity and frequency of attack (Table 17-1).

45. What is the appropriate management of an acute asthma attack?

An acute asthmatic attack is best treated by administration of supplemental O_2 with an inhaled beta-adrenergic agonist (albuterol, 3.0 mL [2.5 mg], in 2 mL of normal saline every 4 to 6 hours, in a nebulizer). If the patient is resistant to beta agonists, theophylline should be considered. Therapy also may include parenteral steroids, such as methylprednisolone (50 to 250 mg over 4 to 6 hours). In a severe asthmatic attack that is unresponsive to the above, administer 0.3 mg of 1:1000 epinephrine subcutaneously.

46. What clinical information is relevant for patients with COPD to risk-stratify prior to surgery?

- Smoking history: number of packs per days and duration in years
- Clinical symptoms: dyspnea, wheezing, cough
- Functional capacity: assessment of metabolic equivalents (METs). Those who cannot tolerate >4 METs (i.e., climbing ≥1 flight of stairs, walking one to two blocks uphill, golf) are considered increased risk.
- Hospitalizations: previous intubations/need for mechanical ventilation
- Medications: home O_2 therapy and flow-rate? Need for systemic steroids?
- Infections: any recent exacerbations, pulmonary infections
- Weight loss: may be related to end-stage lung disease or cancer

47. What is emphysema?

Emphysema is an inflammatory response in the lungs due to continuous exposure to irritants such as air pollution and smoking. This causes narrowing of small airways and breakdown of the lung tissue resulting in destruction of airspaces. The resultant fibrosis results in air trapping (hyperinflation) and ventilation-perfusion mismatch. Patients compensate through hyperventilation and prolonged expiratory periods to maintain oxygen saturation >90% (i.e., pink puffer). Physical examination reveals use of accessory muscles, hyperinflated lung fields that are hyperresonant to percussion, with distant, diminished breath sounds.

Table 17-1. Classifying the Severity of an Asthma Attack

SEVERITY	SYMPTOM FREQUENCY	NIGHTTIME SYMPTOMS	% FEV$_1$ OF PREDICTED	SHORT-ACTING BETA-AGONIST USE
Intermittent	≤2/week	≤2/month	≥80%	≤2 days/week
Mild persistent	>2/week	3-4/month	≥80%	>2 days/week
Moderate persistent	Daily	>1/week	60-80%	Daily
Severe persistent	Continuously	Frequent (7/week)	<60%	≥2/day

48. **What is chronic bronchitis?**

Chronic productive cough lasting at least 3 months over a minimum of 2 years that is highly associated with smoking. It is characterized by hypertrophy of bronchial mucinous glands. This hypertrophy leads to increased thickness of mucus glands relative to overall bronchial wall thickness (Reid index increases to >50%; normal is <40%). The clinical signs are a productive cough (due to excessive mucus production) and cyanosis (blue bloaters). The excess mucus causes mucous plugs, trapping carbon dioxide, increasing $PaCO_2$, and decreasing PaO_2, resulting in an increased risk of infection and cor pulmonale.

49. **What is bronchiectasis?**

Bronchiectasis is a condition in which the bronchi are abnormally and irreversibly dilated due to destruction of the muscle and elasticity of the lung parenchyma secondary to inflammation. The disorder can be associated with congenital lung diseases or the result of a variety of pulmonary insults including aspiration or severe infection. The resultant dilation and destruction causes the lung to inadequately clear secretions and become colonized with pathogenic bacteria, resulting in recurrent pulmonary infections.

50. **What is adult respiratory distress syndrome (ARDS)?**

ARDS is a C5a-induced neutrophil aggregation in the lung. This aggregation is one of the major mechanisms of pathology of ARDS. The damaged capillaries leak protein-rich fluid into the interstitium, which leads to changes in pulmonary function.

51. **What causes ARDS?**

ARDS usually results from an injury to the alveolar-capillary membrane. It also can be caused by an existing underlying disease, such as systemic sepsis, fat embolism, head injury, aspiration, pancreatitis, or inhalation injury. Patients typically show severe dyspnea and hypoxemia refractory to supplemental O_2 with diffuse pulmonary infiltrates on chest radiograph.

52. **What is the appropriate management of ARDS?**

Management of ARDS includes immediate transfer to an intensive care unit and placement of a pulmonary artery catheter with mechanical ventilation to maintain the pulse oximetry (SpO_2) >90%, which corresponds to PO_2 >60 mm Hg. In addition, the pulmonary capillary pressure should be kept in the range of 12 to 15 mm Hg, and the cardiac index should be maintained above 3 L/min/m2. Treatment of ARDS is generally supportive to achieve O_2 saturation of 90% while minimizing barotrauma and oxygen toxicity.

53. **What are the features of ARDS?**

- History of major insult
- Increased respiratory distress
- Diffuse infiltration on chest X-ray
- Hypoxemia (PaO_2 <60 mm Hg with FiO_2 >0.6)
- Respiratory alkalosis
- Normal pulmonary capillary wedge pressure (PCWP)
- Decreased pulmonary compliance
- Increased shunt function
- Increased dead space and ventilation

54. **How often does aspiration occur, and what are the complications?**

Aspiration is a relatively rare occurrence affecting approximately 1 out of every 10,000 patients undergoing general anesthesia. In the outpatient setting, deep sedation without a secure airway has also been shown to be safe without a significant increased risk for aspiration. Complications include bronchospasm, pneumonitis, pneumonia, acute respiratory distress syndrome, lung abscess, and empyema conferring an increased risk of mortality.

55. **What are common risk factors for aspiration?**

- Inadequate NPO status (emergent cases) or failure to follow NPO guidelines for anesthesia
- Extremes of age (twice as common in children and elderly)
- Medications that decrease level of consciousness (sedative/hypnotics/anxiolytics) and blunt protective reflexes
- Head trauma
- Stroke

- Presence of a nasogastric tube
- Prolonged supine position

56. **What is the appropriate management of aspiration?**

A baseline chest radiograph should be obtained for any patient suspected of aspiration. After immediate suctioning, supportive care is the mainstay of treatment and includes supplemental oxygen and monitoring of oxygen saturation in an inpatient setting. Ventilatory support should be initiated if concern for respiratory failure arises (see question 12 above). Antibiotics should not be initiated unless the event leads to pneumonia and cultures can be tailored to target specific organisms. Classically, aspirated material consists of gram-negative or anaerobic organisms (oral/gastrointestinal flora). Aspiration of gastric contents can lead to chemical pneumonitis and also requires supportive care.

57. **How can aspiration risk be decreased?**

By recognizing surgical patients who are high risk, adjunctive steps and medication can be taken to minimize the overall risk. Adhering to standard fasting protocols prior to any procedure will optimize gastric emptying. Gastric acids can be neutralized with antacids or histamine receptor antagonists. Logically, pro-motility agents such as metoclopramide will aid in gastric emptying; however, no data supports this. Aspiration can be prevented in critically ill patients by maintaining the head-of-bed ≥30 degrees, minimizing sedatives, and avoiding bolus feeds in high-risk patients.

58. **What drugs interfere (interact) with aminophylline?**

The most commonly cited drug is erythromycin, which increases serum levels of aminophylline. Cimetidine also increases serum levels of aminophylline.

59. **What are the signs and symptoms of pulmonary embolism (PE)?**

PE can present with acute onset of pleuritic chest pain, dyspnea, syncope, or leg pain and swelling. Many patients may have no symptoms. Signs of a PE include tachypnea, hypoxemia, rales, unexplained tachycardia, elevated jugular venous pressure, and low-grade fever. Risk factors for PE include stasis (immobility, obesity), recent endothelial injury (trauma, surgery, recent fracture, and deep vein thrombosis), and hypercoagulable state (pregnancy, oral contraceptive use, malignancy).

60. **How is the pre-test probability of deep vein thrombosis (DVT) determined?**

The Well's criteria is a method of determining the likelihood of DVT. It is based on major and minor criteria. Major criteria include active cancer, immobilization, bed rest >3 days, major surgery within 4 weeks, swelling of the thigh and calf, family history of DVT. Minor criteria include recent trauma to symptomatic extremity within 60 days, pitting edema, dilated superficial veins, erythema, and recent hospitalization within 6 months. If more than three major criteria or two major and two minor criteria are met, then there is a high likelihood that DVT/PE can be present (~85% + DVT).

61. **How is PE diagnosed?**

Immediate ABG, electrocardiogram (ECG), and chest X-ray should be obtained. The ABG will reveal hypoxemia, hypocapnia, and respiratory alkalosis with an increased A–a gradient. An ECG may reveal sinus tachycardia or atrial fibrillation with signs of right ventricular strain (e.g., right bundle branch block with t-wave inversions in leads V1-V4). Chest X-ray may show atelectasis, effusion, and a raised diaphragm. With a large PE, the chest X-ray may have a Hamptom's hump, a wedge-shaped density abutting the pleura, or Westermark sign, which sharply cuts off of a vessel distal to the embolus. D-dimer levels can be assessed with high sensitivity but poor specificity. If the patient is experiencing any asymmetric swelling in any extremity, then DVT should be ruled out with an ultrasound. Bypassing these laboratory tests and obtaining CT angiography may be warranted.

62. **What is the appropriate management of postoperative PE?**

Once the patient has been stabilized, treatment includes acute anticoagulation with intravenous or subcutaneous heparin or a low molecular weight heparin. If given intravenously, heparin should be titrated to a goal PTT of 60 to 85 seconds. Once suitable acute anticoagulation has occurred and PTT is therapeutic, the patient is transitioned to anticoagulation with warfarin (goal INR of 2 to 3 for 3 to 6 months post event). With a contraindication for anticoagulation, an inferior vena cava filter should be placed. For large proximal PE with hemodynamic compromise, thrombectomy may be considered.

BIBLIOGRAPHY

Barash P, Cullen B, Stoelting R, et al.: *Clinical anesthesia*, ed 2, Philadelphia, 1996, Lippincott-Raven.

Bates B, Bickley L, Hoekelman R: The thorax and lungs. In Bates B, editor: *A guide to physical examination and history taking*, ed 6, Philadelphia, 1995, J.B. Lippincott.

Bradley TD, Rutherford R, Grossman RF, et al.: Role of daytime hypoxemia in the pathogenesis of right heart failure in the obstructive sleep apnea syndrome, *Am Rev Respir Dis* 131:835, 1985.

Chung F, Yang Y, Liao P: Predictive performance of the STOP-Bang score for identifying obstructive sleep apnea in obese patients, *Obes Surg* 23(12):2050–2057, December 2013.

Cohen MM, Duncan PG, Pope WD, Wolkenstein C: A survey of 112,000 anaesthetics at one teaching hospital (1975–83), *Can Anaesth Soc J* 33:22–31, 1986.

Dean G, Jacobs AR, Goldstein RC, Gevirtz CM, Paul ME: The safety of deep sedation without intubation for abortion in the outpatient setting, *J Clin Anes* 23:437–442, 2011.

Gottlieb DJ, Yenokyan G, Newman AB, et al.: Prospective study of obstructive sleep apnea and incident coronary heart disease and heart failure: the sleep heart health study, *Circulation* 122:352, 2010.

Kearney DJ, Lee TH, Reilly JJ, et al.: Assessment of operative risk in patients undergoing lung resection, importance of predicted pulmonary function, *Chest* 105:753–759, 1994.

Kispert JF, Kazmers A, Roiman L: Preoperative spiromtery predicts predicts perioperative pulmonary complications after major vascular surgery, *Ann Surg* 58:491–495, 1992.

Kollef M, Goodenberger D: Critical care and medical emergencies. In Ewald G, McKenzie C, editors: *The Washington manual of medical therapeutics*, Boston, 1995, Little, Brown.

Li KK: Maxillomandibular Advancement for obstructive sleep apnea, *J Oral Maxillofac Surg* 69(3):687–694, March 2011. Epub December 24, 2010.

Martínez-García MA, Campos-Rodríguez F, Catalán-Serra P, et al.: Cardiovascular mortality in obstructive sleep apnea in the elderly: role of long-term continuous positive airway pressure treatment: a prospective observational study, *Am J Respir Crit Care Med* 186:909, 2012.

Miller R, Stoelting R: Acid-base and blood gas analysis. In Miller R, editor: *Basics of anesthesia*, ed 3, New York, 1994, Churchill Livingstone.

Miller WP: Cardiac arrhythmias and conduction disturbances in the sleep apnea syndrome. Prevalence and significance, *Am J Med* 73:317, 1982.

Murray MJ, Coursin DB, Pearl RG, Prough DS: *Critical care medicine perioperative management*, ed 2, Philadelphia, 2002, Lippincott.

National Asthma Education and Prevention Program: *Expert panel report III: guidelines for the diagnosis and management of asthma*, Bethesda, MD, 2007, National Heart, Lung, and Blood Institute (NIH publication no. 08-4051). www.nhlbi.nih.gov/guidelines/asthma/asthgdln.htm.

Olsson GL, Hallen B, Hambraeus-Jonzon K: Aspiration during anaesthesia: a computer-aided study of 185,358 anaesthetics, *Acta Anaesthesiol Scand* 30:84–92, 1986.

Pettit TW, Cobb JP: Critical care. In Doherty GM, Wells SA, Baumann DS, et al.: *The Washington manual of surgery*, Boston, 1997, Little, Brown.

Punjabi NM, Caffo BS, Goodwin JL, et al.: Sleep-disordered breathing and mortality: a prospective cohort study, *PLoS Med* 6:e1000132, 2009.

Roser SM: Management of the medically compromised patient. In Kwon P, Laskin D, editors: *Clinician's manual of oral and maxillofacial surgery*, ed 2, Chicago, 1997, Quintessence.

Vana KD, Silva GE, Goldberg R: Predictive abilities of the STOP-Bang and Epworth Sleepiness Scale in iden-tifying sleep clinic patients at high risk for obstructive sleep apnea, *Res Nurs Health* 36:84–94, 2013, http://dx.doi.org/10.1002/nur.21512.

Wells PS, et al.: Derivation of a simple clinical model to categorize patients with a probability of pulmonary embolism: increasing the models utility with the SimpliRED D-dimer, *Thromb Haemost* 83(3):416–420, 2000.

Wells PS, et al.: Excluding pulmonary embolism at the bedside without diagnostic imaging: management of patients with suspected pulmonary embolism presenting to the emergency department by using a simple clinical model and d-dimer, *Ann Intern Med* 135(2):98–107, 2001.

West JB: *Respiratory physiology: the essentials*, ed 9, Baltimore, 2012, Lippincott, Williams, and Wilkins.

West JB: *Pulmonary pathophysiology: the essentials*, ed 8, Baltimore, 2012, Lippincott, Williams, and Wilkins.

Young T, Finn L, Peppard PE, et al.: Sleep disordered breathing and mortality: eighteen-year follow-up of the Wisconsin sleep cohort, *Sleep* 31:1071, 2008.

CHAPTER 18

MANAGEMENT OF PATIENTS WITH LIVER DISEASES AND HEMATOLOGICAL DISEASES

Roman G. Meyliker, Helen Giannakopoulos, Osama Soliman

MANAGEMENT OF PATIENTS WITH LIVER DISEASES*

1. What functions does the liver perform?
   - Stores glycogen
   - Gluconeogenesis
   - Maintains blood glucose levels
   - Deamination of amino acids
   - Beta-oxidation of fatty acids
   - Excretes bile salts
   - Synthesizes plasma proteins
   - Metabolizes endogenous and exogenous compounds
   - Phagocytizes bacteria
   - Excretes bilirubin

2. What are the common risk factors for developing liver disease?
   - Intravenous drug abuse
   - Multiple sexual contacts
   - Cocaine use
   - Diabetes
   - Contact with blood
   - Family history of liver disease
   - Blood transfusion before 1989
   - Intake of certain medications and food supplements
   - Alcohol abuse

3. What are the signs and symptoms of hepatocellular disease?
   Depending on the cause, severity, and chronicity of liver dysfunction, the following may be present:
   - Malaise
   - Anorexia
   - Pruritus
   - Low-grade fever
   - Right upper quadrant (RUQ) discomfort
   - Dark urine
   - Jaundice
   - Amenorrhea
   - Tender, enlarged liver or hepatomegaly
   - Splenomegaly
   - Spider telangiectasias
   - Palmar erythema
   - Ascites
   - Gynecomastia
   - Testicular atrophy
   - Asterixis

---

*Written by Helen Giannakopoulos and Osama Soliman.

4. What are the signs and symptoms of biliary obstruction?
   - Colicky RUQ pain
   - Weight loss (suggesting carcinoma)
   - Jaundice
   - Dark urine
   - Light-colored stools

5. What are the orofacial features of patients with chronic alcoholism?
   - Poor oral hygiene
   - Impaired healing
   - Jaundice of the oral mucosa
   - Candidiasis
   - Glossitis
   - Bruxism
   - Parotid gland enlargement
   - Petechiae
   - Angular cheilosis
   - Xerostomia

6. Which laboratory studies make up the liver function tests (LFTs), and how are they used to evaluate liver disease?
   LFTs are a collective group of blood tests that indicate the overall health of the liver in terms of enzymatic activity, synthetic capability, and detoxifying capacity.
   Elevated serum aminotransferases (AST, ALT) result from direct injury to the liver manifesting as hepatocellular necrosis or inflammation. ALT is more specific for the liver than AST. AST is also found in the heart, skeletal muscle, pancreas, kidney, and red blood cells.
   Elevated alkaline phosphatase levels suggest cholestasis, obstructive or infiltrative liver disease (i.e., tumor, abscess, granuloma). Alkaline phosphatase elevation due specifically to liver disease will result in concomitant elevation of gamma-glutamyl transpeptidase (GGT).
   Elevated bilirubin (conjugated and unconjugated) is present in the cholestatic pattern of disease.

7. What is a MELD score, and how should it influence the surgical plan?
   MELD is an acronym for model for end-stage liver disease and was originally created to predict the 3-month mortality rate of patients. It has become a standard in evaluating patients for liver transplant. It utilizes a patient's creatinine, bilirubin, and international normalized ratio (INR) with the final number ranging from 6 to 40. A higher score is indicative of more advanced disease.
   The MELD score has been used to determine a patient's suitability for surgery as follows:
   - <10 = Patients are suitable for all types of surgery.
   - 10 to 15 = The surgeon is to utilize caution and only perform necessary surgeries.
   - >15 = No elective surgeries should be performed.

8. What class of drugs can cause spasm of the choledochoduodenal sphincter (sphincter of Oddi)?
   Opioids. Only approximately 3% of patients receiving opioids experience sphincter spasm and intrabiliary pressure.

9. Which inhaled anesthetic is best for maintaining hepatic blood flow and hepatocyte oxygenation?
   Isoflurane.

10. What is the effect of inhaled anesthetics on hepatic blood flow?
    A 20% to 30% decrease in hepatic blood flow results from decreased perfusion pressure. The metabolites of inhalational anesthetics can cause inflammation or death of hepatocytes by direct toxicity and result in an asymptomatic transient elevation of AST and ALT.

11. What is the effect of positive pressure ventilation on hepatic blood flow?
    Decreased hepatic blood flow secondary to increased central venous pressure decreases hepatic perfusion pressure.

12. **Which muscle relaxants are the best choices to use in a patient with liver dysfunction?**
Cisatracurium, atacurium, and mivacurium, because they are metabolized via a process known as Hofmann elimination and therefore are independent of liver function.

13. **How does liver dysfunction affect metabolism of procaine?**
The liver is responsible for the production of pseudocholinesterase, which metabolizes procaine (and other ester anesthetics). Decreased production can result in prolonged half-life of these drugs.

14. **What mechanism is responsible for metabolism of amide anesthetics?**
Hepatic microsomal enzymes have the major role in metabolism of amide local anesthetics. A decrease in liver function can therefore prolong the plasma half-life of amide anesthetics.

15. **How is drug protein binding affected by liver disease?**
Decreased albumin production by the liver results in a decreased number of protein-binding sites. The amount of unbound, pharmacologically active drug is, in turn, increased.

16. **What are the most common drugs used in the dental office that are metabolized primarily by the liver?**
Local anesthetics, including articaine (Septocaine), lidocaine (Xylocaine), mepivacaine (Carbocaine), prilocaine (Citanest), and bupivacaine (Marcaine) are metabolized by the liver. Analgesics that are metabolized in the liver include aspirin, acetaminophen (Tylenol), codeine, meperidine (Demerol), and ibuprofen (Motrin). Commonly used sedation drugs that are metabolized in the liver include diazepam (Valium) and midazolam (Versed). Valium is metabolized into the active metabolites desmethyldiazepam and oxazepam, thereby prolonging its effects on the central nervous system. Antibiotics that are metabolized in the liver include ampicillin, penicillin, clindamycin, erythromycin, and tetracycline. Erythromycin inhibits substrates CYP1A2 and 3A4, thereby increasing plasma concentrations of many other drugs. Because of this, close scrutiny of other medicines a person may be taking is required when prescribing erythromycin.

17. **What are the signs of acetaminophen toxicity, and how should it be treated?**
The maximum recommended dose of acetaminophen is 80 mg/kg in children and 4 grams over 24 hours in adults. Typically patients will remain asymptomatic until levels of 250 mg/kg or 12 grams over 24 hours are seen. In the first 24 hours (stage 1) after ingestion, signs and symptoms can be vague and often consist of nausea, vomiting, diaphoresis, pallor, lethargy, and malaise. Over the following 48 hours (stage 2), patients will often show clinical improvement while their LFTs rise, and RUQ pain with hepatomegaly is seen, indicating true liver damage. Over the next 24 hours (stage 3), the patient will typically experience jaundice, hepatic encephalopathy, hyperammonemia, and bleeding diathesis. If the patient survives stage 3, then he or she enters stage 4, which is roughly 2 weeks of healing in which the liver actually returns to normal function.
  If a patient presents within 4 hours of ingestion, it may be beneficial to undergo GI decontamination with activated charcoal (maximum of 50 g). According to the 20-hour IV protocol, administering N-acetylcysteine 150 mg/kg over 60 minutes followed by a 4-hour infusion at 12.5 mg/kg per hour and then finally a 16-hour infusion at 6.25 mg/kg per hour is recommended.

18. **How is drug metabolism affected by liver cirrhosis?**
Fibrosis leads to decreases in blood flow from the hepatic artery to the most distal areas of the liver. These areas are concentrated with the cytochrome P450 system, which is important in metabolizing many drugs. Prolonged plasma half-life of these drugs is a consequence of cirrhosis.

19. **Which are the Vitamin K–dependent clotting factors?**
Factors II, VII, IX, and X, and proteins S and C.

20. **How can liver disease affect the bleeding time?**
The bleeding time may be increased in patients with portal hypertension by splenic sequestration of platelets leading to thrombocytopenia.

21. **What lab values will be affected by a deficiency in the factors produced by the liver?**
Prothrombin time (PT) and partial thromboplastin time (PTT).

22. **What is the treatment for bleeding diathesis from liver disease?**
    Fresh frozen plasma (FFP). If the patient is thrombocytopenic, he or she may need platelet transfusion as well. Vitamin K–dependent clotting factors alone are not sufficient because they do not include factor V, which is also produced in the liver.

23. **How are each of the hepatitis viruses transmitted?**
    - Hepatitis A virus (HAV): fecal-oral route resulting from contaminated food or water
    - Hepatitis B virus (HBV): inoculation of infected blood or blood products or by sexual contact
    - Delta agent: causes hepatitis only in association with hepatitis B infection
    - Hepatitis C virus (HCV): parenteral route as seen with IV drug abuse
    - Hepatitis E virus: enteral route

24. **What are the differences among the various viral hepatitides?**
    HAV is a 28-nm RNA virus whose mode of transmission is primarily fecal-oral from contaminated food or water. The diagnostic marker for hepatitis A is anti-HAV. Hepatitis A is an acute disease and does not exist in a chronic state. Antivirus IgM marks active infection, while the antivirus IgG is protective, and its presence indicates prior infection or immunization. A vaccine is available for HAV.
        HBV is a 42-nm DNA virus whose mode of transmission is predominately parenteral (blood or blood products) or through sexual contact. Diagnostic markers for HBV include immunoglobulin M (IgM) anti-HBc (acute), HBsAg (acute/chronic/infective), HBeAg (infectious), anti-HBs (recovery/immunity), and anti-HBcIg (ongoing or past infection). Infections result in chronic disease approximately 20% of the time. Infected patients are treated with hepatitis B immunoglobulin and will develop lifetime immunity. A vaccine is available for HBV.
        HCV is a 38- to 50-nm RNA virus whose mode of transmission is predominantly parenteral. Diagnostic markers include anti-HCV (recovery/immunity) and HCV RNA (infectivity). Infections are mainly chronic in nature. Patients with chronic hepatitis C, who develop cirrhosis, have a twentyfold greater risk of developing hepatocellular carcinoma. Immunity following infection is weak and ineffective, and no cure currently exists. There have been new treatment methods, including interferon therapy and most recently a class of drugs called direct-acting antivirals (DAAs), which interfere with the enzymes the HCV needs to multiply. Genotype 1 HCV is the most common infection, accounting for approximately 70% to 75% of all hepatitis C infections.
        Hepatitis D virus (HDV) is a viral infection that occurs only in patients with preexisting HBV. This co-infection often causes marked decline in hepatic function and may cause fulminate hepatic failure. HDV is usually transmitted by needles in drug users.
        Hepatitis E virus (HEV) is a 32-nm RNA virus whose mode of transmission is predominately fecal-oral. The diagnostic marker used is anti-HEV (recovery). No treatment is currently used for infected patients. Infected patients will develop lifetime immunity, but no vaccine is currently available for HEV. HEV infection in pregnant women is associated with fulminant hepatitis (liver failure with massive liver necrosis).

25. **What causes jaundice?**
    Jaundice results from the accumulation of bilirubin, a product of heme metabolism, in the body tissue. It is typically first noted in the sclera.

26. **What is the difference between unconjugated and conjugated bilirubin?**
    - Unconjugated (indirect): This is a breakdown product of hemolysis that is generated by reticuloendothelial cells of the spleen. This form of bilirubin is very insoluble and utilizes albumin for transportation through the blood. Unconjugated hyperbilirubinemia may result from overproduction of bilirubin because of hemolysis, impaired hepatic uptake of bilirubin due to certain drugs, hyperthyroidism, or impaired glucoronidation of bilirubin as seen in Gilbert's syndrome.
    - Conjugated (direct): When unconjugated bilirubin is delivered to the liver, it dissociates from albumin and is conjugated with glucoronide. It is then water soluble. Conjugated hyperbilirubinemia is seen with hepatocellular disease, drugs, sepsis, or extrahepatic biliary obstruction.

27. **What is Gilbert's syndrome?**
    Gilbert's syndrome, the most common cause of idiopathic hyperbilirubinemia, is an autosomal dominant trait with variable penetrance. Decreased bilirubin uptake by hepatocytes results in increased plasma concentration of unconjugated bilirubin.

28. **What is the definitive study that determines the cause and severity of the hepatocellular dysfunction or infiltrative liver disease?**
    Percutaneous liver biopsy is performed with ultrasound or CT guidance.

29. **What is hepatic encephalopathy, and how is it treated?**
Hepatic encephalopathy is altered mental status (ranging from subtle to severe) due to the accumulation of neurotoxic substances traditionally cleared by a healthy liver. The most commonly associated toxin is ammonia that bypasses the hepatocytes and ends up in the astrocytes of the brain. Here, the ammonia increases GABA and decreases glutamate for an overall inhibitory action on the CNS. The laxative lactulose is typically used for elimination of by-products until the precipitating factor is brought under control.

30. **How is cardiovascular function affected in a patient with liver disease?**
Cardiovascular function is characterized by a hyperdynamic circulatory state.
   - Increased cardiac output
   - Decreased systemic vascular resistance
   - Increased blood volume
   - Unchanged blood pressure and heart rate
   - Decreased portal vein blood flow
   - Maintained or decreased hepatic artery blood flow
   - Maintained or decreased renal blood flow
   - Presence of arteriovenous fistulas in many sites
   - Possible cardiomyopathy

31. **What is hepatorenal syndrome?**
Hepatorenal syndrome is a progressive renal failure that occurs in patients with severe liver disease. It is considered a functional renal failure since the kidneys are morphologically normal and resume normal function when transplanted into recipients who don't have a history of liver dysfunction.

32. **What are contraindications to surgery in the patient with liver disease?**
   - Acute liver failure
   - Acute renal failure
   - Acute viral hepatitis
   - Alcoholic hepatitis
   - Cardiomyopathy
   - Hypoxemia
   - Severe coagulopathy (despite treatment)
   - MELD score >15

33. **What precautions should be taken before oral and maxillofacial surgery in a patient with viral hepatitis?**
The patient's liver function status should be determined by means of liver function enzymes (AST, ALT, and ALP). Drug choice and dosage should be determined with these lab values in mind. The patient's bleeding tendency should also be assessed by PT, PTT, INR, and bleeding time. For patients undergoing major surgical procedures, if the PT or PTT is more than 1.5 times > control values or if the INR is ≥3.0, transfusion of FFP should be considered. This supplies the patient with factors II, VII, IX, X, XI, XII, and XIII and heat-labile factors V and VII. In patients with a platelet count of <50,000/mm^3, platelet administration to a level above 50,000 mm^3 is indicated. Universal precautions should also be taken to prevent hepatitis exposure to the surgeon and assistants.

34. **What is the preoperative therapy for patients with liver disease?**
Preoperative maximization of liver function in patients with liver disease should include evaluating and optimizing the nutritional status and correcting electrolyte and coagulation abnormalities. The patient should stop alcohol intake and increase protein intake. If the patient has active hepatitis, all elective surgeries should be postponed until the hepatitis has resolved completely. Defects in coagulation should be corrected with FFP. If the patient is taking steroids, intravenous corticosteroids should be given. Finally, preoperative or operative sedation should be done to a degree that is compatible with the patient's decreased ability to metabolize drugs by the liver, especially benzodiazepines, barbiturates, and other sedatives.

35. **How can bleeding diathesis due to liver disease be corrected?**
Increased PT/INR.
   - Vitamin K and FFP (vitamin K alone does not increase factor V levels and requires 12 to 48 hours to synthesize)
Decreased platelets/increased bleeding time.
   - Transfusion of platelets ± DDAVP if impaired von Willebrand factor

36. **What are the intraoperative considerations in patients with liver disease?**
    It is important to maintain adequate liver perfusion during surgery by maintaining adequate blood pressure. This can be done by infusing saline, FFP, and platelets if there is thrombocytopenia. If the patient swallowed blood, the stomach should be evacuated to prevent protein loading and false-positive blood in the stool. If the patient is taking corticosteroids, supplemental steroids should be given.

37. **What are the surgical considerations in post-liver transplant patients?**
    During the first 3 months of the postoperative period, and in patients with chronic rejection of the graft, only emergency oral surgical procedures should be rendered. Such procedures should be performed only after consultation with the patient's transplant service, and whenever possible, antibiotic prophylaxis should be given to prevent bacterial endarteritis. After the first 3 months, the patient is usually on immunosuppressants. If the patient has a stable functional graft, good liver function is established. However, there is still the risk of acquired infection including influenza, fungal infections, and post-transplant viral infections. In these patients, prevention and treatment of any possible infection is important, and consideration must be given to the patient's immunosuppressant doses, supplementation of steroids (if necessary), and use of effective infection control measures.

MANAGEMENT OF PATIENTS WITH HEMATOLOGICAL DISEASES†

38. **Which blood clotting factors are dependent on vitamin K for their synthesis?**
    Factors II, VII, IX, and X.

39. **Which blood test is used to monitor the effect of warfarin?**
    Prothrombin time (PT) test.

40. **What is the international normalized ratio (INR)?**
    The INR is a calculated value developed to normalize the reporting of PT.

$$\textbf{INR} = \left(\frac{\text{patient protime}}{\text{mean of the normal range}} \right) \text{ISI}$$

The ISI is the International Sensitivity Index value assigned by the manufacturer to each lot of thromboplastin calibrated to the World Health Organization reference material. The INR standardizes reporting of anticoagulation activity and monitors patients on stabilized oral anticoagulant therapy only. The therapeutic INR range is 2.0 to 3.0 for most clinical situations. Patients with mechanical prosthetic heart valves are maintained at 2.5 to 3.5.

41. **What are the three phases of hemostasis?**
    Vascular, platelet, and coagulation phases.

42. **What effect can long-term antibiotic therapy have on hemostasis?**
    Long-term antibiotic therapy can suppress the normal flora in the gastrointestinal tract that are necessary for the synthesis of vitamin K. Clotting factors II, VII, IX, and X require vitamin K for their synthesis.

43. **What is the mechanism of action of warfarin?**
    Warfarin is a vitamin K antagonist that leads to a decrease in factors II, VII, IX, and X proteins C and S. Warfarin is used for long-term anticoagulation and is monitored by frequent INR and PT.

44. **If warfarin (Coumadin) is to be discontinued before oral surgery, how soon should this occur before the planned procedure?**
    Although dose dependent, in general, the duration of action for warfarin is 3 to 5 days with an onset in 12 to 24 hours. The half-life is 1.5 to 2.5 days. Warfarin should be discontinued at least 3 days before the procedure, and a PT test should be done within 24 hours of the surgery.

45. **How does administering vitamin K affect warfarin?**
    Vitamin K reverses the action of warfarin; however, the process takes about 6 to 14 hours. In the event of severe and acute blood loss, transfusions (e.g., FFP) may be necessary to replenish missing factors.

---

†Written by Roman G. Meyliker.

Once vitamin K is administered, the patient may be resistant to further anticoagulation with warfarin for a few days. In addition, certain patients may have an underlying thrombotic tendency that puts them at risk for thrombosis and embolic complications should the effects of the anticoagulant be stopped abruptly. Therefore administering vitamin K or abruptly stopping warfarin medication can be harmful to some patients.

46. **How does heparin affect blood clotting?**
Heparin potentiates antithrombin III, and, as a result, clotting factors IIa, IXa, Xa, XIa, and XIIa are inhibited. Factors IIa and Xa are more sensitive to the heparin and antithrombin III complex and are considered to be more clinically relevant than the remaining factors listed above.

47. **Why are PT and PTT not used to monitor low molecular weight heparin (LMWH)?**
LMWH binds to antithrombin III and potentiates its inhibition of factor Xa; unlike in heparin, the effect on factor IIa is significantly less. Therefore PT and PTT are unreliable for monitoring LMWH.

48. **How can the effects of heparin be reversed?**
Protamine sulfate is used to reverse the effects of heparin. Protamine, which itself is an anticoagulant, must be administered with caution. When protamine is given with heparin, the anticoagulant effect of both drugs is lost. Careful control of the protamine dosing is necessary to prevent bleeding from an overdose. Too rapid administration of protamine can result in hypertensive and anaphylactoid reactions.

49. **What is the pathophysiology of heparin-induced thrombocytopenia (HIT)?**
Heparin bound to platelet binding protein 4 on platelets can form antigenic complexes that induce the formation of IgG antibodies. These antibodies cause the formation of cross-bridges that result in platelet aggregation, which causes a decrease in platelet count.

50. **What is a major complication of heparin-induced thrombocytopenia (HIT)?**
Thrombosis occurs in up to 75% of cases of HIT.

51. **How does aspirin affect blood coagulation?**
Aspirin (acetylsalicylic acid [ASA]) and other nonsteroidal antiinflammatory drugs (NSAIDs) affect the platelet phase of coagulation. These drugs alter cyclooxygenase activity within platelets. Cyclooxygenase controls the release of the adhesive proteins from platelets that are necessary for them to aggregate and stick together in response to trauma. Inhibition of cyclooxygenase activity by either aspirin or another NSAID will cause the development of an ineffective platelet plug, resulting in prolonged bleeding. This side effect of ASA has led to its accepted controlled use as a prophylactic measure against coronary and cerebral vessel thrombosis.

52. **What are the components of the extrinsic, intrinsic, and common pathways of the coagulation cascade?**
The components of the intrinsic pathway are factors VIII, IX, XI, and XII. The components of the extrinsic pathways include tissue factors and factor VII. The common pathway involves factors X and XIII, prothrombin, thrombin, fibrinogen, and fibrin.

53. **Which factors are measured by PT, and which ones are measured by PTT?**
PT measures factors II, VII, IX, and X, and fibrinogen. PTT measures the integrity of the intrinsic pathways before the activation of factor X and the activity of factors I, II, V, VIII, IX, X, XI, and XII, and fibrinogen.

54. **What is anemia?**
A decrease in the oxygen-carrying capacity of the blood. General symptoms include weakness, fatigue, palpitations, tingling, and numbness of the fingers and toes, a burning tongue, bone pain, and shortness of breath. Clinical signs of anemia include pallor, spooning and brittle nails, and a smooth, red tongue caused by loss of filiform papillae.

55. **What causes iron deficiency anemia?**
Iron deficiency anemia is most commonly caused by low dietary iron intake or blood loss. When blood loss is suspected in men or non-menstruating females, the most likely source is the gastrointestinal tract and further investigation for a source is necessary. In patients with dietary deficiency, oral iron replacement with ferrous sulfate is an effective treatment.

56. **What is pernicious anemia?**
Normally, vitamin B12 binds to intrinsic factor, which is necessary for its absorption in the ileum. The intrinsic factor is a glycoprotein that is secreted by the parietal cells in the stomach. In patients

with pernicious anemia, there is autoimmune destruction of parietal cells leading to malabsorption of vitamin B12 and subsequent formation of fragile megaloblastic erythrocytes.

57. **What causes sickle cell anemia?**
The inherent defect causing sickle cell anemia is the substitution of valine for glutamine on the beta chain of the hemoglobin molecule. This defective hemoglobin, now called hemoglobin S, ultimately causes the RBCs to become sickle shaped when exposed to low oxygen tension.

58. **What is the perioperative management of a patient with sickle cell disease?**
Perioperative management of a sickle cell anemia patient involves avoiding all possible precipitating factors, which include hypoxia, dehydration, stress, and infection. This can be done with intravenous (IV) fluids, sedation, oxygen supplementation, and all measures that prevent infection, including antibiotic coverage. In patients with severe sickle cell disease who are undergoing major surgical procedures, exchange transfusions may be used to dilute the defective RBCs by 50%, keeping the hematocrit under 35%. Treatment of sickle cell crisis involves maintenance of hydration, administration of oxygen, and analgesics.

59. **What is the result of a deficiency of glucose-6 phosphate dehydrogenase (G6PD)?**
The enzyme glucose-6 phosphate dehydrogenase is largely responsible for maintaining intracellular levels of NADPH and consequently protecting the erythrocyte from oxidative damage. In states of oxidative stress, these patients are at high risk for hemolytic anemia.
   Some of the known substances that can precipitate an exacerbation are aspirin, fava beans, sulfonamides, nitrofurantoin, and dimercaprol. Infections have also been linked with inducing hemolysis.

60. **Which variant of G6PD is potentially fatal?**
There are two types of G6PD deficiency. The Mediterranean type can be acute and fatal; the A form is mild and self-limiting.

61. **What is the normal WBC count?**
Between 4500 and 11,000/mm^3. An increase in WBCs is termed leukocytosis, and a decrease is leukopenia.

62. **Which form of leukemia is most often associated with the Philadelphia chromosome?**
Chronic myelogenous leukemia. This marker can be found in the metaphase and is associated with a poor prognosis.

63. **Can you list risk factors associated with non-Hodgkin lymphoma?**
   - HIV/AIDS
   - Sjogren's syndrome
   - Hashimoto thyroiditis
   - *Helicobacter pylori* gastritis
   - Epstein-Barr virus (EBV)
   - Human T-cell lymphotropic virus type 1 (HTLV-1)
   - Organ transplant
   - Immunosuppression

64. **Reed-Sternberg cells are found in which disease?**
Hodgkin Disease.

65. **Bence Jones proteins are found in which diseases?**
Multiple myeloma and Waldenström macroglobulinemia.

66. **What is von Willebrand disease?**
Von Willebrand disease is an inherited disorder in which von Willebrand factor, required for platelet adhesion, is either deficient or defective.

67. **What are the known functions of von Willebrand factor (vWF)?**
   1. Enhances platelet aggregation
   2. Stabilizes factor VIII
   3. Contributes to the ability of platelets to attach to injured vascular endothelium

68. What are the four hereditary types of von Willebrand disease (vWD)?
    - **Type 1 vWD:** quantitative defect that is heterozygous for the defective gene. The production of von Willebrand factor (vWF) is decreased.
    - **Type 2 vWD:** a qualitative defect; four subtypes exist (2A, 2B, 2M, and 2N):
        - 2A: This is a qualitative defect in the vWF resulting in a decreased ability to bind to platelet glycoprotein1 (GP1) as well as a decreased capability at multimerization.
        - 2B: This is a qualitative defect in the vWF resulting in abnormally enhanced binding to the GP1 receptor on the platelet membrane, leading to its spontaneous binding to platelets and subsequent rapid clearance of the bound platelets and of the large vWF multimers. DDAVP is contraindicated for this type.
        - 2M: This is a qualitative defect of vWF characterized by its decreased ability to bind to the GP1 receptor on the platelet membrane, and it retains a normal capability at multimerization.
        - 2N: This is characterized by a normal quantity of vWF but a deficiency of the binding of vWF to coagulation factor VIII. This results in low levels of factor VIII due to lack of vWF stabilization from proteolytic degradation.
    - **Type 3 vWD:** complete absence of production of vWF, resulting in low factor VIII levels from lack of vWF to prevent proteolytic degradation. This is the most severe type of vWD and can be life threatening.
    - **Platelet-type vWD:** vWF is qualitatively normal, and the vWF protein lacks any mutational alteration. The defect lies in the altered GP1 receptor on the platelet membrane, which increases its affinity to bind to vWF.

69. How can hemophilia A and B be differentiated?
    Hemophilia A is an X-linked recessive disorder in which factor VIII is deficient, whereas the affected serine protease in type B is factor IX.

70. Which hemostatic agents can be used to manage hemophilia patients prior to surgery?
    Patients with hemophilia A are managed according to the severity of their disorder and anticipated blood loss. Patients with severe hemophilia should receive replacement of factor VIII with factor VIII concentrate. For mild hemophiliacs, desmopressin (DDAVP) can boost plasma levels of factor VIII, and vWF and can be used safely in these patients. FFP and cryoprecipitate is not recommended due to potential adverse effects and should only be reserved when no other modalities are available.

71. What is the replacement therapy for hemophilia B?
    Purified factor IX.

72. What is DIC?
    Disseminated intravascular coagulation (DIC) is the consequence of intravascular activation of both the coagulation and fibrinolytic systems. DIC is characterized by widespread microvascular thrombosis and severe coagulopathy due to deletion of platelets and coagulation factors.

73. What is Plummer-Vinson syndrome?
    Plummer-Vinson syndrome occurs with iron deficiency anemia and is a predisposing factor to oral carcinoma. It is found primarily in women in the fourth and fifth decades of life. Clinical signs include cracking at the lip commissure; lemon-tinted pallor; smooth, red, painful tongue with atrophy of the filiform; and, later, fungiform papillae. A characteristic esophageal webbing or stricture is also identified. Iron deficiency anemia responds well to iron replacement therapy.

74. What is tranexamic acid, and how is it used?
    Tranexamic acid is an antifibrinolytic agent that is used to promote stability of a formed blood clot. The final phase in the common pathway to blood clot formation is the activation of fibrinogen to fibrin in the presence of thrombin. Fibrin forms the basis for the blood clot. Fibrinolysis or clot breakdown begins in the presence of plasmin that is formed from activated plasminogen. Tranexamic acid inhibits the activation of plasminogen, thereby promoting stability of the blood clot.

75. Can you list adverse events associated with erythrocyte transfusions?
    - Acute hemolytic reaction
    - Acute lung injury

- Urticaria
- Anaphylaxis and anaphylactic shock
- Non-hemolytic fever
- Bacterial and viral infections
- Transfusion errors such as incompatible transfusion or wrong person

76. **What is the mechanism of action of dabigatran etexilate?**
Dabigatran etexilate is a low molecular weight prodrug that exhibits no pharmacological activity. After oral administration, dabigatran etexilate is converted to its active form, dabigatran, a potent, competitive, and reversible direct inhibitor of the active site of thrombin.

77. **What is the mechanism of action of Rivaroxaban?**
Rivaroxaban is an orally active, direct-acting factor Xa inhibitor.

BIBLIOGRAPHY

Management of Patients with Liver Diseases

Asthana S, Kneteman N: Operating on a patient with hepatitis C, *Can J Surg* 52(4):337–342, 2009.

Cerulli MA: Management of the patient with liver diseases, *Oral Maxillofac Surg Clin North Am* 10:465–470, 1998.

Douglas LR, Douglas JB, Sieck JO, et al.: Oral management of the patient with end-stage liver disease and the liver transplant patient, *Oral Surg Oral Med Oral Pathol Oral Radiol Endod* 86:55–64, 1998.

Duke J: Renal function and anesthesia. In Duke J, editor: *Anesthesia secrets*, ed 3, Philadelphia, 2006, Mosby.

Friedman LS: The risk of surgery in patients with liver disease, *Hepatology* 29:1617, 1999.

Friedman LS, Maddrey WC: Surgery in the patient with liver disease, *Med Clin N Am* 71:453–476, 1987.

Lee WM: Drug-induced hepatotoxicity, *N Eng J Med* 333:1118, 1995.

Muir AJ: Surgical clearance for the patient with chronic liver disease, *Clin Liver Dis* 16(2):421–433, 2012.

Oghalai MA: Liver diseases. In Abubaker AO, Benson KJ, editors: *Oral and maxillofacial surgery secrets*, ed 2, Philadelphia, 2007, Elsevier/Mosby.

Sherlock S: Alcoholic liver disease, *Lancet* 345:227, 1995.

Stoelting RK, Dierdorf SF: Diseases of the liver and biliary tract. In Stoelting RK, Dierdorf SF, editors: *Anesthesia and co-existing disease*, ed 2, London, 1993, Churchill Livingstone.

Stoelting RK, Miller RD: Liver and biliary tract disease. In Stoelting RK, Miller RD, editors: *Basics of anesthesia*, ed 3, New York, 1994, Churchill Livingstone.

Teh SH, Nagorney DM, Stevens SR: Risk factors for mortality after surgery in patients with cirrhosis, *Gastroenterology* 132:1261–1299, 2007.

Ziccardi VB, Abubaker AO, Sotereanos GC, et al.: Maxillofacial considerations in orthotopic liver transplant patient, *Oral Surg Oral Med Oral Pathol* 71:21–26, 1991.

Management of Patients with Hematological Diseases

Beirne O, Koehler J: Surgical management of patients on warfarin sodium, *J Oral Maxillofac Surg* 54:1115–1118, 1996.

Eriksson BI, Quinlan DJ, Weitz JI: Comparative pharmacodynamics and pharmacokinetics of oral direct thrombin and Factor xa inhibitors in development, *Clin Pharmacokinet* 48(1):1–22, 2009.

Giglio JA, Doriot RE: Hematology. In Abubaker AO, Benson KJ, editors: *Oral and maxillofacial surgery secrets,* ed 2, Philadelphia, 2007, Elsevier/Mosby.

Gordeuk VR: Abnormalities of hemostasis. In Fishman MC, Hoffman AR, Klausner RD, Thaler MS, editors: *Medicine*, ed 5, Philadelphia, 2004, Lippincott Williams and Wilkins.

Gordeuk VR, McDonald-Pinkett SR: Anemia. In Fishman MC, Hoffman AR, Klausner RD, Thaler MS, editors: *Medicine*, ed 5, Philadelphia, 2004, Lippincott Williams and Wilkins.

Hankey GJ, Eikelboom JW: Dabigatran etexilate: a new oral thrombin inhibitor, *Circulation* 123:1436–1450, 2011.

Herman W, Konzelman J, Sutley S: Current perspectives on dental patients receiving Coumadin anticoagulant therapy, *J Am Dent Assoc* 128:327–335, 1997.

Hirsch J, Raschke R: Heparin and low-molecular-weight heparin: the seventh ACCP Conference on Antithrombotic and Thrombolytic Therapy, *Chest* 126(suppl):188S–203S, 2004.

Lew D: Blood and blood products. In Kwon PH, Laskin DM, editors: *Clinician's manual of oral and maxillofacial surgery*, ed 2, Carol Stream, IL, 1997, Quintessence.

Little J, Falace D, Miller C, et al.: *Dental management of the medically compromised patient*, ed 6, St Louis, 2002, Mosby.

Pinto HA: Leukemia, lymphoma and multiple myeloma. In Fishman MC, Hoffman AR, Klausner RD, Thaler MS, editors: *Medicine*, ed 5, Philadelphia, 2004, Lippincott Williams and Wilkins.

Provan D, Singer CRJ, Baglin T, Dokal I: *Oxford handbooks: Oxford handbook of clinical haematology*, ed 3, New York, 2009, Oxford University Press.

Todd DW, Roman A: Outpatient use of low-molecular-weight heparin in an anticoagulated patient requiring oral surgery: case report, *J Oral Maxillofac Surg* 59:1090–1092, 2001.

CHAPTER 19

MANAGEMENT OF PATIENTS WITH RENAL DISEASES

Samir Singh, Mark A. Oghalai

1. What are the six main functions of the kidney?
   1. Elimination of metabolic waste (foreign substances, drugs, urea, uric acid)
   2. Maintenance of fluid balance
   3. Maintenance of electrolyte balance
   4. Maintenance of acid and base balance
   5. Endocrine and metabolic functions (erythropoietin secretion and vitamin D conversion)
   6. Regulation of blood pressure

2. What are the three basic processes that take place in the nephron (functional unit of the kidney)?
   Filtration, reabsorption, and secretion.

3. Which compound is used as a sensitive, indirect measurement of glomerular filtration rate (GFR)?
   Creatinine is a natural product of the body (breakdown product of creatinine phosphate found in muscle). It is used because it is freely filtered by the glomeruli and minimally secreted by peritubular capillaries. It can result in an overestimation of GFR by 10% to 20%, which is clinically acceptable.

4. What is renal failure?
   Renal failure is defined as impairment in renal function, as measured by the GFR. It is classified as either acute or chronic.

5. What is acute renal failure (ARF) or acute kidney injury (AKI)?
   This syndrome is characterized by sudden decline in renal function, resulting in retention of nitrogenous waste with corresponding elevations of serum creatinine (relative increase of 50% or absolute increase of 0.5 to 1.0 mg/dL) and blood urea nitrogen (BUN).

6. What is the RIFLE criteria?
   It is one method of staging AKI.
   Risk: 1.5-fold increase in serum creatinine or GFR decrease by 25% or urine output <0.5 mL/kg/hr for 6 hours
   Injury: Twofold increase in serum creatinine or GFR decrease by 50% or urine output <0.5 mL/kg/hr for 12 hours
   Failure: Threefold increase in serum creatinine or GFR decrease by 75% or urine output <0.5 mL/kg/hr for 24 hours or anuria for 12 hours
   Loss: Complete loss of kidney function (requiring dialysis) for more than 4 weeks
   End-stage renal disease: Complete loss of kidney function (requiring dialysis) for more than 3 months

7. What are the major classes of ARF/AKI?
   - **Prerenal.** Renal blood flow decreases enough to lower the GFR, which leads to decreased clearance of metabolites (BUN, creatinine, uremic toxins). This class is the most common type and is associated with insufficient renal perfusion. Examples include hypovolemia, hypotension, impaired cardiac function (CHF), cirrhosis and hepatorenal syndrome, decreased renal perfusion with concomitant NSAID, ACE inhibitor, and/or cyclosporine use, and sepsis. It is potentially reversible.
   - **Renal.** Kidney tissue is damaged such that glomerular filtration and tubular function are significantly impaired. The kidneys are unable to concentrate urine effectively. Glomerular diseases (acute glomerulonephritis, Goodpasture's syndrome, Wegener's granulomatosis, poststreptococcal glomerulonephritis, lupus), acute tubular necrosis (ischemic AKI, nephrotoxic AKI), and acute interstitial nephritis (allergic interstitial nephritis) fall under this classification.

- **Postrenal.** Least common cause of AKI. Obstruction of any segment of the urinary tract causes increased tubular pressure that leads to decreased GFR. Urine is produced but cannot be excreted. Benign Prostate Hypertrophy is the most common cause of urethral obstruction. Other possible causes include nephrolithiasis, neoplasm, retroperitoneal fibrosis and ureteral obstruction.

8. What is FENa? How is it used to determine which type of ARF/AKI is present?
   Fraction of excreted sodium (FENa) is the percentage of sodium filtered by the kidney that is excreted in urine. It is calculated as follows:

   $$[(Urine\ Na)/(Plasma\ Na)/(Urine\ creatinine)/(plasma\ creatinine)] \times 100$$

   FENa below 1% suggests prerenal etiology. FENa above 2% to 3% suggests ATN or other kidney damage.

9. What are some of the urinalysis findings in ARF/AKI?
   - Prerenal: benign sediment, few hyaline casts, absence of protein and blood
   - Renal:
     - ATN: muddy-brown casts, renal tubular cells/casts, granular casts, trace protein, absence of blood
     - Acute glomerulonephritis: dysmorphic RBCs, RBCs with casts, WBCs with casts, fatty casts, 4+ protein, 3+ blood
     - Acute interstitial nephritis: RBCs, WBCs, WBCs with casts, eosinophils, 1+ protein, 2+ blood
   - Postrenal: benign, may or may not see RBCs, WBCs, absence of protein and blood

10. How is ARF/AKI managed?
    General measures include avoiding medications that decrease renal blood flow, adjusting medication doses for level of renal function, correcting fluid imbalance, correcting electrolyte abnormalities, and optimizing cardiac output.
    - Prerenal: Treat the underlying disorder, give normal saline to maintain euvolemia and restore blood pressure, stop antihypertensive medications, and give dialysis if symptomatic uremia, intractable acidemia, hyperkalemia, or volume overload develops.
    - Renal: Supportive therapy. Remove offending agent/cause. If patient is oliguric, a trial of furosemide may help increase urine flow.
    - Postrenal: A bladder catheter may decompress the urinary tract.

11. What is chronic renal failure (CRF) or chronic kidney disease (CKD)?
    It is defined as either decreased kidney function (GFR <60 mL/min) or kidney damage (structural or functional) for at least 3 months regardless of cause. CRF/CKD is an irreversible, advanced, and progressive renal insufficiency.

12. What are the stages of CRF/CKD?
    There are five stages that are defined by the estimated GFR. Therapy is guided by the stage of CRF/CKD.
    Stage 1 (normal): GFR 90 mL/min
    Stage 2: GFR 60 to 89 mL/min
    Stage 3: GFR 30 to 59 mL/min
    Stage 4: GFR 15 to 29 mL/min
    Stage 5: GFR <15 mL/min

13. What are some causes of CRF/CKD?
    - Diabetic nephropathy (most common cause, 30% of all cases)
    - Hypertension (25% of cases)
    - Chronic glomerulonephritis (15% of cases)
    - Interstitial nephritis, polycystic kidney disease, obstructive uropathy
    - Untreated ARF/AKI

14. What are the clinical manifestations of CRF and end-stage renal disease (ESRD)?
    The clinical manifestations of CRF and ESRD depend on the stage of the disease and include:
    - Fluid and electrolyte disturbances (hyperkalemia due to decreased urinary secretion, hypermagnesemia due to reduced urinary loss, hyerphosphatemia)
    - Peripheral neuropathy

- Hypertension and pericarditis
- Anemia and thrombocytopenia (due to uremia, platelets do not degranulate in uremic environment)
- Uremia and uremic osteodystrophy
- Nausea and vomiting
- Tiredness and insomnia
- Pruritus and hyperpigmentation
- Sexual/reproductive system disturbances (decreased testosterone in men; amenorrhea, infertility, and hyperprolactinemia in women)

15. How is CRF/CKD managed, and what are some complications?

Dietary restrictions (low protein, low salt, restricted potassium magnesium and phosphate intake), ACE inhibitors (dilate efferent arteriole of glomerulus), control of BP, glycemic control, correction of electrolyte and acid/base abnormalities, supplementation with oral calcium and vitamin D to prevent secondary hyperparathyroidism, management of pulmonary edema (diuretics and dialysis).

Life-threatening complications of CRF/CKD include hyperkalemia, pulmonary edema (from volume overload), and infection (pneumonia, urinary tract infection, sepsis).

16. What are the main treatment options for ESRD?

- Peritoneal dialysis
- Hemodialysis
- Renal transplant

17. What are the absolute indications for dialysis?

Absolute indications can be remembered by the mnemonic AEIOU:

A: Acidosis that is intractable and severe
E: Electrolyte disturbances that are persistent
I: Intoxications (methanol, eythylene glycol, lithium, aspirin, NSAIDs)
O: Overload (hypervolemia) unmanaged by other therapy
U: Uremia (severe)

18. What is secondary hyperparathyroidism?

As the kidneys lose their ability to convert vitamin D, intestinal absorption of calcium decreases, causing hyperparathyroidism.

19. What are the oral manifestations of renal disease?

Patients with renal disease or CRF often demonstrate orofacial signs and symptoms that are not necessarily specific for ESRD but are related to the systemic manifestations of the disease. The most common of these manifestations are:

- Enamel hypoplasia and staining of teeth
- Halitosis and metallic taste
- Stomatitis and xerostomia secondary to fluid intake restriction
- Gingival bleeding, ecchymosis, petechiae, and pale and inflamed gingiva
- Osteolytic bone defects in the mandible, mandibular condyles, and maxilla; loss of lamina dura; and decreased trabeculation of bone
- Skeletal facial deformities secondary to altered growth
- Accelerated dental calculus accumulation

20. What are the lab findings in patients with CRF/CKD?

- Elevated BUN and creatinine resulting from decreased glomerular filtration
- Metabolic acidosis secondary to impaired tubular function, causing an accumulation of ammonia
- Multiple electrolyte abnormalities, including hyperkalemia, hypocalcemia, and hypermagnesemia
- Anemia from decreased renal production of erythropoietin
- Thrombocytopenia (due to uremia)

21. How does renal disease affect the pharmacodynamics of administered drugs?

The effects of drugs may be potentiated by increased volume of distribution, decreased protein binding, and decreased glomerular filtration and renal tubular secretion. Renal failure may modify drug bioavailability, distribution, pharmacologic action, or elimination when the kidney excretes the drug or its metabolites. For the ESRD patient, most drugs are administered in an initial loading dose to provide therapeutic blood concentrations. Sustained effects are controlled by dosage adjustments and time-interval alterations and are based on serum drug levels.

22. **How do nonsteroidal antiinflammatory drugs (NSAIDs) affect renal function?**
NSAIDs inhibit prostaglandin synthesis and, therefore, decrease prostaglandin-associated intrinsic renal vasodilatation. The net result is renal afferent arteriole constriction and eventual decrease in renal perfusion pressure.

23. **What classes of drugs should be avoided in patients with renal disease?**
    • Nephrotoxic drugs, including NSAIDs, aminoglycosides, and intravenous (IV) dyes
    • Drugs that are converted to toxic metabolites, including morphine, meperidine, and propoxyphene
    • Drugs that contain excessive electrolytes, including penicillin G and magnesium citrate

24. **What analgesics should be avoided in patients with renal disease?**
    • Aspirin
    • Acetaminophen
    • NSAIDs
    • Meperidine (accumulation of meperidine can result in seizures)
    • Morphine (dose decreased secondary to accumulation of morphine-6-glucuronide)

25. **What antibiotics should be avoided in patients with renal disease?**
    • Cephalosporins
    • Tetracycline
    • Erythromycin
    • Aminoglycosides

26. **In severe renal dysfunction patients, are metabolic end products from local anesthetics contraindicated?**
No. Local anesthetics are metabolized in the liver and plasma and then excreted. Therefore anesthetics can accumulate and not be a factor in patients with renal disease.

27. **What effect might general anesthetics have on renal blood flow and GFR?**
General anesthetics that can cause myocardial depression also can cause decreased renal blood flow and a GFR that is proportional to the depth of anesthesia. Methoxyflurane is no longer in use because of fluoride-induced nephrotoxicity. Halothane, enflurane, and isoflurane produce much lower fluoride levels and are safer to use with regard to nephrotoxicity. Therefore, it is important to choose the type of agent and the appropriate level of anesthesia in renal failure patients to minimize further injury and likelihood of renal failure.

28. **What is Compound A? Which volatile anesthetic produces it?**
Compound A (trifluoroethyl vinyl ether) is produced from the breakdown of sevoflurane. It is nephrotoxic with prolonged exposure and low fresh gas flows (<2 L/min). The package insert recommends fresh gas flows >2 L/min.

29. **Which metabolites from halogenated general anesthetics can lead to nephrotoxic renal failure?**
Inorganic fluoride from the metabolism of methoxyflurane. Sevoflurane also increases inorganic fluoride, and its use is controversial in patients with renal disease.

30. **Which halogenated general anesthetics do not significantly increase plasma inorganic fluoride concentrations?**
Isoflurane, halothane, and desflurane.

31. **At what time before and after surgery should dialysis be performed?**
One day before surgery and 1 to 2 days after surgery to correct potassium and fluid balance while minimizing bleeding complications.

32. **What lab tests should be performed for renal failure patients before surgery?**
CRF patients should have bleeding time, prothrombin time (PT), partial thromboplastin time (PTT), platelet count, complete blood cell count (CBC), and a basic metabolic panel (BMP). Bleeding time is the most sensitive test for a bleeding tendency in CRF patients. If the bleeding time is elevated, the patient should receive vigorous dialysis and, if necessary, deamino-D-arginine vasopressin (DDAVP) intravenously or nasally, at a dose of 0.3 μg/kg, 30 minutes before surgery. Hyperkalemia also can be corrected with preoperative dialysis. If surgery is emergent and dialysis cannot be performed preoperatively, hyperkalemia should be treated aggressively to decrease the arrhythmogenic effect

of hyperkalemia. This can be done by IV infusion of calcium chloride to stabilize the myocardium, glucose to prevent hyoglycemia, and insulin to drive potassium intracellularly.

33. **What is the cause of CRF-induced anemia?**
Decreased erythropoietin production from the kidneys.

34. **What is the treatment for CRF-induced anemia before surgery?**
Anemia in CRF patients should be treated with administration of recombinant human erythropoietin until the patient's hematocrit is raised to at least 30% to 33%.

35. **What is the difference between peritoneal dialysis and hemodialysis?**
In peritoneal dialysis, a hypertonic solution is placed into the peritoneal cavity via an implanted catheter or a temporary catheter, and removed a short time later. The peritoneum serves as the dialysis membrane. During the removal process, dissolved solutes such as urea are drawn out. Peritoneal dialysis does not require anticoagulation, the patient can learn to perform dialysis on his or her own, and it is less expensive than hemodialysis. However, peritoneal dialysis requires more frequent sessions than hemodialysis, is less effective, and has a higher incidence of complications such as infection, hyperglycemia, hypertriglyceridemia, peritonitis, hypoglycemia, and protein loss. The most common use for peritoneal dialysis is the treatment of patients with ARF/AKI.

Hemodialysis is the most commonly used method of dialysis for CRF/CKD/ESRD and is performed at 2- to 3-day intervals. Surgical placement of a permanent arteriovenous (AV) fistula for large-bore cannulation is required; the patient's blood is filtered through a dialysis machine and returned to the patient via the AV fistula. Administering heparin prevents clotting. Hemodialysis may also be performed through a central line dialysis catheter or a tunneled central line dialysis catheter. Hemodialysis is considered to be more efficient than peritoneal dialysis and shortens the time of dialysis. Patients receiving hemodialysis are at risk for contracting hepatitis B, hepatitis C, and HIV because of multiple blood exposures. They may be predisposed to developing hypotension due to rapid removal of intravascular volume and hypo-osmolality due to solute removal. In addition, these patients are at risk for infection of their AV shunts, which predisposes them to septic emboli, septicemia, infective endarteritis, and infective endocarditis.

Alternatives to traditional hemodialysis include continuous arteriovenous hemodialysis (CAVHD) and continuous venovenous hemodialysis (CVVHD). These are often used in hemodynamically unstable patients with ARF/AKI. Lower flow rates of blood and dialysate enable dialysis to occur while minimizing rapid shifts in volume and osmolality.

36. **What steps should be taken before surgical procedures in ESRD patients?**
   - Review lab values to detect possible bleeding diathesis (bleeding time, platelet count, PT, PTT) and electrolyte abnormalities.
   - Monitor blood pressure.
   - Avoid nephrotoxic drugs such as acyclovir, aspirin, NSAIDs, and high-dose acetaminophen.
   - Decrease dosage of drugs metabolized by the kidney.
   - Aggressively manage orofacial infections.
   - Ensure that patients receiving hemodialysis do not undergo surgery for at least 4 hours after hemodialysis to avoid heparin-induced bleeding.

37. **What pre-surgical adjustments need to be made in drug dosing or interval in patients with CRF?**
See Table 19-1.

38. **What medical considerations should be given to patients receiving dialysis before oral surgical procedures?**
No adjustments are required for patients receiving peritoneal dialysis, but there are several concerns for patients receiving hemodialysis. Surgically created bacteremia can cause infection of the AV fistula. Because graft endothelialization takes up to 3 to 6 months after placement, standard American Heart Association antibiotic prophylaxis is strongly recommended for the first 6 months after fistula placement and may be beneficial for all graft patients undergoing oral surgery. The arm that contains the AV shunt should not be used for blood pressure recording because the shunt could collapse. Likewise, IV administration of medications should be avoided in the arm because clot formation could jeopardize the shunt. The quality of the AV thrill should be assessed initially and then periodically during surgery. During long surgeries, the use of a circulating heating pack over the arm is advocated.

Table 19-1. Pre-surgical Drug Adjustments Made in Chronic Renal Failure Patients

DRUG	PRE-SURGERY ADJUSTMENT
Aspirin	Increase interval between doses and avoid drug completely if glomerular filtration rate is low
Acetaminophen	Increase interval between doses and avoid drug completely in cases of severe failure
Penicillin V, cephalexin, tetracycline	Increase interval between doses in severe failure
Ketoconazole	Reduce dose
Lidocaine, codeine, erythromycin, clindamycin, metronidazole	No adjustment necessary

Patients should be screened for bleeding tendencies because hemodialysis destroys platelets. Surgery should be delayed for at least 4 hours after hemodialysis to prevent heparin-induced bleeding. Patients should be screened periodically for hepatitis B, hepatitis C, and HIV. Universal precautions should be followed by the surgical team when treating any patient undergoing hemodialysis. The positioning of the access site must be observed during surgery to avoid pressure on the site.

39. What physical finding is associated with a functioning AV fistula?
    Palpable thrill due to high-velocity flow.

40. How are bleeding problems prevented and managed in patients with renal failure?
    Bleeding encountered in patients with renal failure is best managed initially with local hemostatic procedures, such as good surgical technique, primary wound closure, hemostatic agents and topical thrombin, and electrocautery. Preoperative IV ($0.3\,\mu g/kg$) or intranasal ($3.0\,\mu g/kg$) DDAVP temporarily corrects the increase in bleeding time in uremic patients for up to 4 hours. It also may be useful as a therapeutic modality in acute postsurgical hemorrhage. Cryoprecipitate has a peak effect in 4 to 12 hours and duration of 24 to 36 hours but generally is reserved for acute bleeding that is not easily managed. Conjugated estrogen, which has a duration of up to 30 days and peak effects in approximately 2 to 5 days, also may be used.

BIBLIOGRAPHY

Agabegi SS, Agabegi ED, Ring AC: *Step-up to medicine*, ed 3, Baltimore, 2013, Lippincott Williams & Wilkins.
Bennett WM, Muther RS, Parker RA, et al.: Drug therapy in renal failure: dosing guidelines for adults. Part I: antimicrobial agents, analgesics, *Ann Intern Med* 93:62–89, 1980.
Carl W, Wood RH: The dental patient with chronic renal failure, *Quintessence Int* 7:9–15, 1976.
Cooper DH, Krainik AJ, Lubner SJ, Reno HE, Micek ST: *Washington manual of medical therapeutics*, ed 32, St Louis, 2007, Lippincott Williams & Wilkins.
Duke J: Renal function and anesthesia. In Duke J, editor: *Anesthesia secrets*, ed 3, Philadelphia, 2006, Mosby.
Little JW, Falace DA: Chronic renal failure and dialysis. In Little JW, Falace DA, editors: *Dental management of the medically compromised patient*, ed 6, St Louis, 2002, Mosby.
Oghalai MA: Renal patient. In Abubaker AO, Benson KJ, editors: *Oral and maxillofacial surgery secrets*, ed 2, Philadelphia, 2007, Mosby/Elsevier.
Silverstein KE, Adams MC, Fonseca RJ: Evaluation and management of the renal failure and dialysis patient, *Oral Maxillofac Surg Clin North Am* 10:417–427, 1998.
Silverthorn DU: *Human physiology: an integrated approach*, ed 4, San Francisco, 2007, Benjamin Cummings.
Stoelting RK, Dierdorf SF: Renal disease. In Stoelting RK, Dierdorf SF, editors: *Anesthesia and co-existing disease*, ed 3, London, 1993, Churchill Livingstone.
Stoelting RK, Miller RD: Renal disease. In Stoelting RK, Miller RD, editors: *Basics of anesthesia*, ed 3, Philadelphia, 1994, Churchill Livingstone.
Swell SB: Dental care for patients with renal failure and renal transplants, *J Am Dent Assoc* 104:171–177, 1982.
Westbrook DS: Dental management in patients receiving hemodialysis and kidney transplants, *J Am Dental Assoc* 96:464–468, 1978.
Ziccardi VB, Saini J, Demas PN, et al.: Management of the oral and maxillofacial surgery patient with end-stage renal disease, *J Oral Maxillofac Surg* 50:1207–1212, 1992.

CHAPTER 20

MANAGEMENT CONSIDERATIONS TO PATIENTS WITH ENDOCRINE DISEASES AND THE PREGNANT PATIENTS

Sidney Eisig, Vincent Carrao

MANAGEMENT CONSIDERATIONS TO PATIENTS WITH ENDOCRINE DISEASES

1. What is the embryologic migratory path of the thyroid gland?

   The thyroid gland develops during the third week of gestation and courses down a path along the thyroglossal duct originating from the floor of the primitive pharynx. This holds particular interest for oral and maxillofacial surgeons due to the fact that it is possible to trap ectopic thyroid tissue at the base of the tongue and/or generate thyroglossal duct cysts along its migratory path.

2. What is the role of iodine in thyroid function?

   Iodine is crucial for thyroid function; iodine is bound to albumin in the blood and is readily and efficiently taken up by the thyroid. The iodine is then used to synthesize thyroid hormone. Without iodine availability there would be no production of thyroid hormone.

   Dietary intake of iodine is therefore crucial for thyroid function and homeostasis. The most common cause of hypothyroidism is due to poor dietary intake of iodine.

3. What is Hashimoto's thyroiditis?

   Hashimoto's thyroiditis is a form of hypothyroidism caused by an autoimmune process. The autoimmune process produces atrophy of the thyroid follicles due to large infiltrates of lymphocytes producing germinal centers.

   The result is a decrease in thyroid hormone production, and therefore an increase in thyroid stimulating hormone (TSH) expression from the anterior pituitary attempting to stimulate the nonfunctional atrophic thyroid follicles.

4. What is the relationship between T3 and T4?

   T4 is more abundant than T3. T4 is converted to T3 by the converting enzyme deiodinase (I, II, or III). T4 and T3 are bound by various proteins in the blood. The unbound hormone in the blood regulates the expression of TSH that stimulates the thyroid gland to secrete thyroid hormone. Although there is less T3 production compared to T4, T3 has a much greater receptor affinity at the various tissue receptors, and thus greater systemic effect.

5. What is thyrotoxicosis?

   Thyrotoxicosis is a state of excess thyroid hormone; hyperthyroidism is defined as an increase in thyroid function. They are often associated with one another but not always.

   Graves disease is the most common form of thyrotoxicosis.

6. What are the signs and symptoms of thyrotoxicosis?

   Some of the common signs of thyrotoxicosis are increased weight loss, nervousness, hyperactivity, irritability, hyperreflexia, sinus tachycardia, osteopenia, and atrial fibrillation.

   Some of the common symptoms include warm skin, sweating, heat intolerance, fine hair, alopecia, oligomenorrhea, amenorrhea, diarrhea, and eyelid retraction (proptotic appearance).

7. What lab thyroid function test and findings characterize sick euthyroid syndrome?

   Sick euthyroid syndrome is a euthyroid condition common in the critically ill patient. It is due to excessive conversion of thyroxine (T4) to reverse triiodothyronine (rT3) instead of its more potent isomer, T3, and possibly hypothalamic suppression of TSH. These patients are clinically euthyroid. Lab findings include a normal to low TSH, low to normal T4, and low free T4 index. Direct free T4 by equilibrium dialysis, however, is normal. Reverse T3 is high, and T3 is low.

8. **What common postoperative complication is associated with subclinical hypothyroidism?**
   Significant respiratory suppression with inability to wean from a respirator can be seen in patients who have even mild untreated hypothyroidism that is otherwise asymptomatic. Thyroid function tests alone may be needed to make this diagnosis. Preoperative TSH is the best screening test. This test would be elevated even in mild hypothyroidism.

9. **What is the most common cardiac arrhythmia present in the elderly with hyperthyroidism?**
   Hyperthyroidism in the elderly may be of the clinical form or the apathetic form. In the latter, patients rarely present with classic signs and symptoms, such as anxiety, sweating, weight loss, or palpitations. Rather, they may present with depressed mood or somnolence, cognitive impairment, or poor appetite. A TSH that is suppressed is the most sensitive indicator of hyperthyroidism. Even patients who are elderly and symptomatic are at a significantly increased risk for cardiac arrhythmia—most commonly atrial fibrillation.

10. **What is the function of the parathyroid hormone (PTH)?**
    The parathyroid gland is made up of four separate glands that are anatomically positioned behind the thyroid. The function of the parathyroid is to regulate serum calcium balance. The system for which calcium balance is achieved results from PTH release related to calcium levels. PTH acts upon the bone, kidneys, and gastrointestinal tract. In the example of calcium deficiency, PTH will be released to allow for increased bone resorption, decreased renal excretion of calcium, and increased dietary absorption of calcium.
    A common cause of hypercalcemia is hyperparathyroidism.

11. **What is the significance of hypercalcemia?**
    Hypercalcemia can cause a short QT interval, arrhythmias, nausea, vomiting, fatigue, constipation, and renal tubular defects.
    Hypercalcemia is a significant finding on routine laboratory testing. It is most often caused by hyperparathyroidism, but it is important to rule out a malignancy associated with an increase in serum calcium.

12. **What is calcitonin?**
    Calcitonin is a hormone mostly produced by the thyroid gland. It is somewhat of an antagonist to PTH due to its prevention of osteoclastic activity. This activity plays little to no role in calcium homeostasis in humans.

13. **What is the embryologic path of the pituitary gland?**
    The developmental path of migration of the pituitary gland is of particular importance to oral and maxillofacial surgeons. The gland travels along the midline cell migration of the nasopharyngeal Rathke's pouch; therefore a craniofacial midline cleft or deformity may also result in pituitary dysplasia.

14. **What hormones are produced by the anterior and posterior pituitary?**
    The anterior pituitary produces six major hormones: thyroid stimulating hormone (TSH), luteinizing hormone (LH), follicle stimulating hormone (FSH), prolactin (PRL), adrenocorticotropic hormone (ACTH), and growth hormone (GH).
    The posterior pituitary produces two major hormones: oxytocin and antidiuretic hormone (ADH).

15. **What is a pituitary adenoma?**
    A pituitary adenoma is a benign tumor of the pituitary gland. It is the most common cause of hypersecretion or hyposecretion of the pituitary gland. The selective hormone deficiency or excess depends on the one of the six hormone-producing tissue responsible for the adenoma. It makes up approximately 15% of all intracranial tumors.
    An MRI is the preferred imaging modality for identification of a pituitary tumor.

16. **What is McCune-Albright syndrome?**
    McCune-Albright syndrome is a disorder associated with fibrous dysplasia, café au lait spots, precocious puberty, and a variety of endocrine anomalies including acromegaly, ovarian dysfunction, and adrenal adenomas. This syndrome is of particular concern to the oral and maxillofacial surgeon secondary to facial bone expansion. These patients may need osseous recontouring surgery or simple observation, always keeping in mind the possible need for further work-up from an endocrine perspective.

17. What is acromegaly?

Acromegaly is a condition of excess growth hormone, often hypersecretion of a pituitary adenoma. It is characterized by an increase in linear growth of both hard and soft tissues.

18. What are the clinical features of acromegaly?

The typical clinical features are hand and foot enlargement, frontal bossing, coarse facial features, class three skeletal facial deformity, and malocclusion.

19. What is the difference between acromegaly and gigantism?

Both disease entities are caused by an excess of GH and are often due to hypersecretion for a pituitary tumor. In gigantism, the excess circulating GH occurs before closure of the epiphyses, thus causing great stature, in contrast to acromegaly, in which the presence of excess GH occurs after the growth plates have closed.

20. What are the three kind of steroids produced by the adrenal cortex?

1. Glucocorticoids (e.g., cortisol)
2. Mineralocorticoid (e.g., aldosterone)
3. Androgen precursors (e.g., dehydroepiandrosterone [DHEA])

21. What is the regulatory control over adrenal cortex steroid production?

Glucocorticoid and androgen precursors are under the control of the hypothalamus pituitary adrenal axis (HPA).

Mineral corticoids are regulated by the renal angiotensin adrenal system (RAA).

22. What is the function of aldosterone?

Aldosterone increases sodium retention and increases potassium excretion. It also regulates the release of renin by increasing renal arterial perfusion pressure.

The release of renin from the juxtaglomerular cells of the kidney converts angiotensinogen to angiotensin I in the liver. ACE converts angiotensin I to angiotensin II, thus activating aldosterone release.

23. What is Cushing's syndrome?

Cushing's syndrome is defined by excess production of cortisol, which is a glucocorticoid. The signs and symptoms include abdominal obesity, diabetes, hypertension, hirsutism, and hypokalemia.

ACTH is secreted from the anterior pituitary following circadian rhythms, which can be altered by exercise, acute illness, hypoglycemia, physical stress, and psychological stress.

The adrenal-hypothalamic-pituitary feedback loop is governed by the amount of circulating glucocorticoid; therefore the higher the glucocorticoid, the less ACTH release, thus decreasing the demand on the adrenal gland to produce more glucocorticoid.

The overproduction of glucocorticoid can be due to a tumor, a genetic translocation, or local adrenal gland dysfunction.

24. Describe adrenal insufficiency.

The two types are primary and secondary adrenal insufficiency.

Primary adrenal insufficiency can have multiple etiologies resulting in loss of both glucocorticoids and mineral corticoid secretion.

Secondary adrenal insufficiency can also have different etiologies resulting in a decrease or loss of glucocorticoid secretion only.

25. What is adrenal crisis?

Adrenal crisis is a life-threatening physiological state brought about by insufficient cortisol production in the presence of an increase in physiologic demand. It is usually brought about in response to major physical stress, such as major surgery, trauma, or sepsis.

26. What is the clinical presentation of adrenal crisis?

The acute presentation consists of severe circulatory collapse resulting in profound refractory hypotension even in the face of vasopressors. The other possible symptoms can be delirium, confusion, lethargy, and severe abdominal pain.

27. What is the syndrome of inappropriate antidiuretic hormone (SIADH)?

SIADH is essentially an increase in secretion of ADH due to increase in activity of the posterior pituitary gland. The hypersecretion of the gland can be due to a variety of reasons resulting in hyponatremia and increased water retention.

28. **What are the causes of SIADH?**
    The common causes include small cell lung carcinoma, tuberculosis, pneumonia, meningitis, and head trauma. Other causes include pharmacologic agents such as clofibrate, cyclophosphamide, and the oral hypoglycemic chlorpropamide. Less common causes include mechanical ventilation, narcotics, and hypercarbia.

29. **What is the clinical presentation for patients with SIADH?**
    A few of the most common presenting clinical signs are seizures, headache, nausea, vomiting, coma, and delirium. The concomitant lab findings are hyponatremia, increase of urine concentration, and low blood urea nitrogen.

30. **How is SIADH diagnosed?**
    A **clinical exam** may reveal weakness, lethargy, seizure, confusion, and coma. **Lab findings** usually show persistent hyponatremia, serum hyposmolarity > plasma, and an inappropriately concentrated urine and abnormally high Na. Dehydration must be ruled out before diagnosis of SIADH can be made.

31. **What is the treatment for SIADH?**
    Treatment for SIADH depends on the symptoms. Mild to moderate symptoms are treated with fluid restriction (500 to 1000 mL/24 hr). Severe water intoxication (symptomatically severe hyponatremia) requires hypertonic saline (3%, 200 mL) in addition to free water restriction. Water restriction is effective in most cases of chronic SIADH. Demeclocycline, which inhibits ADH action at the renal tubular cell, can also be used.

32. **Which hormone is also known as vasopressin, and where is it produced and released?**
    Antidiuretic hormone (ADH). ADH is produced and released in the posterior pituitary.

33. **What causes ADH release?**
    ADH is released in response to changes in the serum osmolality detected by the hypothalamus. Osmolality that decreases to about 295 mOsm/kg initiates release.

34. **What effect does an increased release of ADH have on urine concentration?**
    Because ADH affects the renal collecting tubule's permeability, water will be reabsorbed, resulting in a more concentrated urine.

35. **Where are angiotensin I and II produced, and how does angiotensin II affect blood pressure?**
    Angiotensin I and II are produced in the kidney. Angiotensin II actively increases vascular tone, stimulates catecholamine release, and increases Na reabsorption (at the distal tubule). It also stimulates release of aldosterone from the zona glomerulosa of the adrenal cortex.

36. **What is azotemia?**
    Nitrogen retention resulting from factors other than primary renal disease.

37. **What is a pheochromocytoma?**
    A pheochromocytoma is a tumor that produces catecholamines that have significant effects on blood pressure. There are various blood assays and urine analyses that can be utilized to identify high levels of circulating catecholamines. They vary in their sensitivities and can occasionally produce false positives. Preferred imaging for a pheochromocytoma is an MRI T2 weighted with gadolinium, although a CT scan with contrast is also acceptable.
    Treatment is surgical removal.

38. **What is the rule of tens concerning a pheochromocytoma?**
    - 10% intraadrenal
    - 10% extraadrenal
    - 10% malignant

39. **What are the common symptoms of a pheochromocytoma?**
    The classic triad of symptoms is palpitations, sweating, and headache.
    Hypertension is the mainstay of the disease process; however other clinical findings may include anxiety, arrhythmias, pulmonary edema, heart failure, and intracranial bleeding.
    A few other processes can mimic these symptoms and clinical findings: the use of amphetamines or cocaine, essential hypertension, anxiety, and intracranial lesions.

40. **What syndromes are associated with a pheochromocytoma?**
Various syndromes can be associated with a pheochromocytoma; thus, once diagnosed, a further work-up may be necessary. If one of the syndromes is diagnosed, the possibility of a pheochromocytoma may need to be explored.
Possible associated syndromes are neurofibromatosis, MEN 2a, MEN 2b, von Hippel-Lindau syndrome, and para-glanduloma syndromes.

41. **What is multiple endocrine neoplasia (MEN) syndrome?**
This is a syndrome by which at least two hormone-producing organs or tissues contain neoplasms. These findings are usually associated with several members of the same family.

42. **What are the different types of MEN?**
MEN 1 (Wermer's syndrome) is the most common MEN syndrome characterized by tumors of the parathyroid, pituitary, and pancreas.
MEN 2a is characterized by medullary thyroid carcinoma, hyperparathyroidism, and pheochromocytoma.
MEN 2b is characterized by medullary thyroid carcinoma, pheochromocytoma, and mucosal neuromas.
Treatment in general for all types of MEN can be complicated and requires a team approach. The modalities of treatment usually are strategically planned surgery and medial management of the various hormonal imbalances and consequences.

43. **What is diabetes insipidus?**
Diabetes insipidus is characterized by a decrease in ADH (vasopressin), causing a decreased ability to concentrate urine at the renal tubules, therefore leading to excessive water loss. This results in a large amount of excreted dilute urine.
The three potential sites of alteration in ADH are the pituitary, the neurohypophysis, and the kidney.
The symptoms of diabetes insipidus are polyuria and polydipsia, which mimic some symptoms of diabetes mellitus. It is important not to confuse the two disease entities.

44. **What are the two types of diabetes insipidus (DI)?**
   1. Central DI is a decrease in the production of ADH, which can be caused by some of the following: head trauma, tumors, surgery, autoimmune disorders, and Langerhans histiocytosis X.
   2. Nephrogenic DI is a decrease in the kidney response to circulating ADH, which can be caused by chronic renal disease and sickle cell anemia.

45. **How is DI diagnosed?**
DI is characterized by diluted urine with increased serum osmolality. The diagnosis is made by fluid restriction for 6 to 10 hours. A patient with an intact neurohypophyseal axis will increase urine osmolality up to 500 to 1400 mEq/L while keeping serum osmolality <295 mEq/L. A patient with full-blown DI cannot protect his or her serum osmolality. As a result, levels of serum osmolality >320 with a urine osmolality <200 may be seen. When this patient is given parenteral ADH, the urine osmolality rises significantly.

46. **How is central DI treated?**
Treatment for central DI depends on etiology. DI due to trauma or surgery is often transient and self-limited. DDAVP (1-deamino-8-D-arginine vasopressin), an ADH analogue with an antidiuretic pressor activity ratio of 2000:1, is the treatment of choice for DI from other etiologies. Duration of action is 6 to 20 hours when taken intranasally or subcutaneously. It requires once- or twice-daily dosing.

MANAGEMENT CONSIDERATIONS TO THE PREGNANT PATIENT

47. **What is the normal human gestation time?**
Pregnancy lasts approximately 275 days, or 40 weeks divided into trimesters.

48. **A 22-week pregnant woman is in which trimester?**
She is in her second trimester. The trimester system is:
   - First trimester (0 to 14 weeks)
   - Second trimester (14 to 27 weeks)
   - Third trimester (28 to 40 weeks)

49. What are the development milestones for a normally developing fetus?
    - 24 weeks: Low end of fetal survival
    - 34 weeks: Lung maturation; fetal survival increases exponentially. Mortality is equal to 37 weeks; however, there is a much higher morbidity. Common fetal complications include feeding and temperature control issues, as well as an increased risk of neonatal jaundice.
    - 37 weeks: Fetal mortality same as at 40 weeks; therefore this is considered a term pregnancy.
    - 39 weeks: Fetal morbidity is so low as to permit elective delivery.

50. When does organogenesis take place?
    Weeks 3 to 14.
    - Weeks 1 to 2: Embryo implantations—all or no response to embryo insult
    - Weeks 3 to 14: Organogenesis—extremely sensitive to exogenous insults
    - Weeks 14 to 27: Fetus less sensitive to exogenous insult. Fetal heart sound can be heard for first time.
    - Weeks 28 to 40: Fetus becomes sensitive to transplacental carcinogens.

51. What are the FDA categories for pregnant and lactating patients?
    A: Controlled studies in humans have failed to demonstrate a risk to the fetus, and the possibility of fetal harm seems remote.
    B: Animal studies have not indicated fetal risk, and there are no human studies; or animal studies have shown a risk, but controlled human studies have not.
    C: Animal studies have shown a risk, but there are no controlled human studies; or no studies are available in humans or animals.
    D: Evidence of human fetal risk exists, but in certain situations, the drug may be used despite its risk.
    X: Evidence of fetal abnormalities or fetal risk based on human experience exists. The risk outweighs any possible benefit for use during pregnancy.

52. What are the FDA drug classes for antibiotics commonly used by oral and maxillofacial surgeons (OMFS)?
    Class B: penicillin, erythromycin, clindamycin, cephalosporins, metronidazole
    Class D: tetracycline, quinolones

53. What are the FDA drug classes for analgesics?
    Class B:
    - Acetaminophen
    - Ibuprofen (It can be given in first 32 weeks; past that, theoretical risk of premature closure of the patent ductus arteriosus [PDA]. This is true of all nonsteroidal antiinflammatory drugs [NSAIDs].)
    - Oxycodone
    - Morphine
    - Fentanyl
    - Meperidine
    - Hydrocodone
    There is concern for fetal dependence with any opioid, as well as respiratory depression in the newborn recently exposed to opioids.
    Class C:
    - Codeine: associated with first trimester malformations; can use in second or third trimester
    - Aspirin: associated with late-term intrauterine growth restriction

54. What are the FDA drug classes for common sedatives used in OMFS?
    Both benzodiazepines and barbiturates pose a risk for fetal craniofacial anomalies and are FDA Class D drugs.

55. What are the FDA drug classes for common local anesthetics used in OMFS?

Category B	*Category C*
Lidocaine	Articaine
Prilocaine	Bupivacaine
Etidocaine	Mepivacaine

56. What is the effect of pregnancy on the cardiovascular system?
    The physiologic state of pregnancy increases demand on the cardiovascular system. Gravid women have a need for increased blood volume and increased cardiac output to allow for additional blood

supply needed for fetal perfusion. This increase in volume can lead to a dilutional anemia and possibly an extra heart sound (S_3 or systolic murmur).

Fetal size and uterine position can also lead to aortocaval compression especially in the supine position, therefore increasing pressure and decreasing venous return.

57. **How is the respiratory system compromised with pregnancy?**
The gravid patient will have an increase in O_2 demand and O_2 consumption. These patients also exhibit a decrease in functional residual capacity, a low PCO_2, thus resulting in an increased in minute ventilation.

58. **What is the hypercoagulable state of pregnancy?**
Pregnancy has a global effect on the gravid woman, leading to an increase in thrombin, coagulation factors, and hemoglobin. The other important change is a mechanical compression of the venous system from the uterus, causing venous stasis. This combination ultimately leads to an increased risk of deep venous thrombosis (DVT) and pulmonary embolus (PE).

59. **How do you treat a gravid woman with a DVT?**
The usual treatment of a DVT is the administration of heparin. Heparin is preferred over Coumadin for treatment due to the fact that heparin does not cross the placenta due to its increased molecular size. The fear of fetal toxicity with Coumadin is always a concern. There is no good data to show which form of heparin is more advantageous—either low molecular weight heparin or unfractionated heparin.

60. **Which clotting factors are altered during pregnancy?**
Factors XI and XII are increased during pregnancy.

61. **What are the elements of Virchow's triad?**
A hypercoagulable state, venous stasis, and endothelial wall damage.

62. **Can pregnant women demonstrate a physiologic leukocytosis?**
In the pregnancy state, there is an increase in cortisol and release of catecholamines that can lead to an increase in circulating white blood cells due to demarginaton of the endothelium.

63. **When is the best time to treat a pregnant woman surgically?**
The second trimester is the best time for treatment; however it is still suggested to wait until the woman is postpartum for elective procedures.

64. **Why is GERD a common symptom in pregnancy?**
There is little evidence to support any change in gastric volume or pH during pregnancy. However, gastroesophageal sphincter tone is decreased leading to GERD. The actual reason for a decrease in sphincter tone is unclear, as no underlying causality is agreed upon in the literature.

65. **Is kidney function altered during pregnancy?**
The gravid woman has an increase in blood volume and an increase in cardiac output, and therefore an increase in renal plasma flow. This ultimately causes an increase in glomerular filtration rate (GFR). This increase in GFR can lead to increased clearance of creatinine and urea.

66. **Why is local anesthesia administration with epinephrine a concern in a pregnant patient?**
Local anesthetic is often prepared with a vasoconstrictor, such as epinephrine, to increase the longevity and effectiveness of the anesthetic. The concern in pregnancy is the risk of uterine artery constriction, thus decreasing fetal blood flow, if the epinephrine is injected intravascular.

67. **What are the potential effects of nitrous oxide during pregnancy?**
Animal models have shown that nitrous oxide will have an effect on uterine blood flow by vasoconstriction and increasing the androgenic tone of the uterus. The consequences of this physiologic action are abortion and congenital anomalies.

68. **What are the major concerns of general anesthesia during pregnancy?**
It is acceptable to have general anesthesia during pregnancy as long as the preoperative and intraoperative management are understood and followed closely.

The major concerns are hypoglycemia, hypotension, hypothermia, and hypoxia. If these factors are controlled, there is no data that supports a risk of fetal anomalies, miscarriage, or preterm labor during surgery.

69. **Do antibiotics have an effect on the fetus in utero?**
Most antibiotics are acceptable during pregnancy; however some antibiotics are not considered safe during pregnancy. Sulfonamides given late in gestation can cause hyperbilirubinemia and kernicterus. Tetracycline given after the fifth month of gestation can stain the bone. Chloramphenicol can produce neonatal toxicity. Amino glycosides can cause fetal ototoxicity and nephrotoxicity. Fluoroquinolones can carry risk of arthropathy.

70. **Why is it recommended to restrict the use of NSAIDS during pregnancy?**
The restriction of NSAIDS is recommended to prevent premature closure of the fetal ductus arteriosus, which is necessary for fetal circulation. Other possible concerns in the last trimester with the use of ibuprofen are low amniotic fluid and inhibition of labor.

71. **Why are benzodiazepines not recommended during pregnancy?**
Benzodiazepines are considered to be teratogenic.

72. **Can a gravid woman be prescribed narcotics?**
Narcotics given for a short period of time are considered safe for the fetus even though they cross the placenta.

73. **Why should the supine position be avoided when treating a gravid woman?**
Placing a pregnant woman in the supine position will increase the pressure on the aorta and vena cava by the gravid uterus. This position will increase blood pressure and decrease venous return.

74. **What is placental abruption?**
Abruption is a traumatic separation of the placenta from the uterine wall, resulting in uncontrollable bleeding. This state of excessive bleeding can lead to preterm delivery, fetal death, DIC, and possible maternal death.

75. **What are the clinical hallmarks of abruption?**
The typical hallmarks of abruption are vaginal bleeding, uterine bleeding that leads to uterine hypertonicity, and fetal distress.

76. **Is general anesthesia safe in the pregnant patient?**
If possible, it is best to treat a pregnant patient in the second trimester. In the preoperative stage, the practitioner should consider aspiration prophylaxis with antacid or h2 antagonist. During intubation it is important to remember the pregnant patient's airway is more edematous and vascular, which may lead to bleeding or could decrease the view of the cords. Intra-operatively, it is important to control fluid administration, blood pressure control, and good oxygenation. If possible, fetal monitoring is recommended. There is no evidence as to what anesthetic is best for the pregnant patient.

77. **What is the benefit of regional anesthetic techniques versus general anesthesia?**
Regional anesthetics have the advantage of decreasing fetal exposure of various inhalation or intravenous drugs. If the patient is awake, the patient can respond and report symptoms of preterm labor, fetal heart rate should have little variability, and the patient will be mobilized more quickly. Early mobilization will decrease the risk of a thromboembolic event.

78. **What is the leading cause of maternal death?**
The leading cause of maternal death is major trauma. Fetal loss in this situation is directly related to the timing of maternal death and fetal maturity at the time of the traumatic event.

79. **What are the reasons for emergent caesarean section?**
The reasons for emergent C-section are:
- A stable mother with fetal distress
- Uterine rupture
- Gravid uterus size preventing necessary abdominal surgery
- A gravid mother's life is in danger and cannot be saved (e.g., trauma)

80. **Is it possible to prevent HIV transmission to the fetus from an HIV positive gravid mother?**
Yes. Combination medical therapy throughout pregnancy is recommended to prevent transmission to the fetus.

81. **What is the percentage of pregnant patients who undergo nonobstetric surgery?**
The statistics show approximately 0.2% to 1% of pregnant patients will undergo a surgical procedure unrelated to pregnancy.

82. **What are the most common nonobstetric surgeries performed on a pregnant woman?**
The most common nonobstetric procedure performed on a pregnant woman is an appendectomy, followed by cholecystectomy.

83. **What is considered the maximum fetal radiation exposure?**
The maximum amount of radiation exposure considered safe for a fetus is 5.0 rad.

84. **What is the amount of background fetal radiation exposure during a 9-month pregnancy?**
The average amount of background fetal radiation during 9 months of pregnancy is approximately 0.3 to 0.9 rad.

85. **What are the possible or potential concerns with excess fetal radiation?**
The theoretical concerns with excess fetal radiation are abortion, birth defects, and future risk of cancer throughout life. These concerns make it important to use radiation as a diagnostic modality only if completely necessary.

86. **What amount of radiation is associated with fetal loss?**
The cause of fetal loss seems to be an absolute threshold phenomenon. If a fetus receives 10 rad of radiation or greater during the first 8 weeks of gestation, it will result in the loss of the fetus.
Most diagnostic imaging exposes fetus with 0.0007 (Chest X-ray) to 0.4 rad (Arteriogram) of radiation. (A head CT exposes the fetus to 0.0013 rads.)

87. **Do ultrasounds or MRI have any deleterious effects on the fetus?**
MRI and ultrasound are considered safe imaging modalities during pregnancy. When performing an MRI, gadolinium should be avoided due to its uptake in the amniotic fluid. This uptake may have an effect on the fetus; however the possible effect is unknown.

BIBLIOGRAPHY

Management Considerations to Patients with Endocrine Diseases

Arlt W: Disorders of the adrenal cortex (Chapter 342). In Longo DL, Fauci AS, Kasper DL, Hauser SL, Jameson J, Loscalzo J, editors: *Harrison's principles of internal medicine, ed 18*, New York, 2012, McGraw-Hill.

Clark OH: Thyroid & parathyroid (Chapter 16). In Doherty GM, editor: *Current diagnosis & treatment: surgery, ed 13*, New York, 2010, McGraw-Hill.

Favus MJ, Vokes TJ: Paget's disease and other dysplasias of bone (Chapter 355). In Longo DL, Fauci AS, Kasper DL, Hauser SL, Jameson J, Loscalzo J, editors: *Harrison's principles of internal medicine, ed 18*, New York, 2012, McGraw-Hill.

Fitzgerald PA: Endocrine disorders (Chapter 26). In Papadakis MA, McPhee SJ, Rabow MW, editors: *Current medical diagnosis & treatment 2014*, New York, 2014, McGraw-Hill.

Idrose A: Adrenal insufficiency and adrenal crisis (Chapter 225). In Tintinalli JE, Stapczynski J, Ma O, Cline DM, Cydulka RK, Meckler GD, editors: *Tintinalli's emergency medicine: a comprehensive study guide, ed 7*, New York, 2011, McGraw-Hill.

Jameson J, Weetman AP: Disorders of the thyroid gland (Chapter 341). In Longo DL, Fauci AS, Kasper DL, Hauser SL, Jameson J, Loscalzo J, editors: *Harrison's principles of internal medicine, ed 18*, New York, 2012, McGraw-Hill.

Melmed S, Jameson J: Disorders of the anterior pituitary and hypothalamus (Chapter 339). In Longo DL, Fauci AS, Kasper DL, Hauser SL, Jameson J, Loscalzo J, editors: *Harrison's principles of internal medicine, ed 18*, New York, 2012, McGraw-Hill.

Neumann HH: Pheochromocytoma (Chapter 343). In Longo DL, Fauci AS, Kasper DL, Hauser SL, Jameson J, Loscalzo J, editors: *Harrison's principles of internal medicine, ed 18*, New York, 2012, McGraw-Hill.

Potts Jr JT, Jüppner H: Disorders of the parathyroid gland and calcium homeostasis (Chapter 353). In Longo DL, Fauci AS, Kasper DL, Hauser SL, Jameson J, Loscalzo J, editors: *Harrison's principles of internal medicine, ed 18*, New York, 2012, McGraw-Hill.

Robertson GL: Disorders of the neurohypophysis (Chapter 340). In Longo DL, Fauci AS, Kasper DL, Hauser SL, Jameson J, Loscalzo J, editors: *Harrison's principles of internal medicine, ed 18*, New York, 2012, McGraw-Hill.

Vasquez C, Gagel RF: Disorders affecting multiple endocrine systems (Chapter 351). In Longo DL, Fauci AS, Kasper DL, Hauser SL, Jameson J, Loscalzo J, editors: *Harrison's principles of internal medicine, ed 18*, New York, 2012, McGraw-Hill.

Endocrine pathology (Chapter 18). In Kemp WL, Burns DK, Brown TG, editors: *Pathology: the big picture*, New York, 2008, McGraw-Hill.

Acromegaly (Chapter 228). In Usatine RP, Smith MA, Chumley HS, Mayeaux Jr EJ, editors: *The color atlas of family medicine, ed 2*, New York, 2013, McGraw-Hill.

Management Considerations to the Pregnant Patient

Ananth CV, Kinzler WL, Sheiner E: *Placental abruption; bleeding during pregnancy*, New York, 2011, Book Section Springer. pp 119–133.

Brookie M: *Best; clinical pharmacology during pregnancy, Chapter 13 clinical pharmacology of anti-infectives during pregnancy*, Elsevier, 2013.

Che Yaakob CA, Dzarr AA, Ismail AA, Zuky Nik Lah NA, Ho JJ: Anticoagulant therapy for deep vein thrombosis (DVT) inpregnancy, *Cochrane Database Syst Rev*, 2010, http://dx.doi.org/10.1002/14651858.CD007801.pub2. Issue 6. Art. No.: CD007801.

Giglio DDS, MEd JA, Lanni MD SM: *Oral health care for the pregnant patient*, Laskin, Daniel M, DDS, MS; Gigilo, Nancy W, CNM. Dental Assistant 82.6. November/December 2013. 38, 40, 42, 44–45, 47.

Hawkins JLMD: In Schwartz MD, MSEd AJ, Gross MD JB, Matjasko MD MJ, editors: *Anesthesia for the pregnant patient undergoing nonobstetric surgeryasa; refresher courses in anesthesiology:* vol. 33(1), 2005, pp 137–144.

Katz PO: *Curbside consultation in GERD, 49 clinical questions; question 41: how does pregnancy affect GERD? Is GERD in pregnancy a risk for long-term reflux?* Thorofare: Slack incorporated, 2008. 137-xiii; 4 pages.

Lawrenz DR, Whitley BD, Helfrick JF: Considerations in the management of maxillofacial infections in the pregnant patient, *J Oral Maxillofac Surg* 54(4):474–485, April 1996.

Lewis B, Carson G, Michael P, Cohn E, Steven L: *Perioperative medicine: the pregnant surgical patient; book section*, London, 2011, Springer. pp 395-407, 2011–01-01.

Kizer MD, MSCI Norat, Powell MD MA: *Surgery in the pregnant patient clinical obstetrics and gynecology*, Lippincott Williams & Wilkins, 2011. Vol 54(4), pp 633–641.

Pradel C: The pregnant oral and maxillofacial surgery patient, *Oral Maxillofac Surg Clin North Am* 10:471–489, 1998.

Theodorou D, Larentzakis A, Velmahos GC, et al.: *The pregnant patient; penetrating trauma a practical guide on operative technique and peri-operative management [chapter]69*, 2012, pp. 529–535.

Turner M, Aziz S: Management of the pregnant oral and maxillofacial surgery patient, *J Oral Maxillofac Surg* 60: 1479–1488, 2002.

CHAPTER 21

MANAGEMENT OF THE DIABETIC PATIENT

Samir Singh, Bradley A. Gregory

1. What is diabetes?

   Diabetes is a chronic metabolic disorder resulting in hyperglycemia from defects in insulin secretion, insulin action, or both. Diabetes creates a physiologic predisposition for developing generalized microvascular, macrovascular, and neuropathic complications.

2. How is glucose normally metabolized?

   Glucose absorbed after a meal enters the circulation of the hepatic portal system and is taken to the liver where about 30% of all ingested glucose is metabolized. The remaining glucose continues in the bloodstream for distribution to other organs and tissues. Blood glucose levels are normally maintained between 60 and 130 mg/dL. Excess glucose is converted to glycogen (glycogenesis) stored mostly in liver and muscle and triglycerides stored in adipose tissue (lipogenesis). If plasma glucose concentrations decrease, the body breaks down glycogen to glucose (glycogenolysis).

   During energy deprivation states, triglycerides (omega-3 fatty acids attached to glycerol) are broken down into glycerol and fatty acids (lipolysis), which are converted to glucose. Amino acids can be converted to glucose in the liver through gluconeogenesis.

3. How does insulin facilitate uptake of glucose into cells?

   Insulin is released in a rapid surge during the first 10 to 30 minutes after a meal. This is followed by a second phase of a slower, sustained release of insulin. Insulin receptors in the cell membrane have alpha and beta subunits. Insulin binds to subunit alpha, which causes a change in subunit beta. Subunit beta promotes the activity of the enzyme tyrosine kinase that phosphorylates intracellular insulin receptors (insulin-receptor substrates). This activates second messenger pathways that alter existing protein and protein synthesis. The net result is a change in cell metabolism that brings glucose into the cell via GLUT transporters.

4. From where is insulin secreted?

   Insulin is secreted from the beta cells of the endocrine pancreas during the fed state when blood glucose concentrations rise above 100 mg/dL or with increased parasympathetic activity.

5. How does insulin lower the plasma glucose?

   - Insulin promotes glucose uptake into most tissues. Target tissues for insulin are the liver, adipose tissue, and skeletal muscles. Other tissues, including the brain and transporting epithelia of the kidney and intestine, do **not** require insulin for glucose uptake and metabolism.
   - Insulin enhances cellular utilization (glycolysis), storage of glucose (glycogenesis), and fat synthesis (lipogenesis). Insulin simultaneously inhibits glycogen breakdown (glycogenolysis), glucose synthesis in the liver (gluconeogenesis), and fat breakdown (lipolysis).
   - Insulin enhances utilization of amino acids in protein synthesis and inhibits protein breakdown.
   - Insulin promotes fat synthesis by inhibiting beta oxidation of fatty acids and promoting conversion into triglycerides (lipogenesis).

6. From where is glucagon secreted?

   Glucagon is secreted from alpha cells of the endocrine pancreas during the fasted state when blood glucose concentrations fall below 100 mg/dL or with increased sympathetic activity. It is also found in the alpha cells of the stomach.

7. What metabolic effects does glucagon regulate?

   The metabolic effects exerted on the liver, muscle, and adipose tissue are antagonistic to those of insulin. Glucagon mobilizes stored energy by promoting glycogenolysis (especially at the liver), gluconeogenesis, and lipolysis by activating hormone-sensitive lipase. Other effects of glucagon include stimulating the secretion of insulin by increasing plasma glucose and stimulating the secretion of growth hormone.

8. **How is cortisol secreted and regulated?**
Cortisol is a glucocorticoid released in response to stress and low blood glucose. The control pathway for cortisol secretion is known as the hypothalamic-pituitary-adrenal (HPA) pathway. Corticotropin-releasing hormone (CRH) is released from the hypothalamus. CRH stimulates the release of adrenocorticotropic hormone (ACTH) from the anterior pituitary gland. ACTH stimulates cortisol release from the zona fasciculata of the adrenal cortex, which in turn causes negative feedback to CRH and ACTH.

9. **What metabolic role does cortisol play in glucose metabolism?**
Overall cortisol is catabolic and prevents hypoglycemia. It promotes gluconeogenesis in the liver, breakdown of skeletal muscle proteins into pyruvate and lactate, which facilitate gluconeogenesis, and enhances lipolysis. The glycerol from fatty acids can be used for gluconeogenesis.

10. **How does epinephrine exert its metabolic controls?**
Effects are mediated through both alpha-1 and beta-2 receptors. Alpha-1 receptors of the pancreas promote glucagon release from the alpha cells of the pancreas and inhibit insulin secretion at the beta cells of the pancreas. Beta-2 receptor agonism results in lipolysis, gluconeogenesis, and glycogenolysis.

11. **What is the role of epinephrine in glucose regulation?**
The overall goal of epinephrine is to protect plasma glucose levels. In the muscle and liver, it promotes glycogenolysis and gluconeogenesis as well. Additionally, it will inhibit insulin release and stimulate glucagon release through alpha-1 receptors in the pancreas. In the bloodstream, it will inhibit glucose uptake. Finally, epinephrine stimulates hormone-sensitive lipase to facilitate lipolysis in muscle and adipose tissue.

12. **What is the role of growth hormone in glucose regulation?**
Growth hormone is an anabolic hormone secreted by cells in the anterior pituitary gland. It is secreted by stimuli such as exercise-induced hypoglycemia, fasting, and stress from trauma, fever, and surgery. Growth hormone counteracts, in general, the effects of insulin on glucose and lipid metabolism. Growth hormone release is inhibited by glucose and free fatty acids. Growth hormone also increases plasma glucose, mobilizes free fatty acids and protein stores, lipolysis, glycogenolysis, and inhibits glucose uptake by muscle and adipose tissue.

13. **What is the role of thyroid hormone in glucose regulation?**
Triiodothyronine (T3), which is the metabolically active form of thyroid hormone, and thyroxine (T4), which is the prohormone, both act to raise blood glucose. They do so by enhancing glycogenolysis and by enhancing protein metabolism and absorption of glucose from the intestines.

14. **What are the four different types of diabetes mellitus?**
   - **Type 1 diabetes (insulin-dependent diabetes mellitus or IDDM).** Characterized by a severe deficiency of insulin due to autoimmune destruction of beta cells of the pancreas. This form accounts for <10% of all cases of diabetes mellitus. It is usually associated with young people, but can occur at any age. These patients require insulin to maintain glucose homeostasis.
   - **Type 2 diabetes (noninsulin-dependent diabetes mellitus or NIDDM).** Initially characterized by insulin resistance secondary to environmental and genetic factors, followed by failure of beta cells of the pancreas to compensate for the increased insulin requirements. It accounts for >90% of all cases of diabetes mellitus. It is usually a disease of adulthood; however, it is being increasingly diagnosed in younger age groups. Therefore their muscle and adipose cells cannot transport glucose.
   - **Gestational diabetes.** Complicates up to 4% of all pregnancies. It typically resolves after delivery; however, up to 40% of women with gestational diabetes will develop type 2 diabetes within 10 years of developing gestational diabetes.
   - **Secondary diabetes.** Diabetes that results from genetic defects in insulin secretion or action, exocrine pancreatic disease, pancreatectomy, endocrinopathies (e.g., Cushing's syndrome, acromegaly), drugs, and other syndromes.

15. **What are the hallmark symptoms of diabetes?**
Polyuria (excessive urination), polydipsia (excessive thirst), and polyphagia (excessive eating/hunger). Other symptoms may include fatigue, weight loss, blurred vision, fungal infections, and neuropathy of hands and feet.

16. What is the pathogenesis of type 1 diabetes?
    Overt signs of type 1 diabetes do not typically appear until about 90% of beta cells are destroyed.
    - A **genetic susceptibility** predisposes some people to autoimmunity against beta cells of the pancreas.
    - **Autoimmunity** develops spontaneously or, more commonly, is stimulated by an environmental agent.
    - **Environmental injury** can damage beta cells, which are then recognized as foreign by the immune defenses.

17. What is the pathogenesis of type 2 diabetes?
    - Obesity is the greatest risk factor. It does not cause diabetes but can unmask it. It is associated with increased plasma levels of free fatty acids, which make muscles more insulin resistant, causing decreased glucose uptake.
    - Insulin production decreases with age.
    - Genetics plays a significant but poorly understood role.
    - Lack of compensation in type 2 diabetics from failure of free fatty acids to stimulate pancreatic insulin secretion. Therefore, compensation does not occur, and hyperglycemia develops. Beta cells become desensitized to glucose, leading to decreased insulin secretion.

18. What metabolic abnormalities are associated with type 1 diabetes?
    Abnormalities are classified into those of carbohydrate, protein, and lipid metabolism.
    - Type 1 patients generally have a combination of glucose underutilization and excessive glucose production resembling the fasting state. Glucose is unable to get into certain tissues, which causes the renal threshold to be surpassed, resulting in polyuria. Polyuria leads to dehydration, which triggers polydipsia. In addition, because cells are not getting nourishment, patients experience polyphagia.
    - These patients break down protein from muscle to make glucose. Proteins are required for antibody production, white blood cell production, and healing of wounds. Deficiency of these proteins leads to susceptibility of infections and poor wound healing.
    - Insulin deficiency leads to lipolysis of triglycerides into free fatty acids. Excessive fatty acid breakdown leads to beta oxidation in the liver, creating acidic ketone bodies (acetoacetic acid and beta-hydroxybutyric acid). Ketone bodies enter the blood and cause a type of metabolic acidosis.

19. What metabolic abnormalities are associated with type 2 diabetes?
    The metabolic abnormalities are classified as insulin resistance, loss of sensitivity of cells to insulin, and a decrease in insulin secretion. Insulin is unable to get into cells because either a post-receptor defect prevents uptake or there is a problem of insulin binding to target cells in the liver, muscle, and adipose tissue. In addition, type 2 diabetics may have a gradual decrease in basal levels of insulin secretion because the pancreas loses sensitivity to glucose level changes.

20. What is diabetic ketoacidosis?
    Diabetic ketoacidosis (DKA) is an acute, life-threatening medical emergency that can occur in type 1 and type 2 diabetic patients (more commonly in type 1). DKA is the result of severe insulin deficiency coupled with an absolute or relative increase of glucagon, which contribute to accelerated ketogenesis and severe hyperglycemia. Diagnostic criteria of DKA include blood glucose levels >450 mg/dL, metabolic acidosis (pH <7.3), serum bicarbonate <15 mEq/L, ketonemia, and ketonuria. Clinical manifestations include nausea and vomiting, Kussmaul respirations (rapid, deep breathing) to reduce carbon dioxide levels in blood, abdominal pain, fruity acetone breath odor, altered mental status/coma, dehydration, and tachycardia. Goals of treatment are fluid replacement initially using 0.9% normal saline intravenously (add 5% glucose once blood glucose reaches 250 mg/dL to prevent hypoglycemia) and administration of insulin after confirming patient is **not** hypokalemic (0.1 u/kg of regular insulin followed by infusion of 0.1 units/kg/hr); monitor and replace potassium, magnesium, and phosphate within 1 to 2 hours of starting insulin. Bicarbonate replacement is controversial and not necessary in most cases.
    Complications of treatment of DKA include cerebral edema if glucose levels decease too rapidly, hyperchloremic non-gap metabolic acidosis due to rapid infusion of normal saline, cardiac arrhythmias, and death.

21. What is hyperosmolar hyperglycemic nonketotic coma?
    Hyperosmolar hyperglycemic nonketotic coma (HHNS) is a state of severe hyperglycemia (>600 mg/dL), hyperosmolarity (>320 mOsm/L) and dehydration. It usually occurs in patients who are type 2 diabetics, age 65 or older. It is less common than DKA, but it carries a higher mortality rate.

Low insulin levels lead to hyperglycemia, causing osmotic diuresis and dehydration. Ketogenesis is minimal because a small amount of insulin is released to blunt counterregulatory hormone release (glucagon). Ketosis and acidosis are typically minimal or absent. The symptoms may go unrecognized for weeks. Key features of HHNS are severe hyperosmolarity (>320 mOsm/L), hyperglycemia (>600 mg/dL), dehydration, and the absence of acidosis and ketosis (unlike DKA). BUN is usually elevated with other laboratory findings consistent with prerenal azotemia. The treatment involves fluid replacement with normal saline (1 L in the first hour followed by another liter in the next 2 hours. Switch to 5% glucose in one-half normal saline once blood glucose reaches 250 mg/dL) and administration of insulin (initial bolus of 5 to 10 units intravenously, followed by a low-dose infusion of 2 to 4 units/hour). Complications include cerebral edema from rapid lowering of glucose, exacerbation of CHF in predisposed patients, cardiac arrhythmias, and death.

22. **What tissues do not require insulin for glucose transport?**
    - Nervous tissue
    - Brain
    - Lens of the eye
    - Blood vessels
    - Kidney tubules

23. **What are the major chronic complications of diabetes?**
    - Neuropathy (peripheral neuropathy [feet and hands], cranial nerve complications [most often involves CN III, IV, VI], mononeuropathies [median nerve, ulnar nerve, common peroneal], and autonomic neuropathy [impotence, neurogenic bladder, gastroparesis, constipation, postural hypotension])
    - Retinopathy (nonproliferative retinopathy most common [funduscopic exam shows hemorrhages, exudates, microaneurysms, and venous dilation] and proliferative retinopathy [shows neovascularization and scarring, can lead to retinal detachment, vitreal hemorrhage, and blindness])
    - Macroangiopathy (accelerated atherosclerosis, stroke, myocardial infarction, peripheral vascular disease)
    - Nephropathy (nodular glomerular sclerosis [**Kimmelstiel-Wilson syndrome**], diffuse glomerular sclerosis, isolated glomerular basement membrane thickening, microalbuminuria/proteinuria)
    - Increased susceptibility to infection (impaired WBC function, reduced blood supply, and neuropathy; increased risk of cellulitis, candidiasis, pneumonia, osteomyelitis, and polymicrobial foot ulcers)

24. **What are some of the ocular problems manifested in diabetic patients?**
    Cataracts, retinopathy, and glaucoma. Diabetic retinopathy is the leading cause of blindness in the United States.

25. **What biochemical pathways are suspected of contributing to diabetic complications?**
    The suspected pathways are enzymatic glycosylation and the buildup of sorbitol. *Enzymatic glycosylation* is the process by which glucose attaches to proteins throughout the body at a rate proportional to the plasma glucose concentration. The proteins glycosylated include serum albumin, collagen, basic myelin protein, and low-density lipoproteins (LDLs). The function of the proteins is altered.
    Hyperglycemia leads to buildup of glucose in tissues that do not require insulin for uptake. Excess glucose is metabolized to sorbitol, which creates an osmotic gradient favoring water diffusing into the cell.

26. **What is the enzyme that is responsible for the breakdown of glucose into sorbitol?**
    Aldose reductase.

27. **How do advanced glycosylation end-products (AGEs) contribute to diabetic complications?**
    AGEs are the result of enzymatic glycosylation. They get incorporated into the collagen that comprises the basement membranes of capillaries located in the eye, kidney, nerves, and skin. This results in thickening of basement membranes and a reduction in production of relaxing factors by the endothelium, causing vasoconstriction and, ultimately, hypertension. In addition, AGEs irreversibly attach to collagen walls in larger vessels. This impedes the normal efflux of LDLs entering the vessel wall and promotes cholesterol deposition.

28. How does sorbitol accumulation lead to diabetic complications?

Cells of the tissues that do not require insulin for glucose transport (see question 22) become hypertonic. In Schwann's cells, the hypertonicity causes loss of feeling in extremities and a decrease in sensation. In the lens of the eye, water accumulation leads to cataracts, macular edema, and glaucoma. Damage to endothelial cells leads to thickening of basement membranes, resulting in microangiopathies of the retina, arterioles of the kidneys, and small vessels of the skin.

29. What is the importance of nonenzymatic glycosylation of hemoglobin?

The degree of nonenzymatic glycosylation is dependent on the amount of plasma glucose levels. Therefore high levels result in more glycosylation of hemoglobin. The normal hemoglobin A1c is 4% to 6%. In diabetics, levels may reach 16% to 20%. Because the lifespan of a red blood cell is about 120 days and the glycosylation occurs continuously over that span, hemoglobin A1c concentrations provide an index of the average blood glucose over the preceding 60 to 90 days.

30. How does glycosylation of platelets affect microvascular disease?

Glycosylation of platelets increases platelet adhesiveness. This allows platelets to produce excessive thromboxane, which makes the platelets hypercoagulable. This hypercoagulable state predisposes a diabetic to microvascular disease.

31. What are the criteria for the diagnosis of diabetes mellitus?

The diagnosis is made based on one or more of the following criteria (perform tests on *two separate days*):
- Signs and symptoms plus a random plasma glucose concentration ≥200 mg/dL
- A fasting plasma glucose ≥126 mg/dL on two occasions
- Oral glucose tolerance test with a 2-hour postprandial glucose concentration ≥200 mg/dL and a time 0 serum glucose level >126 mg/dL; hemoglobin A1c >6.5

32. What considerations should be taken in diabetic patients who require contrast imaging?

Patients with diabetes are susceptible to developing radiocontrast-induced acute renal failure. If IV contrast is necessary, give generous hydration before administering contrast agent. If the patient is on metformin, hold it for 48 hours after contrast is given to prevent renal damage. Make sure renal function has returned to baseline before resuming it.

33. What test is accepted by the American Diabetes Association for diagnosing diabetes?

The fasting plasma glucose test is a diagnostic marker for diabetes. The patient fasts overnight for at least 8 hours, and the test is performed the next morning. This test is performed only on non-pregnant adults who are not taking any medications and do not have any other metabolic conditions that would lead to abnormal results. A normal fasting plasma glucose is usually 65 to 110 mg/dL.

34. What is the oral glucose tolerance test, and how is it performed?

This test measures a person's ability to handle a glucose load over a period of time. The patient fasts overnight. In the morning, the fasting blood glucose is determined. The patient then ingests a 75-g glucose load. In children and non-pregnant adults, the blood glucose is tested every 30 minutes for 2 hours. The test is considered normal if the fasting blood glucose is <110 mg/dL and the 2-hour postprandial blood glucose is <140 mg/dL.

35. What are the different categories of hypoglycemia?

Categories of hypoglycemia can be broken down depending on the level of plasma glucose and associated signs and symptoms (Table 21-1).

Table 21-1. Categories of Hypoglycemia

	PLASMA GLUCOSE LEVEL	SIGNS/SYMPTOMS
Mild	60-70 mg/dL	Tachycardia, palpitations, pallor, shakiness, irritability
Moderate	50-60 mg/dL	Impaired central nervous system function: confusion, inability to concentrate, slurred speech, blurred vision
Severe	>40-50 mg/dL	Loss of consciousness, difficulty awakening, seizures

36. **How do you treat mild to moderate hypoglycemia?**
    Initially, treat with 10 to 15 g of carbohydrates. Give the patient one-half cup of orange juice or a regular soft drink, three to five hard candies, one cup of milk, three glucose tablets, *or* two tbsp. of raisins. Evaluate plasma glucose levels as soon as possible. If symptoms do not improve in 15 minutes, treat with an additional 10 to 15 g of a carbohydrate source.

37. **How do you treat severe hypoglycemia?**
    If a glucagon kit is available, the patient should be given a subcutaneous injection of glucagon. The adult dose is 1 mg; children younger than age 5 years, 0.5 mg; and infants younger than 1 year, 0.25 mg. If no kit is available and the patient can swallow without risk of aspiration, 15 to 50 g of a carbohydrate source can be given on the inside of the cheek. Sources include glucose gel, 1 to 4 tsp of honey (except in infants), syrup, *or* jelly. When the patient is more alert, follow with a liquid such as orange juice.

38. **What is the best route to administer agents to stimulate insulin release?**
    Oral glucose and amino acids have a greater stimulatory effect on insulin than intravenously administered solutions because of stimulation of intestinal hormones by ingested substances. These hormones include gastric inhibitory peptide, cholecystokinin (CCK), glucagon, and gastrin. All are stimulators of insulin secretion.

39. **What are the different insulin preparations?**
    See Table 21-2.

40. **What are the effects of surgery on glucose control?**
    Surgery and general anesthesia cause a stress response with release of epinephrine, glucagon, cortisol, growth hormone, interleukin-6, and tumor necrosis factor alpha. These neurohormonal changes result in insulin resistance, decreased peripheral glucose utilization, impaired insulin secretion, increased lipolysis, and protein catabolism. These effects can lead to hyperglycemia and ketosis in some cases.

41. **How do you manage a patient with diabetes that is controlled by diet only?**
    If plasma glucose levels exceed and remain above 250 mg/dL as a consequence of surgical stress or infection, sliding-scale short-acting insulin therapy should be instituted.

42. **How do you manage a surgical patient who controls diabetes with oral hypoglycemic agents?**
    Short-acting sulfonylureas and oral agents should be withheld on the operative day. Metformin and long-acting sulfonylureas (Chlorpropamide) should be held 1 day before planned surgical procedures. Metformin is typically held 48 hours postoperatively. Renal function should be normal prior to resuming treatment. Glucose values should be checked regularly postoperatively, and elevated levels >180 mg/dL may be treated with short-acting sliding-scale insulin.

43. **What is the management of a patient with insulin-controlled diabetes who is undergoing major surgery?**
    Basal insulin is required *at all times*. Most diabetic patients who receive insulin use a combination of intermediate-acting (NPH) and regular insulin. The formulation is 70% NPH and 30% regular insulin. In these patients, total insulin dosage is usually given in the morning or divided between morning and afternoon. Typically two-thirds of the NPH and regular insulin formulation is given in the morning and one-third is given in the afternoon.

Table 21-2. Insulin Preparations

	TYPE OF INSULIN	ONSET	PEAK	DURATION
Short-acting	Regular	0.5-1 hr	2-4 hr	5-7 hr
Intermediate-acting	Isophane (NPH)	1-2 hr	6-14 hr	18-24 hr
	Lente	1-2 hr	6-14 hr	18-24 hr
Long-acting	Ultralente	6 hr	18-26 hr	36+ hr

For short procedures (<2 hours):
> If breakfast is delayed, patients may delay taking their usual short-acting insulin until after surgery and before eating. Those who take long-acting insulin may continue basal insulin without any change to the usual regimen.

For intermediate procedures (breakfast and lunch are delayed/missed):
- Omit any short-acting insulin on the morning of surgery.
- For patients who take two types of insulin (intermediate/long-acting and rapid/short-acting), only in the morning, give one-half to two-thirds of their usual total morning insulin dose (both types).
- For patients who take insulin (intermediate/long-acting and rapid/short-acting) two or more times a day, give one-third to one-half of the total morning dose (both types of insulin).
- Start dextrose containing intravenous solution to provide 3.75 to 6.25 g glucose/hour to avoid metabolic changes of starvation.
- For patients who develop hyperglycemia, supplemental short-acting insulin may be administered subcutaneously.
- During surgery, plasma glucose, serum electrolytes, and arterial blood gases (ABGs) should be monitored.
- Once the patient has resumed oral intake, NPH insulin is started. The patient's plasma glucose is monitored, and the insulin dosage is adjusted with regular insulin as needed.

For long and complex procedures:
> IV insulin is usually required. Blood glucose and electrolytes should be closely monitored (no less than hourly). Generally, insulin infusions should be started early in the morning prior to surgery to allow time to achieve glycemic control. The most common infusion is the glucose insulin potassium (GIK) infusion. It contains 10% dextrose, 10 mmol of potassium chloride, and 15 units of short-acting insulin.

44. What is an example of an order for typical sliding-scale insulin?
    See Table 21-3.

45. What are the classes of oral diabetic agents?
    See Table 21-4.

Table 21-3. Typical Sliding-Scale Insulin (Regular Insulin)

BLOOD GLUCOSE	INSULIN DOSE
150-200	2 units
201-250	4 units
251-300	6 units
301-350	8 units
351-400	10 units
>400	Notify provider (10-14 units and adjust SSI)

Table 21-4. Classes of Oral Diabetic Agents

TYPE	MECHANISM OF ACTION	SITE OF ACTION
Biguanides	Enhances insulin sensitivity Decreases GI absorption Decreases hepatic glucose production	Liver, GI tract
Sulfonylureas	Stimulates pancreas to produce more insulin	Pancreas
Alpha-glucosidase inhibitor	Reduces glucose absorption from gut by reducing enzymes required for carbohydrate breakdown	GI tract
Thiazolidinediones	Reduces insulin resistance	Fat, muscle

46. Which oral hypoglycemic is categorized as a biguanide?

Metformin (Glucophage) reduces hepatic glucose production, decreases GI glucose absorption, and increases target cell insulin sensitivity.

47. What is the pharmacology of the sulfonylureas?

These type 2 diabetic agents acutely increase insulin secretion from the beta cells and potentiate insulin action on several extrahepatic tissues. Long-term sulfonylureas increase peripheral utilization of glucose, suppress hepatic gluconeogenesis, and possibly increase the sensitivity or number of peripheral insulin receptors.

48. What drugs make up the sulfonylureas?

See Table 21-5.

49. What are the contraindications to the use of metformin in type 2 diabetes?

Metformin therapy is strictly contraindicated in alcoholics, patients with significant renal insufficiency or failure (serum creatinine >1.5 and >1.4 for women), and patients with liver disease. These conditions considerably increase the risk of lactic acidosis, a fatal side effect. Patients who are older than age 70 and those with low cardiac ejection fractions also are not candidates for metformin therapy. Patients who are about to receive iodine contrast dye, such as before cardiac catheterization, or who are to undergo major surgery should discontinue metformin 48 to 72 hours before the procedure.

50. What is the pharmacology of the meglitinides?

These type 2 diabetic agents quickly stimulate insulin release by the beta cells of the pancreas to reduce postprandial hyperglycemia. These drugs are taken before each of three meals.

51. What drugs make up the meglitinides?

See Table 21-6.

52. What is the pharmacology of the thiazolidinediones?

These type 2 diabetic drugs lower blood glucose by improving the target cell response to insulin in muscle and fat. At the same time, they do not increase pancreatic secretion of insulin. The thiazolidinediones are taken once or twice a day with food. These drugs can be used by themselves or in combination with sulfonylureas, metformin, or insulin. However, thiazolidinediones can have a rare but serious effect on liver function requiring regular liver function tests. This could affect the length of time that the amide local anesthetics are in circulation.

Table 21-5. Sulfonylureas

DRUG	BRAND NAME	DOSE	DURATION
Tolbutamide	Orinase	2 g	6-12 hr
Tolazamide	Tolinase	250 mg	10-18 hr
Glipizide	Glucotrol	10-15 mg	12 hr
Glyburide	Micronase	5-10 mg	16 hr
Acetohexamide	Dymelor	1 g	8-12 hr
Chlorpropamide	Diabinese	250 mg	1-3 days

Table 21-6. Meglitinides

DRUG	TRADE NAME	DOSE	ONSET OF ACTION	DURATION
Repaglinide	Prandin	0.5-2 mg bid	15-60 minutes	4-6 h
Mitiglinide	Starlix	120 mg bid 1-30 minutes before meals	20 minutes	4 h

bid, Twice a day.

53. **What drugs make up the thiazolidinediones?**
    See Table 21-7.

54. **What is the pharmacology of the alpha-glucosidase inhibitors?**
    These type 2 diabetic agents help the body to lower blood glucose levels by competitively inhibiting pancreatic alpha-amylase and intestinal brush border alpha-glucoside, resulting in delayed break-down of ingested complex carbohydrates, therefore slowing the absorption of glucose. These drugs should be taken with the first bite of a meal. The alpha-glucosidase inhibitors can be used alone or in combination with a sulfonylurea metformin or insulin.

55. **What drugs make up the alpha-glucosidase inhibitors?**
    Acarbose (Precase) and miglitol (Glyset). These drugs have <2% absorption as active drug because they work in the gastrointestinal tract. The metabolism is exclusively via the gastrointestinal tract.

56. **What is the oral combination drug Avandamet?**
    Avandamet is a combination of biguanide and thiazolidinediones, such as metformin and Avandia. It is used to treat type 2 diabetics who are not adequately controlled with metformin alone. The dosage is determined by starting Avandia 4 mg/day and adding it to the current metformin dose. If the patient is already taking Avandia, then add metformin so that the patient is getting l000 mg/day.

57. **What is the oral combination drug Metaglip?**
    Metaglip is the combination of sulfonylurea and biguanide, such as glipizide (Glucotrol) and metformin. This drug can be used as initial therapy for management of type 2 diabetes when hyperglycemia cannot be controlled with diet and exercise, or as second-line treatment when neither drug by itself controls hyperglycemia. Dosages are expressed as glipizide/metformin components. When used as initial therapy, 1.25 mg/250 mg is taken daily or twice daily with meals. As second-line therapy, 2.5 mg/500 mg or 5 mg/500 mg is given twice daily with meals.

58. **What is the oral combination drug Glucovance?**
    Glucovance is the combination of sulfonylurea and biguanide, such as glyburide and metformin. It can be used for initial management of type 2 diabetes, or as second-line therapy when a sulfonylurea or metformin alone cannot control hyperglycemia. In addition, Glucovance with a thiazolidinedione may be required to achieve adequate control.
    Glucovance dosages are expressed as glyburide/metformin components. When used as initial therapy, 1.25 mg/250 mg is taken with a meal once daily. Patients with an HgA1c >9% or fasting plasma glucose >200 mg/dL are started at 1.25 mg/250 mg twice daily. The maximum dose is not to exceed 10 mg/2000 mg. For those patients previously treated with a sulfonylurea or metformin alone, the initial dose is 2.5 mg/500 mg or 5 mg/500 mg twice a day.

59. **What is pramlintide?**
    Its brand name is Symlin, and it is a synthetic form of the hormone amylin, which is produced in the beta cells of the pancreas. It slows gastric emptying, suppresses glucagon, and regulates appetite. It is an injectable drug that has been recently approved by the FDA. Pramlintide has been approved for type 1 diabetics who are not achieving their A1c goal levels, and for type 2 diabetics using insulin and unable to achieve their A1c goals. It has been shown to modestly improve HgA1c levels, as well as promote modest weight loss without causing increased hypoglycemia.

60. **What is exenatide?**
    Exenatide (Byetta) is a glucagon-like peptide-1 agonist that mimics incretin and promotes insulin secretion, suppresses glucagon, and slows gastric emptying. It is an injectable drug approved

Table 21-7. Thiazolidinediones

DRUG	TRADE NAME	DOSE	ONSET OF ACTION	DURATION
Rosiglitazone	Avandia	4-8 mg qd or bid	Delayed	12 weeks
Pioglitazone	Actos	14-45 mg qd	Delayed	Several weeks
Troglitazone	Rezulin	Not available	Not available	Not available

bid, Twice a day; *qd*, daily.

by the FDA for the treatment of type 2 diabetics who have not been able to achieve their target HgA1c levels using metformin, a sulfonylurea, or a combination drug. As with pramlintide, exenatide is injected with meals, and patients using it have experienced improved HgA1c levels and modest weight loss.

61. **How do insulin pumps work?**
Insulin pumps deliver short-acting insulin 24 hours a day through a catheter placed subcutaneously. Insulin doses are separated into basal rates, boluses, and doses to correct glucose levels.

62. **What is a basal rate and a bolus?**
A basal rate is a constant rate of insulin delivered over 24 hours, keeping blood glucose levels in range between meals and overnight. The rate of insulin can be programmed to deliver different amounts of insulin at different times of the day and night. A bolus amount of insulin is used to cover the carbohydrate in each meal or snack. There are buttons on the insulin pump that will deliver the bolus if the meal is larger than planned, and a larger bolus of insulin can be programmed to cover it.

63. **What are the differences between type 1 and type 2 diabetes?**
Type 1:
- Sudden onset
- Occurs at any age (typically young)
- Body habitus is usually thin
- Ketosis is common
- Autoantibodies are present in most cases
- Endogenous insulin is low or absent

Type 2:
- Gradual onset
- Occurs mostly in adults
- Patients are frequently obese
- Ketosis is rare
- Autoantibodies are absent
- Endogenous insulin can be normal, decreased, or increased

64. **What is the response of insulin and glucagon to dietary protein?**
An increase in both hormones.

65. **Which hormones are considered ketogenic? Why?**
Epinephrine, glucocorticoids, glucagon, and growth hormone because they promote lipolysis.

66. **What is the response by insulin to parasympathetic stimulation?**
Insulin release will be increased.

67. **How will epinephrine that is released from the adrenal medulla affect plasma glucose?**
Epinephrine decreases glycogen synthesis in the liver. In addition, its release is increased in response to hypoglycemia.

68. **Where is the major site of action for glucagon?**
The breakdown of hepatic glycogen to glucose.

69. **What hormones antagonize the action of insulin on blood sugar?**
- Growth hormone
- Glucagon
- Cortisol
- Epinephrine

70. **What are the most common types of infections in diabetics and why?**
Diabetic patients have enhanced susceptibility to infections of the skin, tuberculosis, pneumonia, and pyelonephritis. Together, these infections cause the death of about 5% of diabetics. In addition, diabetics are very susceptible to fungal infections. The susceptibility to infections is a combination of impaired leukocyte function, inability to make antibodies against the bacteria, and vascular insufficiency.

BIBLIOGRAPHY

Agabegi SS, Agabegi ED: *Ring AC: step-up to medicine*, ed 3, Baltimore, 2013, Lippincott Williams & Wilkins.

Cada DJ, Covington TR, Hebel SK, editors: *Drug facts and comparisons*, St Louis, 1998, Wolters Kluwer.

Cooper DH, Krainik AJ, Lubner SJ, Reno HE, Micek ST: *Washington manual of medical therapeutics*, ed 32, St Louis, 2007, Lippincott Williams & Wilkins.

Gregory BA: Diabetes. In Abubaker AO, Benson KJ, editors: *Oral and maxillofacial surgery secrets*, ed 2, Philadelphia, 2007, Mosby/Elsevier.

Khan NA, Ghali WA, Cagliero E: *Perioperative management of blood glucose in adults with diabetes mellitus*, UpToDate, 2014, Wolters Kluwer.

Kumar V, Abbas A, Fausto N: *Robbins & Cotran pathologic basis of disease*, ed 7, Philadelphia, 2005, Saunders.

Roser M: Management of the medically compromised patient. In Kwon PH, Laskin DM, editors: *Clinician's manual of oral and maxillofacial surgery*, Carol Stream, IL, 1997, Quintessence.

Silverthorn DU: *Human physiology: an integrated approach*, ed 4, San Francisco, 2007, Benjamin Cummings.

Steil CF: Diabetes: an overview. In *CVS pharmacy pharmaceutical care module—diabetes*, Woonsocket, RI, 1998, CVS Pharmacy.

CHAPTER 22

THE IMMUNOCOMPROMISED SURGICAL PATIENT

Ludmils Antonos Jr., Osama Soliman, Noah Sandler, A. Omar Abubaker

1. **What are the major components of our immune system, and how do they function?**
   The immune system is the body's main way of fighting infections. Our immune system is composed of both an innate and adaptive system. The innate components are congenital, and the adaptive immunity develops throughout one's life. Adaptive immunity can be further divided into humoral and cellular immunity. The innate immune system is composed of the skin (which acts as a barrier to prevent invasion from foreign organisms), phagocytes, the complement system, and interferons. The humoral portion of the adaptive system is composed of B-cells that produce antibodies (immunoglobulins) that attach themselves to the surface of invading cells or organisms that help phagocytes detect them and then engulf them. B-cells also help activate the complements system. Humoral immunity is a very important component for attacking bacteria. The cellular portion of adaptive immunity is more useful in the defense against viruses, parasites, and cancer cells. Cellular immunity is a T-cell-mediated response. There are two types of T-cells: the helper T-lymphocytes and the killer T-cells. The helper T-cells recognize and flag the invading organism to the killer T-cells, which in turn destroy the target organism.

2. **What are the main organs involved in providing immunity?**
   The major human immune system is composed of several organs including the skin, spleen, tonsils, bone marrow, and lymph nodes.

3. **What is the main problem with immunocompromised patients?**
   Immunocompromised patients usually suffer from one or more types of immunodeficiency disorders that decrease the patient's immune system's ability to mount an adequate immune response to various immunological assaults. This in turn makes patients more susceptible to develop viral and bacterial infections as well as malignancies.

4. **What are the types of immunodeficiency?**
   Immunodeficiency can be either **primary** or **acquired** (secondary). Primary immunodeficiency is usually caused by a defect in a specific aspect of the immune system, such as a specific immunoglobulin. Acquired immunodeficiency can be secondary to disease or iatrogenic causes, such as the result of chemotherapy, and may involve more than one aspect of the immune system.

5. **Which types of immunodeficiency disorders are more common?**
   Acquired (secondary) immunodeficiency disorders are much more common than hereditary (primary) ones.

6. **What are the types of primary immunodeficiency disorders?**
   The WHO lists over 150 different primary immunodeficiency disorders. They are all categorized in one of five categories: B-cell deficiencies, T-cell and combined T-cell and B-cell deficiencies, phagocyte deficiencies, complement deficiencies, and periodic fevers.
   See Box 22-1 for common specific disorders.

7. **What are the common causes of acquired (secondary) immunosuppression and immunodeficiency in hospitalized patients?**
   Acquired (secondary) immunodeficiency can be caused by any of several factors, including:
   - Malnutrition: Most common cause worldwide
   - Drugs: Especially cytotoxic drugs (chemotherapy)
   - Iatrogenic causes: Such as post-transplant drug immunosuppression

Box 22-1. Common Immunodeficiency Disorders

B-cell Deficiencies
- X-linked agammaglobulinaemia (Bruton's Disease), (XLA)
- Common variable immunodeficiency (CVID)
- Selective IgA deficiency
- IgG subclass deficiency
- Immunodeficiency with thymoma (good syndrome)
- Transient hypoagammaglobulinaemia of infancy (THI)
- Hyper-IgM syndrome.- ar (Autosomal Recessive)

T-cell and Combined T- and B-cell Deficiencies
- Severe combined immunodeficiency (SCID, several forms)
- Catch 22 syndrome (DiGeorge syndrome, DGS)
- X-linked lymphoproliferative syndrome (Duncan's syndrome)
- Hyper-IgM syndrome: xl (cd40 ligand deficiency)
- MHC class II deficiency (bare lymphocytes)
- Ataxia-teleangiectasia (Louis Bar's syndrome)
- Wiskott-Aldrich's syndrome
- IPEX
- Hyper-IgM syndromes, autosomal recessive (AR)-Forms
- Chronic mucocutaneous candidiasis

Phagocyte Deficiencies
- Chronic granulomatous disease (CDG)
- Interferon g/interleukin 12, and receptors, deficiencies
- Familial hemophagocytic lymphohistiocytosis (FHI)
- Congenital agranulocytousis (Kostmann's syndrome)
- Cyclic neutropenia
- Leukocyte adhesion deficiency (LAD)
- Chédiak-higashi's syndrome
- Griscelli's syndrome (GS)
- Hyper-IgE syndrome (HIES)

Complement Deficiencies
- Properdin deficiency
- Mannan-binding lectin deficiency (MBL)
- Hereditary angioedema (HAE)
- And deficiencies of all other complements

Periodic Fevers
- Traps (tumor necrotic factor receptor associated periodic syndrome)
- Familial Mediterranean fever (FMF)
- Hyper-IgD syndrome (HIDS)
- PFAPA and others
  http://www.ipopi.org//index.php?mact=News,cntnt01,detail,0&cntnt01articleid=117&cntnt01returnid=38

- Viruses: HIV, CMV
- Lymphoreticular malignancy
- Protein loss: Due to nephrotic syndrome
- Advanced age
- Burns
- Organ failure, for example, renal disease requiring peritoneal dialysis
- Diabetes
- Radiation
- Surgery
- Trauma

8. **What are the different classes of systemic immunity?**
   Systemic immunity can be classified into an **antigen-specific** or **nonspecific immunity**. Antigen-specific can be either humoral or cell-mediated immunity. Parts of the nonspecific immunity system are the phagocytes and complement cascade.

9. **What is the effect of deficiency in cell-mediated immunity, and what are the appropriate methods of testing for such deficiency?**
   Deficiencies in cell-mediated immunity predispose the patient to infection from gram-negative organisms, mycobacteria, viruses, *Pneumocystis jiroveci* pneumonia (PJP) (formerly known as *Pneumocystis carinii* pneumonia [PCP]—the most common opportunistic infection in persons with HIV infection), and *Toxoplasma*. The best test for cell-mediated immunity is delayed-type hypersensitivity (DTH) skin testing, in which patients' reactions to intradermal injections of *Candida*, tuberculin, *Trichophyton*, and other antigens are observed. Direct measurement of T-cell function by the use of monoclonal antibodies is, however, a more specific test. The ratio of helper T-cells (CD4) to suppressor T-cells (CD8) (normally 1.8:2.2) is often used as a measure of this immune-type function.

10. **How is deficiency in humoral immunity manifested, and what are the appropriate methods of testing for humoral immunity?**
    Deficiency in humoral immunity predisposes patients to infection from pyogenic bacteria, hepatitis viruses, *Cytomegalovirus*, parasites, and *P. jiroveci*. Measuring serum immunoglobulin levels tests humoral immunity. Testing for the presence of antibodies to previous vaccination or infections can also indicate the status of the patient's humoral immunity. Other tests for humoral immunity, such as circulating B-cell count and in vitro B-cell testing, can also be performed.

11. **What infections are caused by deficiency in polymorphonuclear neutrophils (PMNs)?**
    Deficiencies of neutrophilic leukocytes (leukopenia) predispose patients to infections from *staphylococci*, *Serratia*, *Escherichia coli*, *Pseudomonas*, *Proteus*, *Enterobacter*, *Salmonella*, *Candida*, and *Aspergillus*. Absolute neutrophil count (ANC) and most functions of polymorphonuclear leukocytes can be tested by obtaining a CBC with differential and an absolute neutrophil count test.

12. **What is the effect of deficiency in complement, and how can complement functions be tested?**
    Deficiency in complement predisposes patients to infections from *Neisseria* and viruses. The status of complement cascade can be measured by the C'H50 (50% hemolyzing dose of complement) assay and by individual assay or C3 and C4 levels.

13. **What are the possible complications of immunosuppressive drugs in transplant patients?**
    Although newer immunosuppressive medications have reduced the amount and severity of acute transplant rejection, these new regimens are not without consequences. An increased risk of infection is seen in these patients secondary to decreased host resistance, with an increased risk for graft rejection in patients with severe infection. Infection is also the leading cause of death in transplant patients. Therefore, any transplant patients with active infections should be treated aggressively. Another risk for transplant patients is the increased incidence of de novo cancer. There may be a 100-fold increased incidence of cancer in the transplant patient. The most prevalent neoplasms are lymphoma and squamous cell carcinoma of the lips and skin. The incidence of tumors such as non-Hodgkin's lymphoma is approximately 2%, and this risk increases with the duration of immunosuppressive therapy. Most of these lesions occur in the head and neck, gastrointestinal tract, and transplanted allograft. These lesions are seen primarily with the use of cyclosporine and tacrolimus and are believed to be related to the inhibition of Epstein-Barr virus (EBV) cytotoxic T-cells. Transplant patients on immunosuppressive therapy, therefore, should be examined carefully for lip and skin lesions, nonhealing ulcers, and lymphadenopathy, and questionable lesions should undergo biopsy.

14. **What are the most common types of orofacial infection seen in immunocompromised patients?**
    T-cell deficiency is commonly found in post-transplant patients on immunosuppressive therapy, in AIDS patients, in some patients with certain forms of carcinoma, and in patients receiving treatment for cancer. Viral and fungal infections are more common in these patients. Viral infections are most

often produced by the *Herpesviridae* family (i.e., herpes simplex, varicella zoster virus, and cytomegalovirus). The clinical presentation of these infections is typically an acute, vesiculobullous lesion with a lack of inflammatory response in leukopenic patients. If not treated aggressively with antiviral agents, such as acyclovir, valaciclovir (Valtrex), or ganciclovir, these infections can lead to significant local and possible systemic morbidity.

Among fungal infections, *Candida albicans* is the most common fungal pathogen, but others such as *Aspergillus* and *Cryptococcus* are commonly encountered. The more aggressive fungi show an invasive behavior that often involves deeper tissues. Patients should be monitored carefully for signs of local tissue trauma that may predispose them to viral or fungal colonization.

15. **What are the characteristics of bacterial oral infections in immunocompromised patients?**

Oral infections in immunocompromised patients typically occur with significant local symptoms and may spread to involve adjacent or distant anatomic sites. These infections tend to progress more rapidly and may produce systemic symptoms or local osteomyelitis. Infections may be caused by gram-negative enteric flora secondary to colonization of these organisms in the oral cavity. These bacteria are often resistant to penicillin and cephalosporins. Broad-spectrum antibiotic prophylaxis should be used empirically before definitive identification of the causative microorganism in immunocompromised patients with evidence of infection.

16. **What are the general principles of the preoperative evaluation of immunocompromised patients?**

Immunosuppression is not in itself a contraindication to well-planned surgery. The general approach to the care of these patients when they are to undergo surgery is to increase host resistance to infection and to maximize wound healing. The patient's immune status should be evaluated by means of a history, physical exam, and lab studies. The history should include questions about the patient's underlying disease, previous infections, use of medications and other therapy, previous anesthesia, and trauma. The physical exam should also determine the patient's nutritional status and include a search for signs of existing infection and lymphadenopathy.

High-risk patients should have elective procedures scheduled at the beginning of the day. The possibility of reducing the dosages of immunosuppressive drugs must be weighed against the effect this might have on the reason why the patient is being treated with these agents. Other considerations include the removal of any infected foreign bodies; assessment of the need of invasive devices; restoration of cardiac and renal function, including tissue perfusion; correction of nutritional deficiencies, if present; assessment of the patient's need for vaccinations; and administration of prophylactic antibiotics. Also, regardless of the etiology, hemostasis should be achieved with pressure, packing, or suturing, and if the platelet count is below 50,000/mm^3, platelet transfusion should be considered. In the case of dental extractions, alveolectomy and primary closure are recommended. If platelet counts are <40,000/mm^3, platelets should be transfused 30 minutes before surgery to achieve platelet levels of more than 40,000/mm^3. One unit (pack) of platelets typically raises the platelet count by 10,000/mm^3. Although correcting the patient's immunodeficiency is usually difficult or impossible, defects in B-cell function may be partially treated by administering immunoglobulin.

17. **What preoperative lab studies should be included in evaluation of immunocompromised patients?**

- Chest radiograph
- Urinalysis
- Serum albumin determination
- Liver and kidney function tests
- Culture of material from any infected sites

Because some of these patients may present with neutropenia as well as thrombocytopenia, other tests include:

- Complete blood count with platelet count
- Absolute neutrophil count (ANC)
- Prothrombin time (PT)
- Partial thromboplastin time (PTT)

Specific testing of the patient's T-cells, B-cells, PMNs, and complement should be checked before surgery.

18. **What are the effects of chemotherapeutic and immunosuppressant drugs on the immune system?**
    The effects of these drugs vary from agent to agent. For example, chemotherapeutic agents depress the number and activity of the neutrophilic leukocytes (leukopenia). The nadir of white cell counts varies with the agents used but generally occurs 10-20 days after administration. The patient is susceptible to infection when the ANC falls below $1500/mm^3$. The susceptibility increases significantly when the count falls below $500/mm^3$. Corticosteroids, on the other hand, decrease the leukocyte response to inflamed tissue and depress T-cell function. Wound healing is slowed, and the ability to localize infection is reduced. Cyclosporine has almost no effect on the local inflammatory reaction but causes the initiation of interleukin-2 production and the suppression of T-helper and cytotoxic cells. Antilymphocyte antibodies appear to work by lysing target cells. With all these agents, increased dosage is associated with increased predisposition to infection. These patients should receive prophylactic antibiotics before most surgical procedures.

19. **When should prophylactic antibiotics be used in a chemotherapy patient?**
    Prophylactic antibiotics should be considered if the granulocyte count is $<2000/mm^3$. Surgery generally should be performed at least 3 days before chemotherapy is initiated in cancer patients because granulocyte levels may fall below $500/mm^3$ one week after the initiation of many types of chemotherapeutic agents. When surgery needs to be performed during severe neutropenia (granulocyte counts $< 500/mm^3$), it is recommended that the procedure be performed in a hospital setting with broad-spectrum antibiotic prophylaxis administered during the perioperative period.

20. **What type of virus is HIV, and what is its cell target?**
    Human immunodeficiency viruses (HIVs) are a group of retroviruses that can be acquired by the transmission of body fluids, including transfusions, and through the infection of infants by infected mothers. The specific target of the virus is the CD4 T-cell lymphocytes. The virus multiplies in the cell and eventually destroys it. Cell-mediated immunity is thereby severely affected.

21. **What are the general categories of HIV-infected patients?**
    - Asymptomatic patients with evidence of HIV infection demonstrated by the presence of HIV antibodies in the serum or in the secretions of these patients
    - Patients with AIDS-related complex (ARC), manifested by the presence of symptoms including lymphadenopathy, unexplained fever, weight loss, and hematologic and neurologic abnormalities
    - Patients with AIDS as defined by the Centers for Disease Control and Prevention (CDC) (i.e., HIV infection and CD4 lymphocyte count <200)

22. **What are the lab tests to determine the status of the HIV patient?**
    Diagnosis of HIV infection is made by detection of antibodies to HIV. Antibodies to HIV are determined by the enzyme-linked immunosorbent assay (ELISA) method or by the Western blot method; both tests require the patient's consent in many states.
    The status of patients with HIV infection and potential risk of surgery are evaluated by assessing the viral load and the CD4+ lymphocyte count. The viral load, determined by the HIV RNA, should ideally be undetectable. The CD4+ lymphocyte count should be greater than 200 and ideally greater than 400. Information regarding the overall physical status of the patient and the patient's symptomatic and physical manifestations of HIV-related diseases are also helpful in assessing the HIV patient's risk for surgery.
    Viral load measurements give an indication of the amount of current viral activity and have been shown to correlate with disease progression. Studies have demonstrated that viral loads of more than 30,000-50,000 HIV RNA copies/mL of plasma correlate with a poor prognosis, whereas viral loads of <5000 copies/mL correlate with better short-term prognosis.
    The CD4+ lymphocyte gives an indication of the degree of immunologic destruction. Lab findings in patients with AIDS include low lymphocyte counts and depressed CD4 T-cells, with the CD4-to-CD8 ratio of 1:0 or less (normally 1.8:2.2).

23. **What are the clinical manifestations of AIDS?**

Signs and Symptoms	Opportunistic Infections
Lymphadenopathy	*P. jiroveci* (pulmonary)
Weight loss	Toxoplasmosis (cerebral)
Diarrhea	Cryptosporidiosis (diarrhea)

Signs and Symptoms	*Opportunistic Infections*
Thrombocytopenia	Candidiasis (esophageal)
Anemia	*Cryptococcus* (meningitis)
Leukopenia	Herpes
Neurologic abnormalities	Varicella viruses (skin)
Dementia	Histoplasmosis
Encephalopathy	Tuberculosis
Central nervous system toxoplasmosis	**Neoplasms**
Lymphoma	Kaposi's sarcoma
	Lymphoma

24. **What are the principles of drug therapy of AIDS patients?**
The major goal of therapy of patients with AIDS is treatment of the opportunistic infections, including antiviral therapy. Prophylaxis is essential for all persons with symptomatic HIV disease, AIDS, or CD4+ counts <200/μL. Survival has also been prolonged in HIV-positive patients by prophylaxis against opportunistic infections such as *P. jiroveci* pneumonia (PJP), the *mycobacterium avium* complex (MAC), and other fungal infections. PJP prophylaxis commonly is with trimethoprim-sulfamethoxazole, although dapsone-trimethoprim or clindamycin-primaquine may be used alternately. Prophylaxis for MAC usually consists of a macrolide antibiotic, clarithromycin, or azithromycin and is recommended when the CD4+ cell count falls below 75 or 50/mL. Prophylaxis against *Candida* or other fungal diseases is currently not recommended, although many immunocompromised patients may be taking an antifungal medication, such as fluconazole or another azole, when they have manifestations of fungal infection. Current antiretroviral therapies have been shown to reduce viral counts and slow disease progression, and they can be effective in raising the CD4+ lymphocyte counts considerably. The most effective antiretroviral treatment strategies are multiple drug therapies that combine nucleoside analogue drugs with protease inhibitors and, when patients are able to tolerate these regimens, triple drug therapy with two nucleoside analogue drugs plus a protease inhibitor.

25. **What are the considerations in the surgical treatment of an HIV-infected person?**
Patients with early HIV infection and with no immunologic impairment generally tolerate elective oral surgical procedures well, and recent studies have demonstrated no increased incidence in infection, bleeding, or dry socket in extractions. In fact, routine prophylactic antibiotics are not indicated for these patients and may even further predispose them to candidiasis or drug reactions. In contrast, patients with AIDS and ARC are not good surgical candidates because of their hematologic abnormalities and predisposition to AIDS infection. Patients with mandibular fractures who have AIDS infection have an increased incidence of postoperative infections compared with asymptomatic HIV-positive patients. Accordingly, it is recommended that patients with AIDS (as defined by CD4+ count of <200 cells/mL or history of AIDS-defining illness such as lymphoma, tuberculosis, or *P. jiroveci*) should not undergo elective surgery. When urgent and emergency surgery is necessary, these patients should receive broad-spectrum prophylactic antibiotics before undergoing any surgical procedure, and proper attention to the prevention of wound infection must be given to prevent transmission of the virus to personnel caring for the patient.

26. **What are the potential drug interactions in HIV-infected patients?**
See Table 22-1.

27. **What is the management of health care workers exposed to HIV-infected blood or body fluids?**
The rate of seroconversion of health care workers exposed to HIV-infected blood or body fluid has been reported to be 0.42%. The management of occupational exposures of contaminated or suspected contaminated fluids is controversial. Currently, the CDC recommends that, after informed consent is obtained, the patient should be tested for HIV. If the patient is HIV-positive, the exposed health care worker should undergo HIV testing immediately and then at 6 weeks, 12 weeks, and 6 months. Initiation of zidovudine prophylaxis after exposure remains controversial because of its yet unproven efficacy.

Table 22-1. Potential Interactions of Drugs Used by HIV-Infected Patients

DRUG	DRUG USED TO TREAT HIV	MECHANISM OF INTERACTION	EFFECT	RECOMMENDATION
Benzodiazepines	Ritonavir, indinavir (protease inhibitors)	Inhibition of hepatic metabolism	↑ Concentration of benzodiazepines	Adjust benzodiazepine dosage, use alternate agent, or monitor closely for toxicity
Cisapride	Azole antifungals, clarithromycin, ritonavir, indinavir	Inhibition of hepatic metabolism	Cardiotoxic effects (including fatal arrhythmias)	Avoid concomitant use
Clarithromycin	Ritonavir, indinavir	Inhibition of hepatic metabolism	↑ Concentration of clarithromycin	Dosage reduction not required for patients with normal renal function
Didanosine (nucleoside analogue)	Oral ganciclovir	Unknown	↑ Didanosine	Monitor for didanosine toxicity; dosage reduction may be required
Ganciclovir	Zidovudine (thymidine analogue)	Pharmacodynamic interaction	Enhanced bone marrow toxicity	May require decreased dose of zidovudine or concomitant G-CSF
Ketoconazole	Saquinavir (protease inhibitor)	Inhibition of hepatic metabolism	↑ Saquinavir concentration	Under investigation to maximize saquinavir exposure
Metronidazole	Ritonavir (liquid only)	Alcohol in liquid formulation	Disulfiram-like reaction	Monitor for toxicity; change form of ritonavir
Opiate analgesics (especially meperidine, propoxyphene, fentanyl)	Ritonavir	Inhibition of hepatic metabolism	↑ Opiate concentration	Use alternate pain medication; monitor for toxicity
Terfenadine, astemizole (H1 antihistamines)	Azole antifungals, clarithromycin, ritonavir	Inhibition of hepatic metabolism	Accumulation of cardiotoxic unmetabolized antihistamine	Avoid concomitant use

G-CSF, Granulocyte colony-stimulating factor.
Adapted from Sandler NA, Braun TW: Current surgical management of the immunocompromised patient, *Oral Maxillofac Surg Clin North Am* 10:445–455, 1998.

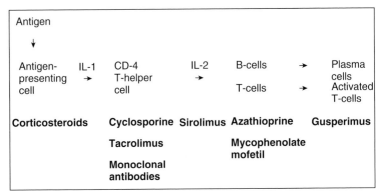

Figure 22-1. Sites of action of immunosuppressive drugs used in transplant patients. *IL,* Interleukin. *(Modified from Sandler NA, Braun TW: Current surgical management of the immunocompromised patient,* Oral Maxillofac Surg Clin North Am *10:445–455, 1998.)*

28. **What is the mechanism of action of immunosuppressive agents used in transplant patients?**
The drugs listed in Figure 22-1 suppress the immune system at sites complementary to traditional immunosuppressive medications. Many transplant patients currently are on two or more of these drugs in an attempt to prevent rejection. This may predispose the patient to overimmunosuppression or potential drug interactions.

29. **What is graft-versus-host disease (GVHD)?**
GVHD results when immune cells or tissues transplanted from a donor act toward the transplant recipient as foreign, thereby initiating an immune reaction that causes disease in the transplant recipient. It is primarily a T-cell-mediated immune process.

30. **What are the common immunosuppressive agents used to treat GVHD?**
Medications used for the prevention and treatment of GVHD include immunosuppressive drugs, such as corticosteroids and methotrexate, as well as more specific T-cell immunosuppressive drugs, such as cyclosporine and tacrolimus. Corticosteroids are the most widely used front-line therapy for the treatment of clinical GVHD, commonly administered in combination with therapeutic doses of cyclosporine or tacrolimus.

31. **What oral manifestation may indicate an overdosage of methotrexate in patients being treated for GVHD?**
Grade III/IV mucositis.

32. **What are some of the common post-transplantation immunosuppressive drugs?**
Post-transplantation immunosuppressive drugs are several and include:
Nonspecific
- **Corticosteroids:** The most commonly utilized corticosteroid is methylprednisolone.
- **Methotrexate:** An antimetabolite with primary goal to cause cell death. It can induce tolerance following marrow transplantation.
Specific T-Cell Immunosuppressive Drugs
- **Cyclosporine:** Blocks the calcium-dependent signal transduction pathways distal to engagement of the T-cell receptor. This block interrupts the activation of T-cells.
- **Tacrolimus:** This is a macrolide antibiotic. It inhibits the signaling through the T-cell receptor. See question 33 for more details.
- **Sirolimus:** (rapamycin) is a lipophilic macrolide antibiotic.
- **Mycophenolate:** Mycophenolate Mofetil (MMF, CellCept) is a morpholinoethyl ester of mycophenolic acid (MPA).
Antibodies
- Most of the promising results have come from studies using selected monoclonal antibodies. Directed **Muromonab-CD3 (OKT3)** is a monoclonal mouse antibody licensed for the therapy of allograft rejection. High incidences of infection have discouraged the use of this antibody.

Table 22-2. Side Effects of Immunosuppressive Drugs Used in Transplant Patients

MEDICATION	POTENTIAL SIDE EFFECTS
Corticosteroids	Cushing's syndrome, adrenal insufficiency
Azathioprine	Myelodepression (leukopenia, thrombocytopenia)
Cyclosporine	Nephrotoxicity, neurotoxicity, hypertension, hepatotoxicity
Tacrolimus	Nephrotoxicity, neurotoxicity, diabetogenic effects
Mycophenolate mofetil	Myelodepression (leukopenia, anemia), gastrointestinal (diarrhea, emesis)
Sirolimus	Myelodepression (leukopenia, thrombocytopenia), potential nephrotoxicity
Gusperimus	Myelodepression (leukopenia, anemia, thrombocytopenia)
Monoclonal antibodies	Central nervous system (seizure, encephalopathy, psychosis)*

*Increased risk of encephalopathy and psychosis reported with indomethacin use.
Adapted from Sandler NA, Braun TW: Current surgical management of the immunocompromised patient, *Oral Maxillofac Surg Clin North Am* 10:445–455, 1998.

- **Antithymocyte globulin** is a polyclonal immunoglobulin prepared by injecting various cellular preparations into animals. The antibodies produced are capable of destroying human leukocytes.
- **Rituximab** is an anti-CD20 monoclonal antibody used to decrease allogeneic donor B-cell immunity.

Thalidomide
- **Thalidomide** is an immunomodulator that lacks a global inhibitory effect upon lymphocyte proliferation and does not impair DTH.

Novel Agents
- **Anti-cytokines** to TNF-alpha, IL-1, and gamma-interferon
- **Induction of anergy**
- **Other approaches:** Drugs or nonpharmacological treatment options that appear to be promising include clofazimine, psoralen and ultraviolet light A (PUVA), photopheresis, radiation therapy, and novel molecules such as a fusion immunotoxin directed against CD3.

33. What are the side effects of immunosuppressive drugs in transplant patients?
    See Table 22-2.

34. What are the oral manifestations of cyclosporine use?
    Cyclosporine is associated with gingival hyperplasia in the dental papillae of the anterior teeth, which typically occurs after 3-6 months of immunosuppressant therapy. Studies suggest that approximately 30% of patients medicated with cyclosporine alone experience significant gingival changes. Calcium channel blocking agents that may be prescribed to counter the hypertension caused by cyclosporine may also induce gingival hyperplasia with an additive effect to that of cyclosporine. When the two drugs are used simultaneously, they can result in a nearly 40% incidence of gingival hyperplasia. Other significant risk factors that influence gingival overgrowth include age and sex (with younger men having an increased susceptibility), duration of therapy, serum creatinine levels, and the HLA-B37 haplotype.

35. How is cyclosporine-induced gingival hyperplasia treated?
    Decreases in the dosage of the drug or discontinuing the drug early may result in reversal of this side effect. However, surgical intervention that consists of gingivectomy and tissue re-contouring is often necessary to improve aesthetics and function.

36. What are the different drug interactions of cyclosporine/tacrolimus?
    See Table 22-3.

37. What is tacrolimus, and what are its major side effects?
    Tacrolimus (FK-506) is a macrolide immunosuppressant isolated from *Streptomyces tsukubaensis* in 1984. This drug is 50-100 times more potent than cyclosporine. Initially used during episodes of severe graft rejection, it is now used for baseline immunosuppression.
    The principal adverse effects associated with tacrolimus are similar to those of cyclosporine and include nephrotoxicity and neurotoxicity. In addition, diabetogenic effects are seen. The mechanism

Table 22-3. Drug Interactions of Cyclosporine and Tacrolimus

DRUG	CLASS	MECHANISM
Increased Cyclosporine		
Metoclopramide	Prokinetic	↑ cyclosporine absorption
Cisapride	Prokinetic	↑ cyclosporine absorption
Erythromycin	Macrolide antibiotic	Mechanism unclear
Increased Cyclosporine/Tacrolimus		
Clotrimazole	Imidazole	Inhibit cytochrome P450
Fluconazole	Antifungal	Inhibit cytochrome P450
Corticosterone	Corticosteroid	Inhibit cytochrome P450
Dexamethasone	Corticosteroid	Inhibit cytochrome P450
Bromocriptine	Dopamine agonist	Inhibit cytochrome P450
Cyclosporine/tacrolimus	Immunosuppressant	Inhibit cytochrome P450
Ergotamine	Alpha blocker	Inhibit cytochrome P450
Nifedipine	Ca channel blocker	Inhibit cytochrome P450
Diltiazem	Ca channel blocker	Inhibit cytochrome P450
Verapamil	Ca channel blocker	Inhibit cytochrome P450
Cimetidine	H2 blocker	Inhibit cytochrome P450
Omeprazole	H/K ATPase blocker	Inhibit cytochrome P450
Increased Tacrolimus		
Danazol	Androgen	↑ Renal impairment
Grapefruit juice		Inhibit intestinal cytochrome P450
Decreased Cyclosporine/Tacrolimus		
Rifampin	Antibiotic	↑ Cytochrome P450 activity
Phenytoin	Anticonvulsant	↑ Cytochrome P450 activity
Phenobarbital	Anticonvulsant	↑ Cytochrome P450 activity
Decreased Cyclosporine		
Sulfadimidine	Antibiotic	↑ Cytochrome P450 activity
Trimethoprim	Antibiotic	↑ Cytochrome P450 activity
Decreased Tacrolimus		
Carbamazepine	Anticonvulsant	↑ Cytochrome P450 activity
Primidone	Anticonvulsant	↑ Cytochrome P450 activity

ATPase, Adenosine triphosphatase.
Adapted from Sandler NA, Braun TW: Current surgical management of the immunocompromised patient, *Oral Maxillofac Surg Clin North Am* 10:445–455, 1998.

by which tacrolimus causes nephrotoxicity is related to an alteration of prostaglandin metabolism, by inducing vasoconstriction, and reduction in renal blood flow and a resultant decreased glomerular filtration rate. With the addition of a nonsteroidal antiinflammatory drug (NSAID), the renal blood flow can become even more impaired. Therefore, the routine prescription of NSAIDs to patients on tacrolimus should be avoided. Drugs that may induce nephrotoxicity and contribute to renal impairment, such as aminoglycosides, trimethoprim-sulfamethoxazole, amphotericin B, and acyclovir, also should be avoided in patients who are taking tacrolimus.

38. **Does tacrolimus interact with any drugs that are routinely used in oral and maxillofacial surgery patients?**
    Yes. Tacrolimus is eliminated in the liver by cytochrome P450 isoenzymes and, therefore, may show a rise in concentration with the concomitant use of macrolide antibiotics, such as erythromycin

or clarithromycin, azole antifungal agents, or corticosteroids. Also, the antihistamines terfenadine (Seldane) and astemizole (Hismanal) have been associated with cardiac arrhythmias after coadministration with tacrolimus or cyclosporine. Concurrent use of NSAIDs or nephrotoxic antibiotics and tacrolimus also increases the potential for nephrotoxicity.

39. **What are the oral manifestations of GVHD in the transplant patient?**
The oral cavity can be affected, along with the liver, skin, and gastrointestinal tract. More than 80% of patients with GVHD have oral lesions, which in many cases may be the first symptom. The clinical presentation of oral GVHD resembles that of other collagen vascular diseases, such as systemic lupus erythematosus or lichen planus. The oral mucosa may show erythema, ulceration, white striations, atrophy, or a pseudomembranous covering. Symptoms may range from mild discomfort to burning and severe pain and salivary dysfunction. GVHD is treated by augmenting immunosuppressive therapy. Careful monitoring of the patient for signs of overimmunosuppression should also be performed during this period.

40. **What are the perioperative considerations of post-splenectomy patients?**
Post-splenectomy patients have the potential to develop overwhelming sepsis with shock and disseminated intravascular coagulation (DIC). The most common organisms causing such infections are *Pneumococcus, Meningococcus,* and *Haemophilus*. Therefore, before splenectomy, patients should receive vaccination with pneumococcal polysaccharide. Prophylactic antibiotics should be given before surgical procedures in contaminated sites, such as the oral cavity. Early aggressive treatment of infections in these patients is recommended.

BIBLIOGRAPHY

Abubaker AO, Sandler N: The immunocompromised surgical patient. In Abubaker AO, Benson KJ, editors: *Oral and maxillofacial surgery secrets,* ed 2, Philadelphia, 2007, Mosby/Elsiever.

Bleyer WA: Methotrexate: clinical pharmacology, current status and therapeutic guidelines, *Cancer Treat Rev* 4:87, 1977.

Carpenter CC, Fischl MA, Hammer SM, et al.: Antiretroviral therapy for HIV infection in 1996: recommendations of an international panel. International AIDS Society-USA, *JAMA* 276:146–164, 1996.

Centers for Disease Control and Prevention: USPHA/IDSA guidelines for the prevention of opportunistic infections in persons infected with human immunodeficiency virus: a summary, *MMWR Morb Mortal Wkly Rep* 44:1–34, 1995.

Chao NJ, Schmidt GM, Niland JC, et al.: Cyclosporine, methotrexate, and prednisone compared with cyclosporine and prednisone for prophylaxis of acute graft-versus-host disease, *N Engl J Med* 329:1225, 1993.

Chao NJ, Snyder DS, Jain M, et al.: Equivalence of 2 effective graft-versus-host disease prophylaxis regimens: results of a prospective double-blind randomized trial, *Biol Blood Marrow Transplant* 6:254, 2000.

Deeks SG, Smith M, Holodniy M, et al.: HIV-1 protease inhibitors: a review for clinicians, *JAMA* 277:145–153, 1997.

Dodson TB, Parrott DH, Nguyen T, et al.: HIV status and the risk of postoperative complications, *J Oral Maxillofac Surg* 49(Suppl 1):81–82, 1991.

Fernandez J: Overview of immunodeficiency disorders. In Porter S, editor: *Merck manual,* ed 19, New Jersey, 2013, Merck & Co.

Fernandez, MD: Overview of immunodeficiency disorders. Merck manual, 2013.

Ferrara JL, Deeg HJ: Graft-versus-host disease, *N Engl J Medu* 324:667, 1991.

Grant D, Wall W, Duff J, et al.: Adverse effects of cyclosporine therapy following liver transplantation, *Transplant Proc* 19:3463–3465, 1987.

Ho M, Dummer JS: Risk factors and approach to infections in transplant recipients. In Mandell GL, Douglas RG, Bennett JE, editors: *Principles and practices of infectious diseases,* ed 4, New York, 1995, Churchill Livingstone.

Holler E, Kolb HJ, Wilmanns W: Treatment of GVHD–TNF-antibodies and related antagonists, *Bone Marrow Transplant* 12(Suppl 3):S29, 1993.

Lockhart PB, Sonis ST: Relationship of oral complications to peripheral blood leukocyte and platelet counts in patients receiving cancer chemotherapy, *Oral Surg Oral Med Oral Pathol* 48:21–28, 1979.

Martinez-Gimeno C, Acero-Sanz J, Martin-Sastra R, et al.: Maxillofacial trauma: influence of HIV infection, *J Craniomaxillofac Surg* 20:297–302, 1992.

Matsuda H, Iwasaki K, Shiriga T, et al.: Interactions of FK506 (tacrolimus) with clinically important drugs, *Res Commun Mol Pathol Pharmacol* 91:57–64, 1996.

Maxymiw WG, Wood RE: The role of dentistry in patients undergoing bone marrow transplantation, *Br Dent J* 167:229–234, 1989.

Mignat C: Clinically significant drug interactions with new immunosuppressive agents, *Drug Saf* 16:267–278, 1997.

Pernu HE, Pernu LM, Huttunen K, et al.: Gingival overgrowth among renal transplant recipients and uremic patients, *Nephrol Dial Transplant* 8:1254–1258, 1993.

Peterson DE, Sonis ST: Oral complications of cancer chemotherapy: present status and future studies, *Cancer Treat Rep* 66:1251–1256, 1982.

Portery SR, Scully C, Luker J: Complications of dental surgery in persons with HIV disease, *Oral Surg Oral Med Oral Pathol* 75:165–167, 1993.

Reichart PA, Gelderblom HR, Becker J, et al.: AIDS and the oral cavity. The HIV-infection virology, etiology, origin, immunology, precautions and clinical observation in 110 patients, *Int J Oral Maxillofac Surg* 16:129–153, 1987.

Robinson PG, Cooper H, Hatt J: Healing after dental extractions in men with HIV infections, *Oral Surg Oral Med Oral Pathol* 74:426–430, 1992.

Roser SM: Management of the medically compromised patient. In Kwon PH, Laskin DM, editors: *Clinician manual of oral and maxillofacial surgery*, ed 2, Chicago, 1996, Quintessence.

Samaranayake LP: Oral mycoses in HIV infection, *Oral Surg Oral Med Oral Pathol* 73:171–180, 1992.

Schmidt B, Kearns G, Parrott D, et al.: Infection following treatment of mandibular fractures in human immunodeficiency virus in seropositive patients, *J Oral Maxillofac Surg* 53:1134–1139, 1995.

Storb R, Deeg HJ, Fisher L, et al.: Cyclosporine v methotrexate for graft-v-host disease prevention in patients given marrow grafts for leukemia: long-term follow-up of three controlled trials, *Blood* 71:293, 1988.

Storb R, Deeg HJ, Whitehead J, et al.: Methotrexate and cyclosporine compared with cyclosporine alone for prophylaxis of acute graft versus host disease after marrow transplant for leukemia, *N Engl J Med* 314:729, 1986.

Thomason JM, Seymour RA, Rice N: Determinants of gingival overgrowth severity in organ transplant patients. An examination of the role of HLA phenotype, *J Clin Periodontol* 23:628–634, 1996.

Thomason JM, Seymour RA, Rice N: The prevalence and severity of cyclosporine and nifedipine-induced gingival overgrowth, *J Clin Periodontol* 20:37–40, 1993.

Wysocki GP, Gretzinger HA, Laupacis A, et al.: Fibrous hyperplasia of the gingiva: a side effect of cyclosporine A therapy, *Oral Surg Oral Med Oral Pathol* 55:274–278, 1983.

Yee J, Christou NV: Perioperative care of the immunocompromised patient, *World J Surg* 17:207–214, 1993.

http://www.uptodate.com/contents/overview-of-immunosuppressive-agents-used-for-prevention-and-treatment-of-graft-versus-host disease?

V

ORAL AND MAXILLOFACIAL SURGERY

CHAPTER 23

APPLIED OROFACIAL ANATOMY

A. Omar Abubaker, Kenneth J. Benson

THE NOSE AND PARANASAL SINUSES

1. Which five bones make up the nose?
   1. Maxilla: frontal process of maxilla
   2. Frontal bone: nasal process of frontal bone
   3. Nasal bones
   4. Vomer: contributes to the septum
   5. Ethmoid: perpendicular plate of the ethmoid also contributes to the septum

2. What embryologic structures form the external nose?
   The **maxillary processes**, which originate from the dorsal ends of the first (mandibular) arch and the lateral nasal processes, grow toward the midline to merge with the downward-growing frontonasal process to form the external nose. The **frontonasal process** then continues to elongate, forming the median nasal process and fetal philtrum. The lateral nasal processes form the lateral portion of the adult nose (i.e., lower lateral cartilage and lobule). The **olfactory placode**, an ectodermal thickening, invaginates as a pit between the medial portion of the frontonasal process and the lateral nasal process. The olfactory placode finally comes to rest high in the nose as the analogue of the olfactory epithelium.

3. What nasal bones and cartilages make up the external nasal skeleton?
   Several bones and cartilages make up the external nose and give it its characteristic pyramidal shape (Fig. 23-1). The nasal bones articulate with the nasal part of the frontal bone superiorly and the nasal process of the maxilla laterally. The nasal bones are attached at their inferior aspect to the upper lateral cartilages. The upper lateral cartilages in turn attach their inferior portion to the lower lateral cartilages and, medially, to the cartilaginous septum.

   Small rudimentary cartilages known as *sesamoid cartilages*, or *alar cartilages*, give additional support to the lateral nasal ala, where the lower lateral cartilage extends to meet the cheek. The fibrofatty tissue of the lower lateral cartilage, which contains the sesamoid cartilages, is known as the *lobule*.

   The nasal septum is made up of quadrangle cartilage that continues with the lateral nasal cartilage toward the bridge of the nose, forming the cartilaginous portion of the septum. Posteriorly and above, the septal cartilage with the perpendicular plate of the ethmoid and the inferior edge of the septum fits into a groove on the vomer and the nasal crest.

4. What is the vascular supply to the nose?
   Branches from both the external and internal carotid arteries supply the nose. The external nose is supplied by the dorsal nasal of the ophthalmic artery superiorly, and the septal and lateral nasal of the angular artery inferiorly. The lower part of the dorsum of the nose is supplied by the external nasal, from the anterior ethmoidal artery.

   The external carotid artery via the terminal branches of the internal maxillary artery, namely the sphenopalatine and greater palatine arteries, supplies the posterior inferior part of the internal nose. Branches from the anterior and posterior ethmoid arteries of the ophthalmic artery supply the anterior inferior nasal cavity, which is a branch of the internal carotid artery. Venous drainage of the nose corresponds to the arterial nomenclature and occurs through the sphenopalatine, ophthalmic, and anterior facial veins.

5. How is the sensory nerve supply to the nose mapped?
   - Olfactory fibers are located in the superior portion of the internal nose and serve the sensory function of smell.
   - The sensory innervation of the skin of the root of the nose is derived from the supratrochlear and infratrochlear branches of the ophthalmic nerve.

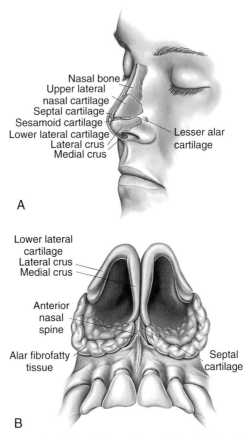

Figure 23-1. A, Normal anatomy and underlying soft tissues of the nose. **B,** Normal position of the nasal septum and nasal spine. *(From Bertz JE: Nasal injuries. In Fonseca RJ, editor: Oral and maxillofacial surgery, vol 3, Philadelphia, 2000, Saunders.)*

- Branches of the infraorbital nerve supply the skin on the lower half of the nose's side.
- Nasociliary branches of the ophthalmic nerve supply the skin over the lower dorsum of the nose down to the tip.
- The trigeminal nerve supplies general sensory innervation to the anterior internal nose through the anterior ethmoidal, external, and internal nasal branches.
- The lateral posterior superior, pharyngeal, and lateral posterior inferior branches of the maxillary nerve supply the posterior portion.
- The terminal branches of the infraorbital nerve supply the lining of the nasal vestibule.
- The internal nasal (anterior ethmoidal) and medial posterior superior branches supply the septum anterior and posterior portions, respectively.

6. How is the motor nerve supply to the nose mapped?
   - The autonomic nerve supply of the nose controls the secretory function of the mucous glands.
   - The preganglionic sympathetic innervation originates from the hypothalamus, passes through the thoracolumbar region of the spinal cord, and synapses in the superior cervical ganglion in the neck.
   - Postganglionic sympathetic fibers then pass through the sphenopalatine ganglion to reach the nasal glands along the posterior nasal nerves.

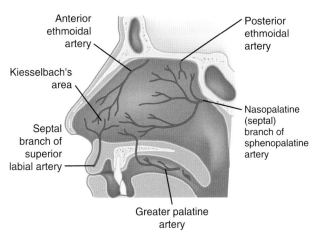

Figure 23-2. Vessels that make up Kiesselbach's plexus. *(From Marx JA: Rosen's Emergency Medicine: Concepts and Clinical Practice, 8th ed, Philadelphia, 2014, Saunders.)*

- The parasympathetic nerve supply to the nose originates in the superior salvatory nucleus of the midbrain to reach the sphenopalatine ganglion through the greater petrosal nerve.
- The postganglionic fibers are carried out along the vidian nerve to finally reach the nose via the posterior nasal nerve.
- The motor nerve supply to all the muscles of the external nose is by way of the facial nerve.

7. What are the most common vessels involved with anterior epistaxis?
   Kiesselbach's plexus of septum arterioles is the source of 90% of nosebleeds. Four anastomosed arteries make up this plexus: the sphenopalatine, anterior ethmoidal, greater palatine, and superior labial arteries. The nasopalatine branch of the descending palatine artery anastomoses with septal branches of the sphenopalatine artery, the anterior ethmoidal artery, and superior lateral branches of the superior labial branch of the facial artery. Traumatic nasal bleeding can be caused by laceration of the nasal mucosa, and any of the nasal vessels can be the source of the bleeding (Fig. 23-2).

8. How does lymphatic drainage of the nose occur?
   The lymphatics of the nose arise from the superficial portion of the mucous membrane and travel posteriorly to the retropharyngeal lymph nodes. Anteriorly, the lymphatics drain into the submandibular lymph nodes or the upper deep cervical nodes.

9. Where do the paranasal sinuses drain?
   The sphenoid sinus drains into the sphenoethmoidal recess. The posterior ethmoid sinus drains into the superior nasal meatus, and the nasolacrimal duct drains into the inferior nasal meatus. All other sinuses (maxillary, frontal, and anterior and middle ethmoidal) drain into the middle nasal meatus.

THE EAR AND LARYNX

10. What other nerves supply the ear?
    The auriculotemporal nerve (CN V3) supplies the root helix, crus, tragus, and canal, whereas the auricular branch off the facial nerve (CN VII) supplies the concha and canal. Thus, in all, four cranial nerves (V, VII, IX, and X) provide sensory innervation for the ear.

11. What are Arnold's and Jacobson's nerves? Which organ do they supply?
    Both nerves provide sensory innervation to the ear. Arnold's nerve is a branch of the vagus nerve (CN X) and supplies the concha and auditory canal. Jacobson's nerve is a branch of the glossopharyngeal nerve (CN IX) and supplies the concha, canal, and middle ear.

12. **What is the sensory innervation to the larynx?**

The vagus nerve innervates the larynx via two laryngeal branches, the *internal laryngeal* and the *recurrent laryngeal*. The internal laryngeal branch provides sensory innervation to the mucous membrane above the vocal fold, whereas the recurrent laryngeal nerve provides sensory innervation to the mucous membrane below the vocal fold.

Motor function of the laryngeal muscles and vocal cords also is provided by the laryngeal branches of the vagus nerve (fibers of CN XI traveling with CN X). The *external laryngeal* branch innervates the cricothyroid muscle, and the recurrent laryngeal branch innervates all other intrinsic muscles.

ORBITAL ANATOMY

13. **Which bones form the orbital cavity?**
    - Lacrimal
    - Sphenoid
    - Ethmoid
    - Zygomatic
    - Palatine
    - Maxillary
    - Frontal

14. **What is Whitnall's orbital tubercle?**

Whitnall's orbital tubercle is a bony protuberance present at the lateral orbital wall approximately 5 mm behind the lateral orbital rim. The tubercle is the area for attachment of the lateral horn of the levator aponeurosis, lateral palpebral ligament, and lateral check ligament. The attachment of these structures is in that order, from anterior to posterior.

15. **Which orbital voluntary muscle does *not* originate at the orbital apex?**

The inferior oblique muscle arises from the medial portion of the floor of the orbit just posterior to the orbital rim. The muscle then passes laterally and inserts on the posterolateral sclera.

16. **What is the anatomy, nerve supply, and function of the extraocular muscles?**

See Table 23-1.

17. **What are the distance limits from the lateral, inferior, superior, and medial orbital rims for safe posterior dissection?**

Although the distance from the orbital rim to the orbital apex is 4 to 4.5 cm, subperiosteal dissection along the orbital walls can be safely extended only up to 25 mm posteriorly from the inferior orbital rim and 25 mm from the lateral orbital rim. From the anterior lacrimal crest, dissection can be extended 25 mm posteriorly with minimal danger to the posterior orbital contents. From the superior orbital rim, dissection can be extended 30 mm. However, because most traumatic forces tend to displace all or part of these rims posteriorly, this displacement should be considered when carrying out posterior dissection in the orbit (Fig. 23-3).

18. **What occurs during the autonomic nerve supply to the pupil?**

Postganglionic sympathetic fibers have their cell bodies in the superior cervical ganglion. These nerves reach the dilator pupil muscles via the **short and long ciliary nerves**. Preganglionic parasympathetic fibers have their cell bodies in the Edinger-Westphal nucleus in the brain and travel to the ciliary ganglion in the orbit via the oculomotor nerve. The short ciliary nerves from the ciliary ganglion to the sphincter pupillary muscles carry the postganglionic fibers. Parasympathetic fibers contribute to pupillary constriction; the sympathetic supply activates pupillary dilator muscles.

19. **What are the sebaceous and sweat glands of the eyelids called?**

The sebaceous glands of the eyelid are called the *glands of Zeis*. The sweat glands of the eyelid are called the *glands of Moll*.

20. **What is the anulus of Zinn?**

The anulus of Zinn, or common tendinous ring in the orbit, is the fibrous thickening of the periosteum from which the recti muscles originate.

Table 23-1. Anatomy, Nerve Supply, and Function of the Extraocular Muscles

MUSCLE	ORIGIN	INSERTION	NERVE SUPPLY	FUNCTION
Levator palpebrae superioris	Lesser wing of sphenoid	Anterior surface and upper border of superior tarsal plate		
• Voluntary portion			Oculomotor nerve	Raises upper eyelid
• Involuntary portion			Sympathetic nerves	
Superior rectus	Common tendinous ring	Sclera 6 mm behind corneal margin	Oculomotor nerve	Raises and medially rotates cornea
Inferior rectus	Common tendinous ring	Sclera 6 mm behind corneal margin	Oculomotor nerve	Depresses cornea, medially rotates cornea
Lateral rectus	Common tendinous ring	Sclera 6 mm behind corneal margin	Abducent nerve	Moves cornea laterally
Medial rectus	Common tendinous ring	Sclera 6 mm behind corneal margin	Oculomotor nerve	Moves cornea medially
Superior oblique	Body of sphenoid	By way of pulley and attached to sclera behind coronal equator of eyeball; line of pull of tendon passes medial to vertical axis	Trochlear nerve	Moves cornea downward and laterally
Inferior oblique	Anterior part of floor of orbit	Attached to sclera behind coronal equator; line of pull of tendon passes medial to vertical axis	Oculomotor nerve	Moves cornea upward and laterally

Adapted from Snell RS: *Clinical Anatomy for Medical Students*, ed 5, Boston, 1996, Little, Brown.

21. What are the functions of the extraocular muscles?
   - **Lateral rectus muscle:** abduction
   - **Medial rectus muscle:** adduction
   - **Inferior rectus muscle:** depression, adduction, and extorsion (extorsion—the superior pole of the globe moves laterally)
   - **Superior rectus muscle:** elevation, adduction, and intorsion (intorsion—the superior pole of the globe moves medially)
   - **Superior oblique muscle:** depression, abduction, and intorsion
   - **Inferior oblique muscle:** elevation, abduction, and extorsion

22. Which bony structures surround the orbit and protect its contents?
   - **Superiorly:** The supraorbital rim is formed by the supraorbital arch of the frontal bone.
   - **Inferiorly:** The thick infraorbital rim is formed by the zygoma laterally and the maxilla medially.
   - **Medially:** The nasal spine of the frontal bone and the frontal process of the maxilla constitute the anteromedial orbital wall.
   - **Laterally:** The frontal process of the zygoma and the zygomatic process of the frontal bone constitute the lateral orbital rim.

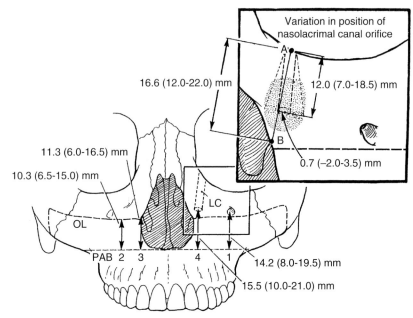

Figure 23-3. The relationship of the nasolacrimal duct to the nasal floor and turbinates. Heights (means and ranges) are from the piriform aperture base (PAB) to the infraorbital foramen (1), the simulated osteotomy (2), the anterior attachment of the inferior turbinate (3), and the inferior orifice of the nasolacrimal canal (4). **A,** The inset illustrates the variation in position of the nasolacrimal canal orifice relative to the x line drawn between the lacrimal fossa and **B,** the anterior attachment of the inferior turbinate. *LC,* Nasolacrimal canal; *OL,* simulated high-level Le Fort I osteotomy. *(Modified from You-ZH, Bell WH, Finn RA: Location of the nasolacrimal canal in relation to the high Le Forte I osteotomy, J Oral Maxillofac Surg 50:1075–1080, 1992.)*

23. How many bones form the orbit? Which bones?
    Seven bones form the orbit.
        The **roof** is composed mainly of the orbital plate of the frontal bone. Posteriorly it receives a minor contribution from the lesser wing of the sphenoid.
        The **orbital floor** is composed of the orbital plate of the maxilla, the zygomatic bone anterolaterally, and the orbital process of the palatine bone posteriorly. The orbital floor is equivalent to the roof of the maxillary sinus.
        The **lateral wall** is formed primarily by the orbital surface of the zygomatic bone and the greater wing of the sphenoid bone. The sphenoid portion of the lateral wall is separated from the roof by the superior orbital fissure and from the floor by the inferior orbital fissure.
        The **medial wall** is quadrangular in shape and composed of four bones: (1) the ethmoid bone centrally; (2) the frontal bone superoanteriorly; (3) the lacrimal bone inferoanteriorly; and (4) the sphenoid bone posteriorly. The medial wall is made of a very thin plate, with the largest component being the ethmoidal portion, which is called the lamina papyracea (paperlike).

24. Which is the only bone that exists entirely within the orbital confines?
    The lacrimal bone.

25. Which bone is the keystone of the orbit?
    The sphenoid bone. All neurovascular structures to the orbit pass through this bone.

26. Where is the superior orbital fissure located? Which structures pass through it?
    The superior orbital fissure is a 22-mm cleft that runs outward, forward, and upward from the apex of the orbit. This fissure, which separates the greater and lesser wings of the sphenoid and lies between the optic foramen and the foramen rotundum, provides passage to the three motor nerves

to the extraocular muscles of the orbit—the oculomotor nerve (CN III), trochlear nerve (CN IV), and abducens nerve (CN VI). The ophthalmic division of the trigeminal nerve (CN V1) also enters the orbit through this fissure.

27. **What structures pass through the inferior orbital fissure?**
The inferior orbital fissure, which separates the greater sphenoid wing portion of the lateral wall from the floor, permits passage of (1) the maxillary division of the trigeminal nerve (CN V2) and its branches (including the infraorbital nerve); (2) the infraorbital artery; (3) branches of the sphenopalatine ganglion; and (4) branches of the inferior ophthalmic vein to the pterygoid plexus.

28. **What is Tenon's capsule?**
Tenon's capsule is a fascial structure that subdivides the orbital cavity into two halves: an anterior (or precapsular) segment and a posterior (or retrocapsular) segment. The ocular globe occupies only the anterior half of the orbital cavity. The posterior half of the orbital cavity is filled with fat, muscles, vessels, and nerves that supply the ocular globe and extraocular muscles and provide sensation to the soft tissue surrounding the orbit.

29. **Distinguish between intraconal and extraconal fat. Which is important for globe support?**
The orbital fat can be divided into anterior and posterior portions. The anterior, extraocular fat is largely **extraconal**, which means that it exists outside the muscle cone. Posteriorly, only fine fascial communications separate the extraconal from the intraconal fat compartments. **Intraconal** fat constitutes three-fourths of the fat in the posterior orbit and may be displaced outside the muscle cone, contributing to a loss of globe support from loss of soft tissue volume. The fat on the anterior portion of the orbital floor is extraconal and does not contribute to globe support.

30. **What is the interval between open eyelids called?**
The palpebral fissure (rima).

31. **What is the average height of the inferior and superior tarsi?**
The superior tarsus is 8 to 12 mm; the inferior tarsus is 5 to 7 mm.

32. **What is the autonomic innervation to the lacrimal gland?**
Preganglionic parasympathetic fibers originate at the superior salivatory nucleus and are carried along the facial nerve to reach the sphenopalatine ganglion by the greater petrosal nerve. The postganglionic parasympathetic fibers travel through the zygomatic nerve to reach the lacrimal gland along the lacrimal nerve. Postganglionic sympathetic fibers from the superior cervical sympathetic ganglion travel through the deep petrosal nerve to reach the lacrimal gland in the same fashion as the parasympathetic fibers.

33. **What are the components of the lacrimal drainage system?**
Approximately 12 small ducts under the outer corner of the upper eyelid drain tears onto the conjunctiva. From the superior and inferior puncta at the upper and lower eyelids at the medial canthus, the **lacrimal canaliculi** travel first vertically, then medially and downward (of the superior canaliculi), and finally upward and medially (of the inferior canaliculi) to converge at the **lacrimal sac**. The canaliculi length is approximately 8 mm. Often the canaliculi converge before the lacrimal sac and create a small dilation called the **sinus of Maier**. The lacrimal sac is 12 mm long and is found in the anterior aspect of the medial orbital wall. The **lacrimal crest** is covered by periosteum. The medial palpebral ligament lies anterior and superior to the sac. The lacrimal sac empties into the nasolacrimal duct, which drains into the inferior nasal meatus of the nose.

34. **What is the relationship of the nasolacrimal duct to the nasal cavity and maxillary sinus?**
The nasolacrimal duct lies within the thin, bony wall between the maxillary sinus and the nasal cavity. The duct ends at the inferior nasal meatus through the valve of Hasner. The position of the nasolacrimal duct beneath the inferior turbinate is 11 to 14 mm posterior to the piriform aperture and 11 to 17 mm above the nasal floor (Fig. 23-4).

35. **What are crocodile tears?**
This condition results after injury to the fibers of the facial nerve carrying parasympathetic secretory fibers that normally innervate the salivary gland. The injury causes the fibers to heal in contact with fibers supplying the lacrimal gland, leading to crying when the patient eats.

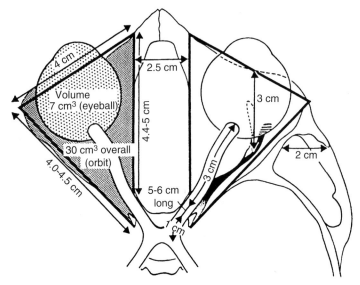

Figure 23-4. Major orbital dimensions and relationships. *(Modified from Ochs M, Buckley M: Anatomy of the orbit,* Oral Maxillofac Surg Clin *5:420, 1993.)*

THE SCALP, FACE, AND TEMPORAL REGION

36. **What are the layers of the scalp?**
    The scalp is made up of five tissue layers, the first three of which are intimately bound together and move as one unit called the scalp proper. The layers are:
    - **S**kin
    - **C**onnective tissue layer
    - **A**poneurosis
    - **L**oose areolar tissue occupying the subgaleal space
    - **P**eriosteum or pericranium

    The aponeurosis is the tendinous sheet that connects the frontalis muscles to the occipitalis posteriorly and auricularis muscles and superficial temporal fascia laterally. Because the aponeurosis layer is the most distinct layer and covers the cranium like a helmet, it is also called the *galea*, which is Latin for helmet.

37. **How does blood supply and nerve supply to the scalp occur?**
    The scalp has a rich network of nerve and blood supply. Both the sensory nerves and the arteries of the scalp run in a radial fashion anterior to posterior, posterior to anterior, and laterally to the midline from both sides. All these vessels and nerves meet at the vertex of the cranium, providing an even richer network of nerves and vessels in this region.

    The **sensory nerves** supplying the cranium are a pair of supratrochlear and supraorbital nerves anteriorly (V1); the greater and third occipital nerves posteriorly (from the cervical); and the zygomaticotemporal (V2), auriculotemporal (V3), and lesser occipital nerves (C2-C3) laterally. The arterial supply consists of the supratrochlear and supraorbital arteries anteriorly (from the internal carotid); the occipital artery posteriorly; and the zygomaticotemporal, superficial temporal, and posterior auricular laterally (all from the external carotid) (Fig. 23-5).

    The **motor nerves** to the muscles of the scalp (frontalis, occipitalis, and auricularis muscles) are supplied by the temporal and posterior auricular branches of the facial nerve.

38. **What is the extension of the galea of the scalp into the temporal region?**
    The musculoaponeurotic layer covering the cranium is made of fascia (galea) in some locations and of muscles (frontalis, occipitals, and auricularis) in others. When this layer reaches the temporal region it is called the *superficial temporal fascia* or the *temporoparietal fascia.*

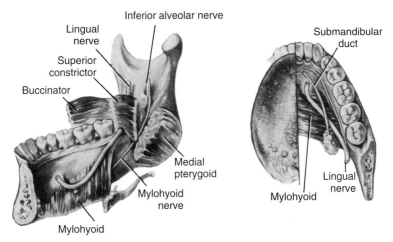

Figure 23-5. The course and relationships of the submandibular gland duct. *(From Sinnatamby CS:* Last's anatomy: regional and applied, *ed 12, Edinburgh, 1999, Churchill Livingstone.)*

39. **What is the extension of the temporoparietal fascia in the face?**
The temporoparietal fascia in the temporal region of the face is confluent with the superficial muscu-loaponeurotic system (SMAS). This system consists of muscles of facial expression in some locations, and in other locations where there are no muscles, it consists of a dense fascial layer.

40. **What are the other fascial layers of the temporal region?**
In the temporal region, the temporalis fascia (the deep temporal fascia) becomes the extension of the pericranium, forming the periosteum covering the skull. In the preauricular region, roughly 2 cm superior to the zygomatic arch, the temporalis fascia splits into two layers (or leaflets): superficial and deep. These fascial layers form a pocket that contains the temporal fat pad. The two layers attach to the zygomatic arch and fuse with its periosteum (Fig. 23-6).

41. **What is the extension of the temporalis fascia below the level of the zygomatic arch?**
The temporalis fascia extends below the zygomatic arch to invest muscles of mastication and adjacent structures, namely the masseter muscle and parotid gland. This layer is called *parotideomas-seteric fascia.*

42. **What is the superficial musculoaponeurotic system (SMAS)?**
The SMAS is a layer of tissue that includes the platysma, risorius, triangularis, and auricularis muscles. Some authors also include the frontalis and the other muscles of facial expression in this tissue layer. The SMAS is connected to the dermis by a dense network of fibrous septae. These septae allow for movement of the overlying skin when the muscles in this tissue layer contract, giving rise to changes in facial expression. The skin can be dissected from the underlying SMAS by transection of these connecting fibrous septa, such as during rhytidectomy. The significance of the SMAS is related to its relationship to the nerves in the face: facial motor nerves deep to it, and sensory nerves more superficial to it (Fig. 23-7).

43. **What are the extensions of the SMAS and parotideomasseteric fascia in the neck?**
In the neck, the extension of the SMAS is the superficial cervical fascia, which is similar to the SMAS in containing the muscle of facial expression of the neck, the *platysma*. This layer is loose in most areas, but is bound firmly to the underlying structures in a few places. The continuation of the parotideomasseteric fascia in the neck is the deep cervical fascia. This fascia also varies in thickness and splits in various sites to enclose the muscles of the neck, the submandibular gland, and the thyroid glands.

44. What is the relationship of the facial nerve to the parotideomasseteric fascia?

    As the facial nerve branches leave the parotid gland, the parotideomasseteric fascia covers them. The SMAS is located superficial to this layer.

45. What is the blood supply to the temporalis muscle and the temporalis fascia?

    The muscle is supplied primarily by the anterior and posterior deep temporal arteries (branches of the internal maxillary artery) and to a lesser extent by the superficial temporal artery.

    The middle temporal artery, a branch of the superficial temporal artery, is the main supply to the fascia.

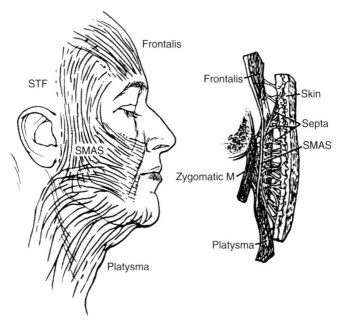

Figure 23-6. Anatomy of the superficial musculoaponeurotic system (SMAS). *STF,* Superficial temporal fascia. *(From Rees TD, Aston SJ, Thorne CHM: Blepharoplasty and fascioplasty. In McCarthy JG, editor:* Plastic surgery, *Philadelphia, 1990, Saunders.)*

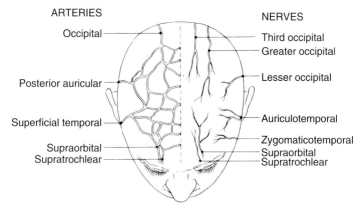

Figure 23-7. Nerve and blood supply of the scalp. *(From Welch TB, Boyne PJ: The management of traumatic scalp injuries: report of cases,* J Oral Maxillofacial Surg *49:1007–1014, 1991.)*

46. **What is the blood supply to the temporal fat pad?**
    The blood supply to the temporal fat pad is from the middle temporal artery, which is a branch of the superficial temporal artery.

47. **What is the function and foramina of the 12 cranial nerves?**
    See Table 23-2.

48. **At what distance from the stylomastoid foramen does the facial nerve bifurcate?**
    The nerve bifurcates into two main trunks (the zygomatico facial and the mandibular cervical) at variable distances after the nerve exits the skull, but on the average this distance is 1.3 cm.

49. **At what distance from the external auditory canal does the facial nerve bifurcate?**
    The point of bifurcation of the facial nerve is located 1.5 to 2.8 cm inferior to the lowest concavity of the bony external auditory canal.

50. **What is the danger zone for the frontal branch of the facial nerve as it crosses the zygomatic arch?**
    The frontal branch of the facial nerve crosses superficial to the zygomatic arch in an area that lies 0.8 to 3.5 cm anterior to the anterior concavity of the bony external auditory canal (an average of 2 cm anterior to the canal). A danger zone for injuring the frontal branch of the facial nerve during surgical

Table 23-2. Cranial Nerve Components, Function, and Foramen of Exit from the Cranium

NERVE	COMPONENTS	FUNCTION	SKULL OPENING
1. Olfactory	Sensory	Smell	Opening in cribriform plate of ethmoid
2. Optic	Sensory	Vision	Optic canal
3. Oculomotor	Motor	Lifts upper eyelid; turns eyeball upward, downward, and medially; constricts pupil; accommodates eye	Superior orbital fissure
4. Trochlear	Motor	Assists in turning eyeball downward and laterally	Superior orbital fissure
5. Trigeminal			
• Ophthalmic division	Sensory	Cornea, skin of forehead, scalp, eyelids, and nose; also mucous membrane of paranasal sinuses and nasal cavity	Superior orbital fissure
• Maxillary division	Sensory	Skin of face over maxilla and the upper lip; teeth of upper jaw; mucous membrane of nose, the maxillary air sinus, and palate	Foramen rotundum
• Mandibular division	Motor	Muscles of mastication, mylohyoid, anterior belly of digastric, tensor veli palatini, and tensor tympani	Foramen ovale
	Sensory	Skin of cheek, skin over mandible, lower lip, and side of head; teeth of lower jaw and temporomandibular joint; mucous membrane of mouth and anterior two-thirds of tongue	
6. Abducent	Motor	Lateral rectus muscle; turns eyeball laterally	Superior orbital fissure

Continued on following page

Table 23-2. Cranial Nerve Components, Function, and Foramen of Exit from the Cranium—*(continued)*

NERVE	COMPONENTS	FUNCTION	SKULL OPENING
7. Facial	Motor	Muscles of face, the cheek, and scalp; stapedius muscle of middle ear; stylohyoid; posterior belly of digastric	Internal acoustic meatus, facial canal, stylomastoid foramen
	Sensory	Taste from anterior two-thirds of tongue; floor of mouth and palate	
	Secretomotor parasympathetic	Submandibular and sublingual salivary glands, the lacrimal gland, and glands of nose and palate	
8. Vestibulocochlear			
• Vestibular	Sensory	Position and movement of head	Internal acoustic meatus
• Cochlear	Sensory	Hearing	
9. Glossopharyngeal assists swallowing	Motor	Stylopharyngeus muscle:	
	Secretomotor parasympathetic	Parotid salivary gland	Jugular foramen
	Sensory	General sensation and taste from posterior third of tongue and pharynx; carotid sinus and carotid body	
10. Vagus	Motor	Constrictor muscles of pharynx and intrinsic muscles of larynx; involuntary muscles of trachea and bronchi, heart, and alimentary tract from pharynx to splenic flexure of colon; liver and pancreas	Jugular foramen
	Sensory	Taste from epiglottis and valecula and afferent fibers from structures named above	
11. Accessory			
• Cranial root	Motor	Muscles of soft palate, pharynx, and larynx	Jugular foramen
• Spinal root	Motor	Sternocleidomastoid and trapezius muscles	
12. Hypoglossal	Motor	Muscles of tongue controlling its shape and movement (except palatoglossus)	Hypoglossal canal

Adapted from Snell RS: *Clinical anatomy for medical students,* ed 5, Boston, 1996, Little, Brown.

procedures in the temporal and preauricular regions is located between two parallel lines drawn in the temporal region. The anterior line is drawn from the inferior attachment of the earlobe to the most lateral extension of the eyebrow. The posterior line is drawn from a midpoint on the tragus of the ear to the most superior forehead crease of the forehead, or at least 2 cm from the first line or 2 cm above the supraorbital regions.

51. **What is the danger zone for the marginal mandibular branch of the facial nerve?**
The mandibular branch of the facial nerve courses in an area where incisions to approach the mandible and mandibular condyle are commonly placed. Accordingly, this area is considered a danger zone for injury to this branch. The zone is located between the inferior border of the mandible and a line in the retromandibular and submandibular region. This line extends from anterior to posterior and is 2 cm (1 thumb-breadth) behind the gonion and posterior border of the ascending ramus, 2 cm below the gonion, extending forward 2 cm below the inferior border of the mandible as far anteriorly to the level of the second premolar tooth. The anterior border of the zone is located at the intersection of two lines: a horizontal line 2 cm below and parallel to the inferior border of the body of the mandible, and another along the long axis of the lower second premolar.

52. **How can the main trunk of the facial nerve be located during a parotidectomy?**
As the facial nerve trunk travels from the stylomastoid foramen to the parotid gland, it passes anterior to the posterior belly of the digastric muscle, lateral to the styloid process and the external carotid artery, and posterior to the facial vein. Start a parotidectomy by mobilizing the tail of the parotid superiorly and retracting the anterior border of the sternocleidomastoid laterally, to identify the posterior belly of the digastric muscle. Follow this muscle superiorly toward its insertion at the mastoid tip. After bluntly separating the parotid from its attachment to the cartilage of the external auditory canal, the **tragal pointer** (outer surface of the external auditory cartilage) comes into view. The facial nerve trunk lies approximately 1 cm deep and slightly anteroinferior to the tragal pointer.

53. **What are the branches of the facial nerve?**
The facial nerve trunk has six major branches: temporal, zygomatic, buccal, mandibular, cervical, and auricular. The auricular branch comes off before the facial nerve turns into the parotid body, and innervates the superior auricular, posterior auricular, and occipitalis muscles, as well as provides sensation to the area behind the earlobe. Within the parotid, the facial nerve divides into two main branches, the temporofacial and cervicofacial, which further divide into the temporal, zygomatic, buccal, mandibular, and cervical branches. The stylohyoid and posterior digastric are other minor branches of the nerve.

54. **How do the facial muscles of expression receive their innervation?**
All facial muscles except the mentalis, levator angularis superioris, and buccinator receive their innervation along their deep surfaces. However, because these three muscles are located deep within the facial soft tissue and lie deep to the plane of the facial nerve, they receive their innervation along their superficial surfaces. All other facial muscles of expression are located superficial to the plane of the facial nerve and thus receive their innervation along their deep or posterior surfaces. For example, the platysma, orbicularis oculi, and zygomaticus major and minor are situated superficial to the level of the facial nerve.

55. **What is the relationship of the frontal branch of the facial nerve to the SMAS and temporoparietal fascia?**
Inferior to the zygomatic arch, the frontal branch of the facial nerve travels deep to the SMAS. As it crosses over the zygomatic arch it becomes very superficial. At this point, it is sandwiched between the periosteum (extension of the temporal fascia) and the temporoparietal fascia (extension of the SMAS). Superior to the zygomatic arch, the frontal branch of the facial nerve travels within or on the undersurface of the temporoparietal fascia, but superficial to the outer layer of the temporal fascia.

56. **How do the frontal and mandibular branches of the facial nerve differ from other facial branches?**
Crossover communication between the frontal branch and adjacent branches and between the mandibular branch and adjacent branches is only about 15%. Crossover among the other branches is approximately 70%. Injury to either the frontal or mandibular branches leads to more marked deficit compared with the results of injury to the other branches.

57. **What is the relationship of the frontal and mandibular branch courses of the facial nerve?**
The frontal branch of the facial nerve crosses the zygomatic arch deep to the SMAS and in the temporal region deep to the temporoparietal fascia (superficial temporal fascia). The nerve usually lies within 2 cm from the lateral border of the eyebrow and enters the frontalis muscle from its deep surface.

The mandibular branch courses within 2 cm of the inferior border of the mandible, posterior to the facial artery. The mandibular branch is at risk during an anterior dissection because in this area, it becomes more superficial. It lies deep to the platysma and superficial to the facial artery.

58. **How do you evaluate the five branches of the facial nerve during a physical exam?**

    Test each of the five branches of the nerve in the following manner:
    - Cervical: Contract the platysma muscles.
    - Marginal mandibular: Whistle or pucker the lips.
    - Buccal: Smile or show teeth.
    - Zygomatic: Squeeze eyes shut tightly.
    - Temporal: Raise eyebrows.

59. **What are the most common causes of facial nerve paralysis?**

    Facial nerve paralysis, which may be unilateral or bilateral, can be a manifestation of any of several disease processes. These diseases can be idiopathic, neoplastic, traumatic, infectious, or congenital. The paralysis can also result from a systemic/metabolic process (Box 23-1).

60. **What is the anatomy of taste sensory function?**

    Taste sensory function from the anterior part of the tongue is carried along the chorda tympani of the trigeminal nerve through the submandibular ganglion to reach the facial nerve. From the posterior or pharyngeal part of the tongue, taste sensation is carried along the glossopharyngeal nerve, through the pterygopalatine ganglion, to the major petrosal nerve, and then the facial nerve. From the palatal region, the sensation is carried via the palatine nerves, which also pass through the pterygopalatine ganglion to ultimately reach the facial nerve.

    Along with the facial nerve, taste fibers reach the tractus solitarius, which is concerned with visceral function, including taste. Some textbooks state that taste fibers from the posterior part of the tongue reach the tractus solitarius directly by the glossopharyngeal nerve.

61. **What is the anatomy of the zygoma?**

    The zygoma is a pyramidal bone of the midface. Its anterior convexity gives prominence to the malar eminence of the cheek, and its posterior concavity contributes to the shape of the temporal fossa. The zygoma forms the superolateral and superoanterior portions of the maxillary sinus. It articulates with

---

Box 23-1. Causes of Facial Nerve Paralysis

Idiopathic
- Bell's palsy
- Recurrent facial palsy
- Melkersson-Rosenthal syndrome

Neoplasia
- Cholesteatoma
- Facial neuroma
- Glomus jugulare or tympanicum
- Carcinoma (primary or metastatic)
- Schwannoma of lower cranial nerves
- Meningioma
- Histiocytosis
- Rhabdomyosarcoma
- Leukemia

Trauma
- Temporal bone fractures*
- Birth trauma
- Facial contusions/lacerations
- Penetrating wounds to face and temporal bone
- Iatrogenic injury

Infection
- Herpes zoster oticus (Ramsay-Hunt syndrome)
- Otitis media with effusion
- Acute suppurative otitis media
- Coalescent mastoiditis
- Chronic otitis media
- Malignant otitis externa (*Pseudomonas* osteomyelitis)
- Tuberculosis
- Lyme disease*
- AIDS
- Infectious mononucleosis

Congenital
- Compression injury
- Moebius syndrome*
- Lower lip paralysis

Metabolic and Systemic
- Pregnancy
- Diabetes mellitus
- Sarcoidosis*
- Guillain-Barré syndrome*
- Autoimmune disorders

*May present as bilateral facial paralysis.

Modified from Coker NJ: Acute paralysis of the facial nerve. In Bailey BJ, editor: *Head and neck surgery—otolaryngology*, Philadelphia, 1993, J.B. Lippincott.

the frontal, temporal, maxillary, and sphenoid bones. Superolaterally, the frontal process of the zygoma articulates with the zygomatic process of the frontal bone and forms the lateral orbital wall along with its intraorbital articulation with the sphenoid bone. The temporal process of the zygoma articulates posterolaterally with the zygomatic process of the temporal bone to make the zygomatic arch. The broad articulation inferiorly and medially with the maxilla forms the infraorbital rim and lateral part of the orbital floor. Superiorly and inferiorly, such articulation forms the zygomaticomaxillary buttress, the major buttressing structure between the midface and the cranium.

62. With which bones does the zygoma articulate?
Greater wing of the sphenoid and frontal, temporal, and maxillary bones.

THE NECK

63. What are the contents of the carotid sheath?
The carotid sheath contains the carotid artery, the jugular vein, and the vagus nerve. Within the carotid sheath, the vagus nerve (CN X) lies posterior to the common carotid artery and internal jugular vein.

64. How many branches does the external carotid artery give off? What are they?
The external carotid artery branches from the common carotid artery at the level of the upper border of the thyroid cartilage to be the principal artery supplying the anterior aspect of the neck, face, scalp, oral and nasal cavities, bones of the skull, and dura mater. Note that the orbit and its contents are the only structures that are not supplied by the external carotid. There are eight branches (order of appearance from inferior to superior): (1) the superior thyroid, (2) the ascending pharyngeal, (3) the lingual, (4) the facial, (5) the occipital, (6) the posterior auricular, (7) the internal maxillary, and (8) the superficial temporal.

65. What are the sources for the blood and nerve supply to the sternocleidomastoid muscle (SCM)?
The blood supply to the SCM is provided from two sources. The superior thyroid artery supplies the middle third of the muscle, whereas the occipital artery branches supply the remainder of the muscle. The nerve supply is from the spinal accessory (cranial nerve [CN] XI) and from C2 and C3.

66. What is the course of the facial artery in the submandibular triangle?
The facial artery passes from behind and medial to the submandibular gland, up and over the gland, to emerge from the submandibular space laterally. It then proceeds into the face at the level of the anterior border of the masseter muscle. Thus the facial artery may or may not be encountered in the incision and removal of the gland, and therefore may not require removal, but would have to be located during dissection by pinpointing the two lymph nodes, which overlie it at the level of the inferior border of the mandible.

Superior and deep to these lymph nodes is the marginal mandibular branch of the facial nerve. Posterior to the nodes is the facial vein. Because the vein is lateral to the gland, it is often necessary to ligate and cut this vessel during the dissection to remove the gland.

67. What is the relationship of the lingual nerve to Wharton's duct?
The submandibular gland, or Wharton's duct, is about 5 cm in length, and its lumen is 2 to 4 mm in diameter. It runs anteriorly above the mylohyoid muscle and on the lateral surface of the hyoglossus and genioglossus muscles. At first, the duct lies below the lingual nerve. Then, as the lingual nerve descends, it crosses lateral to the duct. As the duct and lingual nerve pass below the sublingual gland, the lingual nerve passes below the duct and crosses it medially. As the nerve continues toward the genioglossus, the duct continues anteriorly and medially. The duct loops from below upward beneath the lingual nerve at the level of the third molar and then crosses above the lingual nerve at about the level of the second molar. Thus, the nerve loops almost completely around the duct (Fig. 23-8).

68. What are the relationships and the course of the hypoglossal nerves in the sub-mandibular triangle?
The hypoglossal nerve emerges from the hypoglossal canal and passes laterally between the internal jugular vein and the internal and external carotid arteries. It then descends steeply and crosses the stylohyoid and posterior belly of the digastric muscles on their medial surfaces. The hypoglossal nerve courses forward and upward on the lateral surface of the hyoglossus muscle and is accompanied by branches of the sublingual vein entering the oral cavity at the posterior border of the mylohyoid

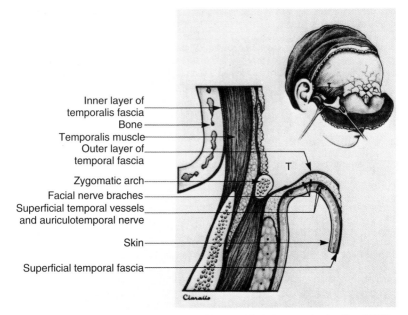

Inner layer of temporalis fascia
Bone
Temporalis muscle
Outer layer of temporal fascia
Zygomatic arch
Facial nerve braches
Superficial temporal vessels and auriculotemporal nerve
Skin
Superficial temporal fascia

T

Figure 23-8. Cross-section showing the level of dissection of the coronal flap in the temporal region. *(From Bell WH: Modern practice in orthognathic and reconstructive surgery, vol 2, Philadelphia, 1992, Saunders.)*

muscle, slightly above the digastric tendon. Here, beneath the tongue, the nerve curves forward and upward on the lateral surface of the genioglossus muscle, splitting into several branches that go into the substance of the tongue. These branches supply all extrinsic and intrinsic muscles of the tongue except the palatoglossus, which is supplied by CN XI via CN X.

69. **What are the boundaries and significance of Lesser's triangle?**
   The triangle is made up by the angle between the tendon of the digastric muscle inferiorly, the hypoglossal nerve superiorly, and the posterior border of the mylohyoid muscle. The hyoglossal and mylohyoid muscles form the floor of this triangle. This triangle is useful in localization and ligation of the artery that lies at the inner surface (beneath) of the hyoglossus muscle deep to the floor of the triangle.

THE MUSCLES OF MASTICATION AND TEMPOROMANDIBULAR JOINT

70. **What are the muscles of mastication?**
   The muscles of mastication can be divided into two groups: primary muscles of mastication and accessory muscles of mastication. Primary muscles of mastication include the temporalis, masseter, and pterygoideus (medial and lateral). Accessory muscles of mastication include the suprahyoid group, infrahyoid group, and platysma. The suprahyoid group includes the digastric, mylohyoid, geniohyoid, and stylohyoid muscles. The infrahyoid group includes the sternohyoid, thyrohyoid, and omohyoid.

71. **How do these muscles act to perform the function of mastication?**
   The muscles of mastication act most of the time as a group during functional movement of the jaw. For example, jaw closing is a coordinated function of the elevator muscles, which are the masseter, medial pterygoid, and temporalis muscles. The jaw closing is a function of the lateral pterygoid and the suprahyoid muscles. The protrusion is a function of the masseter, medial pterygoid, and lateral pterygoid muscles, whereas retrusion is a function of the digastric and temporalis muscles. The infrahyoid

muscles help in the opening of the mouth by fixing the hyoid bone as a stable structure so when the suprahyoid muscles contract, they are able to participate in depressing the anterior portion of the mandible, thus opening the mouth.

72. **What is the origin and insertion of each of the muscles of mastication?**
With few exceptions, for a skeletal muscle to perform its function, it must originate from a fixed structure in the skeleton and insert into another, mobile part. This rule applies to all muscles of mastication, except for the suprahyoid muscle group (as described previously).

MASSETER

Origin: superficial belly from the lower border of the zygomatic arch and the zygomatic process of the maxilla. The deep belly from the posterior third and medial surface of the inferior border of the zygomatic arch.
Insertion: the angle and inferior half of the lateral surface of the ramus of the mandible. The deep portion (belly) of the muscle inserts onto the lateral surface of the coronoid process and superior half of the ramus.

MEDIAL PTERYGOID

Origin: medial surface of the lateral pterygoid plate and pyramidal process of the palatine bone. A small belly of the muscle arises from the lateral surface of the pyramidal process and tuberosity of the maxilla.
Insertion: inferior and posterior part of the medial surface of the ramus and angle of the mandible.

TEMPORALIS

Origin: the temporal fossa of the temporal bone.
Insertion: medial surface, apex, and anterior border of the coronoid process of the mandible.

LATERAL PTERYGOID

Origin: the superior belly arises from the inferior part of the lateral surface of the greater wing of the sphenoid and from the infratemporal fossa. The inferior belly arises from the lateral surface of the lateral pterygoid plate.
Insertion: the superior belly inserts into the anterior margin of the articular disc. The inferior belly inserts into a depression on the anterior portion of the neck of the condyle.

DIGASTRIC

Origin: digastric fossa of the medial side of the lower border of the mandible close to the symphysis. The posterior belly of the muscle arises from the mastoid notch of the temporal bone. Both bellies are united by an intermediate tendon that is connected to the hyoid bone by a loop of fibrous tissue.
The other suprahyoid muscle group originates from different parts of the medial surface of the mandible and inserts into the hyoid bone. The exception is the stylohyoid muscle, which arises from the temporal bone and inserts on the body of the hyoid bone.
Of note is that the origin and insertion of the suprahyoid group (except stylohyoid muscle) are from a mobile origin and insertion. However, because the infrahyoid muscle group functions to stabilize the hyoid bone during mastication, this bone becomes static, allowing the mandible to move when the suprahyoid muscles contract. Inversely, during swallowing, the suprahyoid muscles stabilize the hyoid bone, allowing for swallowing action to be completed with the contraction of the infrahyoid muscles.

73. **How many origins and insertions does each masticatory muscle have?**
For each muscle of mastication, there are two insertions and two origins.

74. **What is the function of the lateral pterygoid muscle?**
The lateral pterygoid muscle is triangular in shape and runs in a slightly inferior and posterior horizontal direction. The muscle has superior and inferior heads. The **superior head** arises from the infratemporal surface of the greater wing of the sphenoid and inserts into the articular capsule and disc. The function of the superior head is to stabilize the condyle and disc during closing movement.
The **inferior head** originates from the lateral surface of the lateral pterygoid plate and inserts into the pterygoid fovea of the neck of the condyle. The inferior head aids in translation of the condyle over the articular eminence during opening of the mouth.

75. **Which muscles make up the pterygomandibular raphe?**
The buccinator muscle anteriorly and the superior constrictor of the pharynx posteriorly make up the pterygomandibular raphe.

76. What are the muscles of the soft palate?

The soft palate is formed by three pair of muscles, all of which fuse at the midline: the uvulus muscle, which runs along the uvula on each side of the midline forming almost one muscle; the levator palatine muscle extending across the midline and forming an arch-shape configuration within the soft palate; and the tensor veli palatine, which loops around the hamulus fusing with the tensor muscle of the opposite side and forming an aponeurosis at the midline.

77. What class of joint is the temporomandibular joint?

The temporomandibular joint is classified as a diarthrodial joint. It has both features of diarthrodial joints which are ginglymus (hinge) and arthrodia (gliding) types. The articular surfaces of the fossa and the condyle are covered by nonvascular fibrous tissue that contains some cartilage cells, designated as fibrocartilage. Because of the incongruity between the articular surfaces of the joint (the mandibular condyle and the glenoid fossa and articular eminence), the joint is subdivided into an upper and lower compartments by a fibrous oval articular disc, the meniscus.

78. What are the sources of the blood and nerve supply to the temporomandibular joint (TMJ)?

The major arterial supply to the TMJ is derived from the superficial temporal artery and from the maxillary artery posteriorly, and from smaller masseteric, posterior deep temporal, and lateral pterygoid arteries anteriorly. The venous drainage is through a diffuse plexus around the capsule and rich venous channels that drain the retrodiscal tissue.

The nerve supply is from the auriculotemporal nerve, which provides the principal sensory innervation to the TMJ. The nerve gives off two or three branches, which enter the capsule inferiorly, medially, and laterally. The masseteric nerve also innervates the capsule from the frontal and medial sides of the joint. The posterior deep temporal nerve supplies the TMJ laterally and anteriorly.

SURGICAL ANATOMY

79. What is the retromandibular approach?

This approach is useful for procedures involving the ramus and areas on or near the condylar neck/head. The incision begins 0.5 cm below the earlobe and continues 3.0 to 3.5 cm inferiorly, approximately 2 cm posterior to the ramus. In some patients, this may limit the direct proximity of the skin incision to the mandible, which is one of the main advantages of this technique. Accordingly, some surgeons recommend placement of the incision more anteriorly at the posterior ramus, just below the earlobe. The deeper dissection of this approach is carried out bluntly through the parotid gland in an anteromedial direction (in the anticipated direction of the facial nerve) toward the posterior border of the mandible. The facial nerve, if identified, is avoided and deeper dissection is continued until the pterygomasseteric sling is identified and incised. The submasseteric dissection is continued to expose the ramus and condyle as needed.

80. Where should the skin incision be placed during a submandibular approach to avoid the mandibular branch of the facial nerve?

The submandibular approach is often referred to as the Risdon approach. It may be used to access the mandibular angle, ramus, condyle, inferior border of the mandibular body, and submandibular gland. The exact location of the skin incision differs, mostly due to the disagreement over the course of the marginal mandibular branch of the facial nerve.

Dingman and Grabb showed, in 192 patients, that this branch is below the inferior border of the mandible, posterior to where the nerve crosses the facial artery. Anterior to that point, the facial nerve is above the inferior border in 100% of patients. In another study, Ziarah and Atkinson found that in 53% of patients the marginal mandible of the facial nerve is below the inferior border of the mandible, posterior to the facial vessels, and in 6% this nerve continues to be below the inferior border anterior to the facial vessels.

Based on these findings, and to err well on the safe side, the recommended placement of the submandibular incision is 1.5 to 2.0 cm (a thumb-breadth) below the inferior border of the mandible.

81. In a patient with a 3-cm vertical laceration of the anterior border of the masseter muscle, what findings are likely?

In such an injury there is a likelihood for paralysis of the frontalis, orbicularis oculi, nasalis muscles, and orbicularis oris. The paralysis of these muscles is due to severance of the frontal, zygomatic, and buccal branches of the facial nerve, respectively. The parotid duct and the parotid gland may also be involved.

82. **What are the structures involved in resection of the mandible from midramus to the mental foramen?**

Composite resection of the body of the mandible usually involves removal of bone, muscles, glands, lymph nodes, and vessels. The muscles involved are the masseter, medial pterygoid, platysma, mylohyoid, buccinator, depressor anguli oris, depressor labii inferioris, superior pharyngeal constrictor, and a small portion of the temporalis. The submandibular gland, sublingual glands, and submandibular lymph nodes surrounding superficial and deep cervical nodes also are removed, depending on the extent of the resection. The facial artery, anterior facial vein, and marginal mandibular branch of the facial nerve also are occasionally removed.

BIBLIOGRAPHY

Abbey SH: Facial nerve disorders. In Jafek BW, Stark AK, editors: *ENT secrets*, Philadelphia, 1996, Hanley & Belfus.

Abubaker AO, Sotereanos GC, Patterson GT: Use of bicoronal approach to treatment of craniofacial fractures, *J Oral Maxillofacial Surg* 48:579–586, 1990.

Anderson JE, editor: *Grant's atlas of anatomy*, Baltimore, 1983, Williams & Wilkins.

Coker NJ: Acute paralysis of the facial nerve. In Bailey BJ, editor: *Head and neck surgery—otolaryngology*, Philadelphia, 1993, J.B. Lippincott.

Cummings CW, Haughey B, Thomas R, et al.: *Otolaryngology: head and neck surgery*, ed 4, St Louis, 2005, Mosby.

Demas PN, Sotereanos GC: Incidence of nasolacrimal injury and turbinectomy-associated atrophic rhinitis with Le Fort I osteotomies, *J Craniomaxillofac Surg* 17:116–118, 1989.

Dingman RO, Grabb WC: Surgical anatomy of the mandibular ramus of the facial nerve, based on the dissection of 100 facial halves, *Plast Reconstr Surg* 29:266–272, 1962.

Ellis E, Zide M: *Surgical approaches to the facial skeleton*, Baltimore, 1984, Williams & Wilkins.

Ermshar Jr CB: Anatomy and neuroanatomy. In Morgan DH, Hall WP, Vamvas SJ, editors: *Diseases of the temporomandibular joint: a multidisciplinary approach*, St Louis, 1977, Mosby.

Frick H, Leanhardt H, Starck D: "The Eye and the Orbit." Human Anatomy. Viscera and Nervous System, Classification of Muscles and Vessels, Organization of Lymphatics and Nerves. 4th ed. Vol. 2. Stuttgart: Georg Thieme, 1991.

Haller J: Trauma to the salivary glands, *Otolaryngol Clin North Am* 32:907–917, 1999.

Hollinstead H: *Anatomy for surgeons: the head and neck*, ed 3, Philadelphia, 1982, Harper & Row.

Last J: Head and neck. In Last J, editor: *Anatomy: regional and applied*, ed 6, New York, 1978, Churchill Livingstone.

Long CD, Granick MS: Head and neck embryology and anatomy. In Weinzweig J, editor: *Plastic surgery secrets*, Philadelphia, 1996, Hanley & Belfus.

Moore KL: *Clinically oriented anatomy*, ed 2, Baltimore, 1984, Williams & Wilkins.

Ochs M, Buckley M: Anatomy of the orbit, *Oral Maxillofac Surg Clin* 5:419–430, 1993.

Pansky B: The facial (VII) nerve. In Pansky B, editor: *Review of gross anatomy*, New York, 1984, Macmillan.

Patrick GH, Bevivino JR: Fractures of the zygoma. In Weinzweig J, editor: *Plastic surgery secrets*, Philadelphia, 1999, Hanley & Belfus.

Pitanguy I, Ramus A: The frontal branch of the facial nerve: the importance of its variation in face lifting, *Plast Reconstr Surg* 38:352–356, 1966.

Rees TD, Aston SJ, Thorne CHM: Blepharoplasty and facioplasty. In McCarthy JG, editor: *Plastic surgery*, Philadelphia, 1990, Saunders.

Schow RS, Miloro M: Diagnosis and management of salivary gland disorders. In Peterson LJ, Ellis 3rd E, Hupp JR, et al.: *Contemporary oral and maxillofacial surgery*, ed 3, St Louis, 1998, Mosby.

Schwember G, Rodriguez A: Anatomic dissection of the extraparotid portion of the facial nerve, *Plast Reconstruct Surg* 81:183–188, 1988.

Sinha U, Ng M: Surgery of the salivary glands, *Otolaryngol Clin North Am* 32:888–905, 1999.

Snell RS: Head and neck anatomy. In Snell RS, editor: *Clinical anatomy for medical students*, ed 5, Boston, 1995, Little, Brown.

Stuzin JM, Wagstrom L, Kawamoto HK, et al.: Anatomy of the frontal branch of the facial nerve: the significance of temporal fat pad, *Plast Reconstr Surg* 83:265–271, 1989.

Weinzweig J, Bartlett SP: Fractures of the orbit. In Weinzweig J, editor: *Plastic surgery secrets*, Philadelphia, 1999, Hanley & Belfus.

You ZH, Bell WH, Finn RA: Location of the nasolacrimal canal in relation to the high Le Fort osteotomy, *J Oral Maxillofac Surg* 50:1075–1080, 1992.

Ziarah HA, Atkinson ME: The surgical anatomy of the mandibular distribution of the facial nerve, *Br J Oral Surg* 19:159–170, 1981.

CHAPTER 24

WOUND HEALING

Din Lam

1. **What are the three phrases of wound healing?**
   1. Inflammatory phase
   2. Proliferative phase
   3. Remodeling phase

2. **What events occur during each phase of wound healing?**
   The inflammatory phase begins at the time of wounding and lasts for 24 to 48 hours. At this stage, platelets release growth factors to attach macrophages and neutrophils to the healing site. The goal for this stage is to remove debris, necrotic tissue, and bacteria from the wound. By day 3, the proliferative phase begins, and at this point, fibroblasts start to produce collagen in a random fashion. This is when the wound starts to gain its initial strength. Moreover, it is also at this stage that angiogenesis begins at the healing site. At the last stage—the remodeling phase—randomly aligned collagen will be replaced by organized collagen that provides stronger strength to the site. This last stage occurs 2 to 3 weeks after wounding and can last for more than a year.

3. **What role do macrophages play in wound healing?**
   Macrophages play a critical role in removing debris and bacteria and, most importantly, secrete growth factors that promote collagen formation by fibroblasts.

4. **What roles do the growth factors PDGF and TGF-β play in wound healing?**
   Platelet Derived Growth Factor (PDGF) is released by platelets during formation of initial thrombus. It is a chemoattractant for macrophages, which are responsible for orchestrating events of healing. Transforming Growth Factor-Beta (TGF-β) is secreted by macrophages, is a chemoattractant for fibroblasts, and stimulates formation of extracellular matrix by fibroblasts.

5. **How does the collagen pattern change during wound healing?**
   During the remodeling phase, fibroblasts and macrophages replace the initial, randomly laid collagen with collagen that is cross-linked and oriented in a more orderly arrangement to the direction of mechanical stress. This new pattern of collagen formation is a lot stronger than those found in initial, randomly laid collagen.

6. **A well-healed wound eventually reaches what percentage of pre-wound strength?**
   In general, well-healed wounds can reach 70% to 80% of prewound strength.

7. **Is collagen makeup different in normal versus newly healing wounds?**
   Type I collagen is the most abundant type of collagen in normal dermis. Type II collagen is the most abundant collagen during the early phase of wound healing. By week 2 of the wound healing process, type III collagen becomes the principal collagen produced by fibroblast until at the remodeling phase, at which type I collagen is replacing type II collagen to restore the normal tissue profile.

8. **What effect does radiation have on wound healing?**
   Radiation causes endothelial cell, capillary, and arteriole damage, which results in progressive and cumulative loss of blood vessels in the affected area. Perfusion to the radiated tissue may be affected, leading to delayed healing. Radiated fibroblasts show decreased proliferation and collagen synthesis, leading to diminished deposition of extracellular matrix. The lymphatic system may also be damaged and lead to prolonged edema and poor clearance of infection in the healing process.

9. **What factors commonly impair wound healing?**
   Nutritional deficiencies, aging, infection, hypoxia, steroids, smoking, diabetes, and radiation.

10. **Why does edema impair wound healing?**
    In normal tissue, cells are in close proximity to the vessels where oxygen and nutrients are diffused to the cells. Edema impairs wound healing by (1) increasing the distance between cells and vessels

that indirectly impair the diffusion process, (2) chronic edema may result in protein deposition in the extracellular matrix, which can act as a diffusion barrier for growth factors and nutrients, and (3) growth factors and nutrients are relatively diluted in the edematous fluid.

11. **What is the mechanism of wound contraction?**
The wound heals by wound contraction, reepithelialization, and scarring. As an integral part of wound healing, myofibroblasts orient themselves along lines of tension and pull collagen fibers together. Scar contracture is an abnormal shortening and thickening of a scar that may cause function or cosmetic deformities.

12. **How much bacteria is needed to cause wound infection?**
A wound with bacterial counts greater than 10^5 organisms per gram of tissue is considered infected and unlikely to heal without further treatment.

13. **What factors are responsible for local wound ischemia?**
Smoking, radiation, edema, diabetes, and peripheral occlusive disease can affect the perfusion and oxygenation of a wound and cause local wound ischemia.

14. **What are the benefits of occlusive dressings?**
Occlusive dressings maintain a moist environment that promotes rapid reepithelization and more effective wound healing than when the wound is allowed to dry out.

15. **What causes hypertrophic/keloid scars? What treatment options are available?**
Excessive inflammatory response during healing is most likely the cause of hypertrophic/keloid scars. No definitive treatment option is available for both. In most cases, multimodal therapies, including intralesional steroid injection, surgical resection, and occlusive dressing are needed to decrease the appearance of the hypertrophic/keloid scars.

16. **What features distinguish between a keloid and hypertrophic scar?**
Keloids usually extend beyond the original incision and become progressively larger. Hypertrophic scars are elevated but do not extend outside the original borders of the wound. Keloids are more common in people with dark skin, whereas hypertrophic scars occur more often in fair-skinned people.

17. **Which layer of a wound repair contributes the most to wound strength?**
The dermal layer contributes the most strength in wound healing. Sutures with prolonged tensile strength should be used to close this layer. Sutures placed in the epidermis that permit fine alignment of the skin edges should be removed within 5 days.

18. **What is the role of immobilization in wound healing?**
By immobilizing the wound, tension across the skin edges is eliminated, yielding a more favorable scar. Immobilization can be achieved by using Steri-Strip and tapes.

19. **What influences the permanent appearance of suture marks?**
- Length of time that skin suture remains in place
- Tension on the wound edges
- Region of the body
- Presence of infection
- Tendency for hypertrophic scarring or keloid formation

20. **How does vacuum-assisted closure help in the wound healing process?**
The application of negative pressure in vacuum-assisted closure removes edema fluid from the wound through suction. This results in increased blood flow to the wound (by causing the blood vessels to dilate) and greater cell proliferation. Another important benefit of fluid removal is the reduction in bacterial colonization of the wound, which decreases the risk of wound infections. Through these effects, vacuum-assisted closure enhances the formation of granulation tissue, an important factor in wound healing and closure.

CHAPTER 25

DENTOALVEOLAR SURGERY AND PREPROSTHETIC SURGERY

Dean M. DeLuke, Vincent J. Perciaccante, James A. Giglio

DENTOALVEOLAR SURGERY

1. **Why is it necessary to use a bite block when removing mandibular teeth?**
   To diminish pressure on the contralateral temporomandibular joint (TMJ).

2. **Why is distilled water not used for irrigation?**
   Distilled water is a hypotonic solution and will enter cells down the osmotic gradient, causing cell lysis and rapid death of bone cells.

3. **Why is buccal to lingual movement not efficient when removing mandibular posterior teeth?**
   Mandibular bone is too dense and does not expand in a fashion similar to that of the maxillary bone.

4. **What anatomic structure can interfere with efficient removal of a maxillary first molar?**
   Root of the zygoma.

5. **What anatomic layers are penetrated or contacted when performing an inferior alveolar nerve block?**
   Mucosa, buccinator muscle, pterygomandibular space, and periosteum.

6. **What muscles insert on the pterygomandibular raphe?**
   The buccinator muscle and the superior pharyngeal constrictor muscle.

7. **What two structures form a V-shaped landmark for an inferior alveolar nerve block?**
   Deep tendon of the temporalis muscle and the superior pharyngeal constrictor.

8. **What is the orthodontic indication for removal of an impacted third molar?**
   To facilitate distal movement of the second molar.

9. **What is the "shift rule" (also called Clark's Rule) as applied to impacted maxillary cuspids?**
   This radiographic technique determines the position of the impacted cuspid. A series of periapical radiographs are made. The film position is kept constant, but the head of the X-ray unit is moved either anteriorly or posteriorly after each exposure. If the impacted tooth seems to move with the X-ray head, it is located on the palate. If it moves opposite to the unit head, it will be found on the buccal. This is also referred to as the SLOB rule: same lingual (palate), opposite buccal.

10. **What is the advantage of an apically positioned mucoperiosteal flap for exposure of a buccally positioned impacted cuspid?**
    This flap design allows for the impacted tooth to erupt into attached mucosa and minimizes the possible development of periodontal defects and pocket formation.

11. **Where is the inferior alveolar nerve most often located in relation to the roots of a mandibular third molar?**
    Buccal to the roots, and slightly apical.

12. **The root of which tooth is most often dislodged into the maxillary sinus during an extraction procedure?**
    Palatal root of the maxillary first molar.

13. While trying to remove a root tip of a mandibular third molar, it disappears from view. Where might it be dislodged?
    - Inferior alveolar canal
    - Cancellous bone space
    - Submandibular space

14. What is the usually recommended sequence for extractions?
    Maxillary teeth before mandibular teeth, and posterior teeth before anterior teeth.

15. What complications are associated with the removal of a freestanding, isolated maxillary molar?
    Alveolar process fracture and fracture of the maxillary tuberosity.

16. How do you minimize the chance of dislodging an impacted maxillary third molar into the infratemporal fossa during its surgical removal?
    Develop a full-thickness mucoperiosteal flap, bringing the incision anterior to the second molar (add a releasing incision if necessary) to improve visualization of the impacted tooth, and place a broad retractor distal to the molar while elevating it.

17. When performing a surgical removal, should you completely section through a mandibular molar?
    No. The lingual plate is often thin, and complete sectioning may perforate the plate and injure the lingual nerve.

18. How is bleeding from pulsating nutrient blood vessels controlled following surgery on alveolar bone?
    - Burnish bone.
    - Crush with rongeurs.
    - Apply bone wax.

19. What are some common causes of postoperative bleeding following dental extractions?
    - Failure to suture
    - Failure to remove all granulation tissue
    - Rebound blood vessel dilation following use of local anesthetic with a vasoconstrictor
    - Torn tissue
    - Torn surgical flaps

20. Why is a mucoperiosteal flap designed with a broad base?
    To ensure an adequate blood supply to the flap margin.

21. What are the two basic flaps used in dentoalveolar surgery?
    1. Full-thickness mucoperiosteal flap
    2. Split-thickness mucoperiosteal flap

22. What are the two basic types of full-thickness mucoperiosteal flaps?
    1. Envelope flap
    2. Envelope flap with a releasing component

23. Where are releasing incisions contraindicated?
    - Palate
    - Through muscle attachments
    - Lingual surface of the mandible
    - In the region of the mental foramen
    - Canine eminence

24. How do absorbable gelatin sponges (Gelfoam) and oxidized regenerated cellulose (Surgicel) assist with homeostasis?
    They form a matrix or scaffold upon which a clot can form. Gelatin sponge does not become as readily incorporated into the clot as does the oxidized regenerated cellulose. Healing is delayed more often with cellulose than with the gelatin sponge, but oxidized regenerated cellulose is the more efficient homeostatic agent.

25. **What is Avitene, and what is its mechanism of action?**
Avitene is microfibrillar collagen. Unlike Gelfoam and surgical, Avitene provides an actual collagen matrix, which then attracts platelets and triggers thrombus formation. It thus assumes an active rather than a passive role in hemostasis.

26. **Why is a conventional dental handpiece that expels forced air contraindicated when performing dentoalveolar surgery?**
Such an instrument can cause tissue emphysema or an air embolism. An air embolism can be fatal.

27. **What are the cardinal signs and symptoms of a localized osteitis (dry socket)?**
1. Throbbing pain (often radiating)
2. Bad taste
3. Fetid odor
4. A poorly healed extraction site, with clot loss and exposure of bone

28. **Why is it contraindicated to curette a dry socket to stimulate bleeding?**
Curetting a dry socket can cause the condition to worsen because healing will be further delayed, any natural healing already taking place will be destroyed, and there is a risk of causing the localized inflammatory process to be spread to the adjacent sound bone.

29. **What is the treatment for a localized osteitis?**
Conservative management is indicated. The wound should be irrigated gently with slightly warmed saline, and a sedative dressing should be placed. The dressing should be removed within 48 hours and replaced until the patient becomes asymptomatic. Systemic antibiotics are generally not indicated. Nonsteroidal antiinflammatory analgesics may be prescribed, and narcotic analgesic may also be indicated.

30. **What causes a dry socket?**
The etiology of a dry socket is not absolutely clear, but it is thought to develop because of increased fibrinolytic activity causing accelerated lysis of the blood clot. Smoking, premature mouth rinsing, hot liquids, surgical trauma, and oral contraceptives have all been implicated in the development of a dry socket.

31. **Why should flaps be repositioned and sutured over sound bone?**
Unsupported flaps can collapse into bony defects, causing tension on the sutures. The sutures subsequently will pull through the tissue, allowing the suture line to open and the wound to dehisce.

32. **What percentage of dentoalveolar injuries include the primary maxillary central incisor?**
70%.

33. **How are avulsed primary teeth treated?**
No treatment is necessary; replantation is not indicated for primary teeth.

34. **How is an extruded primary tooth treated?**
If there is gross mobility or interference with the opposing teeth, the tooth should be extracted. In cases of very minor extrusion without significant mobility or occlusal interference, a primary tooth may be repositioned without fixation, or left and kept under observation.

35. **What is the incidence of pulp necrosis after intrusion injuries of teeth?**
With intrusion injuries, the risk of pulp necrosis for a tooth with a closed apex is 95% and with an immature apex is 65%. Accordingly, any form of luxation should be followed with routine clinical and radiographic exams.

36. **How long should dentoalveolar fractures be splinted?**
4 to 6 weeks.

37. **What media can be used to transport avulsed teeth?**
Saliva, fresh milk, or, preferably, Hanks balanced salt solution (HBSS). Water is harmful because, as a hypotonic fluid, it may cause periodontal ligament cell death when it enters cells down the osmotic gradient, causing cell lysis and death.
Any tooth with an extraoral dry time of greater than 60 minutes will have a poor prognosis for long-term success after replantation. Detailed protocols for management (based on dry time and

whether the root apex is open or closed) are available on the website of the International Association of Dental Traumatology.

38. **How long should extruded or avulsed teeth be splinted?**
Up to 2 to 3 weeks.

39. **What are the significant radiologic predictions of a close relationship between the inferior alveolar canal and the impacted mandibular third molar?**
Signs of close proximity of the mandibular third molar to the inferior alveolar canal are mostly radiographic in nature and include:
- Darkening and notching of the root
- Deflected roots at the region of the canal
- Narrowing of the root
- Interruption of canal outlines
- Diversion of canal from its normal course
- Narrowing of canal outlines on the radiograph

40. **What are the most important signs that may increase potential nerve injury with extraction of impacted mandibular third molars?**
Of the previously listed signs of close proximity of the canal to impacted third molar, diversion of canal, interruption of canal borders, and darkening of roots are the most reliable signs.

41. **What are the possible complications of dentoalveolar surgery?**
- Swallowing or aspiration of foreign objects
- Tissue emphysema
- TMJ pain
- Trismus
- Mandibular fracture
- Tuberosity fracture
- Root fracture
- Injuries to adjacent teeth
- Displacement of root and root fragments into the submandibular space, mandibular canal, or maxillary sinus
- Oral-antral communication, bleeding, infection, ecchymosis, and hematoma
- Localized osteitis (dry socket)
- Wound dehiscence
- Inferior alveolar and lingual injuries
Depending on the location and the nature of the surgery, these complications vary in severity and need for treatment.

42. **How are roots or root tips displaced into the submandibular space managed?**
Once displacement of a mandibular molar root into the submandibular space is suspected, manual lateral and upward pressure should be applied immediately on the lingual aspect of the floor of the mouth in an attempt to force the root back into the socket. If the root is visualized again in the socket, it may be retrieved from the socket with a root tip pick. If not, a mucoperiosteal soft tissue flap should be reflected on the lingual aspect of the mandible until the root tip is found; ensure that the mylohyoid muscle is sharply detached from its insertion in the mandible. Antibiotic coverage is indicated postoperatively. If the root is not visualized because of its location or uncontrollable bleeding, recovery is best performed as a secondary procedure when fibrosis occurs and stabilizes the tooth in a firm position, usually 4 to 6 weeks later. The patient should be informed and be placed on a short course of antibiotics.

43. **How are roots or root tips that are displaced into the inferior alveolar canal managed?**
When displacement of a root into the mandibular canal is suspected, periapical and occlusal radiographs or cone beam CT scan should be taken for verification, because the root may be in a large marrow space or beneath the buccal mucosa. If the root is visualized, careful removal is indicated with a small hemostat after adequate alveolar bone removal. If the root is not visualized, delayed removal is recommended. Delayed removal is also indicated during persistent infection and nerve paresthesia. If the root fragment is small and does not become infected preoperatively, leaving the root in place is a viable and less invasive option.

44. How is a root or root fragment that is displaced into the maxillary sinus managed?

Once the root is suspected to be in the sinus, place the patient in an upright position to prevent posterior displacement and obtain a radiograph or CT to determine its location and size. If the fragment is found to be in the sinus, local measures of retrieval should be attempted first, such as:

- Having the patient blow through the nose with the nostrils closed, and observing the perforation for the root to appear in the socket
- Using a fine suction tip to bring the root back into the defect
- Performing antral lavage with sterile isotonic saline in an effort to flush the root out through the defect

If local measures are unsuccessful, direct entry into the maxillary sinus via the Caldwell-Luc approach in the area of the canine fossa should be performed. Postoperative management includes a figure-of-eight suture over the socket (or flap closure if the opening is sizable), sinus precautions, antibiotics, and a nasal spray to keep the sinus ostium open and infection free.

45. How are oral-antral communications managed?

Probing, irrigation, and having the patient blow forcefully with the nostrils occluded are contraindicated because these maneuvers may enlarge an existing opening or create one that did not previously exist. Some will allow patients to blow gently while compressing the nostrils to observe for air bubble formations that will confirm an antral opening. For openings <2 mm, no surgical treatment is necessary, providing adequate hemostasis is achieved. For openings of 2 to 6 mm, conservative treatment is indicated, including placement of a figure-of-eight suture over the tooth socket and sinus precautions (avoid blowing the nose, violent sneezing, sucking on straws, and smoking). For openings >6 mm, primary closure should be obtained with a buccal flap or a palatal flap procedure. Approximation of the gingiva can be facilitated by removal of a small amount of the buccal alveolar plate and scoring or incising the periosteum on the underside of the flap. Placement of a small piece of absorbable gelatin sponge into the occlusal third of the socket when the gingival margins cannot be coapted is not advisable because it introduces a foreign substance and could lead to subsequent breakdown of the clot. Antibiotics and nasal or oral decongestants are prescribed if there is evidence of acute or chronic sinusitis.

46. What steps should be taken for a tooth (maxillary third molar) that is displaced into the infratemporal fossa?

When a maxillary third molar is displaced into the infratemporal fossa, it is usually displaced through the periosteum and located lateral to the lateral pterygoid plate and inferior to the lateral pterygoid muscle with displacement. If there is good access and adequate light, a single cautious effort to retrieve the tooth with a hemostat can be made. If the effort is unsuccessful, or if the tooth is not visualized, the incision should be closed, the patient should be informed, and prophylactic antibiotics should be prescribed. A secondary surgical procedure is performed 4 to 6 weeks later after localization is determined using either lateral and posteroanterior radiographs or, preferably, a cone beam CT scan. After adequate anesthesia, a long needle—usually a spinal needle—is used to locate the tooth. Careful dissection is performed along the needle until the tooth is visualized and subsequently removed. Some surgeons may prefer to perform this removal in the operating room for better access.

If no functional problems exist after displacement, the patient may elect not to have the tooth removed. Proper documentation of this is critical.

47. How can postoperative or secondary bleeding from extraction sites be managed?

The first step in managing postoperative bleeding is to carefully examine and visualize the bleeding site to determine the precise source of bleeding. In the case of simple generalized oozing, a damp gauze is held over the site with firm manual pressure for 5 minutes. If unsuccessful, the area should be anesthetized and examined more closely. If sutures were placed, they should be removed and the existing clot should be curetted from the socket. Hemostatic agents, such as an absorbable gelatin sponge, oxidized cellulose, or Avitene can be placed in the socket and sutured. If hemostasis is not achieved by local measures, lab screening tests should be performed to assist in diagnosis and treatment of the cause.

48. Why is it not indicated to scrape the walls of extraction sites after teeth are removed?

Often, after using local anesthesia with a vasoconstrictor, the extraction site appears "dry" and the void does not readily fill with blood. It is unnecessary and not a good practice to scrape the walls of the extraction site to stimulate bleeding or for any other reasons. This practice will delay healing.

The remnants of the periodontal ligament (PDL) that are attached to the alveolar crypt are the sources of fibroblasts that form fibrin for the rudimentary clot (scaffold) upon which cells necessary for the healing process can migrate. Moreover, the remnants of the PDL provide small capillaries and pluripotential cells that will form osteoblasts necessary for bone formation.

49. What is the proper positioning of a patient for exodontia procedures in the clinic setting?
   For maxillary procedures, patients are positioned in a semireclined position, such that the maxillary occlusal plane is at an angle of about 60 degrees to the floor. This will normally correspond to a chair tilt of about 30 to 45 degrees from vertical or upright. The height of the mouth should be at the operator's elbow level.
   For mandibular extractions, the patient should be more upright, so that the occlusal plane of the mandible is parallel to the floor when the mouth is opened. The patient will also be positioned slightly lower than for maxillary extractions, with the chair at or slightly below the elbow level of the operator.
   Operators who choose to perform exodontia while sitting will need to make appropriate modifications to the standing positions.

50. Where is the location of the lingual nerve in relation to the mandibular third molar?
   The spatial relationship between the lingual nerve and the mandibular third molar region is highly variable. The nerve has been found to be at the level of the lingual plate or higher, in contact with the lingual plate, or intimately attached to the periosteum and the follicular sac of the impacted mandibular third molar.

51. What is the difference between an incisional and excisional biopsy?
   An excisional biopsy entails removal of the entire lesion along with at least 2 mm of normal marginal tissue from the sides of the lesion. This technique is usually used for biopsy of a lesion 1 cm or less. An incisional biopsy removes only a representative portion or portions of a lesion along with a representation of adjacent normal tissue.

52. When a biopsy is being performed, why is it necessary to incise parallel to the long axis of any muscle fibers beneath the lesion?
   Whenever possible, the incisions should be oriented parallel to lines of muscle tension in order to minimize scarring and wound dehiscence. Biopsy incisions on the face should be oriented to follow Langer's lines.

53. What are the indications for performing a partial odontectomy (coronectomy) of an impacted mandibular molar?
   An intentional partial odontectomy is usually performed on an impacted mandibular third molar. This technique is chosen when there is a significant risk of injury to the inferior alveolar nerve or jaw fracture, and in cases where the benefits of root retention outweigh the risks of conventional third molar removal. The roots must be asymptomatic, not associated with pathologic lesions, and must not interfere with future restorative procedures or orthodontic treatment. The technique involves careful sectioning of the crown from the roots at or below the cementoenamel junction. The roots should not be elevated or disturbed as they must remain attached to their apical blood vessels to ensure vitality. The patient must always be informed when this technique is used.

54. On what relationships are the Pell and Gregory impacted mandibular third molar classifications based?
   The Pell and Gregory impacted third molar classifications are based on the third molar's relationship to the anterior border of the ascending ramus and to the occlusal plane. A Pell and Gregory Class 1 impaction implies sufficient space between the ramus and the second molar into which the third molar can erupt. A Class 2 impacted third molar is found to be at least half covered by ramus bone. The Class 3 impacted third molar is entirely within the ramus. With regard to the occlusal plane, a Pell and Gregory Class A impaction implies that the occlusal surfaces of the second and third molars are at or about the same level. The occlusal surface of a Class B third molar impaction is between the occlusal surface and cementoenamel junction of the second molar. The Class C impaction is the deepest impaction where the occlusal surface of the third molar is completely below the neck of the second molar.

55. **What teeth are most commonly impacted?**
The most commonly impacted teeth are the third molars (mandibular more frequently than maxillary), followed in order by maxillary canines, mandibular premolars, and mandibular canines.

56. **What is low molecular weight heparin (LMWH), and how is it used in oral and maxillofacial surgery?**
Standard unfractionated heparin (UFH) is formed from a heterogeneous combination of sulfated mucopolysaccharides. Its anticoagulant activity is unpredictable, so it must be carefully monitored with the partial thromboplastin time (PTT) test. LMWH (fractionated heparin) is formed from depolymerization of heparin into lower molecular weight particles. Because LMWH has increased bioavailability compared with UFH, it can be given as a fixed dose and without the need for monitoring with the PTT.
　　It is useful in oral and maxillofacial surgery for some higher risk patients who cannot discontinue or reduce oral anticoagulation therapy. Patients stop warfarin therapy and the international normalized ratio (INR) is allowed to normalize while the LMWH is administered to maintain anticoagulation therapy. When the INR returns to an acceptable level, the surgery can be performed and scheduled for early in the day. The LMWH is withheld the day of surgery and resumed in the evening. Warfarin can be resumed the following day and the LMWH continued until the INR returns to the desired therapeutic range.

57. **Should patients discontinue aspirin or Plavix (clopidogrel) for routine dentoalveolar surgery?**
While each patient must be evaluated on an individual basis, it is generally not indicated to stop aspirin or Plavix prior to routine dentoalveolar procedures, including multiple extractions. Medical risks of recurrent myocardial infarction or stroke will outweigh the risk of postoperative bleeding in most cases. For more extensive procedures where there is a particular concern for bleeding, low molecular weight heparin (e.g., Lovenox) can be used.

58. **What are the "new oral anticoagulants," and how are they monitored and adjusted for patients undergoing surgery?**
Rivaroxaban (Xarelto) and apixaban (Eliquis) are direct Factor Xa inhibitors, and dabigatran (Pradaxa) is a direct thrombin inhibitor. Neither the INR nor Protime (PT) levels have been shown to have any reliability in monitoring therapy for these patients. Since the half-life of these agents is relatively short, they can be held for one or two days prior to surgery, based on their respective half-life. As a general rule, for drugs given twice daily (shorter half-life) hold for one day prior to surgery. For those given once daily (longer half-life), hold for two days prior to surgery.

PREPROSTHETIC SURGERY

59. **How does the blood supply of the edentulous mandible differ from that of the dentate mandible?**
As edentulous bone loss (EBL) progresses, there is a change in the blood supply to the mandible. The inferior alveolar vessels become smaller. The primary blood supply to the dentate mandible moves **centrifugally** from the inferior alveolar artery. The primary blood supply to the edentulous mandible flows **centripetally** from the periosteum. Elevation of the periosteum on mandibles that have had severe bone loss could compromise blood supply. Therefore, during surgical procedures, elevation of the periosteum should be done judiciously in the edentulous atrophic mandible.

60. **Does alveolar bone resorb more quickly in the mandible or in the maxilla?**
EBL in the maxilla is usually more rapid and severe. This may be due to the lack of muscle attachments to the maxilla and, therefore, the lack of functional stimulus after tooth loss.

61. **What skeletal relationship results from EBL?**
The skeletal relationship that results from EBL is **pseudo Class III**. Most EBL in the maxilla takes place on the lateral and inferior aspects of the ridge; therefore, the crest moves posteriorly and superiorly. As the height and width of the mandibular ridge deteriorate, the crest moves further anteriorly. As vertical dimension collapses, the mandible autorotates forward as well.

62. How are edentulous alveolar ridges classified?

See Table 25-1.

63. What is combination syndrome?

Combination syndrome is excessive resorption of the edentulous alveolar ridge of the anterior maxilla, caused by the forces generated by opposition of natural mandibular anterior teeth.

64. When and how are torus mandibularis and torus palatinus treated?

Mandibular tori usually need to be removed when a mandibular denture is being planned. The denture flange typically will impinge on these exostoses of bone. Palatal tori often do not need to be removed. Dentures often can be constructed over them. However, if a palatal torus is extremely large and fills the vault, extends beyond the dam area, has traumatized mucosal coverage, has deep undercuts, interferes with speech, or poses a psychologic problem for the patient, it should be removed.

The tissue over mandibular tori is extremely thin and friable. Great care should be taken when elevating it. This tissue can be "ballooned" out by injecting some local anesthesia directly under it. The incision should be crestal or lingual circumdental. No releasing incisions should be made. After careful elevation of tissues, a groove can be cut along the intended line of removal with a fissure burr. A mallet and osteotome may be used to cleave the torus in this plane. After the bone has been smoothed and the area thoroughly irrigated, the wound can be closed. Gauze should be placed under the tongue to minimize the chance of hematoma.

Before removing a palatal torus, a stent should be fabricated. This should be done on a study cast that has had the exostosis removed. A double-Y incision should be made over the midline of the torus. After careful elevation of the flaps, the torus should be scored multiple times in the anterior, posterior, and transverse dimensions. An osteotome can be used to remove each of these small portions. This decreases the risk of fracturing into the floor of the nose. A large burr or bone file is used to smooth the area. After thorough irrigation, the wound is closed with horizontal mattress sutures, and the stent is placed.

65. How can an abnormal frenum be excised?

- Z-plasty
- V-Y advancement
- Diamond excision

66. What is the average size of the maxillary sinus?

The average size of the maxillary sinus is 14.75 cc, with a range of 9.5 to 20 cc. On average the width is 2.5 cm; height, 3.75 cm; and depth, 3 cm.

Table 25-1. Classification of Edentulous Ridges

CLASS	DEFINITION
Kent Classification of Edentulous Ridges (1986)	
I	Alveolar ridge is of adequate height but inadequate width, with lateral deficiencies or undercut areas
II	Alveolar ridge deficient in both height and width, with a knife-edge appearance
III	Alveolar ridge has been resorbed to the level of basilar bone, producing a concave form in the posterior areas of the mandible and sharp ridge form with bulbous, mobile soft tissues in the maxilla
IV	Resorption of the basilar bone, producing a pencil-thin, flat mandible or maxilla
Caywood Classification of Edentulous Ridges (1988)	
I	Dentate
II	Immediately postextraction
III	Well-rounded ridge form, adequate in height and width
IV	Knife-edge ridge form, adequate in height but inadequate in width
V	Flat ridge form; inadequate in height and width
VI	Depressed ridge form, with some basilar loss evident

67. **How should tears of the sinus membrane be managed during sinus lift?**
Tears over corticocancellous grafts will heal. Particulate grafts may be lost if they migrate through perforations. Small tears may not pose a problem because the membrane folds over itself as it is lifted. Larger tears should be patched with a material such as Surgicel or Collatape.

68. **How much native bone is required for immediate placement of implants with sinus lift?**
A minimum of 4 to 5 mm of alveolar bone.

69. **What is the proper size of the window for a sinus lift?**
The window for a maxillary sinus lift begins at the anterior aspect of the sinus and continues inferiorly to several millimeters above the sinus floor. The window extends posteriorly approximately 20 mm. The superior osteotomy is approximately 10 to 15 mm above the inferior osteotomy.

70. **What is the desired thickness of a split-thickness skin graft (STSG)?**
STSGs can be of varying thickness. An STSG is composed of the epidermis layer and part of the dermis layer. The STSG can be classified as thin, intermediate, or thick, based on the amount of dermis included. STSGs are between 0.010 and 0.025 inch.

71. **Which types of skin grafts contract the most? The least?**
The thinner a skin graft, the more the contraction. A thin STSG contracts more than an intermediate STSG, which contracts more than a thick STSG. Full-thickness skin grafts hardly contract at all.
    Primary contraction is caused by elastic fibers in the skin graft as soon as it has been cut. This can be overcome when a graft is sutured in place. Secondary contraction begins about postoperative day 10 and continues for up to 6 months.

72. **What is plasmic imbibition?**
Plasmic imbibition is the process by which a skin graft absorbs a plasma-like fluid from its underlying recipient bed. It is absorbed into the capillary network by capillary action. This process is the initial means of survival for a skin graft and continues for approximately 48 hours.

73. **Does grafted skin most resemble the donor site or the recipient site?**
Grafted skin maintains most of its original characteristics, except that sensation and sweating more closely resemble the recipient site.

74. **What are the goals of vestibuloplasty?**
Vestibuloplasty, skin grafting, and floor of the mouth lowering increase the depth of the sulcus, which helps control lateral displacement of a denture. The skin graft also provides attached tissue, which will not be elevated by movement of the lip, cheeks, and tongue, providing a stable denture seating area. Skin grafts provide more comfortable load-bearing tissue than mucosa. The mandibular resorption rate beneath skin is probably slower.

75. **What are the possible graft donor sites for vestibuloplasty?**
- Skin
- Palatal mucosa
- Buccal mucosa

76. **What are the advantages of using a stent to secure a graft in place for a vestibuloplasty?**
A stent can be used to adapt the skin with accuracy to any contour in the labiobuccal area and undercuts in the lingual area. A stent also provides additional graft stabilization and protects the graft from food in the oral cavity.

77. **What are the advantages of suturing a graft in place for a vestibuloplasty?**
Patients are more comfortable without the stent. Stent construction and adaptation materials are not necessary.

78. **What is the lip-switch procedure?**
The lip-switch procedure is a transpositional flap vestibuloplasty. An incision is made in the labial mucosa. A thin mucosal flap is elevated, continuing into a supraperiosteal dissection on the anterior aspect of the mandible to the crest of the ridge. The mucosal flap is sutured to the depth of the vestibule covering the anterior aspect of the mandible, and the denuded tissue on the inner surface of the lip heals by secondary intention. A modification transposes the lingually based mucosal flap with an inferiorly based facial periosteal flap.

79. **What is submucous vestibuloplasty?**

    Submucous vestibuloplasty can be used for improvement of the maxillary vestibule in situations in which the alveolar ridge resorption is not severe but mucosal and muscular attachments exist near the crest of the ridge. Through a midline incision, submucosal and subperiosteal dissections are performed. The tissue between these two tunnels is cut and allowed to retract. A splint is relined and secured in place for 7 to 10 days.

80. **How is floor of the mouth lowering performed?**

    An incision is made on the lingual aspect of the alveolus. A supraperiosteal dissection is carried inferiorly, and the mylohyoid and genioglossus muscles are sharply dissected from their insertions. No more than half the superior aspect of the genioglossus muscle should be released. The mucosal margins are then sutured to the new depth, either with sutures passed externally or in a circummandibular fashion.

81. **What is the minimum distance from the inferior border that the mentalis must remain attached, during vestibuloplasty, to prevent a sagging chin?**

    A minimum of 10 mm of muscular tissue must remain attached to the vestibular periosteum in order to avoid a sagging chin.

BIBLIOGRAPHY

Dentoalveolar Surgery

Alling CC, 3rd (ed) *Dentoalveolar surgery*, Oral and maxillofacial surgery clinics of North America (vol 5). Philadelphia, 1993, Saunders.

Dental trauma guide, International Association of Dental Traumatology, Accessed September 2014. www.dentaltraumaguide.org.

Hupp JR, Ellis E, Tucker MR: *Contemporary oral and maxillofacial surgery*, ed 6, St Louis, 2014, Mosby/Elsevier.

Kiesselbach JE, Chamberlain JG: Clinical and anatomic observations on the relationship of the lingual nerve to the mandibular third molar region, *J Oral Maxillofac Surg* 42:565, 1984.

Laskin DM: *Clinician's handbook of oral and maxillofacial surgery*, Carol Stream, Ill, 2011, Quintessence.

Lew D: Blood and blood products. In Kwon PH, Laskin DM, editors: *Clinician's manual of oral and maxillofacial surgery*, ed 3, Carol Stream, Ill, 2001, Quintessence.

Pogrel MA, Lee JS, Muff DF: Coronectomy: a technique to protect the inferior alveolar nerve, *J Oral Maxillofac Surg* 62:1447, 2004.

Todd DW, Roman A: Outpatient use of low-molecular weight heparin in an anticoagulated patient requiring oral surgery: case report, *J Oral Maxillofac Surg* 59:1090, 2001.

Whitacre R: *Removal of Teeth*, ed 3, Seattle, 1983, Stoma Press.

Preprosthetic Surgery

Davis WH, Sailer HF: Preprosthetic surgery, *Oral Maxillofac Surg Clin North Am* 6:4, 1994.

Fonseca RJ: *Oral and maxillofacial surgery*, vol 7, St Louis, 2000, Saunders.

MacIntosh RB: Autogenous grafting in oral and maxillofacial surgery, *Oral Maxillofac Surg Clin North Am* 5:4, 1993.

Marx RE, Carlson ER, Eichstaedt RM, et al.: Platelet-rich plasma: growth factor enhancement for bone grafts, *Oral Surg Oral Med Oral Pathol Oral Radiol Endod* 85:638–646, 1998.

Marx RE, Morales MJ: Morbidity from bone harvest in major jaw reconstruction: a randomized trial comparing the lateral anterior and posterior approaches to the ilium, *J Oral Maxillofac Surg* 48:196–203, 1988.

Peterson LJ, Indresano AT, Marciani RD, et al.: *Principles of oral and maxillofacial surgery*, Philadelphia, 1992, J.B. Lippincott.

CHAPTER 26

DENTAL IMPLANTS

George R. Deeb, Graham H. Wilson, Kenneth J. Benson

1. **What are the different dental implant categories?**
   Dental implants are divided into three categories based on their relationship to the oral tissues:
   1. Subperiosteal
   2. Endosteal
   3. Transosseous
   Endosteal implants are subdivided into root-form implants and plate-form or blade implants. Root-form implants can be smooth, threaded, perforated, and solid or hollow, vented, coated, or textured. Root-form implants are subdivided into the following categories including cylinder implants, screw-designed implants, or combination of screw and cylinder implants. Currently, the most commonly used implants are root-form implants. Only endosseous and transosseous implants are considered true osseointegrated implants.

2. **What is osseointegration?**
   Several definitions have been proposed over the years to describe a successful dental implant in the human jaw. However, the most inclusive definition to date describes osseointegration as "a process whereby clinically asymptomatic rigid fixation of alloplastic materials is achieved and maintained in bone during functional loading."

3. **What criteria were used to determine the success of an implant before 1986?**
   Before 1986, the criteria for a successful implant were different from those used today. According to the 1978 Harvard–National Institutes of Health (NIH) consensus conference on implantology, an implant was considered successful despite the presence of one or more of the following clinical features:
   • Mobility of <1 mm in any direction
   • Bone loss of no more than one-third of the vertical height of the implant
   • Gingival inflammation amenable to treatment
   • Absence of symptoms, such as infection, numbness, pain, or maxillary sinus or nasal symptoms
   • Implant functional for 5 years in 75% of cases

4. **What became the criteria for successful implants after 1986?**
   In 1986, with the introduction of osseointegration, the criteria for successful implants were revised:
   • Implant clinically immobile
   • No radiographic evidence of any periimplant radiolucency
   • Vertical bone loss of <0.2 mm after the first year of function
   • Absence of any symptoms, such as pain, infection, numbness, or maxillary sinus or nasal symptoms
   • Success rate of 85% after 5 years and 80% after 10 years

5. **When are dental implants indicated?**
   Dental implants are used to achieve rehabilitation of the oral and facial tissue after tooth loss with and without bone loss, after jaw bone loss due to tumor resection, after tooth loss from trauma, and for partially or completely congenitally missing teeth. More specifically, implants are used to achieve one of the following purposes:
   • Fixed restoration of a single tooth or multiple teeth in a partially edentulous jaw
   • Retention of a removable prosthesis in a partially edentulous jaw
   • Retention of a prosthesis in a completely edentulous jaw
   • Retention of a fixed prosthesis in completely edentulous maxilla or mandible
   • Retention of a maxillofacial prosthesis after loss of jawbone from trauma or after tumor resection
   • As a fixture for orthodontic tooth movement when conventional anchorage is not feasible or is cumbersome

6. What are the advantages of a single implant for replacing a single tooth compared to a conventional three-unit bridge?
   - High success rate
   - Decreased risk of caries or tooth loss of abutment teeth
   - Decreased risk of endodontic problems with abutment teeth
   - Better access for hygiene
   Fixed partial denture failure rates may be as high as 20% after 3 years, and 50% at 10 years.

7. What are some advantages to implant-retained/supported prostheses compared to conventional removable prostheses?
   - Maintain bone.
   - Improve phonetics.
   - Improve retention and stability.
   - Improve masticatory performance.
   - Increase prosthesis success.
   - Improve psychological health.

8. What are Brånemark's surgical principles for ensuring osseous integration of implants?
   Brånemark established a set of surgical principles based on animal and human research that, if followed during implant placement, ensures osseointegration of the dental implants:
   - The implant should be placed in direct contact with the bone.
   - Implants should be inserted in bone in a surgically prepared site, using a graded series of drills followed by a tap rotating at 15 rpm.
   - Absolute temperature control at the surgical site should not exceed 47° C to minimize thermal necrosis of bone adjacent to implant.
   - The mucosa should remain sutured over the newly inserted implant, and the implant should remain functionless for 3 to 6 months.
   - At a second stage (3 to 6 months later), the implant is exposed and an abutment and the implant are connected to the prosthesis. Consequently, loading of the implant is done only after the implant is osseointegrated. This last principle has changed in the last few years by successfully loading implants immediately after placement with no impact on the success rate.

9. How much space is needed between implants for successful integration?
   Imagine that a square box is drawn around the implant. In the buccal-lingual dimension, a minimum of 0.5 mm of bone is required around the implant. Therefore for a standard 3.75-mm implant, the operator would need approximately 5 mm of bone in this dimension. Mesiodistally, the same 0.5 mm is required for implant survival. Prosthodontically, at least 3 mm is necessary on both sides of the implant to create the proper emergence profile of a restoration. Consequently, the recommendation for distance between implants for single-tooth restoration is 7 mm from the center of one implant to the other.

10. How much space is observed between implant and bone in an osseointegrated titanium implant?
    The chemical properties and the interface chemistry are determined by the oxide layer and not by the metal of the implant. Therefore the dense oxide film of a titanium implant, for example, is about 100 Å thick.

11. Describe one-stage placement, two-stage placement, and immediate provisionalization of dental implants.
    In two-stage implant placement, the implant is placed and submerged for a period of time, and secondary surgery for uncovering of the implant is necessary. A single-stage implant placement includes placement of a permucosal component, most often a healing abutment, at the time of implant placement. Immediate provisionalization involves placement of the implant, placement of a temporary or permanent abutment, as well as a restoration.

12. How much is the surface area of an implant increased by increasing the diameter of an implant compared with increasing its length?
    For each 0.25-mm increase in implant diameter, there is a 10% increase in surface area. Therefore a 1-mm increase in diameter increases surface area by 40%. Studies have shown that for implants larger than 15 to 18 mm, there is no further significant biomechanical advantage, regardless of implant diameter.

Some authors have shown that increasing the length of an implant to more than 18 mm provides no additional mechanical advantage and possibly increases the incidence of failure rate because of the difficulty of adequately irrigating during the preparation of the site.

13. **What major anatomic structures in the maxilla can affect implant placement? How can these problems be overcome?**
In the posterior maxilla, a pneumatization of the maxillary sinus can result in a decrease in the available bone in this region. This deficiency can be overcome by bone grafting of this region. If the interarch space is adequate for restoration (implant-to-crown ratio), a sinus-lift bone graft procedure is indicated. However, if there is an excessive interarch space, onlay bone graft with or without sinus-lift procedure is a better choice. Distraction osteogenesis both to increase the bone height and to close the interarch space is another option when there is an increased interarch space.

In the anterior maxilla, bony defects are occasionally observed on the buccal surface, caused either by traumatic extraction or by buccal concavity around the apical one-third of the root. These defects must be treated before or during implant placement. Angulation of the implant to engage existing bone often will result in an implant that is unable to receive a direct axial load and will be more prone to failure after a restoration is placed.

14. **What major anatomic structures in the mandible can affect implant placement? How can these problems be overcome?**
In the posterior mandible, the inferior alveolar nerve is one of the most common impediments to implant placement. Frequently, there is insufficient bone height to place even an 11.5-mm implant in the posterior mandible without the risk of nerve injury. Remedies for this problem depend mostly on restoration length and available interarch space. As in the maxilla, if there is sufficient interarch space, the nerve must be surgically repositioned (lateralized) to gain adequate bone length to achieve a proper crown-to-root ratio and anchorage for the implant. If there is excessive interarch space, onlay bone grafting or distraction osteogenesis should be considered to gain vertical bone height and decrease the interarch space before implant placement.

The lingual concavity of the mandible in the posterior and anterior regions is another anatomic area to be considered during placement of mandibular implants. Computed tomography (CT) or plain tomography should be considered if there is any question as to whether an implant can be placed without perforating the concavity and risking implant failure or damage to the lingual nerve.

15. **Is it necessary to have attached gingiva when placing implants?**
Ideally, implants are more easily maintained if an adequate cuff (1 to 2 mm) of attached tissue is left around the restoration. This does not mean, however, that attached tissue is necessary at the time of placement. In the edentulous mandible, there is often a paucity of attached tissue at the time of placement, and most patients have high mentalis muscle attachments that extend to the crest of the remaining alveolus. At the time of placement, or at a later time but before uncovering the implant in a two-stage implant system, measures can be taken to lower these muscle attachments (lip-switch or other vestibuloplasty procedures) to gain immobile tissue.

16. **What are some tests to evaluate osseointegration at the time of implant uncovering?**
Torque testing can be done to test for osseointegration at the time of implant uncovering. Ideally, one should be able to place a force of 10 to 20 Ncm without unscrewing an implant if it is successfully osseointegrated. Other clinical subjective signs of integration are percussion and immobility when placing a fixture mount or impression coping on the implant. When a lateral force of 5 lb is applied, no movement should be seen. Horizontal mobility of >1 mm or movement <500 g of force indicates a failed implant.

Resonance frequency analysis is an easy, reliable, and noninvasive means of measuring implant stability. The resonance frequency value is measured using a transducer that is mounted directly on the fixture and displays the result as the implant stability quotient (ISQ). The ISQ is between 1 and 100, with a higher value indicating increased resonance frequency and stability of the implant.

17. **What methods are used to uncover implants? Can a laser or electrocautery be used?**
Conventional uncovering is done with a scalpel. If there is a minimal band of keratinized tissue, an incision is made to split this band, and the tissue is sutured to either side of the healing abutment. If there is adequate attached immobile tissue, a punch biopsy can be used after localization of the implant with a needle. Lasers can also be used, but care must be taken to avoid reflecting energy off the implant to the adjacent bone, which will cause irreversible thermal damage. Electrocautery can also be used carefully without touching the fixture to avoid transmitting heat throughout the socket.

18. **What preoperative radiographs are necessary for adequate work-up before implant placement?**

    Panoramic and periapical radiographs are helpful and necessary, although they offer no information regarding the internal anatomy of the alveolar process or residual ridge. In addition, they do not permit accurate three-dimensional superimposition of a clinically verified radiopaque template, which can be used as a surgical guide. Multiplanar reformatted CT can be used to obtain this information if it cannot be obtained easily by a combination of conventional radiographic techniques and clinical exam.

19. **Are magnetic resonance imaging (MRI) and CT scans contraindicated in a patient with dental implants?**

    MRI and CT scans are not contraindicated in patients with pure titanium implants. Most CT scanners can subtract titanium and other metals from the image and eliminate the scatter images.

20. **Can you name some risk factors that may increase the failure rate and complications of implant placement?**
    - Smoking
    - Uncontrolled systemic disease such as diabetes and hematologic disorders; also patients who are immunocompromised (e.g., HIV, chemotherapy)
    - Radiation therapy to the region planned for implant placement
    - Use of bisphosphonates or other antiresorptive agents
    - Existing pathology in the area planned for implant placement (e.g., maxillary sinus pathology)
    - Parafunctional habit (e.g., Bruxism)

21. **What are the most common reasons for endosseous dental implant removal?**
    - Lack of integration
    - Surgical malposition
    - Lack of bone support
    - Psychiatric reasons
    - Loss of bone

22. **What are the possible complications of endosseous dental implants?**

    The most commonly reported reasons for dental implant failure are:
    - Infection
    - Perforation of the maxillary sinus and nasal cavity
    - Perforation of the lingual cortex of the mandible, and possible arterial injury. This may result in troublesome hemorrhage that can compromise the airway.
    - Loss of implant
    - Bone resorption and loss of the implant
    - Fracture of the mandible
    - Damage to adjacent teeth
    - Nerve injury

23. **What is the long-term success rate of endosseous implants?**

    The 5-year combined success rate of maxillary and mandibular dental implants is 94.6%. Albrektsson et al. reported maxillary implants with a success rate of 84.9% for 5 to 7 years. For irradiated maxilla, the success rate of implants is 80%; in grafted maxilla, the success rate is 85%.

    In large, long-term studies of mandibular and maxillary endosseous implants, the success rate ranges from 84% to 97%. Specifically, the maxillary implant success rate after 1 year is 88% and after 5 to 12 years is 84%. In the mandible, the 1- to 2-year success rate is 94% to 97%, the 5- to 12-year success rate is 93%, and the 15-year success rate is 91%. The success rate in the mandible posterior region is 91.5% and in the maxillary posterior region is 82.9%, whereas the success rates are higher in the anterior mandible, in the 94% to 97% range.

24. **What is the success rate of endosseous implants placed in an autogenous bone graft site?**

    In a study by Keller et al., 248 commercially pure titanium endosseous implants were placed in 54 consecutive patients who required bone grafting. Types of grafts included cortical, corticocancellous, and particulate bone. All 74 antral sites received a block graft. Endosseous implant success over the 12-year period was 87%, and bone graft success reached 100%. A higher loss of implants occurred in the Le Fort I fracture groups compared with other grafting approaches.

25. When is a transmandibular implant (TMI) indicated?
    A TMI can be placed in a totally edentulous mandible of any bone height. However, a TMI works particularly well in the prosthetic restoration of a severely atrophic mandible (<12 mm of bone vertically). However, with the recent advances in endosseous implants, the need for and use of TMI has almost been eliminated.

26. Is hand tightening of an abutment acceptable for immediate provisionalization?
    Yes. However, hand tightening does have a high incidence of screw loosening. To decrease the number of emergency patients with loose restorations, use of a calibrated mechanical torque wrench is advised to apply appropriate tightening. Most authors recommend applying 35 Ncm to tighten the abutment. In general, following the individual manufacturer's specifications will decrease loosening.

27. What are three key features for successful implant treatment for single-tooth edentulism?
    1. Primary stability
    2. Oxidized implant surfaces
    3. Light centric occlusion only and removal of lateral excursives on the restoration

28. Which type of implant surface has shown better bone healing response: machine or oxidized surface implants?
    Multiple studies show an increased response of bone to oxidized surfaces. This implant feature has allowed quicker secondary stability because osseointegration is quicker.

29. What considerations should be made when planning implants in an irradiated patient?
    As with any other dentoalveolar procedure, one must know the irradiated field and dose, anatomic considerations with amount of bone available, and time period the radiation was delivered. Dose is a key factor, with 55 Gy and greater being an amount that is traditionally the level at which treatment should be given with the most caution (particularly in the mandible).
    Hyperbaric oxygen (HBO) can be used as an adjunctive treatment for implant rehabilitation. The standard HBO protocol (20 dives before implant surgery and 10 dives postimplant placement) provides improved bone healing and turnover with enhanced angiogenesis and neovascularization in the irradiated tissues. Also, one must know where the radiation was delivered, because some areas ultimately have less radiation delivered than others and treatment can be planned accordingly, with more implants delivered in a less radiated area of the mandible/maxilla. Dosimetry reports, which can provide information regarding the dose received in specific areas, can often be obtained from the patient's radiation oncologist. This information is extremely valuable in treatment planning location of implants and prevention of implant failure as well as osteoradionecrosis.
    Many studies indicate successful integration of endosseous implants in irradiated fields even without the use of HBO therapy. A study by Anderson et al. demonstrates a success rate of 97.8% for endosseous implants placed into an irradiated field. This study evaluated 90 implants placed in 15 patients for treatment of malignancies in the maxillofacial region with radiation doses ranging from 44 to 68 cGy. Other studies show similar rates of success without the use of HBO.

30. What variables increase success in immediate implant placement?
    Patients with thick gingival biotype respond with a more predictable final gingival margin level, and their incisions tend to heal with less scarring. Patients with thin gingival biotype tend to respond to surgical insults and bone loss with higher incidence of gingival recession. A flapless technique is advised, and vertical releasing incisions should be avoided, especially in patients with a thin biotype. Cosyn et al. demonstrated a 96% implant survival rate with mean facial gingival margin recession of 0.34 mm over 3 years with immediate implant placement and temporization in the maxilla in patients with a thick gingival biotype and no labial bone defects.
    Adequate crestal bone levels should be verified with preoperative periodontal probing. If there is a defect in the labial bone, grafting should be completed and implant placement delayed until adequate bony architecture is restored.
    Implants in the esthetic zone must engage bone palatal and apical to the extraction socket, especially if immediate provisionalization is planned. The axis of the implants should be along the cingulum or slightly palatal to the incisal edge. Cone beam CT can readily offer information regarding bone apical and palatal to the existing tooth in planning for implant placement, as well as labial bone thickness.

31. What are some key components to planning implants in the esthetic zone?
    - Assessment of the smile line. A greater percentage of females possess a high smile line, posing a greater challenge for successful implant therapy in the esthetic zone.
    - Gingival biotype. Patients with a thin gingival biotype may be considered for connective tissue grafting to achieve a thicker biotype. Gingival biotype has implications on one- versus two-stage surgery, as well as incision design for implant placement.
    - The interdental papilla commonly fills the interproximal space when the vertical distance from the interproximal crown contact to interseptal bone is 5 mm or less. If the distance is increased to 6 mm, then the papilla fails to fill the space 40% of the time.
    - The ideal labial midcrestal bone position should be 2 mm apical to the facial cemento-enamel junction (CEJ) of the adjacent teeth. The implant platform should be 3 mm below the facial free gingival margin. Placement of the platform at this level will allow for development of proper emergence profile, adequate tissue thickness to cover the darker surface of titanium, and prevention of periodontal pocket formation and gingival recession.
    - Implant placement should be at least 1.5 mm from adjacent tooth roots to prevent bone loss on both the implant and tooth related to the microgap or biologic width, as well as to prevent potential problems with interproximal esthetics. The distance between adjacent implants should be a minimum of 3 mm. The faciopalatal width should be at least 2 mm greater than the implant diameter, and ideally at least 1.5 mm of bone on the facial aspect of the implant should be present. Ridge augmentation for increased width can be completed prior to implant placement, or at the time of implant placement with success. Greater success with augmentation at the time of implant placement occurs if there is no dehiscence of the implant.
    - The mesiodistal dimension of the missing tooth must be considered when selecting the proper size implant. The average mesiodistal dimension of a central incisor is 8.6 mm for a man and 8.1 mm for a woman. Prosthodontically, at least 3 mm is necessary on both sides of the implant to create the proper emergence profile of a restoration.

32. What factors should be considered when using cement versus screw-retained provisionals?
    Screw-retained provisionals have the advantage of being easily retrievable and are indicated when abutment height is less than 5 mm where a cemented restoration would not provide adequate resistance and retention. Cemented restorations lack screw holes that can decrease the physical strength of the restoration, as well as compromise esthetics if they are buccally located. Another advantage with cemented provisional restorations is the lack of screw holes in areas of possible opposing occlusal contacts. Screw-retained restorations also pose the risk of screw loosening, stretching, or fracture if there is offset loading of enough magnitude to overcome the retentive force of the screw. There is always the risk of gingival inflammation and infection to any residual cement that is not removed after cementation of the provisional. There is no significant difference in implant survival or crown loss in the use of cemented versus screw-retained restorations.

33. What are indications for zygoma implants, quad zygoma implants, and nasopalatine implants?
    Zygoma implants are threaded titanium implants available in lengths up to 55 mm. Primary stability is achieved by engaging the cortices of the alveolar ridge crest, the maxillary sinus floor and roof, and the superior border of the zygoma. Zygoma implants were initially used for anchorage of obturator prostheses in patients with significant defects after ablative surgery or traumatic injuries and are still used today for this purpose. Zygoma implants were later applied to cases where vertical onlay grafting had failed. Bilateral single zygoma implants in conjunction with anteriorly placed implants have proven to be a successful alternative to extensive onlay grafting of the severely atrophic posterior maxilla, reducing or eliminating donor site morbidity and decreasing treatment and recovery time.

    The recommended protocol is placement of bilateral single zygomatic implants in combination with two to four anteriorly placed, standard endosseous implants. Prosthesis options include an implant-supported, full-arch fixed-removable prosthesis or a fixed prosthesis. The use of the zygomatic implants can reduce the number of implants needed as compared to a conventional eight-implant-supported fixed prosthesis. CT scans should be used to verify appropriate morphologic bone structure in the zygoma, maxillary sinus, and alveolus. Immediate fabrication of a temporary cross-arch–arch bar is necessary at the time of exposure to ensure cross-arch stabilization.

    In the severely atrophic maxilla where there is insufficient bone between the nasal cavity and maxillary sinus and extensive grafting is contraindicated, the use of two zygomatic implants bilaterally can be considered as an alternative option. The anterior zygoma implant may be engaged into the anterior rim of the lateral wall of the orbit.

The incisive canal may be used to insert an implant for added support for an overdenture in the case of an atrophic maxilla. The length of the incisive canal ranges from 4 to 26 mm and is usually 4 to 6 mm in diameter at the crest and 4 mm at the apex. Reflection of palatal tissue and removal of the nasopalatine nerve and branch of the greater palatine artery rarely cause complications with bleeding or significant sensory deficits.

34. **What are some implant options for treatment of the edentulous maxilla and mandible?**
Placement of at least four implants in the anterior maxilla is recommended for an implant-retained overdenture, as fewer than four implants will not resist the forces placed upon them. Implants are ideally placed bilaterally in the canine region and in the second premolar region to provide adequate A-P spread. Additional implants should be considered at the central incisor, lateral incisor, or incisive canal for additional retention, especially given that failure of one out of four implants may likely compromise restorability. Posterior support is provided by the denture base and palatal coverage should be similar to a complete denture. This concept of implants placed anterior to the maxillary sinus eliminates the need for sinus augmentation. Implants should be a minimum of 9 mm in length and 3.5 mm in diameter. Implants at the premolar site may be angled anteriorly to avoid violation of the maxillary sinus but must be within 30 degrees of draw with the other implants. Kiener et al. demonstrated 95.5% implant survival and 95% denture stability with overdentures retained with four to six implants.

If the patient desires a palateless prosthesis, six to eight implants may be placed and restored with a fixed implant-supported or removable prosthesis. Implants must be placed posteriorly for support. Maxillary sinus grafting may be indicated in these patients. Cone Beam CT (CBCT) scans can provide the necessary information including bony architecture, possible need for sinus or ridge augmentation, status of the sinus membrane, and presence of septae. A surgical guide constructed based on both adequate bone to accommodate the implants as well as the design of the planned restoration should be used to facilitate proper placement of the implants.

The edentulous mandible with bilateral posterior vertical alveolar ridge atrophy is a common clinical scenario that makes placement of posterior implants difficult without significant ridge augmentation that is not possible or desired in many cases. A minimum of two implants is necessary for support of an implant-retained, tissue-supported prosthesis. It is best to place these as far apart on the ridge as possible while avoiding the mental nerve. The All-on-4 concept restored with fixed full-arch prostheses has been demonstrated to be a viable treatment option with 94.8% implant survival rate at 10 years, and prostheses survival rate of 99.2%.

35. **Are antibiotics indicated when placing a single implant?**
A single preoperative dose of systemic antibiotic has been shown to reduce implant failure rate when controlled with a placebo group that did not receive an antibiotic. Systemic antibiotics have not, however, demonstrated a significant difference in infection rate. Existing studies have been unable to demonstrate a significant difference in prevention of implant failure or postoperative infection with various postoperative antibiotic regimens.

36. **What are some modalities for management of periimplantitis?**
Periimplantitis is an inflammatory process of the tissues around an osseointegrated implant in function that results in loss of the supporting bone. Presence of plaque, bleeding on probing, periimplant pocketing, radiographic bone loss, and purulent exudate are indicative of periimplantitis. The most common bacteria species found are anaerobic, gram-negative rods. Common organisms include *Porphyromonas gingivalis, Porphyromonas intermedia*, and *Actinobacillus actinomycetemcomitans*.

Commonly used treatment modalities include antiseptic treatment, systemic antibiotics, mechanical debridement, and guided tissue regeneration.

Antiseptic treatment consists of 0.1% to 0.2% chlorhexidine gluconate for 2 to 4 weeks. Systemic antibiotics can be utilized especially if purulence is found and is directed toward the commonly found anaerobic, gram-negative rods. Metronidazole is often the antibiotic of choice and can be combined with Amoxicillin.

There have been several techniques proposed for decontamination of the implant surface during debridement and regenerative procedures. Chlorhexidine gluconate application has been described and has produced variable results. Diode laser decontamination as an adjunct to conventional treatment of periimplantitis has been shown to increase implant survival. The air-powder abrasive technique or grit blasting has also been described in the literature, and several studies have shown no significant difference in success when compared to laser decontamination.

Nd:YAG lasers used at a low pulse energy have demonstrated the ability to decrease bacterial load and result in no damage to the implant surface when cooling devices are used. The LAPIP (Laser Assisted Periimplantitis Procedure) is a modification of the LANAP (Laser Assisted New Attachment Protocol) in that it is applied to implants. The procedure involves use of the laser to removed inflamed sulcular tissue and decontaminate the implant surface, followed by use of EMS piezo scaler. The result is decontamination of the implant surface with a blot clot that seals off the sulcus and prevents epithelial downgrowth.

37. What factors should be considered for immediate loading?
Patients who are transitioning from a dentate to edentulous state may benefit functionally and psychologically from immediately loaded restoration. Factors that cause instability or soreness with conventional dentures such as high muscle attachments, severe gag reflex, retruded tongue, and compromised hard and soft tissue anatomy should alert the clinician to explore the possibility of an immediately loaded restorative option.

Patient-related factors that would compromise either implant stability or wound healing must be considered. Examples of these factors include osteoporosis, diabetes, heavy smoking (>20 cigarettes/day), head and neck radiation, current chemotherapy or steroids, treatment with bisphosphonates or other antiresorptive agents, and parafunctional habits such as bruxism or clenching. Quality of the bone will also determine implant success as the dense type II bone of the anterior mandible increases primary stability and success in immediate loading.

Implants of at least 10 mm in length are recommended when immediate loading is considered. A minimum of four implants in the anterior mandible is required. If only four implants are to be used, the posteriormost implants may be angled posteriorly to avoid the inferior alveolar nerve and increase A-P spread to a minimum of 10 mm, which will prevent rocking of the denture. No posterior cantilevers should be used, as rocking of the prosthesis and resultant torqueing of the implants may occur. If possible, additional implants should be considered as they provide the advantages of superior load distribution among implants, and extra support should one or more of the implants not obtain adequate primary stability at insertion and require submergence or removal that may eliminate the possibility of immediate loading.

A minimum of six implants for a maxillary fixed implant-supported prosthesis is required. Ideally, additional implants are placed given the decreased bone quality found in the maxilla. As with the mandible, posterior cantilevers should be avoided, and additional implants should be included if possible.

Initial implant stability is critical and should ideally measure between 40 and 65 Ncm, and a minimum of 20 Ncm.

38. What are some advantages and disadvantages of wide diameter implants?
Advantages include:
- Can be used as a rescue implant when narrower implant fails to gain adequate stability
- Can be utilized for immediate implants
- Increased loading advantage due to increased surface area and compensate for poor bone density
- Minimize cantilevers for angled implants
- Improve emergence profile
- Decrease screw loosening and minimize component fracture

Disadvantages of wide diameter implants include:
- Increased surgical failure rate
- More easily placed too close to adjacent teeth or implants
- May result in decreased buccal bone thickness that can result in gingival recession or visualization of the dark color of the implant through gingiva

39. What are some challenges and disadvantages of placing a mandibular second molar implant?
- High bite force that can result in increased force on the implant, surrounding bone, abutment, and screw, and the coronal restoration itself
- Relatively higher position of inferior alveolar canal at that site
- Difficult access to perform adequate hygiene
- Limited access for correct implant body position and abutment screw placement
- The second molar contributes a small percentage to overall chewing efficiency.

BIBLIOGRAPHY

Adell R, Lekholm U, Rockller B, et al.: A 15-year study of osseointegrated implants in treatment of the edentulous jaw, *Int J Oral Surg* 18:387–416, 1981.

Albrektsson T, Brånemark P-I, Hansson HA, et al.: Osseointegrated titanium implants. Requirements for ensuring a long-lasting, direct bone-to-implant anchorage in man, *Acta Orthop Scand* 52:155–170, 1981.

Albrektsson T, Dahl E, Enbom L, et al.: Osseointegrated oral implants. A Swedish multicenter study of 8139 consecutively inserted Nobelpharma implants, *J Periodontol* 59:287–296, 1988.

Albrektsson CJ, Sennerby L: What is osseointegration? In Worthington P, Evans JR, editors: *Controversies in oral and maxillofacial surgery*, Philadelphia, 1997, Saunders.

Anderson G, Andreasson L, Bjelkengren G: Oral implant rehabilitation in irradiated patients without adjunctive hyperbaric oxygen, *Int J Oral Maxillofac Implants* 13:647–654, 1998.

Ata-Ali J, Ata-Ali F, Ata-Ali F: Do antibiotics decrease implant failure and postoperative infections? A systematic review and meta-analysis, *International J Oral & Maxillofac Surg* 43(1):68–74, 2014.

Bach G, Neckel C, Mall C, Krekeler G: Conventional versus laser-assisted therapy of periimplantitis: a five-year comparative study, *Implant Dent* 9(3):247–251, 2000.

Bagheri SC, Bell RB, Khan H: *Current therapy in oral and maxillofacial surgery*, St Louis, 2012, Elsevier Saunders.

Becker W, Becker BE, Alsuwyed K, et al.: Long-term evaluation of 282 implants in maxillary and mandibular molar positions. A prospective study, *J Periodontol* 70:896–901, 1999.

Block MS: *Color atlas of dental implant surgery*, ed 3, Maryland Heights, Missouri, 2011, Saunders Elsevier.

Bosker H, Jordon R, Sindet-Pedersen S, et al.: The transmandibular implant: a 13-year survey of its use, *J Oral Maxillofac Surg* 49:482–492, 1991.

Brånemark P-I: Introduction to osseointegration. In Brånemark P-I, Zarb G, Albrektsson T, editors: *Tissue integrated prostheses*, Chicago, 1985, Quintessence.

Brånemark P-I: *Precision, predictability*, Gothenburg, Sweden, 1990, Institute for Applied Biotechnology.

Brånemark P-I: et al.: Zygoma fixture in the management of advanced atrophy of the maxilla: technique and long-term results, *Scandanavian J Plast Reconstr Surg Hand Surg* 38:70–85, 2004.

Cosyn J, Eghbali A, De Bruyn H, et al.: Immediate single-tooth implants in the anterior maxilla: 3-year results of a case series on hard and soft tissue response and aesthetics, *J Clin Periodontol* 38:746–753, 2011.

de Waal YCM, Raghoebar GM, Huddleston SJJR, Meijer HJA, Winkel EG, Jan van WA: Implant decontamination during surgical peri-implantitis treatment: a randomized, double-blind, placebo-controlled trial, *J Clin Periodontol* 40:186–195, 2013.

Giannini R, Vassalli M, Chellini F, Polidori L, Dei R, Giannelli M: Neodymium: Yttrium aluminum garnet laser irradiation with low pulse energy: a potential tool for the treatment of peri-implant disease, *Clin Oral Implants Res* 17(6):638–664, 2006.

Gonçalves F, Zanetti AL, Zanetti RV, et al.: Effectiveness of 980-mm diode and 1064-nm extra-long-pulse neodymium-doped yttrium aluminum garnet lasers in implant disinfection, *Photomed Laser Surg* 28(2):273–280, 2010.

Hebel KS, Gajjar RC: Cement-retained versus screw-retained implant restorations: Achieving optimal occlusion and esthetics in implant dentistry, *J Prosthet Dent* 77(1):28–35, 1997.

Kaufman EG, Coelho DH, Colin L: Factors influencing retention of cemented gold castings, *J Prosthet Dent* 11:487–498, 1961.

Keller EE, Eckert SE, Tolman DE: Maxillary antral and nasal one-stage inlay composite bone graft: preliminary report on 30 recipient sites, *J Oral Maxillofac Surg* 52:438–448, 1994.

Kiener P, Oetterli M, Mericske E, Mericske-stern R: Effectiveness of maxillary overdentures supported by implants: maintenance and prosthetic complications, *Int J Prosthodontics* 14(2):133–140, 2001.

Kourkouta S: Implant therapy in the esthetic zone: smile line assessment, *Int J Periodontics Restorative Dent* 31(2):195–201, 2011.

Malo P, De Araujo Nobre M, Lopes A, Moss SM, Molina GJ: A longitudinal study of the survival of All-on-4 implants in the mandible with up to 10 years of follow-up, *J Am Dent Assoc* 142(3):310–320, 2011.

Misch CE: *Contemporary implant dentistry*, ed 3, St Louis, 2008, Mosby Elsevier.

Mobelli A, Lang NP: The diagnosis and treatment of periimplantitis, *Periodontology 2000* 17:63, 1998.

Noack N, Willer J, Hoffmann J: Long-term results after placement of dental implants: longitudinal study of 1964 implants over 16 years, *Int J Oral Maxillofac Implants* 14:748–755, 1999.

Sadowsky SJ: Immediate load on the edentulous mandible: treatment planning considerations, *J Prosthodontics* 19(8):647–653, 2010.

Scher ELC: Use of the incisive canal as a recipient site for root form implants: preliminary clinical reports, *Implant Dent* 3:38–41, 1994.

Schliephake H, Schmelzeisen R, Husstedt H, et al.: Comparison of the late results of mandibular reconstruction using nonvascularized or vascularized grafts and implants, *J Oral Maxillofac Surg* 57:944–950, 1999.

Schow SR, Parel SM: The zygoma implant. In Miloro M, Larsen P, Ghali GE, et al.: *Peterson's principles of oral and maxillofacial surgery*, ed 2, Hamilton, Ontario, 2004, B.C. Decker.

Sherif S, Susarla HK, Kapos T, Munoz D, Chang B, Wright R: A systematic review of screw- versus cement-retained implant-supported fixed restorations, *J Prosthodontics* 23(1):1–9, 2014.

Steinemann SG, Eulenberger J, Maeusli PA, et al.: Adhesion of bone to titanium, *Adv Biomater* 6:409, 1986.

Zarb G, Albrektsson T: Osseointegration: a requiem for the periodontal ligament? [editorial], *Int J Periodontal Rest Dent* 11:88, 1991.

CHAPTER 27

TRIGEMINAL NERVE INJURY

David W. Lui, A.Omar Abubaker, Kenneth J. Benson

1. What are the three major classifications of nerve injury?
   1. Seddon classification: neuropraxia, axonotmesis, neurotmesis
   2. Sunderland classification: first- to fifth-degree injury
   3. Mackinnon classification: classes 1 to 6

2. Can you describe the Seddon classification of nerve injury?
   See Table 27-1.

3. Can you describe the Sunderland classification of nerve injury?
   - First-degree injury: Damage is confined to within the endoneurium with no axonal degertion.
   - Second-degree injury: Damage extends through and includes the endoneurium with no significant axonal degeneration.
   - Third-degree injury: Damage extends to the perineurium.
   - Forth-degree injury: Damage to the entire fascicle that extends through the perineurium to the epineurium, but the epineurium remains intact. There is axonal, endoneurial, and perineurial damage with degeneration of the fascicles.
   - Fifth-degree injury: Complete or near complete transection of the nerve with epineurial discontinuity and likely neuroma formation.

4. What is a Mackinnon class 6 nerve injury?
   Mixed nerve injury involving a combination of the Sunderland types of nerve injuries.

5. What is Wallerian degeneration?
   Wallerian or anterograde degeneration is a series of molecular and cellular events triggered throughout the distal nerve stump and within a small reactive zone at the tip of the proximal stump. The primary histologic change involves cytoskeletal fragmentation of both axons and myelin.

6. What are the four types of neuroma based on gross morphology?
   Lateral adhesive neuroma, lateral exophytic neuroma, neuroma-in-continuity, and amputation neuroma.

7. What is dysesthesia?
   An unpleasant abnormal sensation that is either spontaneous or provoked.

8. What is the difference between analgesia and anesthesia?
   Analgesia is an absence of pain in response to stimulation that would normally be painful. Anesthesia is the absence of perception of stimulation by any noxious or nonnoxious stimulation of skin or mucosa. It is divided into general (central), regional, and local types.

9. What is allodynia?
   Allodynia is pain due to a stimulus that does not normally provoke pain. Unlike hyperalgesia, hyperpathia, and hyperesthesia, allodynia may include emotionally induced sensations in the nerve-injured patient.

10. What is anesthesia dolorosa?
    Anesthesia dolorosa is pain in an area or region that is anesthetic.

11. What is hyperalgesia?
    Hyperalgesia is an increased response to a stimulus that is normally painful.

12. What is hyperesthesia?
    Hyperesthesia is an increased sensitivity to any noxious or nonnoxious stimulation of skin or mucosa, excluding the special senses; it includes allodynia and hyperalgesia.

Table 27-1. Seddon Classification of Nerve Injury

	NEUROPRAXIA	AXONOTMESIS	NEUROTMESIS
Sunderland	I	II, III, IV	V
Nerve sheath	Intact	Intact	Interrupted
Axons	Intact	Some interrupted	All interrupted
Wallerian degeneration	None	Yes, some axons	Yes, all axons
Conduction failure	Transitory	Prolonged	Permanent
Spontaneous recovery	Complete	Partial	Poor to none
Time of recovery	Within 4 weeks	Months	None, if not begun by 3 months

Adapted from Meyer RA, Bagheri SC: Clinical evaluation of peripheral trigeminal nerve injuries, Atlas Oral Maxillofac Surg North Am 19:15–33, 2011.

13. **What are the symptoms of hyperesthesia?**
Patients describe a shooting, flashing, burning pain produced by normally nonpainful stimuli.

14. **What is hyperpathia?**
Hyperpathia is a painful syndrome characterized by increased reaction to a stimulus and increased threshold for response. It commonly is induced by repetitive mechanical pressures and characterized by faulty identification and localization of stimuli.

15. **What is hypoalgesia?**
Hypoalgesia is diminished pain response to a normally painful stimulus.

16. **What is paresthesia?**
Paresthesia is an abnormal sensation, either evoked or spontaneous, that is not necessarily unpleasant or painful, as in dysesthesia.

17. **What is sympathetically mediated pain (SMP)?**
SMP is throbbing, diffuse, and hyperalgesic pain perpetuated by abnormal reflex activity in sympathetic pathways following peripheral nerve injury. The classic syndromes of complex regional pain syndrome type I and II (formerly known as reflex sympathetic dystrophy and causalgia, respectively) are theorized to involve both peripheral and central mechanisms.

18. **What are the symptoms of SMP?**
The symptoms are often described as burning, hot, lancinating pain. Patients also complain of increased pain intensity during stressful periods.

19. **What is Tinel's sign?**
Tinel's sign is a provocative test of regenerating nerve sprouts in which light percussion over the nerve elicits a distal tingling sensation. It is used as a sign of small fiber recovery but is poorly correlated with functional recovery and easily confused with neuroma formation.

20. **What is deafferentation pain?**
Deafferentation pain is pain in a body region of partial or complete traumatic peripheral nerve deficit in which retrograde central neuropathy has occurred. Deafferentation mechanisms have been implicated in phantom pain, hyperpathia, and allodynia.

21. **How many axons and fascicles are in the inferior alveolar nerve?**
Approximately 7000 to 12,000 axons and 10 to 24 fascicles.

22. **What is the incidence of inferior alveolar and lingual nerve injury during removal of third molars?**
The incidence of inferior alveolar, lingual, and, less frequently, long buccal nerve injury during mandibular third molar removal ranges between 0.6% and 5.0%. In general, the incidence of inferior alveolar nerve (IAN) injuries is higher than that of the lingual nerve; in one study, incidence was 1.2% for the IAN and 0.9% for the lingual nerve. Factors such as age, surgical technique, and proximity of

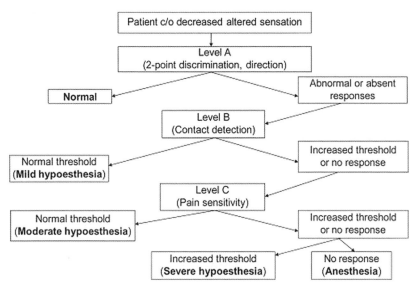

Figure 27-1. Neurosensory testing protocol for nerve injury patients with decreased sensation without dysesthesia. *(Modified from Meyer RA, Bagheri SC: Clinical evaluation of peripheral trigeminal nerve injuries,* Atlas Oral Maxillofac Surg North Am *19:15–33, 2011.)*

the nerve to the tooth influence the incidence of these injuries. More than 96% of patients with lingual nerve injuries recover spontaneously.

23. **What factors are associated with a higher incidence of lingual nerve injury during the course of third molar removal?**
Lingually angled impactions are especially vulnerable to nerve injury during their removal because of the erosion or absence of the lingual cortical plate by infection or cyst exposing the nerve directly to damage during instrumentation to remove the tooth.

24. **What is the average rate of an injured axon's forward growth?**
Approximately 1 to 2 mm/day.

25. **What are the potential clinical manifestations of a trigeminal nerve injury?**
    - Nonpainful anesthesia and hypoesthesia
    - Nonpainful hyperesthesia
    - Painful anesthesia and hypoesthesia
    - Painful hyperesthesia

26. **What is the recommended protocol for neurosensory testing in nerve injury patients with decreased sensation without dysesthesia?**
See Fig. 27-1.

27. **What is the recommended protocol for neurosensory testing in nerve injury patients with painful sensation?**
See Fig. 27-2.

28. **What is the recommended nonsurgical treatment of chronic trigeminal dysfunction and dysesthesia?**
See Fig. 27-3.

29. **How should open nerve injuries be managed?**
If an open injury is observed, it is best managed with immediate primary repair. Delayed primary repair is performed within the first few postoperative days. A delayed secondary repair is performed more than 3 weeks after injury.

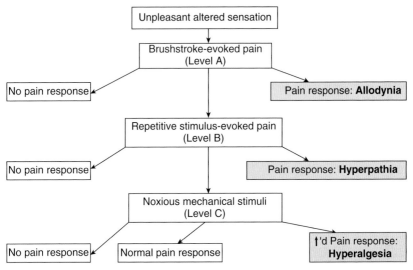

Figure 27-2. Neurosensory testing protocol for nerve injury patients with painful sensation. *(Modified from Meyer RA, Bagheri SC: Clinical evaluation of peripheral trigeminal nerve injuries, Atlas Oral Maxillofac Surg North Am 19:15–33, 2011.)*

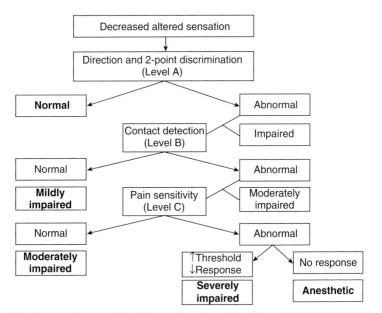

Figure 27-3. Nonsurgical treatment of chronic trigeminal dysfunction and dysesthesia. *NSAIDs,* Nonsteroidal antiinflammatory drugs; *TCAs,* tricyclic antidepressants; *TENS,* transcutaneous electrical neural stimulation. *(Modified from Allig CC, Schwartz E, Campbell RL, et al.: Algorithm for diagnostic assessment and surgical treatment of traumatic trigeminal neuropathies and neuralgias, Oral Maxillofac Surg Clin North Am 4:555, 1992.)*

30. **When should closed (unobserved) nerve injuries be addressed surgically?**
Unobserved nerve injuries should be repaired if the patient has:
- Intolerable anesthesia of more than 3 months
- Painful symptoms that persist more than 4 months that may be relieved with proximal anesthetic block
- Intolerable deterioration of sensation beyond 4 months and no improvement of sensation beyond 4 months

31. **What other method of nerve repair can be done if primary repair is not possible?**
An interpositional free nerve graft and nerve guidance.

32. **What are the general principles of delayed nerve repair?**
Repair must be completed without tension. First, extraneural decompression is performed to remove all irritative, foreign, or compressive forces from nerve contact. Next, the nerve must be inspected for continuity. If nerve continuity is seen, the nerve may be inspected with an epineural incision at the site of injury. Internal decompression (neurolysis) is performed and completed by closing the epineurium. If neuroma-in-continuity is too extensive, excision of neuroma along with part of the nerve is performed. A direct neurorrhaphy is performed in a tension-free manner.

33. **What are the types of nerve repair?**
- Epineural
- Perineural
- Group fascicular

34. **Which type of nerve repair is appropriate for the IAN?**
Mixed motor and sensory nerves are best treated with perineural and group fascicular suturing. The sensory IAN can be treated with the epineural suture technique.

35. **What does coaptation refer to in nerve repair?**
Bringing individual nerve fascicles into the best possible alignment. Direct neurorrhaphy can only be performed when the nerve is tension free.

36. **If a defect is too large for a direct neurorrhaphy of the IAN, which nerves may be considered as donors for free nerve graft?**
The sural, greater auricular, and median antebrachial nerves are considered.

37. **What factors govern the choice of donor site for free nerve repair?**
- Accessibility
- Length required
- Diameter of donor nerve compared with the host nerve
- Patient preference
- Fascicular number and pattern

38. **Which nerve is the best donor site for an interpositional graft for an IAN defect of approximately 25 mm?**
The sural nerve. The sural nerve can provide up to 30 mm of graft harvest. It provides sensation to the posterior and lateral aspects of the leg and foot. It also has up to 50% fewer axons and smaller axonal size than the IAN.

39. **Which free nerve may be used as a donor site for smaller defects (up to 15 mm long) of the IAN?**
The greater auricular nerve can be used for short gaps (up to 15 mm). This nerve graft is a good match with the IAN in terms of axonal size and axonal numbers. However, compared with the host nerve, the greater auricular nerve is half the diameter and has half the fascicles. A cable graft (two parallel strands) may be used to provide a better size match.

40. **How much nerve should be harvested for a nerve graft?**
Because of primary contracture, the length of the harvested nerve should be at least 25% longer than the defect.

41. **When is delayed nerve repair in the maxillofacial region indicated?**
If a wound is grossly contaminated or if the mechanism of injury may cause scarring of the proximal and distal ends. Examples of such injuries are blunt avulsion injuries such as gunshot wounds and injuries sustained in motor vehicle accidents.

Table 27-2. Success Rate of Microsurgical Repairs of Inferior Alveolar and Lingual Nerve Injuries

	PATIENTS	SUCCESS* (%)	RANGE (%)	SEM
Hypoesthetic				
• IAN	N = 192	85.4	66-94	3.68
• Lingual nerve	N = 131	87.0	50-91	5.66
Hyperesthetic				
• IAN	N = 124	55.6	25-80	7.01
• Lingual nerve	N = 74	67.5	50-100	6.82

*Success is defined as (1) minimum recovery of gross touch perception and (2) global pain reduction of >30%. Overall success rate (N = 521) is 76.2%.
SEM, Standard error of the mean; IAN, inferior alveolar nerve.
Adapted from LaBanc JP, Gregg JM: Trigeminal nerve injuries: basic problems, historical perspectives, early success, and remaining challenges, Oral Maxillofac Clin North Am 4:227–283, 1992.

42. **How is the term *anastomosis* applied to nerve injuries?**
    Trick question. *Anastomosis* is not appropriate nomenclature when discussing nerve repair. Vessels are anastomosed, and nerves are repaired or reconstructed.

43. **What type of suture material is most compatible for nerve repair?**
    An inert and nonresorbable suture material, such as 8-0 or 9-0 monofilament nylon (Ethilon) or polypropylene (Prolene).

44. **What potential alloplastic nerve conduits may be used in nerve reconstruction?**
    For guided nerve growth up to 3 mm, the following nerve guides may be used for repair:
    • Type I collagen tubes
    • Expanded polytetrafluoroethylene
    • Polyglycolic acid tubes

45. **What method is used for locating the great auricular nerve?**
    A line is drawn connecting the mastoid process and angle of mandible. A perpendicular line is then drawn to bisect the mastoid-mandible line. The great auricular nerve approximates this second line.

46. **What is the success rate of microsurgical repairs of inferior alveolar and lingual nerve injuries?**
    See Table 27-2.

47. **What is the most significant factor of functional neurosensory recovery?**
    Timing of surgical intervention.

BIBLIOGRAPHY

Allig CC, Schwartz E, Campbell RL, et al.: Algorithm for diagnostic assessment and surgical treatment of traumatic trigeminal neuropathies and neuralgias, Oral Maxillofac Surg Clin North Am 4:555, 1992.

Donoff R: Surgical management of interior alveolar nerve injuries (part 1): case for early repair, J Oral Maxillofac Surg 53:1327–1329, 1995.

Elusten K, Stevens M: Diagnosis and management of interior alveolar nerve injury, Compendium 16:1028–1038, 1995.

Greg J: Neurological complications of surgery for impacted teeth. In Alling CC, Helfric JF, Alling RD, editors: Impacted teeth, Philadelphia, 1993, Saunders.

Gregg J: Surgical management of inferior alveolar nerve injuries (part 2): case for delayed management, J Oral Maxillofac Surg 53:1330–1335, 1995.

Gregg JM: Nonsurgical management of traumatic trigeminal neuralgia and sensory neuropathies, Oral Maxillofac Surg Clin North Am 4:375–392, 1992.

LaBanc J: Reconstructive microneurosurgery of the trigeminal nerve. In Peterson LJ, et al.: Principles of oral and maxillofacial surgery, Philadelphia, 1992, Lippincott.

LaBanc JP, Gregg JM: Glossary, Oral Maxillofac Surg Clin North Am 4:563, 1992.

LaBanc JP, Van Bovan RW: Surgical management of inferior alveolar nerve injuries, Oral Maxillofac Surg Clin North Am 4:425–438, 1992.

Meyer RA, Bagheri SC: Clinical evaluation of peripheral trigeminal nerve injuries, *Atlas Oral Maxillofac Surg North Am* 19:15–33, 2011.

Miloro M: Microneurosurgery. In Miloro M, Gali GE, Larsen PE, Waite PD, editors: *Peterson's principles of oral and maxillofacial surgery*, Hamilton, ON, 2004, BC Decker.

Zuniga JR, Essick GK: A contemporary approach to the clinical evaluation of trigeminal nerve injuries, *Oral Maxillofac Surg Clin North Am* 4:353–367, 1992.

CHAPTER 28

OROFACIAL INFECTIONS AND ANTIBIOTIC USE

A. Omar Abubaker

1. **What is the source of the bacteria that cause the most odontogenic infections, and what is the incidence of these infections?**
Odontogenic infections are caused mostly by indigenous bacteria that normally live on or in the host. When such bacteria gain access to deeper tissues, typically in the majority of cases through decayed or nonvital teeth, they cause odontogenic infection.
    In a recent retrospective study of an 8-year period, the number of patients admitted for treatment of severe odontogenic infection represents 4% of all patients admitted to an OMFS service, with 1.7% requiring intensive medical and surgical therapy and a 0.012% mortality rate.

2. **What are the predominant bacteria found in the oral cavity?**
See Box 28-1.

3. **Which species of bacteria cause odontogenic infection?**
Most of the microorganisms associated with odontogenic infections are gram-negative rods (fusobacteria, bacteroides). Some are gram-positive cocci (streptococci and peptostreptococci), and 25% are aerobic, mostly gram-positive streptococci. About 60% are anaerobic bacteria. Almost all odontogenic infections are caused by multiple bacteria (an average of five species). *Fusobacterium* sp. is associated with severe infections (Fig. 28-1 and Table 28-1). In a recent study, 42 patients were treated with surgical incision and drainage and antibiotics. The specimens from all of these patients were sent for culture and sensitivity tests and for gram-positive and gram-negative aerobes. Forty microorganisms were isolated. There were 28 aerobes and 10 anaerobes. Two fungi were also identified. The most common bacteria isolated were *Staphylococcus aureus*, *Klebsiella*, *Escherichia coli*, and *Peptostreptococcus*. The key takeaway point here is that antibiotics alone cannot resolve odontogenic infection satisfactorily. Quick recovery of patients results from proper basic management including early drainage/decompression, which is equally important.

4. **Which staphylococci are clinically important to orofacial infections?**
Of the 23 species of staphylococci, only three are clinically important to orofacial infections: *Staphylococcus aureus*, *Staphylococcus epidermidis,* and *Staphylococcus saprophyticus.*

5. **What is coagulase? Which Staphylococcus species produces coagulase?**
Coagulase is an enzyme that coats the bacteria with fibrin and reduces the ability of the host cell to phagocytize it. *S. aureus* is the only coagulase-positive staphylococcus.

6. **What is the basis for microbiologic diagnosis of odontogenic infection?**
Initially, an empirical diagnosis of the causative organism of odontogenic infection is made based on the presumption of involvement of bacteria typical for the site (oral flora). The microbiologic diagnosis stems from this presumption and can be confirmed via Gram stain and culture.

7. **What is Gram staining? What is its clinical significance?**
Each specimen obtained from a patient with an infectious process initially should be stained according to the protocol developed by Hans Christian Joachim Gram. The process involves staining, decolorizing, and re-staining the specimen with a different stain. The organisms are categorized into one of four groups based on their stain retention and morphology: gram-positive cocci, gram-negative cocci, gram-negative rods, or gram-positive rods. Because Gram staining can be completed within a few minutes, it usually narrows the list of likely causative organisms immediately, whereas culture and sensitivity testing and biochemical identification may take 1 to 5 days to complete. After the staining process, organisms that retained their initial stain will remain violet (gram-positive), whereas those that lost their initial stain will be re-stained red (gram-negative).

Box 28-1. Predominant Bacteria Found in the Oral Cavity

Aerobes	Anaerobes
Gram-positive rods	Gram-positive rods
Corynebacterium	*Actinomyces*
Rothia	*Lactobacillus*
Diphtheroids	*Propionibacterium acnes*
Gram-negative rods	*Bifidobacterium*
Eikenella corrodens	*Eubacterium*
Haemophilus	*Clostridia*
Enterobacteriaceae	Gram-negative rods
Klebsiella	*Bacteroides*
Pseudomonas	*B. gingivalis*
Escherichia	*B. intermedius*
Gram-positive cocci	*B. endontali*
Streptococcus	*B. oralis*
Alpha-hemolytic	*B. melaninogenicus*
Strep. salivarius	*Fusobacterium*
Strep. mitior	*F. nucleatum*
Strep. sanguis	*Wolinella*
Strep. mutans	*Capnocytophaga*
Strep. milleri	Gram-positive cocci
Beta-hemolytic	*Peptostreptococcus*
Strep. pyogenes	*Streptococcus*
Enterococci	Gram-negative cocci
Staphylococcus	*Veillonella*
Staph. aureus	
Staph. epidermidis	
Gram-negative cocci	
Neisseria	
Branhamella	
Spirochetes	
Treponema	
Fungi	
Candida	

Adapted from Peterson LJ: Microbiology of head and neck infections, *Oral Maxillofac Surg Clin* 3:247–258, 1991.

8. **Are there any factors that predict successful treatment and hospital length of stay (LOS) of odontogenic infection in children?**
   In a recent study of 106 children with odontogenic infection, LOS was significantly shorter in patients who had a tooth extracted within 48 hours versus patients who had a tooth extracted at 48 hours or longer, and LOS was significantly shorter in patients with upper face and left face infections than lower face infections and right face infections, respectively. Patients with a primary first molar infection had the shortest LOS; patients with a white blood cell count less than 10,000 cells/mm^3 had shorter LOS.

9. **How do morphologic findings relate to bacterial categories?**
   See Table 28-2.

10. **What is the pattern of progression of odontogenic infections?**
    Early infection is often initiated by high-virulence aerobic organisms (commonly streptococci), which cause cellulitis, followed by mixed aerobic and anaerobic infections. As the infections become more chronic (abscess stage), the anaerobic bacteria predominate, and eventually the infections become exclusively anaerobic.

11. **What is cellulitis?**
    Cellulitis is a warm, diffuse, erythematous, indurated, and painful swelling of the tissue in an infected area. Cellulitis can be easy to treat but can also be severe and life threatening. Antibiotics and removal of the cause are usually sufficient. Surgical incision and drainage are indicated if no improvement is seen in 2 to 3 days, or if evidence of purulent collection is identified.

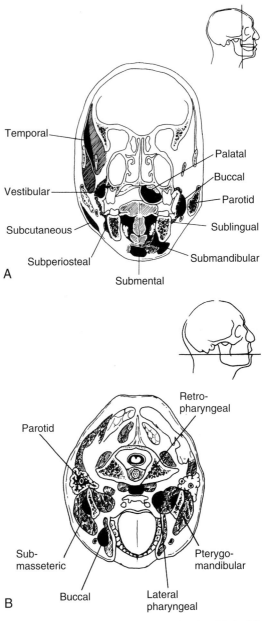

Figure 28-1. Anatomy of the deep space infections. **A,** Coronal, and **B,** Axial sections of the head showing most of the deep fascial spaces of the head and neck. *(Adapted from Eycleshymer AC, Schoemaker DM: Cross-section anatomy, New York, 1911, D. Appleton & Company.)*

Table 28-1. Species of Bacteria Responsible for Odontogenic Infections

ORGANISM	PERCENTAGE
Aerobic*	25
Gram-positive cocci	85
Streptococcus spp.	90
Streptococcus (group D) spp.	2
Staphylococcus spp.	6
Eikenella spp.	2
Gram-negative cocci (*Neisseria* spp.)	2
Gram-positive rods (*Corynebacterium* spp.)	3
Gram-negative rods (*Haemophilus* spp.)	6
Miscellaneous and undifferentiated	4
Anaerobic†	75
Gram-positive cocci	30
Streptococcus spp.	33
Peptococcus spp.	33
Peptostreptococcus spp.	33
Gram-negative cocci (*Veillonella* spp.)	4
Gram-positive rods	14
Eubacterium spp.	
Lactobacillus spp.	
Actinomyces spp.	
Clostridia spp.	
Gram-negative-rods	50
Bacteroides spp.	75
Fusobacterium spp.	25
Miscellaneous	6

*49 different species.
†119 different species.
Adapted from Peterson LJ: Principles of management and prevention of odontogenic infection. In Peterson LJ, Ellis E, Hupp J, et (eds): *Contemporary oral and maxillofacial surgery*, ed 2, St Louis, 1998, Mosby.

12. **What is an abscess?**
   An abscess is a pocket of tissue containing necrotic tissue, bacterial colonies, and dead white cells. The area of infection may or may not be fluctuant. The patient is often febrile at this stage. Cellulitis, which may be associated with abscess formation, is often caused by anaerobic bacteria.

13. **What is the difference between an abscess and cellulitis?**
   See Table 28-3.

14. **What are the signs and symptoms of a serious orofacial infection?**
   Serious infection occurs when the infection extends beyond the local area of infection and presents life-threatening systemic manifestations, including airway compromise, bacteremia, septicemia, fever, lethargy, fatigue, malaise, and dehydration. Swelling, induration, fluctuation, trismus, rapidly progressing infection, involvement of secondary spaces, dysphagia, odynophagia, and drooling are also signs and symptoms of serious orofacial infection.

15. **What factors influence the spread of odontogenic infection?**
   • Thickness of bone adjacent to the offending tooth
   • Virulence of the organism

Table 28-2. The Relation of Morphologic Findings to Bacterial Categories

MORPHOLOGIC FINDINGS	BACTERIAL SPECIES
Gram-positive cocci, single or clumps	*Micrococcus, Peptococcus, Staphylococcus*
Gram-positive cocci, pairs and chains	*Enterococcus, Peptostreptococcus, Streptococcus*
Gram-positive rods, large	*Bacillus, Clostridium*
Gram-positive rods, small	*Arachnia, Bacterionema, Bifidobacterium, Corynebacterium, Erysipelothrix, Eubacterium, Lactobacillus, Listeria, Propionibacterium*
Gram-positive rods, branching	*Actinomyces, Nocardia*
Gram-negative rods, large	Enterobacteriaceae
Gram-negative rods, thin, uniform	*Pseudomonas*
Gram-negative rods, small, coccobacillary	*Bacteroides, Bordetella, Brucella, Capnocytophaga, Cardiobacterium, Eikenella, Fusobacterium, Haemophilus, Pasteurella*
Gram-negative rods, nonspecific morphology	*Alcaligenes, Campylobacter, Cardiobacterium, Flavobacterium, Pectobacterium, Chromobacterium, Helicobacter, Vibrio, Yersinia*
Gram-negative cocci, pairs	*Acinetobacter, Moraxella, Neisseria*
Gram-negative cocci	*Veillonella*

Adapted from Bartlett RC: Laboratory diagnostic techniques. In Tobazian RG, Goldberg MH (eds): *Oral and maxillofacial infections*, ed 3, Philadelphia, 1994, Saunders.

Table 28-3. A Comparison of Cellulitis and Abscess

	CELLULITIS	ABSCESS
Duration	Acute	Chronic
Pain	Severe and generalized	Localized
Size	Large	Small
Localization	Diffuse borders	Well circumscribed
Palpation	Doughy to indurated	Fluctuant
Presence of pus	No	Yes
Degree of seriousness	Greater	Less
Bacteria	Aerobic	Anaerobic

Adapted from Peterson LJ: Principles of management and prevention of odontogenic infection. In Peterson LJ, Ellis E, Hupp J, et (eds): *Contemporary oral and maxillofacial surgery*, ed 2, St Louis, 1998, Mosby.

- Position of muscle attachment in relation to root tip
- Status of patient's immune system

16. **What are the *primary* fascial spaces?**
   The primary spaces are the spaces directly adjacent to the origin of the odontogenic infections. Infections spread from the origin of the infection into these spaces, which are:
   - Buccal
   - Submandibular
   - Canine
   - Submental
   - Sublingual
   - Vestibular

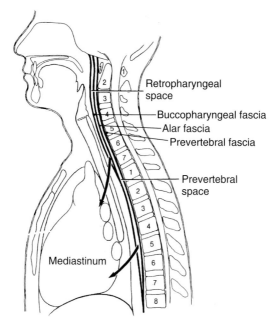

Figure 28-2. Retropharyngeal and prevertebral spaces, with the potential for spread of infection to the mediastinum from these spaces. *(From Peterson LJ: Odontogenic infections. In Cummings CW, Fredrickson JM, Harker LA, et al [eds]: Otolaryngology: head and neck surgery, ed 3, St Louis, 1998, Mosby.)*

17. **What are the *secondary* fascial spaces?**
    Fascial spaces that become involved following spread of infection to the primary spaces (Fig. 28-2). The secondary spaces are:
    - Pterygomandibular
    - Superficial and deep temporal
    - Infratemporal
    - Retropharyngeal
    - Masseteric
    - Masticator
    - Lateral pharyngeal
    - Prevertebral

18. **What is the danger space?**
    Also called space 4 of Grodinsky and Holyoke, it is the potential space between alar and prevertebral fascia. Its superior limit is the skull base, and it extends inferiorly into the posterior mediastinum.

19. **What are the seven spaces of Grodinsky and Holyoke in the head and neck?**
    1. Space 1: between platysma and investing fascia
    2. Space 2: between investing and infrahyoid fascia
    3. Space 2a: space among infrahyoid muscles
    4. Space 3: the pretracheal and retrovisceral spaces
    5. Space 4: danger space and between prevertebral and alar fascia
    6. Space 4a: between prevertebral and investing fascia above clavicle
    7. Space 5: space within prevertebral fascia

20. **Which teeth are likely to be the cause of space infections? What are the surgical approaches for incision and drainage of these spaces?**
    See Table 28-4 and Fig. 28-3.

Table 28-4. Teeth Likely to Cause Fascial Space Infections, with Surgical Approaches

FASCIAL SPACE OF SPACE	ANATOMIC BOUNDARIES OF SPACE	LIKELY SOURCE OF INFECTION	SWELLING SITE	SITE OF I & D
Canine	Between canine fossa, zygomaticus, orbicularis oris, levator labii superioris, and levator anguli oris	Maxillary canines, especially with very long roots and apex situated above attachment of muscles. May also be caused by central, lateral or premolar teeth.	Extraoral swelling just lateral to nose, obliterating nasolabial fold, and may extend upward, causing periorbital cellulitis. May be in labial sulcus.	Intraoral incision in horizontal direction in mucobuccal fold. Rarely, space is drained extraorally.
Buccal	Check area between buccinators and buccopharyngeal fascia medially, overlying skin laterally, zygomatic muscle and despressor muscles anteriorly, zygomatic arch superiorly, lower border of mandible inferiorly, and pterygomandibular raphe posteriorly	Upper premolars, upper molars, and lower premolars	Extraoral swelling over cheek area between inferior border of mandible and zygomatic arch. Typically, if inferior border of mandible palpable, it is buccal space; if inferior border is not palpable, then involved space is submandibular.	Intraoral by a transverse incision to depth of buccinator muscle passing through mucosa, submucosa, and buccinator muscle, avoiding injury to important anatomic structures, such as parotid duct. Drainage also accomplished by extraoral inscision near point of fluctuance below Stensen's duct.
Sublingual	Above mylohyoid muscle. Roof of space is mucosa of floor of mouth; floor is made by mylohyoid, genioglossus, geniohyoid, and styloglossus muscles, tongue, and lingual frenum (medial raphe).	From teeth of root apices above mylohyoid muscle attachment, namely lower premolars and sometimes first molars	Infection spread lingual in floor of mouth causing sublingual swelling involving contralateral side (because barrier between two sides is very weak)	Intraoral incision parallel to Worton's duct and lingual cortex in anteroposterior direction, as close as possible (within 1 cm) to lingual cortical bone because sublingual fold contains sublingual gland and ducts of submandibular gland. Intraoral-extraoral approach may be used.

Space	Boundaries	Source	Clinical features	Incision
Submandibular	Below mylohyoid muscle. Lies inferior to mylohyoid muscle; inferior boundary is anterior and posterior bellies of digastric muscles. Medially, mylohyoid hyoglossus and styloglossus muscles bound space. Lateral boundary is skin, superficial fascia, platysma muscle, superficial layer of deep cervical fascia, and lateral border of mandible.	Lower molars, especially lower second and third molars	Swelling mostly extraoral due to pus accumulation between skin and mylohyoid muscle. Swelling begins by obliterating inferior border of mandible, then extends medially to anterior belly of digastric and posterior to hyoid bone.	Through extraoral incision parallel to inferior border of mandible, kept at least 1 cm from border to avoid injury to mandibular branch of facial nerve, submandibular gland, facial artery, and lingual nerve
Submental	Between hyoid bone and symphysis, at site of attachment of anterior belly of digastric muscle. Roof of space is mylohyoid muscle, floor is skin, laterally is anterior belly of digastric muscle.	Lower incisors and canines, or from trauma such as symphyseal fracture	Mostly extraoral. Chin and submental areas swollen. Pus situated between digastric muscle, mylohyoid muscle, and skin. Rarely, there is submental swelling only. Usually submental and submandibular swelling because boundaries between two spaces are not definitive (only digastric muscle), so pus travels posteriorly to submandibular region.	Extraoral transverse incision midway between symphysis and hyoid bone.

Continued on following page

Table 28-4. Teeth Likely to Cause Fascial Space Infections, with Surgical Approaches—(Continued)

FASCIAL SPACE	ANATOMIC BOUNDARIES OF SPACE	LIKELY SOURCE OF INFECTION	SWELLING SITE	SITE OF I & D
Masseteric	Between outer surface of ascending ramus medially and masseter muscle laterally	Can spread from a buccal space infection site of attachment of buccinators muscle. Also from pericoronitis of lower third molars, or from fracture of angle of mandible.	Extraoral swelling over area occupied by masseter muscles, which is over ascending ramus and angle of mandible. Infection of this space characterized by trismus due to involvement of muscles of mastication.	Approximately 4-cm-long incision made below and behind angle of ascending ramus. Dissection carried through skin, superficial fascia, and platysma muscles. When inserting, artery forceps should remain in contact with outer aspect of ascending ramus. Incision can be used to approach two spaces (masseteric and pterygoid mandibular). Masseteric space can also be drained through an intraoral incision or a combined intraoral-extraoral approach.
Pterygomandibular	Between ascending ramus and medial pterygoid muscle medially; laterally is inner surface of ascending ramus. Superiorly, space bound by lateral pterygoid muscle, posteriorly by parotid gland, and anteriorly by pterygomandibular raphe and superior constrictor of pharynx.	Can result from infection of molar teeth, especially third molar; spread from infratemporal space, which communicates freely with pterygomandibular space; septic inferior dental nerve block with contaminated needle or solution; spread from pericoronitis; spread from submandibular space infection; spread from sublingual space	Intraoral swelling of mucosa over medial aspect of the ascending ramus. Extraorally, swelling is extremely rare, but if seen is found near mandibular angle area. Sometimes no extraoral swelling at all, only trismus due to involvement of medial pterygoid muscle, especially when infection is caused by inferior dental nerve block.	Can be drained extraorally at angle of mandible. When inserting, artery forceps should remain in contact with inner surface of ascending ramus. This space can also be drained through intraoral incision placed just medial to pterygomandibular raphe and by dissecting posteriorly along medial surface of ramus of mandible. Incision can also be used to drain lateral pharyngeal space and inferior portion of infratemporal space.

| Temporal | Muscle divides into two spaces: superficial temporal between temporalis muscle and temporal fascia, and deep temporal space (infratemporal space) between temporalis muscle and bony wall of skull medially. Temporal space is contiguous pterygomandibular and masseteric spaces. | Infection usually originates from upper and lower molars, or from extension of infection from masseteric or pterygo-mandibular spaces through infratemporal space, or from spread of infection from posterior superior alveolar nerve block | Extraoral swelling just behind lateral orbital rim and above zygomatic arch | Infection of this space is almost always associated with trismus; thus is difficult to approach intraorally. Extraoral approach more practical, but intraoral is preferred. Intraoral site for I & D is placed at anterior border of ascending ramus, with forceps inserted on outer aspect of ascend-ing ramus and directed up. Extraoral incision is through transverse incision starting slightly superior to zygomatic arch and extending posteriorly between lateral orbital rim and hairline. Incision is made parallel to it to avoid zygo-matic branch of facial nerve. |

Continued on following page

Table 28-4. Teeth Likely to Cause Fascial Space Infections, with Surgical Approaches—(Continued)

FASCIAL SPACE	ANATOMIC BOUNDARIES OF SPACE	LIKELY SOURCE OF INFECTION	SWELLING SITE	SITE OF I & D
Lateral pharyngeal	Inverted cone shape extending from base of skill to hyoid bone. Situated just medial to pterygomandibular space. Lateral wall made up of medial pterygoid muscle and superior constrictor muscle. Posteriorly, boundary is parotid gland, and anteriorly is pterygomandibular raphe. Medial wall is continuous with carotid sheath. Styloid process divides this space into two compartments: anterior compartment, which contains mainly muscles, and posterior compartment, which contains several important structures, namely carotid sheaths inside which are external carotid artery, internal jugular vein, and CN X. Outside sheaths are CN IX, XI, and XII.	Infection can result from infection of lower and upper molars by way of neighboring spaces, such as submandibular or pterygomandibular spaces. Can also result from nonodontogenic sources, such as palatine tonsils, infected parotid gland, and infected lymph nodes. If infection of this space is not treated at early stage, it can readily spread to retropharyngeal and prevertebral spaces.	Most common site is an intraoral swelling of lateral pharyngeal wall (very characteristic). Medial displacement of uvula and palatal draping may also be present. Extraoral lateral swelling of neck immediately below angle of mandible and anterior to anterior border of sternocleidomastoid muscle also possible.	Intraoral drainage of anterior compartment via a similar incision to that of intraoral incision for drainage of pterygomandibular space. Incision made through mucosa, and dissection directed medially and posteriorly along medial side of medial pterygoid muscle. Extraoral approach through horizontal incision made at level of hyoid bone just anterior to sternocleidomastoid. Dissection made superiorly and medially between submandibular gland and posterior belly of digastric muscle until medial surface of medial pterygoid muscle reached. Dissection carried along surface of muscle into space. Space can also be drained using through-and-through drainage.

| Retropharyngeal | Extending from base of skull superiorly to upper mediastinum inferiorly (level of C6 or T1 behind posterior pharyngeal wall). Anteriorly, space is bounded by posterior wall of pharynx, and posterior to it lies danger space, which communicates with posterior mediastinum. | Spreads from upper and lower molars by extension from lateral pharyngeal space by way of pterygomandibular, submandibular, or sublingual spaces. Retropharyngeal and lateral pharyngeal spaces separated by thin layer of fascia, which can easily rupture and cause spread of infection. Infection of retropharyngeal space may also result from nasal and pharyngeal infection in children, esophageal trauma, foreign bodies, and tuberculosis. | If able to visualize pharynx, bulge of posterior pharyngeal wall will be noticed—usually unilateral. Lateral soft tissue radiographs or CT will better delineate extent of swelling. | Extraoral approach by incision parallel to and along anterior border of sternocleidomastoid muscle below hyoid bone. Muscle and carotid sheath are retracted laterally, and a finger is inserted posterior to inferior constrictor. A soft noncollapsible rubber drain is inserted because of deep location of this space. |

CN, Cranial nerve; CT, computed tomography.

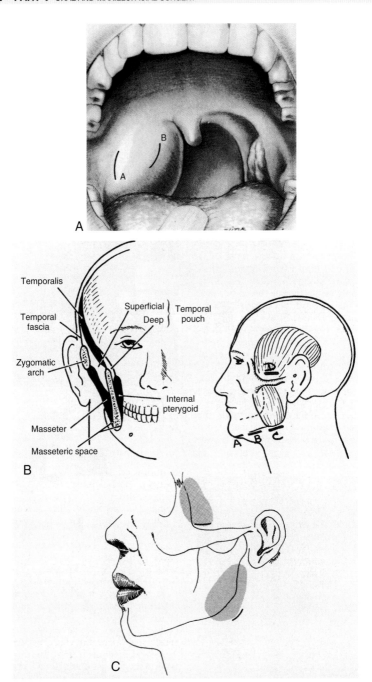

Figure 28-3. Typical sites of incision and drainage for various fascial space infections. **A,** Intraoral drainage of pterygoid compartment of masticator space (A) and lateral pharyngeal space (B). **B,** Masseteric, pterygoid, and temporal compartments of the masticator space. Incisions at B and C can be used to drain the submandibular space. **C,** Suggested locations for incision for extraoral drainage of temporal and lateral pharyngeal space infections. *(From Goldberg MH, Topazian RG: Odontogenic infections and deep fascial space infections of dental origin. In Topazian RG, Goldberg MH, editors: Oral and maxillofacial infections, ed 3, Philadelphia, 1994, Saunders.)*

21. **What imaging and laboratory studies are used for diagnosis of odontogenic infections?**
    - Radiographs are used to identify the cause of infection: periapical, occlusal, and panoramic views.
    - Imaging studies are used to identify the extent of infection and presence of purulent collection. The gold standard is computed tomography (CT) with contrast. In some instances, magnetic resonance imaging (MRI), soft tissue films, and ultrasound can be useful.
    - Lab studies are used to evaluate the immune system, white cell and differential counts, and culture and sensitivity from the infection site.

22. **What are the principles of therapy for odontogenic infection?**
    The important components in treatment of odontogenic infection are:
    - Determining the severity of infection
    - Determining whether the infection is at the cellulitis or abscess stage
    - Evaluating the state of the patient's host defense mechanisms
    Odontogenic infection is treated surgically, pharmacologically, or by medical support of the patient, including removing the source of infection; incision and drainage; and use of antibiotics, fluids, analgesics, and nutritional support.

23. **How is the severity of odontogenic infection determined?**
    By analyzing the history, physical findings, and results of lab and imaging studies.

24. **What are the different methods of drainage of odontogenic infections?**
    - Endodontic treatment
    - Extraction of the offending tooth
    - Incision and drainage of soft tissue collection

25. **What are the surgical principles of incision and drainage?**
    - Before incision, obtain fluid for culture through aspiration of pus using a syringe and needle.
    - Incise the abscess in healthy skin or mucosa and in a cosmetically or functionally acceptable place, using blunt dissection and thorough exploration of the involved space.
    - Use one-way drains in intraoral abscesses; use through-and-through drainage in extraoral cases.
    - Remove the drain gradually from deep sites.

26. **What is the percentage of oral bacteria resistant to commonly used antibiotics for treatment of odontogenic infection?**
    See Table 28-5.

27. **What should be reevaluated during the follow-up appointment after treating a patient for odontogenic infection?**
    - Response to treatment (subjective improvement of pain and other subjective symptoms)
    - Toxicity reactions to antibiotics
    - Recurrence of infection
    - Secondary infection (e.g., *Candida*)
    - Presence of allergic reactions

Table 28-5. Percentage of Oral Bacteria Resistant to Commonly Used Antibiotics

	ORAL BACTEROIDES	FUSOBACTERIA	ANAEROBIC COCCI	ALPHA-STREPTOCOCCI
Penicillin	15-30	6	4	0
Erythromycin	0	85	18	0
Clindamycin	4	0	2	0
Metronidazole	0	0	24	100
Cephalexin	10	0	6	18

Adapted from Peterson LJ: Microbiology of head and neck infections, *Oral Maxillofac Surg Clin* 3:255, 1991.

28. **What are the principles of antibiotic use?**

When choosing a specific antibiotic as part of treatment of odontogenic infection, adhere to the following principles:

- Use the correct and narrow-spectrum antibiotic.
- Use the least toxic drug with the fewest side effects.
- Use bactericidal drugs whenever possible.
- Be aware of drug cost.
- Ensure effective oral administration through the use of proper dose and proper dosage interval.
- Continue the antibiotic for an adequate length of time.
- Administer the antibiotics through the proper route.

29. **What are the most commonly used antibiotic formulations for oral and maxillofacial infections?**

See Table 28-6.

Table 28-6. Formulations for Antibiotics Commonly Used in Oral and Maxillofacial Infections

DRUG	TYPES	FORMULATIONS	UNIT DOSE
Penicillin G			
Potassium	Generic, Pfizerpen	Vial for IM, IV	1-, 5-, and 20-million U
Sodium generic	Vial for IM, IV	5-million U	
Repository	Bicillin CR	Vial for IM	300-600,000 U/mL
Penicillin V	Generic, Betapen	Tablets	250, 500 mg
	VK, Pen Vee K, Veetids	Oral solution	125, 250 mg/5 mL
Ampicillin	Generic, Omnipen,	Capsules	250, 500 mg
	Polycillin,	Oral suspension	250 mg/5 mL
	Principen	Pediatric drops	100 mg/mL
		Vial	125, 250, 500, 1000, 2000 mg
Amoxicillin	Generic, Amoxil,	Capsule	250, 500 mg
	Polymox, Trimox,	Oral suspension	125, 250 mg/5 mL
	Wymox	Pediatric drops	50 mg/mL
Amoxicillin- clavu-lanate	Augmentin	Tablets	250, 500 mg
		Tablets (chewable)	125, 250 mg
		Oral suspension	125, 250 mg/5 mL
Oxacillin	Generic, Prostaphlin	Capsules	250, 500 mg
		Oral solution	250 mg/5 mL
		Vials for IM, IV	250, 500, 1000 mg
Dicloxacillin	Generic, Dynapen,	Capsules	250, 500 mg
	Pathocil	Oral suspension	62.5 mg/5 mL
Cephalexin	Generic, Keflex	Capsules/Pulvules	250, 500 mg
		Tablets	250, 500, 1000 mg
		Oral suspension	125, 250 mg/5 mL
		Pediatric drops	100 mg/mL
Cephradine	Generic, Anspor,	Capsules	250, 500 mg
	Velosef	Oral suspension	125, 250 mg/5 mL
		Vial for IM, IV	250, 500, 1000 mg

Table 28-6. Formulations for Antibiotics Commonly Used in Oral and Maxillofacial Infections

DRUG	TYPES	FORMULATIONS	UNIT DOSE
Cefazolin	Generic, Ancef, Kefzol	Vial for IM, IV	250, 500, 1000 mg
Cefaclor	Ceclor	Pulvules	250, 500 mg
		Oral suspension	125, 250 mg/5 mL
Cefoxitin	Mefoxin	Vial for IM, IV	1000 mg
Erythromycin			
Base	Generic, ERYC, Ilotycin, E-mycin, Ery-Tab	Tablets	250, 500 mg
Estolate	Generic, Ilosone	Tablets	250, 500 mg
		Tablets (chewable)	125 mg
		Oral suspension	125, 250 mg/5 mL
		Pediatric drops	100 mg/mL
Ethylsuccinate	Generic, EES, Ery Ped, Eryzole, Pediamycin	Tablets	400 mg
		Tablets (chewable)	200 mg
		Oral suspension	200, 400 mg/5 mL
		Pediatric drops	100 mg/2.5 mL
Clindamycin	Generic, Cleocin	Capsules	75, 150, 300 mg
		Oral solution	75 mg/5 mL
		Vial for IM, IV	250, 500, 750 mg
Chloramphenicol	Chloromycetin	Capsule	250 mg
		Oral suspension	150 mg/5 mL
		Vial for IV	1000 mg
Vancomycin	Generic, Vancocin	Capsules	125, 250 mg
		Oral solution	250 mg/5 mL
		Vial for IV	500, 1000 mg
Metronidazole	Generic, Flagyl, Protostat	Tablets	250 mg
		Vial for IV	500 mg
Nystatin	Generic, Mycostatin, Nilstat	Tablets	500,000 U
		Oral suspension	100,000 U/mL
		Pastilles	200,000 U
Clotrimazole	Mycelex	Troche	10 mg
Ketoconazole	Nizoral	Tablets	200 mg
Acyclovir	Zovirax	Capsules	200 mg
		Ointment	5% concentration
		Vial for IV	500 mg

IM, Intramuscular; IV, intravenous.
Adapted from Hupp JR: Antibacterial, antiviral, and antifungal agents, *Oral Maxillofac Surg Clin* 3:273–286, 1991.

30. What is the minimal inhibitory concentration (MIC) of antibiotics?

MIC is a measure of sensitivity of bacteria. For an antibiotic to have maximum antibiotic efficacy in treatment of specific infections, the concentration of the antibiotic at the site of infection should be 3 to 4 times the MIC. Concentrations >4 times the MIC are not more effective.

31. What is the beta-lactam group of antibiotics?

These antibiotics, which have in common a beta-lactam ring in their structures, comprise three classes: penicillins, cephalosporins, and carbapenems. Penicillins and cephalosporins encompass many different antibiotics that are commonly used for odontogenic infection. Imipenem is an example of the carbapenems.

32. What was the first carbapenem to be used clinically?

Imipenem was the first clinically available carbapenem. It has the broadest antibacterial activity of any currently used systemic antibiotic and, therefore, is reserved for use in treatment of severe head and neck infections.

33. What is the mode of action of penicillin?

Penicillin affects bacteria by two mechanisms:
1. It inhibits bacterial cell wall synthesis.
2. It activates endogenous bacterial autolytic processes that cause cell lysis. The bacteria must be actively dividing, and the cell wall must contain peptidoglycans for this action. Penicillin inhibits enzymes necessary for cell wall synthesis.

34. How do bacteria build up resistance to antibiotics?

An antibiotic's ability to penetrate cell walls and bind to enzymes plays an essential role in resistance of antibiotics. Specifically, bacteria build resistance by two mechanisms:
1. Alteration in cell wall permeability to prevent antibiotics from inhibiting peptidoglycan synthesis
2. Bacterial production of beta-lactamase that causes beta-lactams to become ineffective

35. What are the pediatric and adult dosages for the most commonly used antibiotics?

See Table 28-7.

36. What is the antimicrobial spectrum of the most common antibiotics used in treatments for oral and maxillofacial infections?

See Table 28-8.

37. When should antibiotics be used?
- Acute-onset infection
- Involvement of fascial spaces
- Diagnosed osteomyelitis of the jaw
- Patients with compromised host defences
- Infection with diffuse swelling
- Severe pericoronitis

38. When are prophylactic antibiotics for prevention of odontogenic infections not necessary?

Antibiotics have minimal or no benefits in the treatment of chronic well-localized abscess, minor vestibular abscess, dry socket, and root canal sterilization.

39. What are the indications for prophylactic antibiotics?
- To prevent local wound infection
- To prevent infection at the surgical site causing local wound infection
- To prevent metastatic infection at a distant susceptible site due to hematogenous bacterial seeding from the oral flora (e.g., subacute bacterial endocarditis, prosthetic joint replacement) following oral surgical procedures

40. When are prophylactic antibiotics indicated for prevention of local wound infection?
- When the procedure to be performed has a high incidence of infection
- When infections may have grave consequences
- When the patient's immune system is compromised
- When the surgical procedure lasts longer than 3 hours
- When the surgical procedure has a high degree of contamination

Table 28-7. Pediatric and Adult Antibiotic Dosages

ANTIBIOTIC	ROUTE(S) OF ADMINISTRATION	ADULT DOSE	PEDIATRIC DOSE/ DAY
Penicillin G	IM, IV	6-12 × 10 U/4 hr	100,000 U/kg ÷ 3
Penicillin V	PO	500 mg qid	50 mg/kg ÷ 3 or 4
Ampicillin	PO, IM, IV	500 mg qid PO	25 mg/kg ÷ 4
Amoxicillin	PO	250 mg qid PO	25 mg/kg ÷ 3
Amoxicillin-clavulanate	PO	250-500 mg tid	20 mg/kg ÷ 3
Oxacillin	IM, IV	500-1000 mg q6h	50-200 mg/kg ÷ 4
Dicloxacillin	PO	250-500 mg q6h	12.5-50 mg/kg ÷ 4 or 5
Cephalexin	PO	500 mg qid	25-50 mg/kg ÷ 4
Cephradine	PO, IV	500 mg qid	25-50 mg/kg ÷ 3
Cefazolin	IM, IV	1 g q8h	25-50 mg/kg ÷ 3 or 4
Cefaclor	PO	500 mg q6h	20 mg/kg ÷ 3
Cefoxitin	IM, IV	500 mg q6h	80-160 mg/kg ÷ 4 or 5
Erythromycin	PO, IV	500 mg qid	40 mg/kg ÷ 4
Clindamycin	PO, IM, IV	300-450 mg q6h	10-20 mg/kg ÷ 4
Chloramphenicol	PO, IV	500-750 mg q6h PO	75-100 mg/kg ÷ 4
Vancomycin	IV	500 mg q6h	50 mg/kg ÷ 4
Metronidazole	PO	500 mg tid	30-40 mg/kg
Nystatin	Topical, PO	0.5-2 million U/day ÷ 2-4	Infants: 800,000 U ÷ 4 Older children: 1.6 million U ÷ 4
Clotrimazole	Topical	10 mg × 5 times/day	<3 yr: Safety not established ≥3 yr: 10 mg × 5 times/day
Ketoconazole	PO	200-400 mg qd	3.3-6.6 mg/kg
Acyclovir	Topical, PO, IV	600 mg ÷ 3 PO 15 mg/kg ÷ 3 IV	Safety in children not established

IM, Intramuscular; IV, intravenous; PO, orally; qid, four times a day; tid, three times a day; q6h, every 6 hours; q8h, every 8 hours; qd, daily.
Adapted from Hupp JR: Antibacterial, antiviral, and antifungal agents, *Oral Maxillofac Surg Clin* 3:273–286, 1991.

41. What is the antibiotic of choice for treatment of odontogenic infection?
    The empiric therapy is **penicillin** or penicillin plus metronidazole, if the patient is not allergic to antibiotics and is not immunocompromised. In patients who are allergic to penicillin, **clindamycin** is an excellent alternative. Definitive antibiotic therapy should be based on culture and sensitivity.

42. What is the mechanism of action, route of excretion, and spectrum of the most commonly used antibiotics for oral and maxillofacial infection?
    See Table 28-9.

43. What are the possible causes of failure of antibiotic therapy?
    • Inadequate surgical treatment
    • Depressed host defences

Table 28-8. Antimicrobial Spectrum of Common Antibiotics Used in the Treatment of Oral and Maxillofacial Infections

ANTIBIOTIC	SPECTRUM	ANTIBIOTIC	SPECTRUM
Penicillin	*Streptococcus* (except group D) *Staphylococcus* (non–beta-lactamase– producing) *Treponema* *Actinomyces* Oral anaerobes	Erythromycin	*Streptococcus* *Staphylococcus* *Mycoplasma* *Haemophilus* *influenzae* *Legionella*
Ampicillin and amoxicillin	Same as penicillin plus: *Escherichia coli* *H. influenzae* *Proteus mirabilis*	Clindamycin	Oral anaerobes *Streptococcus* *Staphylococcus* *Actinomyces* *Bacteroides fragilis*
Amoxicillin plus clavulanate	Same as ampicillin plus: *Klebsiella* *Staphylococcus aureus* *Staphylococcus epidermidis* *Enterococci* *Gonococci*	Chloramphenicol	Oral anaerobes *Streptococcus* *Staphylococcus* *H. influenzae* *E. coli* *Salmonella* *Shigella* *Rickettsia*
Oxacillin and dicloxacillin	Beta-lactamase–producing staphylococci		*Bacteroides fragilis* Oral anaerobes
Cephalexin, cephradine, and cefazolin	*Streptococcus* (except group D) *Staphylococcus* *E. coli* *Proteus mirabilis* *Klebsiella*	Vancomycin	*Streptococcus* *Staphylococcus*
		Metronidazole	Oral anaerobes
Cefaclor	Same as cephalexin plus: *H. influenzae*		
Cefoxitin	Same as cephalexin plus: *Enterobacter* *Bacteroides fragilis* Oral anaerobes		

Adapted from Peterson LJ: Principles of antibiotic therapy. In Tobazian RG, Goldberg MH, editors: *Oral and maxillofacial infections*, ed 3, Philadelphia, 1994, Saunders.

- Presence of foreign body
- Problems associated with use of antibiotics (e.g., patient compliance, inadequate dose, antibiotic-related infection, use of wrong antibiotic)

44. **What is antibiotic-associated colitis (AAC)?**
AAC is a toxic reaction associated with the use of an antibiotic that causes alteration of colonic flora leading to the overgrowth of *Clostridium difficile*. The toxins from *C. difficile* cause pseudomembranous colitis or AAC, which is manifested clinically as profuse, watery diarrhea that may be bloody; cramping; abdominal pain; fever; and leukocytosis.

45. **What are the risk factors for AAC?**
Risk factors associated with AAC are related to the type of antibiotic and patient-related factors. Clindamycin, which originally was thought to be the main antibiotic associated with AAC, has now been recognized to be associated with only one-third of cases. Ampicillin is associated with one-third,

Table 28-9. Profiles of the Most Commonly Used Antibiotics for Oral and Maxillofacial Infection

	PENICILLIN V	ERYTHROMYCIN	CLINDAMYCIN	CEPHALEXIN	CEFADROXIL	METRONIDAZOLE	DOXYCYCLINE	AMOXICILLIN	NYSTATIN
Bactericidal or bacteriostatic	Bactericidal	Bacteriostatic	Both	Bactericidal	Bactericidal	Bactericidal	Bacteriostatic	Bactericidal	Bactericidal
Spectrum	Streptococci, oral anaerobes	Gram-positive cocci, oral anaerobes	Gram-positive cocci, anaerobes	Gram-positive cocci, some gram-negative rods, oral anaerobes	Gram-positive cocci, some gram-negative rods, oral anaerobes	Anaerobes	Gram-positive cocci, some gram-negative rods, oral anaerobes	Gram-positive cocci, *E. coli*, H. influenzae, oral anaerobes	*Candida* organisms
Dose-interval	250-500 mg qid	250-500 mg qid	150-300 mg q6h	500 mg qid	500 mg bid	250 mg qid	100 mg bid	250 mg tid	200,000 U lozenge qid
Metabolized	Kidney	Liver	Liver	Kidney	Kidney	Liver	Liver	Kidney	
Toxicity and side effects	Allergy	Nausea, vomiting, cramping, diarrhea	Nausea, vomiting, cramping, diarrhea, antibiotic-associated colitis	Allergy, antibiotic-associated colitis	Allergy, antibiotic-associated colitis	Nausea, vomiting, cramping, diarrhea, disulfiram-like effect	Teeth coloration, photo-sensitivity, nausea, vomiting, diarrhea	Allergy, antibiotic-associated colitis	
Primary indication	Drug of choice	Useful alternative for mild infection	Useful alternative, especially for resistant anaerobes	Bactericidal drug required	Bactericidal drug required	Only anaerobic bacteria involved	Broad-spectrum in mild infections	Broader spectrum needed	Candidosis

qid, Four times a day; bid, twice a day; q6h, every 6 hours; tid, three times a day.
Adapted from Peterson LJ: Principles of management and prevention of odontogenic infection. In Peterson LJ, Ellis E, Hupp J, et al., editors: *Contemporary oral and maxillofacial surgery*, ed 2, St Louis, 1993, Mosby.

and the cephalosporins are associated with the last third. Patient-related factors for AAC include previous gastrointestinal procedures, medically compromised patients, advanced age, female gender, inflammatory bowel disease, cancer chemotherapy, and renal disease.

46. **What is the diagnosis of and treatment for AAC?**
In addition to the clinical signs and symptoms, the diagnosis of AAC is usually made based on positive *C. difficile* culture and *C. difficile* toxin in the patient's stool. Sigmoidoscopy is occasionally used to confirm the diagnosis. Treatment includes discontinuation of the causative antibiotics, use of alternate antibiotics if necessary, restoration of fluid and electrolyte balance, and administration of anticlostridial antibiotics. The usual choice is oral vancomycin or oral metronidazole.

47. **What is Ludwig's angina?**
Ludwig's angina is bilateral, brawny, board-like induration of the submandibular, sublingual, and submental spaces due to infection of these spaces. The term *angina* is used because of the respiratory distress caused by the airway obstruction. This obstruction can occur suddenly, due to the possible extension of the infection from the sublingual space posteriorly to the epiglottis, causing epiglottis edema.

48. **How is Ludwig's angina treated?**
The principles of treatment of Ludwig's angina are early diagnosis, prompt surgical intervention, and definitive airway management. After securing an airway, surgical drainage of each individual space should begin even before fluctuance becomes palpable externally. Appropriate antibiotics and management of the host defense mechanism are also important.

49. **What is erysipelas?**
Erysipelas is a superficial cellulitis of the skin that is caused by beta-hemolytic streptococci and by group B streptococci. It usually presents with warm, erythematous skin and spreads rapidly from release of hyaluronidase by the bacteria. It is associated with lymphadenopathy and fever and has an abrupt onset with acute swelling. It may affect the skin of the face. Treatment consists of parenteral penicillin.

50. **What is cervicofacial necrotizing fasciitis?**
Cervicofacial necrotizing fasciitis is a very aggressive infection of the skin and superficial fascia of the head and neck and is commonly seen in diabetic and immunocompromised patients. It carries a high mortality rate from sepsis of the dead tissue in the affected area. The etiologic factors of cervicofacial necrotizing fasciitis include odontogenic infections; burns; cuts; abrasions; contusions; peritonsillar abscess and boils of the head and neck region; surgery; and trauma.

51. **Which organisms are involved in necrotizing fasciitis of the head and neck?**
The causative organisms of necrotizing fasciitis include aerobes and obligate anaerobes in synergistic combinations. In a study of 16 patients with necrotizing fasciitis, two distinctive types of bacterial findings were found. Both types had identical clinical presentations. **Type I** patients had anaerobic and facultative anaerobic bacteria, such as Enterobacteriaceae and streptococci other than group A. **Type II** patients had group A streptococci (pyogenous) alone or in combination with anaerobic bacteria. Group A streptococci and staphylococci were not isolated from type I patients.

52. **What are the clinical features of necrotizing fasciitis of the head and neck?**
The initial presentation of necrotizing fasciitis is usually deceivingly benign, although the extent of tissue and fascial destruction far exceeds the external evidence of infection. The rate of infection is usually rapid, and the patient often has a concomitant systemic disease, such as diabetes mellitus, arteriosclerosis, obesity, malnutrition, or alcoholism.
The clinical features of this condition are usually manifested as smooth, tense, and shiny skin, with no sharp demarcation in the area involved. As the disease progresses, the pathognomonic signs of the condition include dusky purplish discoloration of the skin, small purplish patches with ill-defined borders, formation of blisters or bullae, subcutaneous fat, necrosis of the fascia, and gangrene of the overlying skin. Typically, the drainage in these patients yields "dishwater"—a purplish, foul-smelling discharge. Systemic features of necrotizing fasciitis include sepsis, hypotension, hypertension, hyperpyrexia, jaundice, and hemoglobinuria.

53. **What is the treatment for necrotizing fasciitis?**
Treatment for necrotizing fasciitis includes antibiotics, fluid replacement, nutrition, and daily debridement to remove devitalized tissues. However, the cornerstone of treatment is debridement of the necrotic tissue and daily monitoring to assure adequate removal. Appropriate antibiotics and medical

support are also important. Medical support includes fluid and electrolyte replacement, monitoring of the intravascular volume, and management of the underlying medical condition. Hyperbaric oxygen treatment has also been suggested for promotion of vascularization of infected tissue.

After resolution of infection, the resulting soft tissue defect is reconstructed with a skin graft and/or regional or local tissue flaps. Penicillin, clindamycin, and aminoglycosides are effective antimicrobial agents for this condition.

54. **What is the associated morbidity of cervicofacial necrotizing fasciitis?**
The mortality rate of cervicofacial necrotizing fasciitis approaches 28% and when associated with extension into the mediastinum and sepsis, rates as high as 41% and 64% have been reported, respectively. Some of the reported predisposing factors associated with the development of cervicofacial necrotizing fasciitis include diabetes mellitus, poor dental hygiene, obesity, alcoholism, and immunocompromised states.

55. **What are the common granulomatous infections with recognized head and neck manifestations?**
See Table 28-10.

56. **What are the classifications of salivary gland infections?**
Salivary gland infections can be classified based on clinical, microbiologic, or mechanical causes. Accordingly, they are classified as **acute or chronic**, bacterial or viral, and obstructive or nonobstructive (involvement by systemic granulomatous diseases). The **bacterial and viral** infections include mumps and acute, chronic, and recurrent sialadenitis. The **obstructive** infections include sialolithiasis, mucous plugs, stricture/stenosis, and foreign bodies. Systemic granulomatous infections (**nonobstructive**) include tuberculosis, actinomycosis, fungal infections, and sarcoid.

57. **Which studies should be included in evaluation of chronic salivary gland infection?**
Complete blood count with differential, Gram stain, and culture and acid-fast staining of the salivary secretions are all useful in evaluating patients with salivary gland infection. Plain films (occlusal and

Table 28-10. Common Granulomatous Infections with Head and Neck Manifestations

DISEASE	CAUSATIVE ORGANISM	TYPICAL CLINICAL APPEARANCE
Actinomycosis	*Actinomyces israelii* (anaerobic gram-positive bacillus)	Painless, slowly enlarging soft tissue cervicofacial infection with fistulae
Cat scratch disease	Unnamed gram-negative bacillus	Indolent regional lymphadenitis
Glanders	*Pseudomonas mallei* (gram-negative bacillus)	Farcy: draining facial abscesses, lymphadenopathy
Leishmaniasis	Leishmania (protozoal parasite)	Mucocutaneous ulcerations
Leprosy	*Mycobacterium leprae* (acid-alcohol-fast bacillus)	Facial leproma, nasomaxillary destruction, paresthesia of V2 and VII
Scleroma	*Klebsiella rhinoscleromatis* (gram-negative bacillus)	Chronic destructive lesion of nasomaxillary complex
Syphilis (tertiary)	*Treponema pallidum* (spirochete)	Gumma of soft tissue or bone
Tuberculosis	*Mycobacterium tuberculosis* (acid-fast aerobic bacillus)	Scrofula: indolent cervical lymphadenitis, ulcerations of palate or tongue
Tularemia	*Francisella tularensis* (gram-negative coccobacillus)	Oropharyngeal ulcerations

Adapted from Wood RS: Chronic granulomatous infections, *Oral Maxillofac Surg Clin* 3:405–422, 1991.

panoramic view), sialography, CT, MRI, ultrasonography, and scintigraphy of the gland are useful in showing tissue changes of the salivary gland tissue. Chest X-ray, tuberculin test, and salivary gland biopsy may be necessary when involvement of the gland by systemic disease is suspected.

58. **What is the treatment of sialadenitis?**
If stones are present in the submandibular gland duct, a ductoplasty is indicated. If the stones are large, beyond the mylohyoid flexure of the duct, or intraglandular, the gland must be removed. Parotid gland infection is more serious and must be drained or treated by superficial parotidectomy. Antibiotics should be administered to cover *Streptococcus* and *Staphylococcus* spp. *Escherichia coli* and *Haemophilus influenzae* are also occasionally implicated. Hydration with intravenous (IV) fluid, especially in the elderly and children, is often a necessary part of the treatment of acute sialadenitis.

59. **What are the most commonly used antibiotics for treatment of salivary gland infection?**
Empirically, or if Gram stain shows gram-positive cocci, administration of penicillinase-resistant antistaphylococcal antibiotics, such as methicillin, is advisable. In patients who have a history of allergy to penicillin, cephalosporins can be used. Aminoglycosides (gentamicin) could also be used. Antibiotics should be administered in high doses and intravenously in patients who are hospitalized or seriously ill.

60. **Which cranial nerves pass through the cavernous sinus?**
Cranial nerves III, IV, V (ophthalmic division of V), and VI pass through the cavernous sinus.

61. **What is cavernous sinus thrombosis?**
It is an uncommon but potentially lethal extension of odontogenic infection. Valveless veins in the head and neck allow retrograde flow of the infection from the face to the sinus. The pterygoid plexus of veins and angular and ophthalmic veins may contribute to retrograde flow. The first clinical signs of cavernous sinus thrombosis include vascular congestion in periorbital, scleral, and retinal veins. Other clinical signs include periorbital edema, proptosis, thrombosis of the retinal vein, ptosis, dilated pupils, absent corneal reflex, and supraorbital sensory deficits.

62. **What are the pathways of odontogenic infection to the cavernous sinus?**
An orofacial infection can reach the cavernous sinus through two routes: an **anterior route** via the angular and inferior ophthalmic veins, and a **posterior route** via the transverse facial vein and the pterygoid plexus of veins.

63. **What is the flora of acute and chronic sinusitis?**
Acute sinus infections are caused by *Streptococcus pneumoniae* (30% to 50%) and *Haemophilus influenzae* (20% to 40%). Other organisms associated with acute sinusitis include *Moraxella catarrhalis, S. aureus, Streptococcus pyogenes*, and beta- and alpha-hemolytic streptococci.
Chronic sinusitis is due to *S. aureus*, alpha-hemolytic streptococci, *Peptostreptococcus, Pseudomonas, Proteus*, and *Bacteroides*. The flora of chronic sinusitis is usually a mixture of aerobic and anaerobic organisms.

64. **What is the treatment for maxillary sinus infections?**
Treatment for maxillary sinus is based on a combined approach of medical treatment and, if necessary, surgical treatment. The medical treatment includes use of antibiotics, topical or oral decongestants, antihistamines, and topical or oral steroids. Commonly prescribed antibiotics for the treatment of maxillary sinusitis include ampicillin, amoxicillin, amoxicillin plus clavulanic acid, cefaclor, cefuroxime axetil, and trimethoprim-sulfamethoxazole.
Surgical treatment is indicated when the underlying cause of the infection cannot be corrected with medical therapy. The goal is to reestablish drainage and remove the underlying cause (if identified) using minimally invasive techniques, such as functional endoscopic surgery.

65. **What are the most common bacterial and fungal infections affecting patients with diabetes mellitus?**
Mucormycosis (phycomycosis) is the most common infection in patients with diabetes mellitus, especially those with diabetic ketoacidosis. Of patients with rhinocerebral mucormycosis, 75% have ketoacidosis. Mucormycosis is a fungal disease, possibly caused by phycomycetes organisms of the Zygomycetes class.

66. **Which organisms are associated with infections from human and animal bites?**
Approximately 25% of animal bite infections are caused by *Pasteurella multocida*. Approximately 10% are caused by *S. aureus*, 40% are caused by alpha-hemolytic streptococci, and 20% are caused by bacteroides and fusobacteria. About 25% of human bite infections are caused by *S. aureus* from the skin of the victim; 10% are caused by alpha-hemolytic streptococci; 50% are caused by anaerobic bacteria including gram-positive cocci, fusobacteria, and *Bacteroides* species; and 15% are caused by *Eikenella corrodens*. The latter organisms are mostly associated with severe infections.

67. **What is the treatment for animal and human bites?**
Treatment includes antibiotic therapy and surgical intervention. Good surgical technique involves debridement of the devitalized tissue and thorough irrigation with copious quantities of saline. Oral ampicillin and amoxicillin are the antibiotics of choice for both types of bites. Also provide prophylaxis against rabies virus, if deemed necessary.

68. **What is actinomycosis?**
Actinomycosis is a bacterial infection caused by a gram-positive, facultative, anaerobic rod bacteria called *Actinomyces israeli*. The organism is part of the normal oral flora. The infection presents as a hard swelling of the jaw and drainage characterized by sulfur granules. The treatment of actinomycosis includes 10 to 20 million U of penicillin daily for 2 to 4 weeks, followed by 5 to 10 million U for 3 to 4 months. Surgical debridement of the area may accelerate resolution of the infection.

69. **Which diseases are associated with Epstein-Barr virus?**
Mononucleosis, Burkitt's lymphoma, nasopharyngeal carcinoma, and hairy leukoplakia are associated with the Epstein-Barr virus.

70. **What is a Jarisch-Herxheimer reaction?**
It is a transient, increased discomfort in an erythematous skin lesion plus temperature elevation occurring within 2 hours after starting antibiotic therapy in treatment of secondary syphilis and Lyme disease (penicillin or tetracycline).

71. **What are the various fungal infections that may affect the head and neck?**
The various fungal infections of the head and neck include candidiasis, zygomycosis, histoplasmosis, blastomycosis, aspergillosis, and coccidiomycosis.

72. **What are the common *antifungal* agents?**
The most common antifungal agents are nystatin, clotrimazole, ketoconazole, and amphotericin B.

73. **What are the common *antiviral* agents?**
The common antiviral agents are acyclovir, zidovudine, vidarabine (ara-A), and idoxuridine.

74. **What are the most common agents used in HIV-positive patients?**
See Table 28-11.

75. **Is the following statement true or false? Osteomyelitis can be classified into three major groups.**
False. Osteomyelitis is generally classified as two major groups: suppurative and nonsuppurative.

76. **What is the most common classification of osteomyelitis of the jaws?**
Suppurative osteomyelitis is classified as acute, chronic, or infantile osteomyelitis. Nonsuppurative osteomyelitis is classified as chronic sclerosing (focal and diffuse), Garré's sclerosing osteomyelitis, and actinomycotic osteomyelitis.

77. **What is Garré's osteomyelitis?**
Garré's osteomyelitis is characterized by localized, hard, nontender, bony swelling of the lateral and inferior aspects of the mandible. It is primarily present in children and young adults and is usually associated with carious molar and low-grade infection. The radiographic features of Garré's osteomyelitis include a focal area with proliferative periosteal formation, most often seen as a carious mandibular molar opposite the hard bony mass, and periosteal bony outgrowth seen on occlusal films. Treatment of this condition includes extraction of the tooth and removal of potential sources, which leads to gradual remodeling of the area involved. Long-term postoperative antibiotics generally are not necessary.

Table 28-11. Common Drugs Used to Treat HIV-Positive Patients

DRUG	MAIN ACTION	COMPLICATIONS
Immunosuppressive		
Glucocorticoids	Decrease circulating lymphocytes	Infection
		Diabetes mellitus
	Impair delayed hypersensitivity	Adrenal suppression
	Alter lymphocyte–macrophage interaction	Peptic ulcer disease
		Impaired wound healing
	Cause monocytopenia	
	Impair neutrophil chemotaxis	
Azathioprine	Interferes with DNA/RNA synthesis, leading to lymphocytopenia	Hepatitis
		Agranulocytosis
		Infection
Antithymocyte globulin	Lymphocyte-selective immunosuppression	Infection
		Predisposition to tumor development
		Thrombocytopenia
		Hemolysis
		Leukopenia
Cyclosporine	Inhibits T-cell proliferation and activation	Nephrotoxicity
		Hepatotoxicity
		Lymphoma
		Gingival hyperplasia
Cyclophosphamide	Depletes circulating T-lymphocyte pools	Leukopenia
	Inhibits T-cell function and proliferation	

Adapted from Miyasaki SH, Perrott D, Kaban LB: Infections in immunocompromised patients, *Oral Maxillofac Surg Clin* 3:393–402, 1991.

78. **Which conditions are associated with periosteal thickening?**
In addition to Garré's osteomyelitis, infantile osteomyelitis, cortical hyperostoses (Caffey's disease), syphilis, leukemia, Ewing's sarcoma, metabolic neuroblastoma, and fracture callus are all associated with periosteal thickening.

79. **What are the general treatment principles of osteomyelitis of the jaws?**
Treatment of osteomyelitis of the jaws usually includes both surgical intervention and medical management of the patient, as well as sensitivity testing. Medical management involves administration of empirical antibiotics, performing Gram stain, administration of culture-guided antibiotics, use of appropriate imaging to rule out other causes such as tumors, and evaluation and correction of the patient's immune defenses. Surgical treatment includes removal of loose teeth and foreign bodies; sequestrectomy; debridement; decortication; resection; and reconstruction, if necessary.

80. **How does the management of severe odontogenic infections in pregnant patients differ from that in normal patients?**
The principles of treatment of odontogenic infections in pregnant patients are the same and include removal of the source of infection, incision and drainage, antibiotic therapy and medical support. However, the physiologic changes associated with pregnancy as well as the status of the fetus have to be carefully considered and make medical, surgical, and anesthetic management of these infections in the pregnant patient very challenging. Although the details of physiologic changes associated with pregnancy have been discussed elsewhere, it is worth emphasizing that when treating these patients,

such physiologic changes can impact the outcome of the infection treatment as well as the viability of the fetus. Such changes include:

- Cardiovascular: changes in blood pressure, cardiac output, heart rate, etc.
- Respiratory: changes in respiratory drive, tidal volume, respiratory rate, and minute ventilation
- Endocrine: increased incidence of gestational diabetes
- Urinary: changes in kidney output and risk of urinary tract infections
- Hepatic function: changes in serum alkaline phosphate, bilirubin, and peripheral edema
- Hematological: increases in erythrocyte and leukocyte counts and increases in plasma volume with resulting hypercoagulability

81. **What is meant by generations of antibiotics, as in third-generation cephalosporins?**[*]
The earliest antibiotics were bacteriostatic, largely through interference in protein synthesis, so that they might keep a microorganism from reproducing even if they did not kill it. The difference between **infestation** (presence of living microbes in the host) and **infection** (replication and spread of microorganisms in the host) may be useful in understanding how earlier drugs possibly controlled infection but were less capable of eliminating organisms in any brief period of therapy.

Penicillin changed all that. It may be the first antibiotic with a legitimate claim to the title wonder drug, because it has the microbicidal capability of eradicating sensitive organisms. Penicillin was the first generation of the beta-lactam antibiotics, joined by the congener first-generation cephalosporins (e.g., cefazolin). They shared beta-lactam structure and had good gram-positive coverage with less range in any effect over gram-negative microbes.

The second-generation beta-lactam antibiotics (e.g., cefoxitin) covered new classes of microbes beyond gram-positive aerobes, such as many of the *Bacteroides* species, but had little effect on gram-negative aerobic microbes. Because the third-generation cephalosporins covered some of the latter microbes, they were touted as single-agent therapy for all principal-risk flora.

As with penicillin, the original wonder drug, the wonderment waned with failures of the new agents because of rapidly induced antimicrobial resistance. The most easily measured and calculated difference in the generations is cost: wholesale values are about $2.00/g for the first generation, $5.00/g for the second, and $30.00/g for the third. Despite this bracket creep in cost, the higher generations lose some of their potency against the original gram-positive organisms for which the first-generation agents were truly wonderful. Therefore, it takes 2 g of moxalactam to be half as good as 1 g of cefazolin for gram-positive coverage. It does not take a pharmacoeconomist to ask, "What have I got in return for this sixtyfold surcharge?"

82. **Are two prophylactic doses better than one in preventing infection? Are three doses better still?**[1]
Only one dose of prophylactic antibiotic can be proved, beyond statistical or clinical doubt, to be efficacious—the dose in systemic circulation at the time of the inoculum. Whether the dose needs to be repeated one or more times during the 24 hours after the inoculum depends on the blood levels of the drug, which are largely a function of protein binding and clearance rate. We also know for sure that 10 days of the same prophylactic drug that is efficacious if given immediately before the inoculum results in a higher risk of infection than no antibiotic at all.

83. **What factors determine the timing of antibiotic administration under the criteria of prophylaxis?**[1]
The one immutable principle has been set out above—the most important element in timing of prophylaxis is that the drug be **circulating** before the inoculum. When should it stop? When the reduction in infection risk is no longer provable and before continued use will defeat the prophylactic purpose (as explained above). To summarize with an arbitrary rule of thumb: *There is no justification for prophylactic antibiotic 24 hours after the inoculum of an invasive procedure.*

What does this rule imply? Should we not continue prophylaxis for weeks to cover the presence of a prosthetic hip joint? Presumably, the prosthetic hip will be in the patient for many years, but surely you do not argue that the antibiotic should continue on a daily basis as long as the hip is in place. What is "prophylaxed" is not the prosthetic hip but the procedure of implantation. And it is not only implantation that poses a risk to the patient with a prosthesis—so does hemorrhoidectomy done years later, for which prophylaxis is made mandatory by the presence of the hip prosthesis.

The prosthetic or rheumatic heart valve is a risk, but the indication for the use of prophylactic antibiotics is an invasive procedure; a root canal is an example in which an inoculum is unavoidable.

Operations are covered by prophylactic antibiotics; the conditions that are risk factors during the operation are not.

84. To be safe, why not administer prophylactic antibiotics to all patients undergoing any kind of operation?[1]

Can you give me the indication for a prophylactic antibiotic in a patient undergoing a clean elective surgical procedure that implants no prosthesis, such as hernia repair?

"Sure," one of my brighter students once responded, "the patient who has a serious impairment in host response, such as acute granulocytic leukemia in blast crisis."

I responded, "Why on earth are you fixing his hernia? That is a clean error (hopefully not a clean kill) in surgical judgment that has nothing to do with antibiotics at all. A patient with that degree of host impairment does not undergo an elective surgical procedure."

Rule of thumb: If you can provide the indication for a prophylactic antibiotic to cover a clean elective nonprosthetic operation for a patient, you have provided the contraindication for the operation.

85. What is the drug of choice for the treatment of an abscess?*

A knife. Surgically drain the abscess. Abscesses have no circulation of blood within them to deliver an antibiotic. The antibiotic, even if injected directly into the abscess, would be worthless because the abscess contains a soup of dead microorganisms and white blood cells (WBCs). Even if the organisms were barely alive, they would not be reproducing and incorporating the antibiotic. The drug most likely would not work at all at the pH and pKa conditions of the abscess environment.

If there is an indication for an antibiotic, it would be in the circulation around the compressed inflammatory edge of the abscess and the cellulitis (at the vascularized "peel of the orange") and uncontaminated tissue planes through which the necessary drainage must be carried out. A *focal* infection is managed by a *local* treatment, which is both *necessary* in all abscesses and *sufficient* treatment in many. Adjunctive systemic antibiotics are occasionally indicated for protection of the tissues through which drainage is carried out. If it helps to make this fundamental surgical principle clear, here is the rule of thumb for management of abscesses: *Where there is pus, let there be steel.* Perhaps one of the most gratifying procedures in all of medicine is the drainage of pus with immediate relief of local and systemic symptoms (e.g., a perirectal abscess).

86. Are antibiotic drug combinations always superior to a single antibiotic agent?[1]

Monotherapy is superior to combination antibiotic treatment regimens, but this is provable probably only in the highest risk patients. With the carbapenem-class antibiotic agents, a large multicenter clinical trial proved imipenem therapy superior to aminoglycoside and a macrolide antibiotic, with survival demonstrably superior only in the patients with the highest APACHE scores. Ertapenem monotherapy was the equivalent of ceftriaxone and metronidazole in a smaller, more recent trial.

More is not always better, and the R and S on culture reports does not translate directly to the M and M (morbidity and mortality) at the Death and Complications Conference reports. It is not just important that the effective antibiotic regimen kills the bacteria; also important are how this microbicidal effect is carried out and what effect it may have on the patient in quenching or prolonging the systemic inflammatory response.

87. What are triple antibiotics? What are the doses?†

A shotgun approach to potentially life-threatening infections when the patient is seriously ill and the surgeon is seriously concerned:

1. Gram-positive coverage (e.g., ampicillin): 1 g every 6 hours IV in adults; 40 mg/kg every 6 hours IV in children
2. Gram-negative coverage (e.g., gentamicin): 7 mg/kg IV every 24 hours (this single daily dose is less nephrotoxic than 2 mg/kg IV every 8 hours)
3. Anaerobic coverage (e.g., metronidazole [Flagyl]): 500 mg IV every 6 hours in adults; 7.5 mg/kg IV every 6 hours in children. To avoid overgrowth of yeast and resistant bacteria, focus on the culprit bacteria as soon as the cultures define it.

---

*Reprinted from Geelhoed GW: Surgical infectious disease. In Harken AH, Moore EE, editors: *Abernathy's surgical secrets*, ed 5, Philadelphia, 2005, Mosby.

†Reprinted from Harken AH: What does postoperative fever mean? In Harken AH, Moore EE, editors: *Abernathy's surgical secrets*, ed 5, Philadelphia, 2005, Mosby.

88. **How do I use antibiotics correctly to prevent surgical wound infection?***
First by knowing what organism you are targeting, and then by choosing an appropriate antibiotic and delivering it at the appropriate time via the appropriate route. Because you usually will not have a preoperative culture to guide therapy, you need to base your choice of antibiotic on predicted organisms. Staphylococci are the most common skin organisms and the most common etiologic agents in surgical site infections (SSIs). Cefazolin, a first-generation cephalosporin, is usually the recommended antibiotic for prophylaxis in clean surgical procedures. In circumstances in which known contamination has occurred, initial antibiotics should be tailored based on the violated organ's common flora. If the gut was entered, Enterobacteriaceae and anaerobes are common; biliary tract and esophageal incisions yield these organisms plus enterococci. The urinary tract or vagina may contain group D streptococci, Pseudomonas, and Proteus.

89. **If prophylactic antibiotics are used, how and when should they be administered?***
Maximal benefit is obtained when tissue concentrations are therapeutic at the time of contamination. Efficacy is enhanced when prophylactic antibiotics are administered IV 20 to 30 minutes before surgical incision; late administration is similar to no administration. Multiple-dose regimens have no proven benefit over single-dose regimens. Indiscriminate antibiotic selection outside recommended hospital protocols may increase the incidence of SSIs. In special circumstances, administration routes other than IV may be indicated.

90. **What can the patient do to help decrease surgical wound infection?***
Stop smoking. Although obesity, poor nutritional status, advanced age, and diabetes are risk factors for SSIs, cigarette smoking is probably the leading preventable patient factor for SSIs, just like it is the leading preventable cause of death and disability in the United States. Half of all people who smoke eventually die from a smoking-related illness. Smoking not only kills, but also more than triples the risk of incisional wound breakdown; in one study, smoking increased the incidence of SSIs in clean operative procedures sixfold, from 0.6% to 3.6%. Tobacco use results in decreased blood flow and decreased oxygen delivery to the wound. Toxic tobacco by-products also directly impede all stages of wound healing. Despite this knowledge, surgeons continue to operate electively on smokers, and most smokers continue to smoke up until the day of surgery.

BIBLIOGRAPHY

Abubaker AO: Orofacial infections and use of antibiotics. In Abubaker A, Benson KJ, editors: *Oral and maxillofacial surgery secrets*, ed 2, Philadelphia, 2007, Mosby/Elsevier.

Barie PS: Modern surgical antibiotic prophylaxis and therapy: less is more, *Surg Infect* 1:23–29, 2000.

Bartlett RC: Laboratory diagnostic techniques. In Tobazian RG, Goldberg MH, editors: *Oral and maxillofacial infections*, ed 3, Philadelphia, 1991, Saunders.

Ciftci AO, Tanyei FC, Buyukpamukcu N, et al.: Comparative trial of four antibiotic combinations for perforated appendicitis in children, *Eur J Surg* 163:591–596, 1997.

Falagas ME, Barefoot L, Griffith J, et al.: Risk factors leading to clinical failure in the treatment of intraabdominal or skin/soft tissue infections, *Eur J Clin Microbiol Infect Dis* 15:913–921, 1996.

Flynn TR: Anatomy and surgery of deep fascial space infections of the head and neck, *Oral Maxillofac Surg Knowl Update* 1:79–105, 1994.

Geelhoed GW: Surgical infectious disease. In Harken AH, Moore EE, editors: *Surgical secrets*, ed 5, Philadelphia, 2005, Mosby.

Geelhoed GW: Preoperative skin preparation: evaluation of efficacy, timing, convenience, and cost, *Infect Surg* 85:648–669, 1985.

Hupp JR: Antibacterial, antiviral and antifungal agents, *Oral Maxillofac Surg Clin* 3:273–286, 1991.

Kara A, Ozsurekci Y, Tekcicek M, et al.: Length of hospital stay and management of facial cellulitis of odontogenic origin in children, *Pediatr Dent* 36(1):18E–22E, January-February 2014.

Kluytmans J, Voss A: Prevention of postsurgical infections: some like it hot, *Curr Opin Infect Dis* 15:427–432, 2002.

Krueger JK, Rohrich RJ: Clearing the smoke: the scientific rationale for tobacco abstention with plastic surgery, *Plast Reconstr Surg* 108:1063–1073, 2001.

Lieblich SE: Clinical microbiology and taxonomy, *Oral Maxillofac Surg Knowl Update* 1:11–21, 1994.

Miyasaki SH, Perrott DH, Kaban LB: Infections in immunocompromised patients, *Oral Maxillofac Surg Clin* 3:393–402, 1991.

Optiz D, Camerer C, Camerer, et al.: Incidence and management of severe odontogenic infection—a retrospective analysis from 2004 to 2011, *J Craniomaxillofac Surg* 43:285–289, 2015.

Peterson LJ: Microbiology of head and neck infections, *Oral Maxillofac Surg Clin* 3:247–258, 1991.

*Reprinted from Peterson SL: Surgical wound infection. In Harken AH, Moore EE, editors: *Abernathy's surgical secrets*, ed 5, Philadelphia, 2005, Mosby.

Peterson LJ: Principles of management and prevention of odontogenic infection. In Peterson LJ, Ellis E, Hupp J, et al.: *Contemporary oral and maxillofacial surgery*, ed 2, St Louis, 1998, Mosby.

Peterson SL: Surgical wound infection. In Harken AH, Moore EE, editors: *Surgical secrets*, ed 5, Philadelphia, 2005, Mosby.

Rogerson KC: Microbiology of the maxillary sinus antrum: treatment of infections, *Oral Maxillofac Surg Knowl Update* 1:49–60, 1994.

Sarna T, Sengupta T, Miloro M, Kolokythas A: Cervical necrotizing fasciitis with descending mediastinitis: literature review and case report, *J Oral Maxillofac Surg* 70(6):1342–1350, June 2012.

Topazian RG: Osteomyelitis of the jaws. In Topazian R, Goldberg M, editors: *Oral and maxillofacial infections*, ed 3, Philadelphia, 1994, Saunders.

Walia IS, Borle RM, Mehendiratta D, Yadav AO: Microbiology and antibiotic sensitivity of head and neck space infections of odontogenic origin, *J Maxillofac Oral Surg* 13(1):16–21, March 2014.

Wong D, Cheng A, Kunchur R, Lam S, Sambrool PJ, Gossb AN: Management of severe odontogenic infection in pregnancy, *Aus Det J* 57:498–503, 2012.

Wood RS: Chronic granulomatous infections, *Oral Maxillofac Surg Clin* 3:405–422, 1991.

CHAPTER 29

DIAGNOSIS AND MANAGEMENT OF DENTOALVEOLAR INJURIES

Jason A. Jamali, A. Omar Abubaker

1. **What is the prevalence of dentoalveolar injuries?**

   The prevalence of dentoalveolar injuries varies widely depending on factors such as age, the cause of injury, and gender. The general prevalence of these injuries among pediatric patients is reported to be 5% of all facial fractures. Among adolescents with sport-related trauma, the incidence of dentoalveolar injuries is reported to be 36%. Overall, the prevalence of dentoalveolar injuries among children with primary dentition is 11% to 30%, and among children with permanent dentition is 5% to 20% of the time. Boys also are affected almost twice as often as girls with a peak incidence at 2 to 4 years and 8 to 10 years.

2. **Is there a difference between dentoalveolar injuries in children to that in adults?**

   The nature of dentoalveolar fracture varies with age possibly due to the anatomic differences between the teeth and supporting structures of adults and pediatric patients. Such differences are reflected by the fact that trauma to the primary dentition affects mostly the supporting structure (luxation and exarticulation), while trauma to the permanent dentition affects mostly the teeth themselves (causing crown fractures). Trauma to primary dentition result in only 10% of crown or crown-root fractures, and 75% involves luxation or exarticulation of the tooth compared to incidence of mostly crown and crown-root fracture involvement in the permanent dentition.

3. **What is the difference between an injury that is a result of direct trauma to the dentoalveolar structures compared to that of indirect trauma?**

   If the injury is caused by a direct trauma, the most likely teeth to sustain injury are the anterior teeth because of their relatively exposed position. This occurs most commonly to the maxillary incisors when these teeth are protruding, as in patients with Class II division I malocclusion or in patients with insufficient lip closure. Depending on the force of the impacted trauma, direct injury can affect the upper or lower lip, occasionally causing laceration of the lip as well as dental or osseous alveolar fracture (Fig. 29-1). Dentoalveolar injury from indirect trauma usually results from force applied to the chin forcing the mandibular teeth against the maxillary dentition. The impact of this force often results in crown or crown-root fracture, condylar and/or symphyseal mandibular fracture, and anterior intraoral soft tissue and submental lacerations.

4. **What should be included in the history of assessing a dentoalveolar trauma patient?**

   The history obtained from patients with dentoalveolar injury should include the following information:
   - **Biographic and demographic data** of the patient including name, age, sex, race, address, and phone number
   - **When** did the injury occur? The time interval between the injury and presentation to the clinic or emergency room (such time will determine prognosis).
   - **How:** The mechanism of injury—the nature of the accident can provide insight into the type of injury to be suspected.
   - **Where**: The environment where the injury occurred may lead to contamination of the injury site; have the missing teeth been located (aspiration, embedded within tongue/lip)? If missing teeth haven't been accounted for, imaging (CXR, AXR, pan) may be considered.
   - **What:** What treatment has been rendered so far? What type of media teeth have been stored during transfer?
   - **Other:** The patient or parent should also be asked for information regarding any changes in the occlusion as a result of the injury, and a short medical and dental history to delineate any systemic or dental factors that can influence the immediate and later treatment plans. Such factors include the presence of major systemic illnesses, especially those that may influence the treatment such as bleeding disorders and epilepsy.

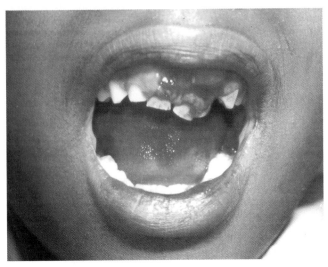

Figure 29-1. Example of an alveolar ridge fracture. *(From Baren JM, Rothrock SG, John Brennan:* Pediatric emergency medicine, *Philadelphia, 2008, Saunders.)*

5. **What should be included in the physical examination of a dentoalveolar injury patient?**
   - An important aspect of the physical examination is the overall evaluation of the physical status of the patient as well as a detailed oral and maxillofacial examination (intraoral and extraoral).
   - The general examination should include measurement of vital signs such as pulse rate, blood pressure, and respiration. Significant changes in these measurements may indicate intracranial injury, cervical spine injury, chest or abdominal injury, or even aspiration of an avulsed tooth. The mental status of the patient should also be assessed by both asking specific questions and by observing the patient's reaction and behavior during the history and examinations.
   - The oral and maxillofacial examination should include extraoral soft tissue examination, intraoral soft tissue examination, examination of the jaws and alveolar bone, examination of the teeth for displacement, and mobility and reaction to percussion.

6. **What physical finding may suggest fracture of the alveolus?**
   During palpation of an involved tooth, movement of adjacent teeth as well may suggest an alveolar fracture.

7. **What is the role of pulp testing immediately after dental trauma?**
   Pulp testing can result in false negative results immediately after injury. Retesting several weeks later is beneficial to determine any need for an endodontic treatment.

8. **What is the role of radiographic examination in evaluation of dentoalveolar fractures?**
   The purpose of radiographic examination is to provide information regarding injuries affecting the root portion of the tooth, periodontal ligaments, and status of the surrounding alveolar and based bone. Such information includes presence of root fracture, root infraction, and root dislocation. It also serves to provide data on the presence of preexisting periapical disease, presence of jaw fracture, degree of extrusion or intrusion, and tooth or tooth fragment or foreign bodies lodged in the soft tissue. In children and young adults, radiographic examination serves to provide information regarding extent of root development, size of the pulp chamber, and root canal and proximity of succedaneous teeth to the injured primary tooth. Because a single radiograph may not be sufficient to show a crown or root fracture, radiographic imaging of dentoalveolar trauma usually consists of more than one radiograph and occasionally more than one projection (periapical, occlusal, and panoramic).

9. **What method can be used to improve detection of the root in dentoalveolar trauma?**
   The beam of X-ray should be parallel with the line of fracture. Multiple angulations should be taken to improve detection. Cone beam CT can be useful for this purpose.

10. **What is the purpose of dentoalveolar injury classification?**
    The purpose of such classification is to provide a comprehensive and universal description of the injury for communication and treatment planning purposes. Many classifications of traumatic injuries to the teeth and supporting structures have been developed. These systems are based on a variety of factors such as etiology, anatomy of injury, pathology, and therapy. All systems of classification of dentoalveolar injuries have advantages or disadvantages. The three most commonly used systems for simple and comprehensive classification of dentoalveolar injuries are those developed by Ellis, by Saunders et al., and by Andreasen.

11. **What is the Ellis classification system of dentoalveolar fractures?**
    - Class I: confined to enamel
    - Class II: enamel and dentin
    - Class III: enamel, dentin, and pulp
    - Class IV: root fracture
    - Also can be described as complicated (involving pulp) and uncomplicated (not involving pulp)

12. **What are the different types of injuries to hard dental tissues and pulp?**
    These injuries include **crown infraction** (an incomplete fracture or crack of the enamel without loss of tooth substance); **uncomplicated crown fracture** (a fracture confined to the enamel or involving the enamel and dentin without exposing the pulp); **complicated crown fracture** (a crown fracture involving enamel and dentin with exposure of the pulp); **uncomplicated crown-root fracture** (a fracture involving enamel, dentin, and cementum without exposure of the pulp); **complicated crown-root fracture** (a fracture involving enamel, dentin, and cementum with exposure of the pulp); and **root fracture** (a fracture involving dentin, cementum, and the pulp).

13. **What are the different types of injuries to the periodontal tissues?**
    These injuries include **concussion** (an injury to the tooth-supporting structures without abnormal loosening or displacement of the tooth, but with marked reaction to percussion); **subluxation (loosening)** (an injury to the tooth-supporting structures with abnormal loosening, but without displacement of the tooth); **intrusive luxation (central dislocation)** (displacement of the tooth into the alveolar bone with comminution or fracture of the alveolar socket); **extrusive luxation (or peripheral dislocation, partial avulsion)** (partial displacement of the tooth out of the alveolar socket); **lateral luxation** (displacement of the tooth in a direction other than axially, accompanied by a comminution or fracture of the alveolar socket); **retained root fracture** (a fracture with retention of the root segment, but loss of the crown segment out of the socket); and **exarticulation (complete avulsion)** (a complete displacement of a tooth out of the alveolar socket).

14. **What are the different injuries to the supporting bone in dentoalveolar injuries?**
    These injuries include **comminution of the alveolar socket** (crushing and comminution of the alveolar socket occurring most commonly with intrusive and lateral luxation); **fracture of the alveolar socket wall** (confined to the facial or lingual socket wall); **fracture of the alveolar process** (which may or may not involve the alveolar socket); and **fractures of the mandible or maxilla** (involving the basal bone of the mandible or maxilla and often the alveolar process).

15. **How does location of the root fracture affect prognosis?**
    In general, the more apical the fracture, the better the prognosis.

16. **What are the treatment options for an intruded tooth with either a closed or open apex?**
    The three options are observation for spontaneous eruption, orthodontic repositioning, and surgical repositioning.
    For an intruded tooth with an open apex, observation should be considered if the tooth is intruded up to 7 mm. Otherwise, surgical versus orthodontic repositioning should be considered.
    For an intruded tooth with a closed apex, observation should be chosen if the amount of intrusion is limited to 3 mm. If there is greater than 3 mm of intrusion with a closed apex, surgical versus orthodontic repositioning should be planned.
    Evaluation for endodontic therapy should be planned at 3 to 4 weeks.

17. **What is the treatment for tooth avulsion?**
    The tooth is replanted and splinted for 2 to 4 weeks in addition to a week of systemic antibiotics. In situations where the extraoral dry time is greater than 60 minutes, a root surface treatment with

2% sodium fluoride solution is applied for 20 minutes. Evaluation for endodontic therapy is done at 7 to 10 days following replantation. In avulsed teeth with a closed apex and a dry time greater than 60 minutes, endodontic therapy can be performed prior to replantation and the necrotic periodontal membrane should be gently cleaned prior to implantation. A soft diet and a week of chlorhexidine is advised in addition to close follow-up.

18. What is the treatment for root fractures?
    The tooth is repositioned and stabilized with a splint for at least 4 weeks. Root fractures closer to the cervical region may require longer splint times (up to 4 months).

19. What are the options available for crown-root fractures in the secondary dentition?
    - If there is no pulpal involvement, the coronal fragment may be removed.
    - With pulpal involvement, the coronal segment is removed, and endodontic therapy is performed. This is then followed by orthodontic versus surgical extrusion or ostectomy with gingivectomy.
    - With vertical crown-root fractures, the tooth should be extracted. Extraction should not be delayed, whereas the other modalities may be delayed for 1 to 2 weeks after bonding of the coronal fragment.

20. What is the treatment for alveolar fractures?
    The alveolar bone is repositioned using manual digital pressure followed by splint therapy for at least 4 weeks. Associated lacerations must be identified and treated.

21. Which injury has highest incidence of pulpal necrosis?
    Intrusion has more pulpal necrosis (65% to 90%), whereas extrusion causes 64% of pulpal necrosis.

22. How are intruded primary teeth managed?
    Intruded deciduous teeth are extracted, as displacement of the root apex may damage the developing secondary tooth. If the root apex of the deciduous is displaced labially, it may be left in place and observed for spontaneous eruption.

23. How are root fractures of deciduous teeth managed?
    Treatment depends on whether the coronal fragment is displaced. If there is no displacement then no treatment is indicated. With displacement the coronal fragment is either splinted or extracted leaving the apical portion in place.

BIBLIOGRAPHY

Abubaker AO, Giglio JA, Murino AP: Diagnosis and management of dentoalveoilar injuries. In Fonseca RJ, editor: *Oral and maxillofacial surgery*, Philadelphia, 2000, W.B. Saunders, pp 54–85.
Andreasen FM, Andreasen JO: Diagnosis of luxation injuries: the importance of standardized clinical, radiographic and photographic techniques in clinical investigations, *Endod Dent Traumatol* 5:160–169, 1985.
Andreasen FM, Andreasen JO, Tsukiboshi M: Examination and diagnosis of dental injuries. In Andreasen JO, Andreasen FM, Andersson L, editors: *Textbook and color atlas of traumatic injuries to the teeth*, ed 4, Oxford, 2007, Blackwell, pp 255–279.
Bakland LK, Andreasen JO: Examination of the dentally traumatized patient, *Calif Dent Ass J* 24:35–44, 1996.

CHAPTER 30

MANDIBULAR TRAUMA

Hani F. Braidy, Vincent B. Ziccardi, A. Omar Abubaker

1. **What are the signs and symptoms that may be associated with mandibular fractures?**

   Signs and symptoms associated with mandibular fractures include pain and tenderness at the fracture site; changes in occlusion; ecchymosis of the floor of the mouth or skin; crepitation on manual palpation; soft tissue bleeding; sensory disturbances (numbness of the lower lip); changes or deviation of the mandible on opening; soft tissue swelling; trismus; flexion or segmental mobility of the mandible; gingival tears and palpable fracture line intraorally or at the inferior border of the mandible.

2. **What is a compound mandible fracture?**

   A compound mandible fracture is a fracture in which there is an external wound involving the skin, mucosa, or periodontal ligament structure (contaminated wound). A compound fracture is at increased risk for infection.

3. **What radiographs are included in a mandible series?**

   The mandible film series includes the right and left lateral oblique views, posteroanterior (PA) cephalogram, and reverse Towne's view. The lateral oblique views are useful to evaluate the body or ramus regions of the mandible. The PA view can assess the symphyseal region and evaluate the buccal-lingual displacement of body or angle fractures. The reverse Towne's view is helpful in assessing the mandibular condyles. Panoramic radiographs remain the gold standard for mandible fracture screening. Because these are seldom available in hospital radiology departments, an additional view that is oriented perpendicular to the lateral cortex can be substituted to accurately assess and diagnose a fracture. A panoramic radiograph combined with a PA or reverse Towne's view is generally adequate for diagnosis. Maxillofacial computed tomograms without contrast are becoming widely available and can be an invaluable adjunct to plain films.

4. **Which mandibular fractures are likely to be missed on panoramic examination?**

   Because panoramic radiograph is a flat view taken by a movable X-ray beam that displays the entire mandible as a flat structure, some overlap and blurring are usually seen in the symphysis-parasymphysis region; therefore, fractures of the mandible in this area are frequently missed. Similarly, and due to the overlap from other cranial and facial structures, fractures of the mandibular condyles can be difficult to detect, and when one is detected, it can be difficult to ascertain the degree of displacement of the fracture. The combination of panoramic examination, Towne's views, and computed tomography (CT) scans helps detect almost all mandibular fractures.

5. **What is the incidence of fractures in different areas of the adult mandible?**

   See Table 30-1.

6. **What is a horizontally favorable fracture?**

   Favorability is determined by the forces exerted by the masticatory muscles on the fracture segments. A favorable fracture is one that is not displaced by masticatory muscle pull, and an unfavorable fracture occurs when the line of fracture permits the fragments to separate. The four muscles of mastication are the temporalis, masseter, medial pterygoid, and lateral pterygoid. After discontinuity of the mandible due to fracture, these muscles exert their actions on the fragments, leading to malocclusion. Horizontal favorability is determined by cephalad-caudad stability as seen on CT or oblique films. An example of a horizontally favorable fracture is a body fracture where the inferior border is displaced superiorly by the pterygomasseteric sling stabilizing the reduction because of fracture orientation.

7. **What is a vertically favorable fracture?**

   Vertical favorability is evaluated in the buccal-lingual plane. A vertically favorable fracture of the angle occurs when oblique fracture lines form a large buccal cortical fragment that prevents medial displacement. Unfavorable vertical mandibular angle fracture as seen on axial CT reveals that a vertically unfavorable

Table 30-1. Fracture Incidences in Different Areas of the Adult Mandible

AREA OF MANDIBLE	PERCENT OF FRACTURE INCIDENTS
Angle	31%
Condyle	18%
Angle (molar) region	15%
Parasymphysis	14%
Symphysis	8%
Cuspid	7%
Ramus	6%
Coronoid process	1%

fracture line extends from a posterolateral point to an anteromedial point. No obstruction counters the action of the lateral pterygoid and mylohyoid muscles, and the posterior fragment is shifted medially.

8. **How does muscle pull affect displacement of mandibular fractures?**
Muscles involved in displacing mandibular fractures include the medial and lateral pterygoid, temporalis, masseter, digastric, geniohyoid, genioglossus, and mylohyoid. The lateral pterygoid displaces the condyle anteriorly and medially because of its insertion on the pterygoid fovea. Muscles attached to the ramus (i.e., temporalis, masseter, and medial pterygoid) result in superior and medial displacement of the proximal segment. As fractures progress anteriorly toward the cuspid region, the digastric, geniohyoid, genioglossus, and mylohyoid exert a posterior-inferior force on the distal segment.

9. **How do pediatric mandibular fractures differ from adult mandibular fractures?**
In general, mandibular fractures are less common in children than in adults. When mandibular fractures occur in children, greenstick fractures of the mandible, particularly in the condylar region, are relatively common. Also, the ossification capability of children allows faster healing and distinguishes them from adult mandible fractures. As a result, many mandibular fractures in children can be treated with immobilization for a shorter period or observation and soft diet compared to adults. Open reduction and internal fixation in children are reserved for severely displaced fractures. Resorbable plates and screws are often used instead of metallic ones when open reduction and internal fixation are indicated. Problems with osteosynthesis in children include the need to avoid damage to developing tooth buds and the need to remove the plates at a later time if resorbable plates are not used. Another common feature of mandibular fractures in children is the occurrence of high and intracapsular condylar fractures.

10. **What are some of the common complications associated with mandibular fracture management?**
    - Infection
    - Delayed union or nonunion, usually resulting from infection or inadequate fixation
    - Malocclusion
    - Facial or trigeminal nerve injury
    - Damage to tooth roots
    - Hematoma
    - Wound dehiscence (most common complication)
    - Tooth injury
    - Osteomyelitis
    Of these, infection is one of the most problematic and is an important cause of nonunion.

11. **What are the risk factors that predispose mandibular fractures to infection?**
Fractures that occur through the tooth-bearing area should be regarded as contaminated. Infected mandibular fractures are often seen in patients who sustain facial trauma and fail to seek immediate treatment. Mucosal tears and fractures extending through the periodontal ligament produce contamination of the fracture by oral flora. Bony sequestra, devitalized teeth, hematoma, and poor oral hygiene also contribute to infection.

The most common cause of postoperative infection, however, is movement at the fracture site due to loose, mobile hardware, such as a loose screw in an otherwise stable plate. This may cause infection and drainage intraorally or extraorally or both until the source of infection is removed. Patients with polysubstance abuse and malnutrition are especially at risk for wound healing complications and osteomyelitis.

12. **What percentage of mandibular fractures are multiple?**
More than 50% of mandibular fractures are multiple. Accordingly, detection of one fracture in the mandible should alert the examiner to the possible presence of additional fractures due to the arch form of the mandible. Radiographic examination should then be directed toward identification of additional fractures.

13. **What percentage of patients with mandibular fractures are associated with concomitant cervical spine injury?**
Approximately 43% of all patients with mandibular fractures have associated other systemic injuries. Cervical spine fractures were found in 11% of this group of patients. It is imperative to rule out cervical neck fractures, especially in patients who are intoxicated or unconscious and in patients who are involved in vehicular accidents. Posteroanterior, lateral films, and CT of the neck should be reviewed with the radiologist before treatment is initiated in these patients.

14. **What potential fatal outcome can result from bilateral mandibular parasymphyseal fractures?**
Bilateral parasymphyseal fractures may result in a free-floating anterior mandibular segment. The genial tubercles to which the genioglossus muscle is attached are located on the lingual surface of the mandible. Lack of stability in this area in the presence of a displaced unstable bilateral symphyseal fracture allows for posterior displacement of the tongue, which can result in airway embarrassment and inferior displacement by the suprahyoid musculature. This is known clinically as "gag bite" and can lead to death. In these types of fractures, serious consideration should be given to securing the patient airway in the early phase of management of these patients. Urgent treatment may be to place interdental wire stabilization or suture through the tongue to allow extension.

15. **What factors contribute to condylar displacement in patients with a condylar fracture?**
The lateral pterygoid is the only muscle that inserts directly on the neck of the mandibular condyle. In subcondylar fractures, the forces of this muscle frequently result in anterior and medial displacement of the condyle. The patient will deviate to the side of the fracture upon opening because of the unopposed action of the contralateral lateral pterygoid muscle. In higher condylar fractures and with intracapsular fractures above the insertion of the lateral pterygoid fractures, the small fragment can occasionally be seen displaced in a pure horizontal or vertical direction.

16. **What surgical techniques are available to treat mandible fractures?**
The most frequently used treatment modalities available for the management of mandible fractures are:
- Closed reduction and maxillomandibular fixation (MMF) with Ivy loops, arch bars, or transalveolar screws
- Closed reduction and fixation with gunning splints secured to stable osseous structures (circummandibular or perialveolar wires)
- External pin fixation, used principally with comminuted and grossly contaminated fractures
- Open reduction with internal fixation using intraoral incisions, extraoral incisions, or endoscopy. With this technique, the segments may be secured across the fracture site with wires, plates, or lag screws with or without concomitant MMF.

17. **What effects do MMF have on the masticatory system?**
- Osteoporosis of bone from disuse atrophy
- Weakness of the muscles of mastication and decreased range of motion
- Capsular and pericapsular fibrosis
- Cartilage thinning
These listed changes are usually reversible once MMF has been discontinued.

18. **What are the indications for external fixation of mandible fractures?**
Indications for external fixation of mandible fractures include:
- Extensive fracture comminution with soft tissue loss (i.e., severe gunshot wounds). In these situations, external fixation may help preserve the vitality of small bony segments and allow the soft tissue to heal prior to definitive treatment.

- Infected fractures when extensive cellulitis and/or osteomyelitis, in combination with abscess drainage and bony debridement. The use of external fixation circumvents extensive extraoral incisions, challenging neck dissections, and placement of internal hardware in grossly infected sites.
- Proximal segment control and space maintenance after severe trauma or resection

19. **What are uniphasic and biphasic external fixation systems?**
A uniphasic system, such as a modified Roger Anderson device, involves two or more percutaneous pins on either side of the fracture connected by a bar. External pin fixation systems are also commercially available using pin fixation, connectors, and carbon rods.
   A biphasic system, such as a Joe Hall Morris device, entails the use of a temporary reduction appliance until a secondary device (usually cold cure acrylic) is placed to connect the pins.

20. **What are the advantages of rigid internal fixation (RIF) in treatment of mandible fractures over other techniques? What are the disadvantages of RIF?**
RIF of mandibular fractures allows early mobilization of the jaws, reducing or eliminating the period of MMF. This is a significant benefit to patients, avoiding the potential sequelae of prolonged immobilization, including temporomandibular joint (TMJ) stiffness after removal of MMF, social inconvenience, phonetic disturbance, loss of effective work time, discomfort, and weight loss. In contrast, open reduction of mandibular fractures with wire osteosynthesis (nonrigid) requires 4 to 8 weeks of MMF for satisfactory healing. Closed reduction with MMF requires the patient to be in MMF for 6 weeks or more, with limitation of diet and function, and difficulty in maintaining good oral hygiene. Disadvantages of RIF include surgery incision with possible scars and nerve injury, anesthesia complications, and higher cost of procedure.

21. **What are the different options for treatment of mandibular angle fractures?**
The treatment of these fractures depends on many factors, including but not limited to the age and medical condition of the patient, severity of the fracture, and displacement. In general, for most angle fractures, superior border plate fixation with a minimum of four screws placed across the fracture line provides adequate stability of the fracture. The patient can be placed in MMF for 1 to 3 weeks, although that is not always necessary. Plates used range from 1.0 to 2.0 mm with monocortical screws that range in length (depending on the thickness of the cortical plate and the positioning of the plate) from 5 to 7 mm. Other treatment options include an inferior border plate or lag screw across the fracture line. If the fracture is nondisplaced, MMF for 3 to 6 weeks represents a viable option for treatment. With comminuted fractures of the angle, treatment options include external pin fixation, reconstruction plate, and/or MMF.

22. **What are the indications for removing a tooth in the line of fracture?**
Because mandibular fractures commonly occur through the dental periodontal ligament space, much debate has been focused on whether to extract teeth in the line of fracture. By definition, a fracture that communicates with the oral cavity through the periodontal ligament space is considered a compound fracture. The literature to date does not provide convincing evidence that infection is more likely to occur if a tooth is retained. Nonetheless, current recommendations for removal of teeth in the line of fracture include:
- Presence of obvious pathology, such as caries or periodontal disease
- Gross mobility of involved teeth
- Teeth that prevent adequate reduction of fractures
- Teeth with fractured roots
- Teeth whose root surfaces or apices are exposed in the fracture site

23. **What are the indications for open reduction and internal fixation of condylar fractures in adults?**
Most fractures of the mandibular condyle are amenable to closed reduction with fixation and immobilization ranging from 7 to 21 days based on age of the patient, displacement of fracture, and number of other concomitant injuries. Intracapsular condylar fractures are generally treated with a short period of MMF (10 to 14 days), followed by physiotherapy to prevent ankylosis of the joint. The mandible will deviate clinically to the side of injury on opening because of unopposed pull of the contralateral lateral pterygoid muscle.
   The indications for open reduction of condylar fractures in adults were well described by Zide and Kent and divided into absolute and relative indications.

Absolute Indications:
- Inability to obtain adequate occlusion using closed reduction techniques
- Displacement of the condyle into the middle cranial fossa
- Severe angulations of the condyle, lateral extracapsular displacement of the condyle or the condyle outside the glenoid fossa
- Removal of foreign body in the joint capsule (e.g., gunshot pellets)

Relative Indications:
- Bilateral condylar fractures with concomitant comminuted midfacial fractures
- Bilateral fractures in an edentulous patient when splints are unavailable or impossible because of severe ridge atrophy
- Displaced condyle fracture in a medically compromised patient (e.g., seizure disorder, psychiatric problems, or alcoholism) with evidence of open bite or retrusion

24. **What are the risks factors for developing TMJ ankylosis following trauma?**
- Intracapsular fracture of the mandibular condyle
- Pediatric population
- Prolonged immobilization (or maxillomandibular fixation) of the fracture
- Intraarticular hemorrhage with subsequent fibrosis of the joint

25. **When treating mandible fractures, what is a tension band?**
During mandibular functioning, stress forces are exerted on the bone in different vectors depending on the location. The superior border is under tension, whereas the inferior border is compressed. A rotational force is found in the parasymphyseal region. A tension band in mandibular fracture management refers to a mechanical means of resisting fracture displacement in the tension zone. This may be accomplished by a superior border plate if teeth are not in the way (i.e., a plate over the external oblique ridge in an angle fracture), an arch bar if stable teeth are present on both sides of the fracture, a superior border wire, or an eccentric dynamic compression plate at the inferior border. Essentially, the tension plate stabilizes the destabilizing forces of the mandible.

26. **What are dynamic compression, eccentric dynamic compression, and passive plating in rigid fixation?**
The concept of rigid internal fixation was designed to allow primary bone healing even under functional loading. In an effort to enhance stability, plates were developed that provide compressive forces across fracture lines. Passive plating provides rigid fixation without compression. Dynamic compression plates compress the fracture site by providing axial guiding inclines for the screw heads to slide down as the screw is tightened. The screws first engage the bone, and as they are tightened, they are moved 0.8 mm toward the fracture site by the guiding incline. This produces a compressive force of approximately 300 kPa. Eccentric dynamic compression plates provide compressive forces in more than one direction by changing the direction of the guiding incline in the outer holes of the plate. This concept is useful when plating mandibular body fractures. A compression plate at both the superior and inferior borders would ideally provide compression throughout the fracture, but is usually not possible because of the presence of teeth superiorly, as well as other vital structures. A single eccentric dynamic compression plate placed at the inferior border serves the same purpose by angling the guiding inclines of the outer holes toward the superior border of the mandible and eliminating the need for a superior border tension plate.

27. **How are atrophic mandibular fractures treated?**
There is considerable controversy over the choice of treatment methods of these fractures. However, many authors agree that the most important element to the success of the treatment of these fractures is adequate and complete stabilization of the fractured segments. Lack of complete immobilization of the fractured segments is likely to account for most of the commonly reported nonunion of these fractures, especially when nonrigid or semirigid fixation is used (such as wires, miniplates, and denture splints). Nonrigid or semirigid plates will not provide adequate and effective stabilization, and will likely fail with function. There is always the concern for devascularization of the bone from open reduction and reflection of the periosteum of the mandible; open reduction and rigid fixation using a reconstruction plate or a titanium mesh with immediate bone graft provide much more predictable results of healing of these types of fractures. Because atrophic mandible fractures are usually observed in the elderly and unhealthy population (often with respiratory and nutritional problems), early and adequate stabilization and resumption of oral intake provide a better chance of primary bony healing of fractures in these patients.

BIBLIOGRAPHY

Aargon SB, Gardner KE: The mandibular fractures. In Jafeck BW, Murrow BW, editors: *ENT secrets*, ed 2, Philadelphia, 2001, Hanley & Belfus.

Aminoff MJ, Greenberg DA, Simon RP: *Clinical neurology*, ed 3, Stamford, Connecticut, 1995, Appleton & Lange.

Assael LA: Maxillofacial trauma. Part 1: applying science to practice, *Oral Maxillofac Surg Clin North Am* 10(4), 1998.

Braidy HF, Ziccardi VB: External fixation for mandible fractures. Atlas of the Oral and Maxillofacial Surgery Clinics 17(1):45–53, 2009.

Deangelis AJ, Backland LK: Traumatic dental injuries: current treatment concepts, *J Am Dent Assoc* 129:1401–1414, 1998.

Ellis III E: Treatment methods for fractures of the mandibular angle, *J Craniomaxillofac Trauma* 2:28–36, 1996.

Fonseca RJ: *Oral and maxillofacial trauma*, ed 4, St Louis, 2012, Saunders.

Polley JW, Flagg JF, Cohen M: Fractures of the mandible. In Weinzweig J, editor: *Plastic surgery secrets*, ed 2, Philadelphia, 1999, Hanley & Belfus.

Posnick, JC: Craniomaxillofacial fractures in children. *Oral Maxillofac Clin North Am.* 1994;1:169.

Smith BR, Ghali GE: Atrophic edentulous mandibular fractures, *Oral and maxillofacial surgery knowledge update*, vol 2. 1998. Tra/29 Chicago, Publisher is AAOMS.

MANAGEMENT OF ZYGOMATICOMAXILLARY COMPLEX AND ORBITAL FRACTURES

CHAPTER 31

Siavash Siv Eftekhari, Tuan Bui, Michael J. Grau Jr., Deepak G. Krishnan

ZYGOMATICOMAXILLARY COMPLEX AND ORBITAL FRACTURES*

1. **What is the anatomy of the zygomaticomaxillary complex?**
   The zygomaticomaxillary complex (ZMC) is part of the midface bony structure contributing to facial width, cheek prominence, and inferior and lateral borders of the orbit. The zygoma has four projections, which create a quadrangular structure, connected to four bones, which include: maxillary bone at the zygomaticomaxillary (ZM) buttress, frontal bone at the zygomaticofrontal (ZF) suture, temporal bone at the zygomaticotemporal (ZT) suture, and sphenoid bone at the zygomaticosphenoid (ZS) suture. The zygomatic arch includes the temporal process of the zygoma and the zygomatic process of the temporal bone. The sensory nerve to the zygoma is the second division of the trigeminal nerve. The zygomatic arch may be fractured independently or as part of this complex. ZM and ZF are part of the vertical buttresses of the midface and correct alignment of these structures is imperative in reestablishing facial projection, facial width, and orbital volume.

2. **What is a tetrapod fracture?**
   The ZMC/zygomatic-orbital-maxillary complex fracture is often referred to also as the tripod fracture. The described fracture in reality involves five bones and four areas of articulation. More accurately, it may be described as a tetrapod fracture with the zygoma relating to the maxilla, frontal bone, greater wing of the sphenoid, and temporal bone.

3. **What are the muscular attachments of zygomatic bone?**
   Muscles of facial expression originating from the zygoma that are innervated by the facial nerve are the zygomaticus major and minor muscles that insert to support the oral commissures and zygomatic head of the levator labii superioris. The masseter muscle inserts along the temporal surface of the zygoma and zygomatic arch. The temporalis muscle and fascia pass beneath the arch and attach to the coronoid process of the mandible. This fascia that attaches to the zygoma produces resistance to inferior displacement of a fractured fragment that is exerted by the downward pull of the masseter muscle.

4. **What are the fracture patterns of the ZMC?**
   ZMC fractures are second only to nasal fractures in frequency of involvement in facial fractures. It is rare to get a true fracture of the zygomatic bone. Fractures usually occur at the suture lines where the zygomatic bone meets the maxilla, frontal, temporal, and sphenoid bones. The zygoma may be separated from its four articulations; this almost always involves the orbital floor as well. These fracture patterns usually lead to posterior and medial positioning of the zygoma that lead to facial flattening and facial widening. Typically, the fracture line travels through the zygomaticofrontal (ZF) suture, into the orbit at the zygomaticosphenoidal suture to the inferior orbital fissure. Anterior to the fissure, the fracture travels through the orbital floor and infraorbital rim, goes through the infraorbital foramen, and continues inferiorly through the zygomaticomaxillary (ZM) buttress. Posteriorly, the fracture extends from the buttress and through the lateral wall of the maxillary sinus. Finally, one of the most

---

*Written by Siavash Siv Eftekhari, Tuan Bui, Michael J. Grau, and Deepak G. Krishnan.

frequent patterns of fractures of the zygoma is isolated arch fracture, which occurs at its weakest point, about 1.5 cm posterior to the zygomaticotemporal suture.

5. **What are the classifications of ZMC fractures?**

Classification pattern assists the surgeon in treatment planning of open versus closed reduction of the fracture and the stability after fixation. There are several classification systems based on anatomic displacement. Perhaps the most popular classification was by Knight and North in 1961. They used the direction of displacement of zygomatic fracture on Waters' view radiographs. With the advent of the CT scan, more modern classification schemes have emerged. Manson and colleagues in 1990 proposed a classification scheme based on pattern of segmentation and displacement, while Gruss and associates proposed a system that stressed the importance of recognizing and treating zygomatic arch fractures in association with the zygomatic body. Zingg et al. in their 1992 review of 1025 zygomatic fractures proposed the following classification:

- Type A: Incomplete low-energy fracture with fracture of only one zygomatic pillar
- Type B: Complete mono-fragment fracture with fracture and displacement along all four articulations
- Type C: Multi-fragmented, comminuted fractures of the zygomatic body

6. **What are the physical findings associated with ZMC fractures?**

The ZMC forms the lateral wall, inferior rim, and floor of the orbit, and consequently, most fractures involving this complex can be considered true orbital fractures. Initial evaluation involves documentation of bony injuries and any injuries to surrounding soft tissue, including eyes, lacrimal apparatus, and canthal tendons. Also important is detailed documentation of any cranial nerve injuries, particularly to cranial nerves V and VII. Visual acuity and status of globe need to be investigated and ophthalmology consulted as needed.

The clinical signs and symptoms of ZMC fractures can include:

- Swelling and flattening of cheek along with periorbital edema/ecchymosis
- Downward displacement of the zygoma, which produces an anti-mongoloid slant to the lateral canthus with accentuation of the supratarsal fold of the upper eyelid. Worm's eye view evaluation of facial symmetry is very useful.
- Subconjunctival hemorrhage
- Step deformity and point tenderness at zygomatic arch, inferior orbital rim, zygomaticofrontal suture, and zygomatic buttress region
- In isolated zygomatic arch fractures, a depression is observed and palpated anterior to the tragus.
- Flattening of the malar prominence or zygomatic arch
- Epistaxis due to involvement of maxillary sinus
- If extensive orbital involvement exists, there is a possibility for presence of changes in globe position, including evidence of vertical dystopia, enophthalmos, and inferior rectus muscle entrapment resulting in restriction in the movement of extraocular muscles especially on upward gaze.
- Visual disturbances such as diplopia, reduced visual acuity, traumatic mydriasis, hyphema, and retinal tears
- Ecchymosis in the maxillary buccal vestibule (Guerin's sign)
- Trismus due to impingement of the coronoid process by collapsed zygoma
- Infraorbital nerve paresthesia due to either direct trauma or impingement from the fractured segments of bone

7. **What ophthalmic injuries may be associated with zygomatic-orbital-maxillary complex fractures?**

ZMC fractures are often accompanied by some degree of ocular injury, whether minor or major. Knowing this, it is imperative that the surgeon performs a thorough ophthalmologic examination and, if deemed necessary, seek consultation with opthalmologist colleagues. Some of these are minor ophthalmic injuries while others are major ones.

- Minor ocular injuries include subconjunctival hemorrhage, iritis, iris sphincter tear, corneal abrasion, commotio retinae, and microhyphema.
- Major ocular injuries include ruptured globe, retinal hemorrhage, retinal detachment, and hyphema.

8. **What degree of vertical dystopia can be compensated secondary to ZMC/orbital fractures before causing binocular diplopia?**

Diplopia following ZMC/orbital fractures is typically secondary to muscle entrapment/edema/fibrosis, hemorrhage, or motor nerve palsies. The brain should be able to accommodate for a vertical dystopia of up to 1 cm without causing diplopia in the primary fields of gaze.

9. **What is enophthalmos?**

   Enophthalmos may be defined as the posterior displacement of the globe that is often due to increase in orbital volume secondary to interruption of the skeletal integrity of the bony orbit. Enophthalmos may present immediately or may be delayed as resolution of edema over the course of the post-injury period exposes underlying abnormalities. Deepening of the supratarsal fold and the presence of a pseudoptosis are common clinical findings. The Hertel exophthalmometer is an instrument that may be used for measuring the position of the globe in an anterior-posterior direction as referenced to the contralateral globe and the lateral orbital rims. A difference of 2 mm is considered to be clinically significant.

10. **What are the radiographic findings associated with ZMC fractures?**

    Radiographic findings of ZMC fractures include the following:
    - Axial and coronal plane CT is the gold standard for radiographic evaluation of zygomatic fractures. It allows for detailed evaluation of buttresses of the midfacial skeleton including the orbit.
    - Waters' view is the single best X-ray for evaluation of ZMC fractures. It is a PA projection with head positioned at a 27-degree angle to the vertical. It provides good visualization of the sinuses, lateral orbits, and infraorbital rims.
    - Submentovertex (jug-handle) X-ray view is helpful for evaluation of the zygomatic arch and malar projections. Waters' and submentovertex-ray views are rarely used. When they are used, it is often in absence of or bypassing CT imaging but rarely in combination with CT.

11. **What are the indications for treatment of ZMC fractures?**

    Surgical treatment is warranted in the presence of displacement, instability, or comminution of the bony fragments. The patient's age, personal desires, and medical status and the status of the globe and of vision on the contralateral side all must be considered. Minimally displaced or nondisplaced fractures often may be observed expectantly and require no acute surgical intervention. Minimally displaced fractures or even moderately displaced fractures may be observed for several weeks for the swelling to resolve while observing for the appearance of cosmetic deformities as edema resides. Factors influencing a decision to surgically intervene are:
    - Facial aesthetics. It is desirable to reestablish the typical contour of the face for a more symmetric look and to prevent complications such as facial dysmorphism, enophthalmos, and orbital dystopia.
    - Protection: The ZMC has a vital absorbent function in the safeguard of the orbit and brain due to its key anatomic location, which would make reestablishing its proper projection important.
    - Functional impairment: Fractures that interfere with ocular function, infraorbital nerve function, or normal mouth opening should be treated.

12. **Is there a role for orbital floor exploration in all ZMC fractures?**

    By definition, ZMC fractures almost always have a variable amount of involvement of the internal orbit. There has been debate over the risks/benefits of performing orbital floor explorations on these injuries. It had been theorized that displaced fractures that had previously been deemed not to need internal orbital exploration/reconstruction might benefit from reconstruction after adequate reduction of the medially displaced and rotated ZMC fracture. Current evidence suggests that status of the internal orbit visualized on preoperative CT scan is a good indicator of the need for reconstruction and that reduction of the displaced ZMC fracture plays little role in increasing this need. The surgeon must treat these injuries on a case by case basis, utilizing physical findings to help guide the decision for internal orbital reconstruction rather than treating all injuries in a standardized manner.

13. **What are the optimal times for treatment of ZMC fractures?**

    ZMC fractures are not emergencies; any associated life-threatening injuries must be addressed first. Open reduction should be performed if indicated before the onset of edema, or after waiting several days for edema to decrease. Such delay is unlikely to compromise the surgical outcome and often results in better surgical results as long as the delay does not extend beyond 2 to 3 weeks.

14. **What are the principles of treatment of ZMC fractures?**

    Conservative treatment is indicated if there is minimal or no displacement of the fractured bones, or in cases involving the elderly or medically compromised patients. The main objectives of surgical treatments are accurate anatomic reduction of the displaced bones and buttresses and, where indicated, stable fixation of reduced fractures to reestablish form and function. Surgical reduction is either by fracture reduction without fixation or by open reduction and internal fixation (ORIF).

   A. Fracture reduction without fixation:

      Some fractures may prove very stable after simple open reduction without fixation using one of two approaches: *Gillies* or *Keen*. These two approaches are commonly used in patients with minimal-to-moderately displaced isolated zygomatic arch fracture. Since fixation is not used for these techniques, relapse rate is relatively high.

   B. Open reduction and internal fixation (ORIF):

      ORIF of fractured ZMC is indicated when there is comminution or fracture instability to reestablish adequate three-dimensional anatomies. It is important to know that a greater amount of fixation will not improve the final results in a fracture that has been poorly reduced in the first place. The intraoperative Keen approach or a transmalar Carroll-Girard screw can be utilized to reposition the zygoma before applying the fixations.

15. **What are the surgical approaches for treatment of ZMC fractures?**

    Any or combinations of the following approaches can be used to reduce and fix ZMC fractures, depending on the patient's age, location of the fractures, and involvement of other facial bones.

- Gillies approach
- Keen approach
- Intraoral maxillary vestibular approach
- Upper eyelid/blephroplasty approach including transconjunctival, subciliary, and subtarsal
- Lateral brow or supraorbital brow
- Extended lower eyelid approach
- Coronal access
- Transconjunctival
- Subciliary
- Subtarsal

16. **What is the sequence for ORIF of ZMC fractures?**

    A systemic approach is helpful to ensure accurate restoration of facial height, width, and projection. More complex ZMC fractures usually require exposure of all three anterior buttresses, which include the zygomaticomaxillary (ZM), zygomaticofrontal (ZF), and inferior orbital rim buttresses. The ZF fracture may be first stabilized temporarily with an interosseous wire. This is followed by fixation of the ZM and the infraorbital rim if indicated. A transmalar Carroll-Girard screw offers great three-dimensional positioning of the zygoma while it is being plated. The temporary wire at the ZF suture line is then replaced with a plate. The orbital floor can then be reconstructed after the zygoma is restored to its correct position. Correct alignment of zygomaticosphenoid suture is a good guide for proper three-dimensional repositioning of the zygoma.

17. **What landmark is most predictable for accurate bony reduction of the ZMC fracture?**

    Adequate reduction of the ZMC fracture depends on precise alignment and appreciation of its ability to be displaced in multiple planes of space. The zygomaticosphenoid suture has often been proposed as one of the key areas for determining adequate reduction due to its large surface area and the inherent stability of the greater wing of the sphenoid. In many situations the orbit itself is not indicated for exploration, due to degree of displacement and integrity of the orbital floor, and in such situations, the risk of possible negative sequelae being unacceptable, one must focus on other areas to guide in accurate reduction. In reality it is not the observation of the one best area but the verification of reduction of multiple areas in concert that will lead to the best results. Checking for reduction at the zygomaticomaxillary buttress and infraorbital rim (both of which can be observed through a vestibular incision) coupled with verification at the zygomaticofrontal suture is often adequate.

18. **What are some of the possible complications of surgical treatment of ZMC fractures?**

    Although complication rates are very low, the surgeon must recognize them to be able to provide appropriate care. Some signs and symptoms include infraorbital paresthesia, malunion and facial asymmetry, infection, enophthalmos, diplopia, traumatic hyphema, traumatic optic neuropathy, superior orbital fissure syndrome, retrobulbar hemorrhage, and trismus.

19. **Does the masseter muscle play a role in post-reduction instability of zygomatic-orbital-maxillary complex fractures?**

    The masseter muscle, having its origin located at the anterior two-thirds of the zygomatic arch, had historically been implicated as a culprit in the post-reduction displacement of ZOMC fractures. That assumption led to debates regarding necessary amount and placement of fixation to resist such forces. Given that the average maximal occlusal bite force approaches 45 kg, it had been proposed that fixation be to a degree to resist such a force. However, it has been found that the post-injury bite force and masseteric force are significantly reduced for four or more weeks postoperatively/post-injury. There is little hard evidence to substantiate claims of masseteric involvement in post-reduction instability; improved results with increased fixation may be explained by the need for increased surgical access and better direct observation of adequate reduction at multiple locations rather than resistance to displacement via muscle pull.

20. **What is the treatment for ankylosis between the zygomatic arch and coronoid process?**

    Coronoidectomy.

21. **What is the incidence of permanent diplopia after zygomatic fracture?**

    Initial transient diplopia is present in up to 10% of patients and is commonly evident on upward, downward, and lateral gaze. Permanent diplopia, evident on upward gaze, remains in 5% of patients.

ORBITAL FRACTURES†

22. **What is the bony anatomy of the orbit?**

    The orbit is composed of seven bones. The floor is formed by the sphenoid bone, the orbital process of the palatine bone, and the orbital process of the maxillary bone. The lateral wall is formed by the greater wing of the sphenoid bone posteriorly and the zygomatic and frontal bones anteriorly. The medial wall is made of the lesser wing of the sphenoid, the ethmoid bone, the lacrimal bone, and the frontal process of the maxilla. The roof of the orbit is composed of the frontal and sphenoid bones.

23. **What are the dimensions of the orbit?**

    By age 5 years, orbital growth is 85% complete, and it is finalized between 7 years of age and puberty. An adult orbit has an average volume of 30 cc with the globe volume being around 7 cc. The height of the orbit is on average around 35 mm, whereas the width is approximately 40 mm as measured at the rims. The child's orbit is rounder, but with age the width increases. From the medial orbital rim to the apex measures approximately 45 mm in length. From the inferior orbital rim going posteriorly, the floor dips slightly inferior for about 15 mm; it then gently curves cephalically to the superior orbital fissure. These measurements and anatomic dimensions and shapes are very important to keep in mind during orbital reconstructions and restoring orbital volume.

24. **What are important foramina, fissures, tubercles, and crests associated with the orbit?**

    - **Inferior orbital fissure:** This is located about 1 cm posterior to the inferolateral oribital rim. It connects the pterygopalatine fossa with the floor of the orbit. Contents include sensory nerves V2 (infraorbital and zygomatic nerves), inferior ophthalmic vein and branches to pterygoid plexus, and parasympathetic branches of the pterygopalatine ganglion. Contents of this fissure are usually reflected for proper inferior orbital floor exposure during surgery.
    - **Superior orbital fissure:** This is located near the apex of the orbit. It serves as a conduit for cranial nerves III, IV, and VI and the first division of cranial nerve V (ophthalmic branch). Additionally, it contains the superior ophthalmic vein and anastomosis of recurrent lacrimal and middle meningeal arteries. Fractures affecting this structure can lead to ophthalmoplegia, upper eyelid ptosis, pupillary dilatation, and forehead anesthesia, also known as superior orbital fissure syndrome.
    - **Optic canal:** This is located at the apex of the orbit, just medial to the superior orbital fissure. It is about 5 mm wide and less than 1 cm long. It houses the optic nerve, meninges, sympathetic fibers, and ophthalmic artery. Fractures involving this canal can lead to blindness. *Orbital apex syndrome* usually results from retrobulbar hematoma with compression of the optic canal and superior orbital fissure. Clinical findings include tense proptosis and periorbital swelling, retroorbital pain, pupillary

---

†Written by Siavash Siv Eftekhari and Tuan Bui.

dilation, ophthalmoplegia, and, most importantly, a change in vision. Fundoscopy reveals a pale disc with cherry red maculae. Prompt surgical decompression via lateral canthotomy is required to prevent permanent vision loss.

- **Anterior and posterior ethmoid foramen:** The anterior ethmoid foramen is located about 25 mm posterior to the medial orbital rim, and the posterior ethmoid foramin is about 30 to 35 mm posterior to the medial orbital rim. They contain the anterior and posterior ethmoidal arteries, respectively. These can be important sources of orbital or nasal bleeds. Nerves within the anterior ethmoid foramen include the anterior ethmoid branches from the nasociliary nerve from the orbit coursing into the nasal cavity. The posterior ethmoid foramen contains, variably, a sphenoethmoidal nerve from the nasociliary nerve. The posterior ethmoid foramen is usually used as a landmark for safe medial posterior extend of dissection.
- **Nasolacrimal canal:** This is located at the inferomedial orbital wall and houses the nasolacrimal duct. Just anterior to the canal is the anterior lacrimal crest that serves as the attachment point for the anterior portion of the medial canthus. The deeper fibers of the medial canthus along with the orbicularis oculi muscle attach to the smaller posterior lacrimal crest.
- **Whitnall's tubercle:** This is located on the lateral orbital wall just below the frontozygomatic suture about 1 cm posterior to the lateral rim. It is a point of attachment for the lateral canthus and other globe suspensory ligaments of significance.

25. What are the layers of the eyelid?
Eyelid layers from superficial to deep include the following: skin, subcutaneous areolar tissue, striated muscle of orbicularis oculi, submuscular areolar tissue (contains the sensory nerves), tarsal plates within a fibrous layer, nonstriated smooth muscle, and conjunctiva.

26. What is the importance of the orbital septum?
The orbital septum is a layer continuous with the orbital periosteum and the periosteum of the facial bones overlying the rims just deep to the orbicularis oculi muscle. It sets the boundary for preseptal versus postseptal/retrobulbar spaces. It is an important layer to consider when dealing with orbital infections or hematomas. It converges with the periosteum about 1 to 2 mm below the inferior orbital rim, forming a periosteal thickening called the *arcus marginalis*. In the subciliary or preseptal transconjunctival approaches to the inferior rim and orbital floor, the orbital septum is an important landmark to keep in mind. Incising below the arcus marginalis prevents orbital contents and fat from herniating into our surgical field, making our subperiosteal dissection much easier to perform.

27. What are the common patterns of orbital fractures?
There are two types of orbital fractures:
1. Fractures involving the internal orbital wall(s) and orbital rim(s). Examples are naso-orbito-ethmoid fractures, zygomatico-orbital fractures, and maxillary Le Fort fractures. These are the most common types of orbital fractures, with the fractures of the zygomatic complex being the most common (30% to 55% of all facial fractures).
2. Pure orbital fractures that involve the orbital walls/floor but do not involve the rims. They account for about 4% to 16% of all facial fractures. Although the bones of the medial orbital wall are the thinnest, they are strengthened by the perpendicular septa of the ethmoid sinus. Therefore, the second thinnest wall of the orbit, which is the orbital floor, is most prone to fractures, especially just medial to the infraorbital canal.

28. What are the clinical findings of orbital fractures?
Common clinical findings in orbital fractures include periorbital edema, subconjunctival ecchymosis, orbital emphysema, infraorbital nerve paresthesia, bony step deformity around the orbital rim with point tenderness, and changes in the globe position in more severe fractures including any evidence of enophthalmous, exophthalmos, or vertical dystopia. A lid retractor such as Desmarres is useful for separating swollen-tight lids during examination. Generally, orbital fractures have an early presentation of exophthalmus due to swelling. Enophthalmos is present within 1 to 3 weeks if the orbital cavity is significantly enlarged and appears as the swelling resolves. Any evidence of proptosis or retrobulbar hematoma should be followed by tonometry examination that indirectly measures intraocular pressure (normal pressures: 10 to 20 mm Hg). An orbital volume enlargement of more than 5% to 10% will most likely require open reduction. Orbital apex syndrome usually results from retrobulbar hematoma with compression of the optic canal and superior orbital fissure. Clinical findings include tense proptosis and periorbital swelling, retroorbital pain, pupillary dilation, ophthalmoplegia, and, most importantly, a change in vision. Funduscopy reveals a pale disc with cherry red maculae. Prompt surgical decompression via lateral canthotomy is required to prevent permanent vision loss.

29. **What are the radiographic imaging needed for evaluating orbtial fractures?**
   CT is the gold standard for assessing the status of the bony orbit. Fine cuts (1 to 2 mm) analyzed through axial and coronal cuts are needed for diagnosis. Sagittal cuts are useful in evaluating the integrity of the orbital floor. A soft tissue window can be used for evaluating any radiographic evidence of muscle entrapment or retrobulbar hematoma. Less optimally, a Waters' view X-ray can be used to show an orbital floor fracture. MRI can be useful to assess soft tissues, extraocular muscle entrapment, or optic nerve damage.

30. **What are the etiologies of monocular versus binocular diplopia?**
   Acute binocular diplopia (double vision) after trauma is usually due to one of three basic mechanisms: (1) orbital edema or hematoma (most common), (2) restricted motility, or (3) neurogenic injury. Binocular diplopia is more common in the traumatic setting and may result from an alteration in globe position, such as proptosis or enophthalmos, or from limitation of globe movement through entrapment of orbital soft tissues. Monocular diplopia is usually due to lens dislocation or opacification or another disturbance in the clear media along the visual axis. These physical findings warrant immediate ophthalmologic consultation. Alternatively, nerve injury may occur intracranially or within the orbit as a result of compression from hematoma or bone fragments. Surgical repair of the bony orbit and decompression of affected nerves usually result in correction of diplopia.

31. **What is the bowstring test, and in what situations should it be utilized?**
   The bowstring test is a means of assessing the status of the medial canthal ligament in more severe orbital fractures involving the Nasoethmoidal (NOE) segments. Commonly, the ligament remains intact and attached to the lacrimal bone, which may be fractured and displaced. The bowstring test is performed by placing gentle lateral traction over the lateral canthus while palpating the medial canthal region to assess mobility. A positive test confirms bony fracture with displacement of the medial canthal ligament or traumatic telecanthus.

32. **How can entrapment of orbital contents be diagnosed in an unconscious patient?**
   Diagnosis of orbital content entrapment is made by performing a forced duction test. The test involves grasping the insertion of a rectus muscle onto the ocular globe with a forceps approximately 7 mm from the limbus. The globe is then gently rotated in all four directions, and any restriction is noted. The inferior rectus muscle is the most commonly tested muscle, although the superior, medial, or lateral recti muscles may be used as well.

33. **What is a Marcus Gunn pupil?**
   It is an afferent pupillary defect resulting from lesions involving the retina or optic nerve back to the chiasm. With this defect, a light shone in the unaffected eye produces normal constriction of the pupils of both eyes (consensual response), but a light shone in the affected eye produces a paradoxical dilation rather than constriction of the affected pupil.

34. **What is the most common site of an isolated intraorbital fracture?**
   The most frequent intraorbital fracture involves the orbital floor just medial to the infraorbital canal and is usually confined to the medial portion of the floor and the lower portion of the medial orbital wall. Depressed fractures of these regions may cause the orbital soft tissue to be displaced into the maxillary and ethmoid sinuses, leading to an increase in orbital volume.

35. **What is the incidence of hypoesthesia or anesthesia in the distribution of infraorbital floor associated with orbital floor fractures?**
   The incidence is 90% to 95%.

36. **What are the indications for operative management of orbital fractures?**
   Indications for surgery can be functional or cosmetic.
      The functional indications include continued diplopia and decreased visual acuity are the most important indications. Any evidence of inferior rectus muscle entrapment, which is most commonly seen in the pediatric population due to the elasticity of their bones, warrants early intervention to free up the tissue and prevent ischemic necrosis or scar contracture.
      The cosmetic deformity indications include enophthalmos or hypo-ophthalmos and result from bony orbital volume increase and/or fat herniation into maxillary sinus in case of orbital floor fractures. Studies show that most patients will notice globe asymmetry once there is 2 to 4 mm of globe malposition. Orbital floor defects of greater than half of the surface area with concomitant CT evidence of orbital content herniation into maxillary sinus generally should be repaired. With minimal floor disturbance (usually less than 50%) and no muscle entrapment or minimal to no orbital content

herniation, observation for 2 weeks is recommended. If a patient develops any functional problems or enophthalmous is greater than 2 mm, then surgery can be offered.

37. **What are the surgical approaches for treating orbital fractures?**
    - Subciliary lower eyelid incision
    - Subtarsal incision
    - Infraorbital approach
    - Transconjunctival incision
    - Lateral brow incision and upper blepharoplasty incision
    - Intraoral maxillary vestibular approach
    - Bicoronal approach

38. **What are important considerations when exposing an orbital floor fracture?**
    Orbital rim fractures need to be adequately reduced prior to repairing any of the orbital walls. No matter which surgical approach is used, the orbital floor dissection is similar in all cases. Pertinent landmarks are the inferior orbital fissure and the infraorbital nerve and its canal. Dissection begins subperiosteally from the inferior orbital rim exposing the orbital floor defect. Medially, the dissection can be carried safely to the level of the posterior ethmoid foramen. At all times, the surgeon needs to keep in mind that the orbital floor ascends at a 30-degree slope from the midaxial plane. The tendency is to dissect into the maxillary sinus unless the surgeon is always ascending as he/she is dissecting posteriorly. The periosteum should be completely dissected off sound bone around the defect. The infraorbital nerve can serve as a guide for the surgeon's path of dissection on the orbital floor. Finally, the most important structure to locate is the posterior ledge of bone on which our reconstruction material can rest. Once we have adequate dissection and exposure, a suitable reconstructive material can be used to span the defect.

39. **What materials are used to reconstruct the orbital floor?**
    Restoring the correct anatomy of the orbit and orbital volume are more important than the material used for restoration as long as the material provides adequate rigidity. The following are some of the materials that have been used for this purpose:
    - Inorganic alloplastic materials (e.g., Medpor, Silastic, Vitallium, stainless steel, Teflon, Supramid, or titanium implants)
    - Autogenous bone grafts (split calvarial, iliac, or split rib)
    - Allogenic bone grafts
    Ideal materials should be thin and rigid, minimal size needed to span the wall defect, properly shaped to restore orbital volume, and placed tension-free and adequately stabilized. Additionally, adequacy of reconstruction should be verified. This can be done by intraoperative versus postoperative CT or use of an intraoperative navigation system.

40. **What is the transantral approach for repairing the orbital floor?**
    The transantral endoscopic approach provides direct access to the orbital floor without any unsightly skin incisions. The approach involves exposing the anterior maxillary sinus wall through an intraoral maxillary vestibular incision and creating a bony window through the anterior portion of maxillary sinus. Through this antrostomy, a 0-degree and 30-degree endoscope can be inserted to evaluate the roof of the sinus that is the orbital floor. Orbital floor blowout fractures can then be reduced. If a trapdoor defect exists, the fracture's bony ledge should be elevated back to the anatomic position with overlap of its edges on the native orbital floor. This may or may not need fixation. Alternatively, a reconstruction plate/mesh can be properly shaped and introduced through the maxillary antral wall defect with adequate curve to support the bony defect back into its proper position with inset into the posterior ledge. Anterior extension of the plate is then brought through the antral window, and the plate is stabilized with two small screws on the anterior maxillary wall.

41. **Which incision has the greatest propensity for ectropion?**
    Scleral show and ectropion are frequent sequelae of the subciliary incision after lower lid surgery and are often due to lid retraction. These conditions improve with time in many patients but may be permanent deformities that result from permanent scarring within the lower eyelid.

42. **What are the most frequent complications of inadequately treated or untreated fractures of the orbital floor?**
    Diplopia and enophthalmos.

43. **What complications are associated with fractures of the orbital roof?**
Fractures of the orbital roof usually involve the supraorbital ridge, frontal bone, and frontal sinus. The trochlea of the superior oblique muscle is often damaged because of its proximity to the surface of the roof, resulting in transitory diplopia. Another sign is globe displacement that occurs in an inferolateral direction and may result in proptosis. Cranial nerve (CN) VI may be traumatized with orbital roof fractures, resulting in paralysis of the lateral rectus muscle and limitation of ocular abduction. Additional complications include dural tears, anterior cranial base injuries, CSF leaks, cerebral herniation, and pulsatile exophthalmos.

44. **What is the mechanism of posttraumatic enophthalmos?**
Enophthalmos results mostly from displacement of a relatively constant volume of orbital soft tissue contents into an enlarged bony orbital volume caused by disruption and displacement of one or more of the orbital walls. Enophthalmos in excess of 5 mm results in a noticeable deformity.
   Diplopia is double vision, which is often transient and present only at the extremes of gaze rather than within a functional field of vision. It is commonly attributed to hematoma or edema that causes muscular imbalance by elevating the ocular globe or to injury of the extraocular musculature and temporary effects on the oculorotary mechanism. Diplopia in itself is rarely an indication for surgery.

45. **What is a blowout fracture of the orbit?**
A blowout fracture of the orbit results from direct trauma to the globe resulting in distortion of the globe and increased intraorbital pressure. The orbital rim generally stays intact, and the force is transmitted to the interior area of the orbital cavity. The force is dissipated by outward fracture of the weaker bones of the orbital floor and medial wall. As force increases, the fractures may extend both posteriorly and circumferentially. A thorough physical exam and diagnostic imaging, specifically CT scanning, are required to evaluate the size of the defect and possible entrapment of orbital structures. Significant defects require operative repair to prevent posttraumatic enophthalmos.

46. **What are the differences between superior orbital fissure syndrome and orbital apex syndrome?**
Superior orbital fissure syndrome results from compression of the contents found in the superior orbital fissure by hematoma or bony fragment. Clinical findings include:
   • Pupillary dilation through dysfunction of CN III innervation of pupillary constrictor muscles
   • Ophthalmoplegia secondary to palsy of CNs III, IV, and VI
   • Upper eyelid ptosis from levator palpebrae paresis
   • Anesthesia of the forehead and loss of corneal reflex from ophthalmic division of the trigeminal nerve compression
   • Proptosis secondary to edema from obstruction of the ophthalmic vein and lymphatic system.
      Orbital apex syndrome usually results from retrobulbar hematoma with compression of the optic canal and superior orbital fissure. Clinical findings include tense proptosis and periorbital swelling, retroorbital pain, pupillary dilation, ophthalmoplegia, and, most importantly, a change in vision. Funduscopy reveals a pale disc with cherry red maculae. Prompt surgical decompression via lateral canthotomy is required to prevent permanent vision loss.

47. **What is the relationship between orbital volume changes as they relate to orbital trauma?**
The normal volume of the bony orbit is approximately 30 cc. Fractures of orbital bones may increase or decrease this volume, with resultant changes in the position of the orbital contents. Fractures that decrease orbital volume compress the orbital contents and may create exophthalmos. Increases in orbital volume provide more room for the globe and may result in dystopia or a change in the vertical position of the globe. Enophthalmos is a change in the anterior-posterior position of the globe. Alterations in globe position as a function of orbital volume change are dependent on two factors: disruption of Lockwood's suspensory ligament and the relationship of the change in volume relative to the axis of the globe. The axis is defined as a line connecting the lateral orbital rim to an area just in front of the lacrimal bone. Volume changes behind this line can produce significant alterations in globe position. It is estimated that 1 mL of volume loss behind the axis produces 1.5 mm of enophthalmos. Anterior orbital floor and medial wall fractures are usually in front of the axis and produce minimal changes in globe position.

48. **What is hyphema, and how is it managed?**
Hyphema is the layering of blood in the anterior chamber of the globe, usually from the tearing of blood vessels at the root of the iris. It may present with pain, blurred vision, and photophobia.

Retinal hemorrhage is also found in more than 50% of hyphemas. Management of hyphema is directed toward prevention of rebleeding, which occurs in 3% to 30% of cases. Rebleeds generally occur 3 to 5 days after injury, are usually more severe than the original injury, and may result in impaired vision, corneal staining, and glaucoma formation. Patients are usually admitted for bed rest and daily ophthalmologic evaluation. An eye patch is applied, and increased intraocular pressure is treated with topical beta blockers and carbonic anhydrase inhibitors or mannitol if necessary. Aspirin is absolutely contraindicated in these patients.

49. **What are the possible etiologies of extraocular movement disorders following trauma?**

Extraocular movements are controlled by the six extraocular muscles. The inferior, superior, medial rectus, and inferior oblique muscles are all innervated by CN III (oculomotor). The superior oblique muscle is innervated by the trochlear nerve (CN IV), and the lateral rectus muscle is supplied by the abducens nerve (CN VI). Traumatic disruption of either muscle or nerve continuity would likely result in a movement disorder manifested by limited gaze in the direction of affected muscle pull and binocular diplopia. Entrapment of muscle in traumatic bony defects (e.g., orbital floor blowout fracture) also may lead to restricted gaze.

50. **What are the causes of traumatic ptosis?**

Ptosis refers to the drooping of the upper eyelid. Normal resting eyelid position is mediated by the sympathetic nervous system by the superior cervical ganglion. The muscle end point of these nerves is Mueller's muscle, a smooth muscle that inserts on the upper tarsal plate. Disruption of the sympathetic fibers (e.g., in Horner's syndrome) leads to ptosis. The levator palpebrae superioris is responsible for voluntary eye opening and is innervated by CN III. Injury to this nerve or muscle also results in ptosis. Alteration in globe position may result in the appearance of ptosis despite full function of related nerves and muscles.

BIBLIOGRAPHY

Zygomaticomaxillary Complex and Orbital Fractures

Abubaker AO, Ziccardi VB, McDonald I: Midfacial fractures: fractures of the nose, zygoma, orbit and maxilla. In Abubaker AO, Benson KJ, editors: *Oral and maxillofacial surgery knowledge update*, vol 3:TRA80-90. 2001, AAOMS.

Carter TG, Bagheri S, Dierks EJ: Towel clip reduction of the depressed zygomatic arch fracture, *J Oral Maxillofac Surg* 63(8):1244–1246, 2005.

Dal Santo F, Ellis III E, et al.: The effects of zygomatic complex fracture on masseteric muscle force, *J Oral Maxillofac Surg* 50:791–799, 1992.

Ellis III E, Kittidumkerng W: Analysis of treatment for isolated zygomaticomaxillary complex fractures, *J Oral Maxillofac Surg* 54:386–400, 1996.

Ellis III E, Reddy L: Status of the internal orbit after reduction of zygomaticomaxillary complex fractures, *J Oral Maxillofac Surg* 62:275–283, 2004.

Haug RH, Bradrick JP, Morgan JP: Complications in the treatment of midface fractures. In Kaban LB, Pogrel MA, Perrott DH, editors: *Complications in oral and maxillofacial surgery*, Philadelphia, 1997, W.B. Saunders, p 153.

Jamal BT, Pfahler SM, et al.: Opthalmic injuries in patients with zygomaticomaxillary complex fractures requiring surgical repair, *J Oral Maxillofac Surg* 67:986–989, 2009.

Knight JS, North JF: The classification of malar fractures: an analysis of displacement as a guide to treatment, *British Journal of Plastic Surg* 13:325–339, 1961.

Kontio R, Lindqvist C: Management of orbital fractures, *Oral Maxillofac Surg Clin NA* 21(2):209–220, 2009.

Lee EI, Mohan K, Koshy JC, Hollier LH: Optimizing the surgical management of zygomaticomaxillary complex fractures, *Semin Plast Surg* 24(4):389–397, 2010.

Long JA, Gutta R: Orbital, periorbital, and ocular reconstruction, *Oral Maxillofac Surg Clin NA* 25:151–166, 2013.

Markiewicz MR, Bell BR: Traditional and contemporary surgical approaches to the orbit, *Oral Maxillofac Surg Clin NA* 24:573–607, 2012.

Markiewicz MR, Gelesko S, Bell BR: Zygoma reconstruction, *Oral Maxillofac Surg Clin NA* 25(2):167–201, 2013.

Miloro M, Ghali GE, Larsen P, Waite P: *Peterson's principles of oral and maxillofacial surgery*, ed 3, Shelton, CT, 2011, PMPH.

Moreira Marinho RO, Freire-Maia B: Management of fractures of the zygomaticomaxillary complex, *Oral Maxillofac Surg Clin NA* 25(4):617–636, 2013.

Ogden GR: The Gillies method for fractured zygomas, *J Oral Maxillofac Surg* 49:23–25, 1991.

Palmieri CF, Ghali GE: Late correction of orbital deformities, *Oral Maxillofac Surg Clin NA* 24:649–663, 2012.

Rhea JT, Noveline RA: How to simplify the CT diagnosis of Lefort fractures, *Am J Roentgenol* 184:1700–1705, 2005.

Turvey TA, Golden BA: Orbital anatomy for the surgeon, *Oral Maxillofac Surg Clin NA* 24(4):525–536, 2012.

Zingg M, Laedrach K, Chen J, et al.: Classification and treatment of zygomatic fractures: a review of 1025 cases, *J Oral Maxillofac Surg* 50:779–790, 1992.

Orbital Fractures

Ellis III E: Orbital trauma, *Oral Maxillofac Surg Clin NA* 24(4):629–648, 2012.

Holmes S: Reoperative orbital trauma: management of posttraumatic enophthalmos and aberrant eye position, *Oral Maxillofac Surg Clin NA* 23(1):17–29, 2011.

Joseph JM, Glavas LP: Orbital fractures: a review, *Clin Opththalmol* 5:95–100, 2011.

Kawamoto HK: Late posttraumatic enophthalmos: a correctable deformity? *Plast Reconstr Surg* 69:423–432, 1992.

Kontio R, Lindqvist C: Management of orbital fractures, *Oral Maxillofac Surg Clin NA* 21(2):209–220, 2009.

Long JA, Gutta R: Oribital, periorbital, and ocular reconstruction, *Oral Maxillofac Surg Clin NA* 25:151–166, 2013.

Manson PN, Iliff N: Management of blow-out fractures of the orbital floor. II. Early repair for selected injuries, *Surv Ophthalmol* 35:280–292, 1991.

Markiewicz MR, Bell BR: Traditional and contemporary surgical approaches to the orbit, *Oral Maxillofac Surg Clin NA* 24:573–607, 2012.

Nguyen PN, Sullivan P: Advances in the management of orbital fractures, *Clin Plast Surg* 19:87–98, 1992.

Palmieri CF, Ghali GE: Late correction of orbital deformities, *Oral Maxillofac Surg Clin NA* 24:649–663, 2012.

Turvey TA, Golden BA: Orbital anatomy for the surgeon, *Oral Maxillofac Surg Clin NA* 24(4):525–536, 2012.

CHAPTER 32

MIDFACIAL FRACTURES: NASAL, NASOETHMOIDAL, AND LE FORT FRACTURES

A. Omar Abubaker, Deepak G. Krishnan, Michael J. Grau Jr.

NASAL FRACTURES*

1. **Where are the most common sites for nasal bones to fracture?**
   Fractures of the nasal bones occur most commonly in the distal nasal bones, which are broad and thin. Direct frontal blows to the nasal dorsum usually result in fracture of the thin lower half of the nasal bones. The proximal nasal bones are stronger and thicker and relatively resistant to fracture. However, when the force of the blow is more severe, the fracture may involve the more proximal nasal bones, the frontal process of the maxilla, and the frontal bone.

2. **What is the role of radiographs in the diagnosis and treatment of nasal fractures?**
   Standard facial radiographs are of limited diagnostic and therapeutic value in the treatment of nasal fractures. However, radiographs can serve as a physical record of a nasal fracture, and computed tomography (CT) scans can accurately determine the degree of displacement of nasal fractures and fractures of the orbitoethmoidal region. Therefore, although radiographic documentation is recommended for medical-legal reasons, physical exam of the nose should provide the basis for whether surgical intervention is indicated.

3. **When is nasal packing indicated after treatment of nasal fractures?**
   After successful reduction of a nasal fracture, intranasal packing is often used to serve the following purposes:
   - To control bleeding and prevent postoperative septal hematoma
   - To splint the nasal septum into position and keep the septal mucosa adapted to the septal cartilage and to provide internal support for reduced bone fragments
   - To prevent synechiae if large areas of mucosa are abraded

4. **What are the indications for posterior nasal packing?**
   A posterior pack is indicated for posterior nasal bleeds. This type of bleeding is often diagnosed when the patient's chief complaint is bleeding into the throat or if a posterior nosebleed is visualized and the bleeding cannot be controlled with a well-placed anterior pack.

5. **How long should a posterior pack be left in place?**
   For 3 to 5 days.

6. **What is the treatment of a severely comminuted nasal fracture?**
   Severely comminuted nasal fractures usually can be reduced primarily and supported with intranasal packing and externally applied splints. Packing is placed underneath the nasal bones so that formation of the bone fragments is sandwiched between and supported by internal and external support mechanisms. The combination of internal and external splinting helps prevent hematoma, compresses and narrows the splayed nasal dorsum, and conserves nasal height. Open reduction of a comminuted nasal fracture early after injury risks loss of bone fragments with little soft tissue attachment and should be used with caution or avoided completely.

---

*Written by A. Omar Abubaker, Vincent B. Ziccardi, and Ian McDonald.

7. **What are the indications for secondary treatment of nasal fractures?**
   Even with adequate reduction, postoperative nasal deformity may still occur, and patients should be informed of such a possibility. Late deformities may include a nasal hump or deviation, loss of dorsal height, septal deviation, and nasal obstruction. Secondary treatment of nasal fractures is indicated when any of these deformities is present, especially in the presence of either functional or cosmetic problems.

8. **How are acute septal hematomas treated?**
   Septal hematomas are treated with an incision along the base or most inferior portion of the hematoma to allow dependent drainage and prevent refilling of the cavity with blood or serum. Bilateral hematomas can be treated with bilateral incisions, maintaining an intact septal cartilage, or with a unilateral incision and resection of a window of cartilage to allow a bilateral communication with the incision. A light nasal packing and prophylactic antibiotics are recommended.

9. **How soon after injury should a nasal fracture be reduced?**
   Nasal fractures should be reduced within the first few hours after injury, if at all possible. If this is not done within this period, edema makes accurate judgment of the degree of deformity and the decision to operate difficult. The next window of opportunity occurs 3 to 14 days after injury, after the edema has resolved but before bony union of the fractured fragments occurs.

10. **What are the late complications of nasal fractures?**
    The following complications may be seen following nasal fractures with and without treatment:
    - Airway obstruction
    - Nasal deformity secondary to saddle deformity or dorsal hump
    - Nasal deviation and septal perforation
    - The formation of synechiae between the septum and turbinates
    - Recurrent epistaxis and recurrent sinusitis and headaches

11. **What is a nasal septal hematoma, and how is it treated?**
    A nasal septal hematoma usually presents as a boggy, blue elevation of the septal mucosa. This finding is significant because it requires drainage to prevent secondary infection and necrosis of the septal cartilage leading to perforation and possible saddle nose deformity. Drainage can be accomplished by either needle aspiration or small mucosal incision. Transseptal resorbable sutures and nasal packing can be placed to prevent re-accumulation of blood.
    Septal hematomas are treated with an incision along the base or its most inferior point to allow dependent drainage and prevent its refilling with blood or serum. Bilateral hematomas can be treated with bilateral incisions, maintaining an intact septal cartilage, or with a unilateral incision and resection of a window of cartilage. Nasal packing and prophylactic antibiotics are recommended.

12. **What is saddle nose deformity?**
    Saddle nose deformity is the concave appearance of the nasal dorsum that sometimes follows significant nasal trauma. It results from fracture and inferior displacement of the nasal bones, resulting in buckling of the cartilaginous septum and disruption of the upper lateral cartilage position. Late effects of the injury that amplify the deformity include septal collapse, which may result from septal hematoma formation, asymmetric septal growth, and scar contractures.

13. **How is epistaxis managed in the emergency department?**
    Anterior nasal epistaxis usually involves Kiesselbach's plexus, which is the confluence of the terminal ends of the superior labial, anterior ethmoid, and sphenopalatine arteries. Packing of this area with phenylephrine-soaked cotton pledgets is frequently successful. Direct visualization with a nasal speculum may allow direct cauterization with either electrocautery or silver nitrate sticks to be performed. Excessive cauterization should be avoided, however, to prevent subsequent septal perforation. Most commonly, sterile petrolatum-impregnated gauze is carefully packed in a layered manner and left in place for 2 to 5 days. Broad-spectrum antibiotic coverage should be initiated to prevent maxillary sinus infections caused by blockage of the middle meatus.
    Posterior nosebleeds are more difficult to manage due to inability to provide adequate pressure with nasal packing. This frequently is managed by placing a Foley urinary catheter into the affected nares, inflating the balloon with saline, and pulling the balloon back to seal the nasopharynx and to allow packing to be placed around the Foley. Tension is maintained on the catheter by placing an umbilical clip on it at the entrance of the nose. Commercially available posterior nasal balloons are also available.

14. **What are the classic clinical findings in a patient with a nasoethmoidal (NOE) fracture?**
The NOE fracture usually results from a direct blow to the bridge of the nose by a blunt object, such as a steering wheel or dashboard during a motor vehicle accident. Patients classically present with a widened nasal bridge, periorbital edema and ecchymosis, epistaxis, cerebrospinal fluid (CSF) rhinorrhea (42%), and traumatic telecanthus (12% to 20%). Epiphora as an early or late finding indicates injury or outflow obstruction to the nasolacrimal apparatus. Treatment goals include restoration of normal intercanthal distance, fixation of the nasal bones, and careful evaluation and possible repair of the bony orbit and nasolacrimal apparatus.

15. **Why is the placement of a nasogastric tube sometimes contraindicated in a midface fracture patient?**
Midface fractures commonly extend through the nasal cavity and may result in soft tissue disruption in the nasopharynx with concomitant cranial injuries and fractures of the cribriform plate. Placement of a nasogastric tube in these patients may result in the inadvertent intracranial placement of the tube or soft tissue dissection in a previously traumatized region.

NASOETHMOIDAL FRACTURES†

16. **What is a nasoethmoidal (NOE) fracture?**
Fractures of the central midface that involve the nasal bones, the medial walls of the orbit, and the ethmoid complex constitute the group of fractures known as nasoethmoidal fractures or NOE fractures, a term coined by Epker in 1973.

17. **How are fractures of the NOE region classified?**
Markowitz and Manson have classified NOE fractures into three patterns of fracture. They are:
- Type I: single-segment central fragment
- Type II: comminuted central fragment with fractures remaining external to the medial canthal tendon insertion
- Type III: comminuted central fragment with fractures extending into bone bearing the canthal insertion. Injuries are further classified as unilateral and bilateral and by their extension into other anatomic areas.

18. **How do you diagnose NOE fractures?**
Diagnosis of NOE fractures is based on physical examination and CT images. A bimanual examination is performed to determine the mobility of the fracture and need for open reduction. On examination, patients typically exhibit telecanthus, severe shortening, and rotation of the distal aspect of the nose. CT imaging produces accurate detail of the hard and soft tissues involved in NOE fractures. Axial and coronal sections are helpful to determine the extent of injury. These sections are especially useful for diagnosing orbital floor and medial orbital blowout fractures. A three-dimensional CT scan can also be helpful to diagnose and plan treatment. CT images can detail the comminuted areas of the central fragment but may not reveal the true extent of the comminution. The most accurate way to evaluate the central fragment is when it is exposed intraoperatively to determine if the canthal attachment is disrupted.

19. **What is the normal intercanthal distance?**
Normal intercanthal distance can be influenced by gender, age, and race. In adults, it can range from 28.6 to 33 mm in women and 28.9 to 34.5 mm in men.

20. **What is the difference between telecanthus and hypertelorism?**
Telecanthus refers to a widening of the distance between the medial canthi, usually traumatic, such as in NOE fractures. **Hypertelorism** is the widening of the orbits themselves and is measured as the interpupillary distance. Hypertelorism is more common in congenital craniofacial anomalies such as craniosynostoses or syndromes.

21. **What is the bowstring test?**
The bowstring test is a simple means of assessing the status of the medial canthal ligament in NOE fractures. Commonly, the ligament remains intact and attached to the lacrimal bone, which

---

†Written by Deepak G. Krishnan and Michael J. Grau Jr.

may be fractured with displacement. The bowstring test is performed by placing gentle lateral traction over the lateral canthus while palpating the medial canthal region to assess mobility. A positive test confirms bony fracture with displacement of the medial canthal ligament or traumatic telecanthus.

22. **What are some surgical approaches to the NOE area?**
Isolated NOE fractures can be approached via a superior surgical approach alone (coronal) or combined with an inferior (transconjunctival) access. A maxillary vestibular incision is used for those fractures extending to the inferior maxilla along the nasal slope. Existing lacerations over the nasal bridge can be utilized but often require extensions. Other skin approaches in the central midface are generally avoided due to poor aesthetics.

23. **How are NOE fractures treated?**
The complexity of reduction and fixation depends on the severity of fracture patterns and associated injuries. Type I and II fractures allow for direct internal fixation of large bone fragments following exposure and reduction. In type III fractures extending through the medial canthal tendon insertion, the bone fragment is isolated by subperiosteal dissection. The canthus is detached to allow for bone reduction. A wire passing bur is used to create two holes **superior and posterior** to the lacrimal crest in the central fragment. A drill guide is helpful to avoid damage to the globe. Care is also taken to prevent damage to the contralateral globe during this procedure. A single 25-gauge wire is secured to the central fragments. A 3-mm vertical incision just medial to the eyelid commissure facilitates passing a permanent suture through the canthus without damage to the lacrimal drainage apparatus. These sutures are placed bilaterally and secured to the transnasal wire. The wire is then tightened until the desired intercanthal narrowing is achieved. Alternatively, a permanent suture may be used for the transnasal reduction.

24. **How does one test for patency of the lacrimal drainage system?**
Impairment of the lacrimal drainage system following NOE injuries can lead to epiphora and symptoms of lacrimal obstruction. Jones tests can be utilized to assess the patency of the lacrimal system. There are two components to the Jones tests. In the Jones 1 test, or the primary dye test, fluorescein dye is applied into the lower cul-de-sac of the affected eye. After adequate time, a cotton tip applicator is placed under the inferior turbinate of the lateral nasal wall on the same side. Failure to see any dye under the inferior turbinate indicates blockage of the nasolacrimal flow.

    The Jones 2 test, or the secondary dye test, helps assess the location of the blockage. The Jones 2 test is performed following irrigation of the inferior cul-de-sac for any remnant dye from the Jones 1 test. The lacrimal punctum is anesthetized, and an irrigation catheter is inserted to allow thorough irrigation of the system. If no fluid at all is detected in the nose, the obstruction is complete. If it is possible to detect some of the fluorescein in the inferior meatus with this flush, then the obstruction is partial. If only clear saline flushes out, this indicates an obstruction of the upper collecting system, because the dye was not collected into the system, but it was possible to irrigate the saline through.

25. **What is dacrocystorhinostomy?**
Dacrocystorhinostomy (DCR) is the repair of the lacrimal drainage system through the creation of a new "ostomy" from the lacrimal canaliculi to the nasal cavity. It can be done via an endonasal approach or an open approach.

LE FORT FRACTURES‡

26. **Who was Le Fort?**
René Le Fort (1869–1951) was a French surgeon little remembered for creating a classification for fractures of the face. In 1901, he published a treatise called *Étude expérimentale sur les fractures de la mâchoire supérieure* involving his experiments with maxillary fractures of the skull. To perform these experiments, Le Fort used intact cadaver heads and delivered blunt forces of varying degrees of magnitude, as well as from different directions. From these tests, he determined that predictable patterns of fractures are the result of certain types of injuries and concluded that there are three predominant types of midface fractures.

---

‡ Written by Deepak G. Krishnan and Michael J. Grau Jr.

27. **What are the types of Le Fort fractures?**

    Le Fort's experiments provided us with a classification system that helps us diagnose and manage injuries of the maxilla, midface.

    - Le Fort I: Maxillary fractures at level I traverse above the alveolar ridge and teeth, from the piriform aperture, along the lateral walls of the maxillary antrum, and extend posteriorly to involve and separate the pterygoid plates. Medially they pass along the lateral nasal wall and the lower third of the septum. These fractures allow the maxillae and hard palate to move as a single block. It is possible to have a unilateral fracture at this level. This would often involve separation along the mid-palate.
    - Le Fort II: Maxillary fractures at level II involve most of the nasal bones, the maxillary bones, the palatine bones, and the lower two-thirds of the nasal septum, the dentoalveolar structures and the pterygoid plates. Le Fort II fractures are referred to as pyramidal fractures. The fracture disconnects superiorly at the nasofrontal junction and continues along the medial inferior third of the orbit and laterally along the zygomaticomaxillary suture and on toward the pterygoid plates. The nasal septum is separated superiorly causing a pyramidal disjunction of the midface.
    - Le Fort III: In this pattern of midface fracture, the fractures run at the midline either across the nasal bones or disjoint at the nasofrontal junction, laterally traversing through the medial orbital wall and the superior orbit extending along the inferior orbital fissure and the lateral orbital wall to the zygomaticofrontal suture. The zygomaticotemporal suture is separated as well. The septum separates at the cribriform ethmoid plate. There is separation of the pterygoid plates causing an entire craniofacial disjunction.

    Le Fort level II fractures are associated with increased mortality. Furthermore, Le Fort II and III fractures are associated with serious intracranial injury, even in the absence of alterations in consciousness. Patients with complex midface fractures were 57% more likely to die.

28. **What are some of the clinical signs of midface fractures?**

    - Mobility of midface: best detected by movement elicited while holding the patient's maxillary anterior teeth with one hand while palpating the nasofrontal junction
    - Pain and edema of the midface
    - Anterior open bite, or other malocclusion
    - Nasal bleeding, subconjunctival ecchymosis, infraorbital nerve hypoesthesia, tenderness along the bony buttresses, step deformities palpable on the face
    - Periorbital ecchymosis (raccoon's eyes)

29. **What is Battle's sign?**

    Battle's sign refers to postauricular ecchymosis. It is indicative of a basilar skull fracture involving the middle cranial fossa that are not infrequently associated with complex midfacial injuries.

30. **What imaging modality is most appropriate for diagnosing Le Fort fractures?**

    Maxillofacial CT scans with axial, coronal, and sagittal cuts are most useful in the diagnostic and preoperative treatment planning phase when midface fractures are suspected. When evaluating for the presence of Le Fort fractures and determining the level, it is helpful to look at certain key areas, and the examiner can either include or exclude the appropriate level of fracture. The pterygoid plates should be visualized first; a fracture of the pterygoid process is almost always indicative of the presence of a Le Fort fracture. Next, the examiner determines the level by visualizing three key areas: (1) the anterolateral margin of the nasal fossa (Le Fort I level); (2) the inferior orbital rim (Le Fort II level); and (3) the zygomatic arch (Le Fort III level). It is important for the examiner to remember that fractures may be present at multiple levels on the ipsilateral or contralateral sides and the presence of one does not exclude that of another.

31. **How can one achieve an airway in patients with midface injuries?**

    Midface fractures can cause extensive soft tissue injuries in the nasopharynx and often with concomitant cranial base injuries. Attempts to place nasotracheal tubes for intubation can cause more injury, bleeding or intracranial perforations, or contamination. The same is applicable when attempting to place nasogastric tubes. If airway is attempted in the field, oral endotracheal intubation is the safest route of intubation. When intubation is not possible, surgical airway such as cricothyrotomy may be attempted. After skull base fractures are ruled out and for purpose of administering anesthesia for management of the fractures, nasotracheal intubation is the preferred airway of choice unless otherwise contraindicated. If a nasal intubation is contraindicated, a tracheotomy or a submental intubation technique may be utilized.

32. **What are the surgical approaches for accessing maxillary fractures?**

Most maxillary fractures (Le Fort I) can be approached using an intraoral maxillary vestibular incision. Wide exposure of the midface superiorly up to the infraorbital rims and laterally beyond the zygomatic buttresses can be achieved through the mouth. Lateral nasal slope fractures and orbital rim fractures can often be reduced and fixated through this approach in combination with orbital rim or sub-conjunctival incisions. However, orbital rim and zygomaticofrontal sutures often need periorbital incisions for access. Existing lacerations can be utilized wherever possible. Nasal bridge and nasofrontal disjunction, zygomatic arches, and zygomaticofrontal fractures as in Le Fort III are best approached via coronal incisions.

33. **What are some of the complications associated with maxillary fractures?**

- Infraorbital nerve paresthesia
- Enophthalmos
- Infection
- Exposed hardware
- Deviated septum
- Nasal obstruction
- Altered vision
- Nonunion
- Malunion or malocclusion
- Epiphora
- Foreign body reactions
- Scarring
- Sinusitis

34. **What is the blood supply to the maxillae and palatine bones?**

The blood supply to the maxilla and palatine bones is through the periosteum, incisive artery, and greater and lesser palatine arteries as well as the ascending pharyngeal and ascending palatine arteries.

35. **How are palatal fractures treated?**

Fractures to the maxilla can be greatly complicated via the involvement of the palate. Fractures involving the palate may occur in varying subtypes and combinations adding varying degrees of difficulty to the restoration of form and function. Failing to appreciate the presence or implications of palatal fractures may lead to less than optimal outcomes including generalized widening of the maxilla and a resultant malocclusion, especially if these fractures occur in combination with mandible fractures that predispose to increasing facial width, that is, symphysis fractures. These injuries are best approached by obtaining preoperative models and performing model surgery with the fabrication of a surgical stent similar to model surgeries that are performed prior to planned osteotomies. The surgical guide may be utilized to establish the planned preinjury occlusion and may be left in place throughout the postoperative healing phase.

BIBLIOGRAPHY

Nasal Fractures

Abubaker AO, Ziccardi VB, McDonald I: Midfacial fractures: fractures of the nose, zygoma, orbit and maxilla. In Abubaker AO, Benson KJ, editors: *Secrets of oral and maxillofacial surgery*, ed 3, Philadelphia, 2007, Mosby and Elsevier.

Colton JJ, Beekhuis GJ: Management of nasal fractures, *Otolaryngol Clin North Am* 19:73–85, 1986.

Dodson BT: Zygomatic, maxillary, and orbital fractures. In Jafek BW, Murrow BW, editors:.

Graper C, Milne M, Stevens MR: The traumatic saddle nose deformity: etiology and treatment, *J Craniomaxillofac Trauma* 2:37–49, 1996.

Harken AH, Moore EE, editors: *Abernathy's surgical secrets*, ed 5, Philadelphia, 2005, Mosby.

Illum P: Long-term results after treatment of nasal fractures, *J Laryngol Otol* 100:273–277, 1986.

Jafek BW: Nasal trauma. In Jafek BW, Murrow BW, editors: *ENT secrets*, ed 3, Philadelphia, 2005, Hanley & Belfus.

Manson PN: Midface fractures. In Georgiade N, Riefhohl R, Barwick W, editors: *Plastic, maxillofacial and reconstructive surgery*, ed 2, Baltimore, 1992, Williams & Wilkins.

Nasoethmoidal Fractures
Le Fort Fractures

Colton JJ, Beekhuis GJ: Management of nasal fractures, *Otolaryngol Clin North Am* 19:73–85, 1986.

Dodson BT: Zygomatic, maxillary, and orbital fractures. In Jafek BW, Murrow BW, editors: *ENT secrets*, ed 3, Philadelphia, 2005, Hanley & Belfus.

Dufresne CR, Manson PN: Pediatric facial trauma. In McCarthy JG, editor: *Plastic surgery*, Philadelphia, 1990, Saunders.

Ellis 3rd E: Fractures of the zygomatic complex and arch. In Fonseca RJ, Walker RV, editors: *Oral and maxillofacial trauma*, Philadelphia, 1991, Saunders.

Evans G, Manson PN, Clark N: Identification and management of minimally displaced nasoethmoidal orbital fractures, *Ann Plast Surg* 35:469–471, 1995.

Fenner GC, Wolfe SA: Maxillary fractures. In Weinzweig J, editor: *Plastic surgery secrets*, Philadelphia, 1999, Hanley & Belfus.

Graper C, Milne M, Stevens MR: The traumatic saddle nose deformity: etiology and treatment, *J Craniomaxillofac Trauma* 2:37–49, 1996.

Harken AH, Moore EE, editors: *Abernathy's surgical secrets*, ed 5, Philadelphia, 2005, Mosby.

Illum P: Long-term results after treatment of nasal fractures, *J Laryngol Otol* 100:273–277, 1986.

Jafek BW: Nasal trauma. In Jafek BW, Murrow BW, editors: *ENT secrets*, ed 3, Philadelphia, 2005, Hanley & Belfus.

Kawamoto HK: Late posttraumatic enophthalmos: a correctable deformity? *Plast Reconstr Surg* 69:423–432, 1992.

Knight JS, North JF: The classification of malar fractures: an analysis of displacement as a guide to treatment, *Br J Plast Surg* 13:325–339, 1961.

Lenhart DE, Dolezal RF: Fractures of the nose. In Weinzweig J, editor: *Plastic surgery secrets*, Philadelphia, 1999, Hanley & Belfus.

Manson PN, Iliff N: Management of blow-out fractures of the orbital floor. II. Early repair for selected injuries, *Surv Ophthalmol* 35:280–292, 1991.

Manson PN, Clark N, Robertson B, et al.: Comprehensive management of panfacial fractures, *J Craniomaxillofac Trauma* 11:43–56, 1995.

Manson PN: Facial injuries. In McCarthy JG, editor: *Plastic surgery*, Philadelphia, 1990, Saunders.

Manson PN: Midface fractures. In Georgiade N, Riefhohl R, Barwick W, editors: *Plastic, maxillofacial and reconstructive surgery*, ed 2, Baltimore, 1992, Williams & Wilkins.

Manson PN: Facial fractures. In Grotting J, editor: *Reoperative aesthetic and reconstructive surgery*, St Louis, 1994, Quality Medical.

Manson PN: Facial fractures. In Aston SJ, Beasley RW, Thorne CHM, editors: *Grabb and smith's plastic surgery*, ed 5, Philadelphia, 1997, Lippincott-Raven.

Markowitz B, Manson P, Sargent L, et al.: Management of the medial canthal ligament in nasoethmoidal orbital fractures, *Plast Reconstr Surg* 87:843–853, 1991.

Nguyen PN, Sullivan P: Advances in the management of orbital fractures, *Clin Plast Surg* 19:87–98, 1992.

Pastrick H, Bevivino BR: Zygomatic fractures. In Weinzweig J, editor: *Plastic surgery secrets*, Philadelphia, 1999, Hanley & Belfus.

Pollock RA: Nasal trauma: pathomechanics and surgical management of acute injuries, *Clin Plast Surg* 19:133–147, 1992.

Romano JJ, Manson PN, Mirvis WE, et al.: Le Fort fractures without mobility, *Plast Reconstr Surg* 85:355–362, 1990.

Schendel SA, editor: *Orbital trauma. Oral and maxillofacial surgery clinics of North America*, vol 5, No. 3. Philadelphia, 1993, Saunders.

Weinzweig J, Bartlett SP: Fractures of the orbit. In Weinzweig J, editor: *Plastic surgery secrets*, Philadelphia, 1999, Hanley & Belfus.

Whitaker L, Yaremchuk M: Secondary reconstruction of posttraumatic orbital deformities, *Ann Plast Surg* 25:440–449, 1990.

Wolfe SA, Baker S: *Facial fractures*, New York, 1993, Thieme.

Wolfe SA, Berkowitz S: Maxilla. In *Plastic surgery of the facial skeleton*, Boston, 1989, Little.

CHAPTER 33

FRONTAL SINUS FRACTURES

A. Omar Abubaker

1. **Describe the functional anatomy of the frontal sinus.**
   The frontal sinus is generally absent at birth, but its growth is complete at about 15 years of age in most individuals. As a result, fractures of the frontal sinus are less common in children than in adults. The anterior table is thicker than the posterior one and more resistant to injury, and that is why it requires greater force to fracture than any other facial bone. The size and shape of the sinus varies among individuals and on the right and left sides in the same individual, the anterior wall of the sinus being stronger than the posterior wall. The frontal sinus drains via a small outflow tract into the ethmoid sinus/nasal cavity tract, which is hourglass shaped with the true ostium at the narrowest portion, the infundibulum. A true frontonasal duct (FND) exists in only 15% of the population, varying from a few millimeters to 1 cm in length. In the remaining 85% of the population, the frontal sinus drains directly into the anterosuperior portion of the middle meatus via an ostium without a true duct or occasionally by a communication through the ethmoids. Because of the lack of duct in these individuals, some authors believe that the significance of FND in frontal sinus fractures is overrated.

2. **What type of epithelium lines the frontal sinus, and how does it relate to its pathology?**
   The frontal sinus is lined with pseudostratified columnar ciliated respiratory epithelium covered by a layer of mucin. Some authors theorize that the frontal sinus drainage is impaired after the nasofrontal duct becomes damaged or obstructed as a result of frontal sinus fracture. The mucus can subsequently build up behind the obstructed duct. A mucocele may develop and act as an expanding tumor. With development of an anaerobic environment in the presence of a mucocele, there is an increased risk of frontal sinusitis involving the intracranial contents. As such, assessment of the patency and subsequent management of the nasofrontal duct are important decision-making elements in the management of frontal sinus injuries.

3. **What is the epidemiology of frontal sinus fractures?**
   The majority of frontal sinus fractures are the result of high-velocity impacts such as motor vehicle accidents, assaults, and sport injuries. These fractures are relatively uncommon fractures (5% to 15% of all maxillofacial ones) with a preponderance of male patients aged 20 to 30.
   The most common fractures involve the combination of the anterior and posterior tables with or without frontal recess involvement (about two-thirds). Isolated anterior wall fractures account for approximately one-third, and isolated posterior table fractures are rare (<1%).

4. **How is the risk for fracture of the frontal sinus in children compared with adults?**
   The frontal sinus starts at birth and begins to appear as a pneumatic expansion at age seven from the nasal cavity, with complete development by ages 18 to 20. The remnants of this embryonic connection between sinuses are the nasofrontal ducts. These bilateral structures (foramina ducts) drain the frontal sinus from its posteromedial aspect, through the ethmoidal air cells and out to the nasal cavity, usually at the middle meatus ducts. Because the frontal sinus is small or nonexistent in children and young adolescents, it is less likely to be involved in a fracture in this age group.

5. **How are frontal sinus fractures classified?**
   Although there are many classifications that describe the pattern of frontal sinus fractures, there is no universally accepted classification of these fractures. Most classifications are based on location, extent of injury, involvement of the nasofrontal duct, and concurrent injury of the dura. Gonty's Classification, which has been adopted by many, combines several previous classifications into one.
   Type 1: Fractures of the anterior wall
   1. Isolated to anterior table
   2. Accompanied by supraorbital rim fractures
   3. Accompanied by nasoethmoidal complex fractures

Type 2: Anterior and posterior table fractures
1. Linear fractures
   - Transverse
   - Vertical
2. Comminuted fractures
   - Involving both tables
   - Accompanied by nasoethmoidal complex fractures

Type 3: Posterior table fractures

Type 4: Very severe comminuted fractures of the whole frontal area, involving the orbit, the nasal base and the ethmoid—Through-and-Through Frontal Sinus Fracture

6. **What are the signs of frontal sinus fracture?**
   History of a blow to the forehead resulting in lacerations, contusions, or hematoma should be suspected to be associated with a possible injury of the frontal sinus. Palpable or visible depression of the brow or the forehead should raise suspicion of frontal sinus involvement, although a visible or palpable depression is not always appreciated initially after injury because of swelling, edema, or hematoma. Supraorbital numbness, subconjunctival hematoma, eyelid ecchymosis, and subcutaneous air crepitus and cerebrospinal rhinorrhea are other signs of possible frontal sinus fracture.

7. **What is the best radiographic modality used for diagnosis of frontal sinus fractures?**
   Although plain radiographs and Waters' view of the skull may show displaced frontal sinus fractures by depicting cortical malalignment or air fluid levels, they frequently miss smaller fractures and involvement of the nasofrontal duct. Conventional radiographs can also fail to show the severity of the fracture or the degree of displacement. The computed tomography (CT) scan has become the standard for evaluation of frontal sinus fractures because it allows for visualization of even small and minimally displaced fractures of the floor, septum, and anterior or posterior tables of the frontal sinus (Fig. 33-1). Direct visualization of the ducts and possible injury to the ducts also can be determined by visualizing fractures of the floor that run near the midline, cross the midline, or involve the nasoethmoidal complex. Coronal CT and three-dimensional reconstruction images may allow direct visualizing of the duct involvement in the fractures.

8. **What are the possible complications associated with frontal sinus fractures?**
   Most authors agree that most of the complications associated with frontal sinus injury are secondary to interference with drainage of the sinus due to obstruction of the nasofrontal duct, entrapment of mucosa in the fracture lines, or dural tears. Most complications of frontal sinus fractures occur in patients in whom such fractures go undetected or untreated. These complications can be divided into early and late complications.
   Early complications: occur within the first 6 months after injury
   - Epistaxis
   - Cerebrospinal fluid (CSF) leakage and fistulae
   - Frontal sinusitis
   - Meningitis
   - Intracranial hematomas and or intracranial abscess
   - Empyema
   - Cavernous sinus thrombosis
   - Concomitant neurologic injuries secondary to penetrating trauma or displacement of the frontal bone into the neurocranium
   - Diplopia to blindness
   - Limitation of extraocular motions
   - Damage of the supraorbital or supratrochlear nerves
   Late complications: occur 6 months or more after the initial injury
   - Mucocele/mucopyocele formation
   - Late frontal sinusitis leading to orbital abscesses
   - Brain abscess secondary to frontal sinus infection
   - Frontal contour defects
   - Osteomyelitis of the frontal bone

9. **What are the overall goals and the basis for management of frontal sinus fractures?**
   The overall goals of management of frontal sinus fracture are to create a safe sinus, restore facial contour, and avoid short- and long-term complications.

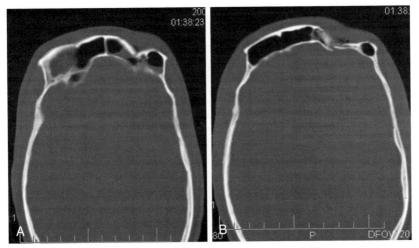

Figure 33-1. Computed tomography scan showing a displaced anterior and posterior table fracture of the left frontal sinus. *(From Fattahi T: Management of frontal sinus fractures. In Fonseca RJ, Marciani RD, Turvey T, editors:* Oral maxillofacial surgery, *vol 2, St Louis, 2009, Saunders.)*

Treatment of frontal sinus fractures is complex and sometimes controversial and often is based on the author's experience and training. However, most authors agree that appropriate treatment rationale should be made based on the clinical and radiographic findings and other clinical variables. Of these variables, assessment of at least five anatomic parameters should be included. These are the presence of:

- An anterior table fracture (A)
- A posterior table fracture (B)
- A nasofrontal recess fracture (C)
- A dural tear (CSF leak) (D)
- Fracture comminution

10. **What are the surgical approaches to exploration and repair of frontal sinus fractures?**
Coronal incision provides the best access to the whole frontal sinus and frontal bone, as well as the ethmoidal, orbital, and intracranial regions, and provides the most cosmetic results. Exploration and reduction of anterior table fractures alone usually can be performed through this approach, allowing unroofing of the remaining anterior table for complete access to the sinus and reduction and fixation of the fractured segments. Posterior table fractures may require a frontal craniotomy in conjunction with a neurosurgical team to assess and repair dural or parenchymal injuries if necessary. If the frontonasal duct is involved, and the sinus needs to be obliterated with material such as fat, muscle, or bone, a coronal approach also provides access to harvest cranial bone, temporalis muscle, fat, or fascia to be used for such purpose. Other approaches to the treatment of frontal sinus fractures include presence of a forehead laceration overlying the fractures and open sky approach. These approaches, however, are mostly useful when only the anterior table is involved. Some surgeons use endoscopic surgery in selected cases for conservative care and sinus preservation.

11. **What are the different management considerations and the treatment options for treatment of frontal sinus fractures?**
Management considerations following frontal sinus fractures include assessment of the following: degree of fracture displacement; injury to the nasofrontal duct; and presence of CSF leak. Treatment options would include:

- Observation
- Open reduction internal fixation (ORIF)

- Obliteration
- Cranialization

Fractures of the anterior table alone without involvement of the nasofrontal duct can be simply reduced and stabilized with microplates to prevent cosmetic deformities.

12. **What is the difference between obliteration and cranialization?**
    - **Obliteration:** Fractures involving the nasofrontal duct have historically been treated with obliteration of the sinus. This procedure consists of removing all sinus mucosa from the sinus and upper duct with a high-speed burr and then packing the duct and the entire sinus with material that encourages scarring and ossification of the sinus and the duct. Many materials have been used, including autologous tissue such as bone, muscle (temporalis), fat (temporal or abdominal), fascia, and periosteal flaps; alloplastic materials such as Gelfoam and synthetic bone have also been used. All methods have been shown to have comparable success, but cancellous iliac bone and abdominal fat remain the two most popular tissues used.
    - **Cranialization:** Fractures that involve a displaced or comminuted posterior table can be associated with dural tear or parenchymal brain injury and may require a craniotomy. Fractures involving only the inner table with no CSF leak are seldom treated. If a CSF leak is present, cranialization and repair of the dura are recommended. In this procedure, after any neurosurgical repair of the dura is completed, the posterior table is removed, the floor is reduced and stabilized, the remaining mucosa and inner cortices of the sinus and duct are burred, and the duct is packed with an appropriate material, as mentioned. The brain is then allowed to resume its proper location in a newly enlarged anterior cranial fossa. Finally, the anterior table is reduced and stabilized with microplates and screws.

13. **What are the indications for surgical intervention in treatment of frontal sinus fractures?**
    Over the years, despite some of the controversy over the management of frontal sinus fractures, most surgeons base the decision to operate to treat frontal sinus fractures, or merely observe these fractures, mostly on degree of displacement of the anterior and posterior tables and the status of the nasofrontal ducts. Some authors developed treatment algorithms for such treatment based on these variables (Figs. 33-2 and 33-3). Nondisplaced or minimally displaced anterior table fractures can be safely observed. However, displaced anterior table fractures may require surgery if the displacement is determined to cause a cosmetic deformity at the time of presentation or later, after the swelling resolves. Similarly, minimally or nondisplaced posterior table fractures can be observed if there is no CSF leak or if the displaced posterior table fracture is less than the thickness of the cortical plate of the sinus wall. Fractures of the posterior wall that are greater than the thickness of the cortical bone, those associated with CSF leak, or those with suspicion of nasofrontal duct injury may merit surgical exploration and reduction.

    Over the past few years, however, with recent large case series publications, there is a strong trend toward changing the management of frontal sinus fracture philosophies into a more conservative approach, and occasionally even nonoperative management of frontal sinus fractures that previously would have been treated surgically by most authors (see next question).

14. **Is there any recent shift in treatment approach to frontal sinus fractures?**
    Although the goals of treatment for frontal sinus injuries have remained relatively constant over the years, the strategies of management and surgical treatments have evolved. For instance, traditional philosophies emphasized either obliteration or cranialization when considering the management of frontal sinus fractures involving possible impairment of outflow of the drainage of the sinus with emphasis on involvement of the frontonasal duct, degree of displacement, and the anterior and posterior tables of the sinus. However, because these treatments are in part based on a concern for long-term complications, there is often a debate as to the exact incidence of these complications. Long-term follow-up is not often possible with these patients and, accordingly, such rational is not considered evidence-based criteria. As a result and by contrast, recent literature is leaning toward a more conservative approach when treating fractures of the frontal sinus, with preservation as much of the form and function of the sinus. A study by Bell et al. of 116 patients with frontal sinus fractures treated over a 10-year period found that in patients who were treated conservatively (nonoperatively, and patients who were treated with preservation of the normal sinus membrane), the protocol resulted in functional sinus preservation for the majority of cases with relatively few significant complications. More recently, Choi et al. and Weathers et al. confirmed the validity of the conservative approach and signaled a shift in treatment of frontal sinus fractures.

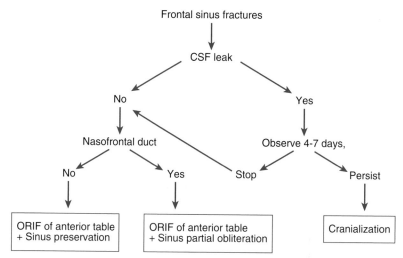

Figure 33-2. Algorithm for the management of frontal sinus fractures. *ORIF,* Open reduction internal fixation; *CSF,* cerebrospinal fluid. *(Adapted from Chen K-Te, Chen C, Mardini S, Tsay P-K, Chen Yu-R: Frontal sinus fractures: a treatment algorithm and assessment of outcomes based on 78 clinical cases, Plast Reconstruct Surg 116:457–468, 2006.)*

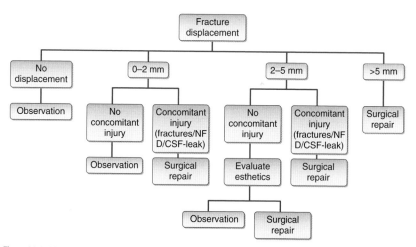

Figure 33-3. Metric-dislocation algorithm for treatment of frontal sinus fractures. *NFD,* Nasofrontal duct; *CSF,* cerebrospinal fluid. *(From Torre DD, Burtscher D, Kloss-Brandstätter A, et al.: Management of frontal sinus fractures–treatment decision based on metric dislocation extent, J Cranio-Maxillo-Fac Surg 42(7):1515–1519, 2014.)*

BIBLIOGRAPHY

Banica B, Ene P, Dabu A, Ene R, Cirstoiu C: Rationale for management of frontal sinus fractures, *Maedica (Buchar)* 8(4):398–403, 2013.

Bell RB, Dierks EJ, Brar P, Potter JK, Potter BE: A protocol for the management of frontal sinus fractures emphasizing sinus preservation, *J Oral Maxillofac Surg* 65(5):825–839, 2007.

Chen KT, Chen CT, Mardini S, Tsay PK, Chen YR: Frontal sinus fractures: a treatment algorithm and assessment of outcomes based on 78 clinical cases, *Plast Reconstr Surg* 118(2):457–468, 2006.

Choi M, Li Y, Shapiro SA, Havlik RJ, Flores RL: A 10-year review of frontal sinus fractures: clinical outcomes of conservative management of posterior table fractures, *Plast Reconstr Surg* 130(2):399–406, 2012.

Disa JD, Robertson BC, Metzinger SE, et al.: Transverse glabellar flap for obliteration/isolation of the nasofrontal duct from the anterior cranial base, *Ann Plast Surg* 36:453–457, 1996.

Guy WM, Brissett AE: Contemporary management of traumatic fractures of the frontal sinus, *Otolaryngol Clin North Am* 46(5):733–748, 2013.

Ioannides C, Freihofer HP, Friens J: Fractures of the frontal sinus: a rationale of treatment, *Br J Plast Surg* 46:208–214, 1993.

Koento T: Current advances in sinus preservation for the management of frontal sinus fractures, *Curr Opin Otolaryngol Head* 20(4):274–279, 2012.

Minniti JG, Harshbarger M: Fractures of the frontal sinus. In Weinzweig J, editor: *Plastic surgery secrets*, Philadelphia, 1999, Hanley & Belfus.

Rodriguez ED, Stanwix MG, Nam AJ, et al.: Twenty-six-year experience treating frontal sinus fractures: a novel algorithm based on anatomical fracture pattern and failure of conventional techniques, Plastic Reconstr Surg, 122: 1850-1866, 2008.

Rohrich RJ, Hollier LH: Management of frontal sinus fractures: changing concepts, *Clin Plast Surg* 19:219–232, 1992.

Rohrich RJ, Mickel TJ: Frontal sinus obliteration: in search of the ideal autogenous material, *Plast Reconstr Surg* 95:580–585, 1995.

Smith TL, Han JK, Loehrl TA, Rhee JS: Endoscopic management of the frontal recess in frontal sinus fractures: a shift in the paradigm? *Laryngoscope* 112(5):784–790, 2002.

Torre DD, Burtscher D, Kloss-Brandstätter A, Rasse M, Kloss F: Management of frontal sinus fractures–treatment decision based on metric dislocation extent, *Journal of Cranio-Maxillo-Facial Surgery* 42:1515–1519, 2014.

Weathers WM, Wolfswinkel EM, Hatef DA, Lee EI, Brown RH, Hollier Jr LH: Frontal sinus fractures: a conservative shift, *Craniomaxillofac Trauma Reconstr* 6(3):155–156, 2013.

Wolfe SA, Johnson P: Frontal sinus injuries: primary care and management of late complications, *Plast Reconstr Surg* 82:781–789, 1988.

MANAGEMENT OF SOFT TISSUE FACIAL INJURIES

Sapna Lohiya, Jasjit Dillon, Bashar Rajab

1. **What are the three important mechanisms involved in protecting the human body against microbiologic invasion?**
   - **Mechanical barrier:** Skin and mucous membranes act as physical barriers against invading microorganisms.
   - **Chemical barrier:** Lipids on the skin surface are hydrophobic and prevent entry of water-soluble substances. Mucosal surfaces provide protection via immunoglobulin (IgA) that neutralizes foreign antigens.
   - **Biological barrier:** Microorganisms activate the kallikrein-kinin system with release of vasoactive amines that increase vascular permeability. This allows for an influx of humoral and cellular immunologic elements, which recognize and phagocytose the microorganisms. Normal flora on skin and oral mucosal surfaces also compete with potential microbial pathogens.

2. **What are the classifications of soft tissue injuries?**
   - Contusions
   - Flap-like lacerations
   - Abrasions
   - Avulsion injuries
   - Lacerations

3. **What are the different types of soft tissue repair?**
   - Primary closure
   - Distance flap
   - Healing by secondary intention
   - Free flap
   - Local flap
   - Specialized flap

4. **What are the types of wound closures?**
   - Primary closure and healing by primary intention
   - Leaving the wound open, treating it with frequent dressing changes, and allowing it to heal by secondary intention and wound contracture
   - Delayed primary closure, in which the wound is splinted in a position of rest with an occlusive dressing and is closed in 3 to 5 days when it is free of infection and necrotic tissue
     The timing of wound closure directly correlates with the risk of infection. Wounds with a high risk of infection should be closed as soon as possible (within the first 6 to 8 hours), whereas wounds with low risk of infection, such as those in the head and neck area, can be closed primarily within the first 18 to 24 hours after injury. After 24 hours, for most wounds, consideration should be given to packing them open and performing a secondary repair 4 to 8 days later. An absolute contraindication to primary wound closure is any evidence of wound infection such as erythema, warmth, swelling, and/or pus drainage.

5. **What factors predispose a wound to infection?**
   Wound factors: (1) size, configuration, and depth of the wound; (2) location of the injury; (3) mechanism of injury; (4) type and amount of contamination, including presence of foreign body; (5) time between injury and wound closure; and (6) care of the wound between injury and definitive care.
   Technical risk factors: (1) inadequate debridement of foreign bodies, bacterial contamination, and presence of devitalized tissues; (2) inadvertent introduction of foreign material into the wound during cleansing; (3) inadequate hemostasis and failure to eliminate dead space, which provides

an environment for bacterial colonization; (4) using an excessive number of sutures to close the wound; and (5) placing excessive tension on the sutures used to approximate the tissue edges and compromising local tissue perfusion.

Host factors: age and systemic condition of the patient including predisposition to diabetes mellitus, peripheral artery disease, malnutrition, chronic renal failure, and use of immunosuppressive agents.

6. **What are the five steps for treating posttraumatic soft tissue wound infection in the head and neck region?**
   1. Early recognition of infection
   2. Rapid resuscitation and initiation of empiric antibiotics
   3. Immediate surgical debridement
   4. Hemodynamic and nutritional support
   5. Early wound closure

7. **How should bleeding from facial injuries be managed?**
   Bleeding is managed initially with compression by direct pressure for up to 15 minutes. If bleeding persists, then local anesthesia with epinephrine can either be injected or directly applied to the wound. Bleeding from arterial vessels may not respond to these measures so hemostasis should be attempted by suturing the laceration or ligating the relevant vessel. Tissue ischemia is unlikely due to the extensive anastomoses among facial arteries. Massive uncontrollable bleeding can be treated with arterial embolization via interventional radiology or ligation of the external carotid artery.

8. **What are anesthetic options available for the repair of facial lacerations?**
   Anesthesia can be achieved using topical gels, local anesthesia, or regional blocks. Regional blocks provide a specific advantage, as wound edges do not become distorted. Regional blocks commonly used for facial soft tissue injuries and their associated areas of anesthesia are as follows:
   - Supraorbital and supratrochlear blocks: forehead, anterior one-third of the scalp
   - Infraorbital block: lower lid, upper lip, and lateral aspect of the nose
   - Mental nerve block: lower lip and chin

9. **In which areas of soft tissue injury should we avoid local anesthesia with vasoconstrictor?**
   In areas of skin or tissue flaps of doubtful viability, where the use of vasoconstrictors might further impair circulation.

10. **What is the role of irrigation with wound preparation?**
    Irrigation is essential in preventing infection as it removes debris, dirt, micro, and devitalized tissue from the wound. High-pressure irrigation with normal saline has been shown to decrease the bacterial count of wounded tissues and decrease the rate of infection. The use of concentrated povidone-iodine, hydrogen peroxide, and detergents may cause significant tissue damage and should be avoided. When available, warmed saline may be more comfortable for the patient than room-temperature saline.

11. **What are the different types of organisms isolated from a bite wound, and what is the optimal therapeutic agent for these injuries?**
    - **Dog bites:** *Pasteurella canis*
    - **Cat bites:** *Pasteurella multocida* and *Pasteurella septica*
    - **Human bites:** *S. aureus, Eikenella corrodens, Haemophilus influenzae*, and beta-lactamase–producing oral anaerobic bacteria

    The optimal therapeutic agents include a combination of beta-lactam antibiotic and beta-lactamase inhibitors. Oral amoxicillin-clavulanic acid will provide adequate coverage of the suspected pathogens particularly in patients presenting 9 to 24 hours after the initial injury. Ertapenem also has an excellent potency against the full range of animal and human bite pathogens.

    For deep or severe wound infections, patients should receive intravenous antibiotics rather than oral antibiotics immediately after injury. Once clinical improvement is seen, the antibiotic regimen can be transitioned to outpatient oral therapy.

12. **In order, what are the layers of the skin? What is the relation of the muscles of facial expression to the layers of the skin?**
    1. The epidermis (stratified squamous epithelium)
       - Stratum corneum
       - Stratum spinosum

- Stratum lucidum
- Stratum germinativum
- Stratum granulosum
2. The dermis
   - Papillary layer
   - Reticular layer

A thin subcutaneous layer supports the facial dermis. The muscles of facial expression are within the subcutaneous layer and insert into the reticular layer of the dermis.

13. **In order, what are the layers of the scalp? What is the appropriate management of scalp lacerations?**
    - S: Skin
    - C: Connective tissue
    - A: (Galea) Aponeurosis
    - L: Loose areolar connective tissue
    - P: Periosteum

    Bleeding can be a serious issue with scalp lacerations, often resulting in significant amounts of blood loss. Direct pressure to the wound and local anesthesia with epinephrine often can provide adequate hemostasis. If not, then the edges of the laceration should be everted and the wound should be closed rapidly with circumferential suture placement. Primary closure up to 48 hours after injury is the treatment of choice for scalp lacerations that extend into or through the dermis. Delayed primary closure may be indicated in wounds that are at a higher risk for infection and present after 24 hours. Hair trimming may be necessary but hair shaving should be avoided. If hemostasis is easily achieved, then the wound should be closed using staples, with staples placed approximately .5 to 1 cm apart. Staples should be removed in 7 to 14 days. Penrose drains can be placed to prevent hematoma formation and eliminated dead space.

14. **What is the interaction of the suture material and tissue healing process?**
    Wound healing is a process that can be divided into three phases:
    1. Initial lag phase (0 to 5 days): There is no gain in wound strength. The wound and the entire burden of tissue approximation are entirely dependent on the suture and epidermal cellular adhesion.
    2. Fibroblastic phase (5 to 15 days): Characterized by a rapid increase in wound strength.
    3. Maturation phase (14 days and onward): There is further connective tissue remodelling during this phase.

    As the tissue reduces the suture strength with time, the relative rates at which the suture material loses strength and the wound gains strength are important in wound healing.

15. **What are the indications of a skin graft for traumatic wounds? Which areas can accept a skin graft?**
    Indications:
    - To limit the amount of contractions and tissue deformity following a large skin loss
    - Temporary coverage before definitive treatment

    Tissues that support a skin graft are muscle, fat, fascia, dura, and periosteum. Tissues that cannot support a skin graft are cortical bone denuded of its periosteum, tendons, nerves, or cartilage.

16. **What are the classification types of free skin grafts?**
    1. Split-thickness grafts, which consist of the epidermis and a portion of the dermis:
       - Thin (0.008 to 0.012 inch)
       - Medium (0.012 to 0.018 inch)
       - Thick (0.018 to 0.030 inch)
    2. Full-thickness skin grafts, which include both the epidermis and the dermis

17. **What are the properties of split-thickness and full-thickness skin grafts?**
    1. Split-thickness skin graft:
       - Thinner graft, which rapidly vascularizes and survives under less optimal conditions. It can be expanded and can be taken from multiple donor sites that will heal with minimal scarring.
       - Thicker split-thickness skin graft closely resembles the color, texture, and limited contractions of a full-thickness graft. This type of graft is usually harvested with a dermatome.
    2. Full-thickness skin graft: Provides a good color and texture match, requires optimal wound conditions, and is less prone to tissue contraction. The graft is usually harvested by dissection and the donor site must be closed primarily.

18. What are the most common causes of graft failure?
    - Hematoma formation
    - Failure of immobilization

19. What are the types of eyelid injury, and how are they managed?
    - **Simple lacerations:** These should be closed in layers, restoring the orientation of the skin, muscle, tarsal, and conjunctival layers. Careful attention should be given to approximating the lid margins to avoid functional or cosmetic defects.
    - **Upper lid lacerations:** These may involve detachment of the levator muscle and Muller's muscle from the tarsal plate. The muscles should be identified and reattached to the tarsal plate to prevent ptosis and to restore levator function.
    - **Laceration of the medial third of the lid:** These may involve the lacrimal canaliculus. The laceration should be explored using a probe and irrigation to rule out involvement of the canaliculi. Lacerations involving the tear drainage system require placement of silicone tubes to maintain patency of the ducts during healing.
    - **Avulsive injuries:** Full-thickness avulsion of <25% of the lid length can be repaired primarily as a simple laceration or by secondary intention. Otherwise, avulsive injures are treated with a full-thickness skin graft from the postauricular region or the contralateral upper eyelid.

20. What is the treatment of an eyelid injury that involves the lacrimal drainage system?
    The lower canaliculus is more commonly injured than the upper canaliculus. The treatment begins with identifying the two segments of the canaliculus. A silicon tube is passed through the punctum and lateral portion of the canaliculus and through the remaining medial canaliculus into the lacrimal sac, nasolacrimal duct, and nasal cavity beneath the inferior turbinate. The other end of the tube is passed into the uninvolved punctum, traveling through the nasolacrimal duct to exit beneath the inferior turbinate. The free ends are then tied and secured in the nose. The tube is left in place for 2 to 3 months or longer if epiphora persists.

21. What are the causes of traumatic transection of the lacrimal system? How is it diagnosed, and how is it treated?
    Traumatic transection of the lacrimal system is usually caused by a laceration in the vicinity of the medial canthus or accompanies Le Fort or nasoethmoidal fractures. The lacrimal punctum may be dilated, and saline may be injected through the punctum into the system. Appearance of saline in the wound is diagnostic of a canalicular laceration.
    These transections are treated by the placement of tubes into the nose, through the lacerated canaliculus to splint the repair. Both upper and lower canalicular lacerations should be explored and repaired if needed. Repair and repositioning of the fracture fragments often permit adequate function of the system. Repair of a chronically obstructed nasal lacrimal duct is accomplished with a dacryocystorhinostomy.

22. What craniofacial injuries are accompanied by facial nerve palsy?
    Fractures of the temporal bone as a part of skull-base fractures may cause facial nerve palsy. In absence of facial laceration, a computed tomography (CT) scan of the temporal bone may show such injury. High-dose steroids and decompression are considered for certain injuries. The prognosis varies with the site of the fracture.

23. What is the course of the parotid duct?
    The duct exits from the anterior portion of the gland and passes inferiorly superficial to the masseter muscle parallel with a plane drawn from the tragus of the ear to the midpoint of the upper lip. One cm anterior to the anterior border of the masseter muscle, the duct turns medially and penetrates the buccinator muscle, opening into the mouth at the level of the second maxillary molar.

24. What are the ways to diagnose a parotid duct injury?
    - Identification of the location of clear fluid in the wound after compressing the gland to express saliva
    - Direct inspection with lacrimal probe cannulation of the distal aspect of the duct and observation if the probe is visible in the wound
    - Injection of methylene blue, saline, or milk into the duct in a retrograde fashion. Of note, methylene blue discolors tissues and may make subsequent visualization of structures more challenging
    - Radiographic examination (sialogram or CT imaging)

25. **How is a parotid duct injury managed?**
    - Place an Intracath stent through the distal portion of the duct from the oral orifice.
    - Identify the proximal portion of the duct, which can be facilitated by massaging the gland to express saliva. The proximal end is then cannulated.
    - Close the ends of the duct over the Intracath with small nylon or Prolene sutures.
    - Secure the Intracath to the buccal mucosa.
    - Layer the closure of the wound and place an external pressure dressing for 24 to 48 hours.
    - Leave the catheter in place for 10 to 14 days.

    Sialocele and salivary fistulas can often be managed with antibiotics, pressure dressings, anticholinergics, and serial aspirations. If the repair of the ductal injury is determined to be impossible, the proximal portion of the duct should be ligated. This will initially result in marked swelling of the gland followed by its secondary physiologic death.

26. **What is the treatment process of parotid duct injury in relation to the location of the injury?**
    - Posterior to the masseter muscle or within the parotid gland: Closure of the parotid capsule and application of pressure dressing.
    - Over the masseter muscle: Primary anastomosis or ligation. If enough length remains, anastomosis should be performed over a silastic stent or an epidural catheter.
    - Anterior to the masseter muscle: If primary anastomosis is impossible, the proximal portion of the duct can be drained directly into the mouth by creating a new opening. If this cannot be achieved without undue tension, then the proximal duct segment should be ligated.

27. **What anatomic structures need to be evaluated in a patient with a large through-and-through laceration of the cheek?**
    Cheek lacerations may involve several underlying vital structures, including the parotid gland and duct, facial nerve branches, facial artery and its branches, and the buccal fat pad. Careful examination of the wound to identify these structures is warranted. Parotid duct laceration requires the placement of a stent and careful suturing of the cut ends with 6.0 nylon suture under magnification to prevent formation of a cutaneous fistula. Overlying tissues are then closed in layers. Gland injuries without duct involvement should be closed routinely and followed for sialocele or parotid fistula formation, which may be treated using pressure dressings or antisialagogues. Facial nerve lacerations proximal to a vertical perpendicular line through the lateral canthus are amenable to surgical repair. The transverse facial artery runs adjacent to the parotid duct and, if injured, does not need to be repaired. The buccal fat should be preserved and replaced, if possible, to prevent cosmetic deformity or cheek hollowing.

28. **What is the etiology and treatment of septal hematomas?**
    Septal hematomas are most frequently associated with trauma to the anterior nasal septum and will present as dark purple or bluish masses against the septum. If left untreated, they can be associated with infection and necrosis.
    Treatment: Incision and expression of the clot should be performed as soon as possible. The nares should then be packed for approximately 2 to 3 days.

29. **What is the etiology and treatment of ear hematomas?**
    The most common etiology of auricular hematoma is blunt trauma. Unevacuated, the extravasated blood is replaced by fibrous tissue or new cartilage, resulting in the cauliflower ear. The hematoma also caries the risk of secondary infection.
    Treatment: Evacuation of the hematoma by needle aspiration soon after the injury, or incision and drainage in late treatment of the hematoma. Application of an external pressure dressing (bolster dressing) after hematoma evacuation will prevent reformation of the hematoma.

30. **What are the ear injury classifications? What are their most common treatments?**
    Simple lacerations: Simple lacerations are classified as those that spare cartilage. These wounds should be closed primarily using simple interrupted stitches with a 6-0 absorbable or nonabsorbable suture. It is important to preserve and maintain all attached tissue due to the rich blood supply to the auricle.
    Split earlobe: Split earlobes most often occur by the pulling through of earrings or by an allergic response to earring metal alloys. These injuries should be closed with subcutaneous placement of 4-0 or 5-0 resorbable sutures and then skin closure with 6-0 absorbable or nonabsorbable sutures.

Complex lacerations: Unlike simple lacerations, these types of injuries expose or extend through cartilage. Sutures should not be passed through the cartilage layer. The deepest layer of closure should be the perichondrium. Often due to the thin overlying skin, stitches will incorporate both the perichondrium and skin layer, which is an accepted method for closure.

Avulsive injuries:
- **Partial avulsion with a wide pedicle:** Use primary closure due to adequate blood supply.
- **Partial avulsions with a narrow pedicle:** In the setting of marginal blood supply, local advancement flaps or other surgical interventions become necessary to preserve the segment.
- **Complete avulsions:**
    - Simple reattachment as a composite graft. The ear is cleansed and sutured directly into the vascular bed. Small incisions are made in the skin to decrease venous congestion. Administration of dextran or heparin to decrease blood viscosity might be helpful. Success of reattachment is greatest within 4 hours of the injury but studies have shown adequate reimplantation results up to 33 hours post-avulsion.
    - The pocket principle. The ear is thoroughly dermabraded, a posterior auricular incision is made, and a pocket is created into which the auricle is tucked. After 10 to 14 days, the auricle is retrieved and allowed to reepithelialize or is raised with the postauricular skin as coverage. The donor site can be closed primarily or by a harvested full-thickness graft from elsewhere.

31. **What management considerations are required in repairing an ear laceration?**
    A complete physical exam evaluating the pinna, external auditory canal, tympanic membrane, and hearing is essential before treatment of external ear injuries. The pinna is the most frequently lacerated component of the ear, consisting of a relatively avascular cartilage layer covered by a thin, but richly vascular, skin layer. Anesthesia should be achieved without the use of vasoconstrictors to prevent disruption of the vascular supply to the ear cartilage. Management then includes irrigation and conservative debridement. Conservative debridement is key as excision of cartilage can lead to notching of the auricular contours and debridement of skin can lead to difficulty in achieving total closure over exposed cartilage. 6-0 nylon skin sutures can then be placed to align known landmarks and to re-approximate the soft tissue envelope. The patient's contralateral ear can be used as a model to reestablish ear anatomy when normal landmarks are otherwise obscured. Suturing the cartilaginous framework is seldom required; however, fine, permanent tacking sutures may be used. Hematoma formation requires drainage, either through fine-needle aspiration or a small incision. Some type of pressure dressing is required in complex lacerations to prevent re-accumulation of blood; this can be most easily accomplished using a transcartilaginous horizontal mattress suture and bolster dressing. The patient should be re-evaluated 24 to 48 hours after repair to assess for hematoma formation or infection. If perichondritis develops, then *Pseudomonas aeruginosa* is the likely offending pathogen, and the infection should be treated with drainage if necessary and oral fluoroquinolones.

32. **What is the appropriate management of tongue lacerations?**
    The tongue has a very rich blood supply that can lead to significant bleeding. Simultaneously, the tongue has a remarkable ability to heal fairly quickly. Therefore, small tongue lacerations, especially in children, often do not warrant primary repair. Indications for repair include: large lacerations (>1 cm) that extend into the muscular layers, lacerations with significant bleeding, and lacerations that may cause dysfunction if healing occurs without repair (anterior split tongue). After local anesthesia is administered via direct local infiltration and inferior alveolar nerve block, the wound should be irrigated and debrided. The laceration should then be closed in layers with interrupted resorbable sutures. Due to the constant motion and muscularity of the tongue, each suture should be tied with at least four square knots. Large lacerations merit a thorough evaluation of the airway because of the possibility of significant swelling and posterior displacement of the tongue. Wounds should be explored and radiographs taken to rule out the presence of foreign bodies, such as dental fragments. Lacerations over 24 hours old should be left to heal by secondary intention.

33. **What is the treatment process of a through-and-through lip laceration?**
    - Regional anesthesia via infraorbital and/or mental nerve blocks
    - Initial irrigation of the wound and closure of the intraoral mucosal layer
    - Copious irrigation of the external wound
    - Re-approximation of the muscular (orbicularis oris) layer
    - Closure of the dermis and subcutaneous layer
    - Skin closure with careful alignment of the vermilion border

34. **What percentage of tissue can be lost without a significant cosmetic defect after primary closure in an avulsive injury of the upper and lower lips?**
    Avulsive injuries involving up to 25% of the upper lip and 35% of the lower lip structure can be closed primarily without significant functional or cosmetic deformity. In these situations, tissue margins should be straightened, with the removal of a tissue wedge for primary closure. Attention must be given to proper alignment of the vermilion border and orbicularis oris muscles. Larger avulsive injuries may be amenable to repair via Abbe or local rotational flaps.

35. **Do facial lacerations require debridement before their repair?**
    Debridement refers to the removal of permanently devitalized tissue within a wound in an effort to prevent future wound infection. Therefore, the zone of contusion should be excised, if permitted by the flexibility and availability of soft tissue. Contraindications to debridement include function and cosmetics. Excision should not be performed in the upper and lower eyelid areas as the eyelids then may not be able to close completely over the globe. In general, excision also should not be performed in nostril rim, ear, or lip margin lacerations because distortion may be noticeable even with minimal tissue deficiency at the suture line. Excisions should be performed in parallel to the relaxed skin tension lines to minimize facial scarring. Once debridement is indicated, then resection of the contused skin allows conversion to a primary surgically created wound with more predictable healing and generally improved appearance. Following this procedure, a layered repair of the facial soft tissue should be performed.

36. **How do animal and human bites differ from other traumatic injuries?**
    Animal and human bites differ from other traumatic injuries because they are contaminated by the oral flora. Thorough cleansing and debridement of the wound with the use of copious normal saline irrigation is essential before closure. Facial wounds can then be closed in routine layered fashion. Wound infections from human bites are frequently caused by *Streptococcus* and *Staphylococcus* organisms. Serious infections may also be associated with *Eikenella*. Unlike human bites, 50% to 75% of infections in animal bites are caused by *P. multocida*. Amoxicillin-clavulanic acid is recommended for prophylaxis in both human and animal bites. Tetanus immunization is required for all bites, and rabies prophylaxis may be required when animals exhibit suspicious behavior.

37. **What are the zones of the neck, and how are they assessed in penetrating neck injuries?**
    Penetrating trauma to the neck carries significant risk of vascular injury. To standardize management, three zones of the neck have been defined. Zone 1 extends from the clavicle to the cricoid cartilage, zone 2 from the cricoid cartilage to the mandibular angle, and zone 3 from the mandibular angle to the base of the skull. Diagnosis of vascular injury by physical examination or exploratory surgery is most easily accomplished in zone 2, whereas zone 1 and 3 injuries often remain obscure. Similarly, surgical repair of zone 2 injuries is frequently successful, whereas repair of zones 1 and 3 is often fraught with danger. Arteriography is useful to locate the site of arterial injury in these zones. Bleeding can then be controlled by intraluminal blockage of the severed artery by embolization.

38. **What distinguishes facial lacerations from other lacerations?***
    Cosmetic appearance is clearly of primary importance. Quality of the final result depends on strict adherence to basic principles of wound management and meticulous surgical technique. Copious irrigation, judicious debridement, gentle tissue handling, adequate hemostasis, minimization of the number of sutures used, and early stitch removal are critical for optimal results. Use of fine sutures, sharp instruments, eversion of the wound margins, layered closure, obliteration of dead space, and tension-free repair are mandatory. As we age, facial skin will develop predictable creases, known as Langer's lines. Lacerations that run parallel to Langer's lines will have less prominent scarring than those that run perpendicular to them.

39. **How are clean lacerations repaired?***
    They should be irrigated with normal saline or Ringer's lactate. Only the surrounding skin should be prepared, and no antiseptic should be introduced into the wound. Regional anesthesia is preferred because of the potential for spread of contamination with direct injection of the wound margin. Epinephrine should be avoided because it devitalizes tissue and may potentiate infection. Wounds should be repaired in layers with absorbable suture in deep tissue. The fewest number of sutures necessary to overcome the natural resting wound tension should be used. Sutures should be removed within 3 to 5 days, and the wound margin should be subsequently supported with Steri-Strips.

40. **How are dirty lacerations repaired?***

    Heavily contaminated wounds should remain open after irrigation and debridement for subsequent delayed closure. Because of cosmetic considerations, however, this approach is unacceptable in the face. Therefore, meticulous debridement of devitalized tissue and removal of all foreign material are essential. The wound should be cultured before copious irrigation, and a broad-spectrum antibiotic should be instituted prophylactically. The patient must be informed of the potential of a post-repair infection.

41. **What factors influence suture selection?***

    Wounds should be closed with sutures when excessive scarring will result if the wound edges are not properly approximated. Suture types are classified by their absorption rates, physical configuration, tensile strength, elasticity, and memory. Absorbable sutures are defined as those that will lose their tensile strength within 60 days. Fast-absorbing gut is recommended for percutaneous closure of facial lacerations while Vicryl and Monocryl sutures are recommended for the dermal closure of deep lacerations. Chromic gut or Vicryl can be used for tongue or oral mucosal wounds. Nonabsorbable sutures include silk, nylon, and Prolene sutures. Since any method of suturing provokes tissue damage, impairs host defense, increases scar proliferation, and invites infection, it is recommended to use as few sutures as possible to close a deep wound. Braided sutures in particular can often harbor bacteria between strands and can result in higher rates of infection.

42. **Can absorbable sutures be used in repair of facial lacerations?**

    Yes. In children, the use of plain catgut absorbable sutures in the repair of traumatic lacerations in general and in facial lacerations in particular is an acceptable alternative to nonabsorbable sutures. Long-term cosmetic outcome seems to be at least as good with no difference in the rate of dehiscence or infection. In a randomized study on repair of facial lacerations in the emergency department, using fast-absorbing catgut or nylon sutures showed no significant differences in the rates of infection, wound dehiscence, keloid formation, and parental satisfaction. In addition, the lack of need to remove the sutures compared to nonabsorbable sutures is less traumatic to the child.

43. **Which wounds are suitable for closure with tissue adhesives?***

    N-butyl-2-cyanoacrylate may suffice for cutaneous closure of <4-cm low-tension lacerations with good wound approximation in children (preferred method) and adults. This adhesive effectively closes low-tension lacerations. This method is fast, relatively painless, and does not require the use of injected local anesthesia. It has a low complication rate and produces excellent cosmetic outcomes. In many instances, if initial wound orientation is against Langer's lines, it may, in fact, offer an advantage over conventional manual suturing. Once applied, maximum bonding strength is obtained within 2.5 minutes; the adhesive will then slough off approximately 5 to 10 days later.

44. **Should eyebrows be shaved when facial lacerations are repaired?***

    No. They provide a landmark for realignment of disrupted tissue edges and do not always grow back. In addition, shaving hair to skin level can deposit particles in the wound bed, increasing the risk of infection. This practice should, therefore, be avoided in all lacerations if possible.

45. **Should skin grafts or flaps be used for primary closure of a wound?***

    Complicated tissue transfer techniques have no place in the acute treatment of facial wounds. Closure should be achieved in the simplest way possible, and complex reconstructive efforts should be deferred until the scar has matured (months). When tissue loss prevents closure, it may be necessary to use a thin split-thickness skin graft for coverage.

46. **When are antibiotics indicated in the treatment of facial lacerations?***

    Copious irrigation, debridement, and gentle tissue handling are more pertinent to the prevention of infection than the use of antibiotics in facial wounds, especially skin wounds. Antibiotic coverage is indicated, however, in crush avulsion injuries, bites, and heavily contaminated injuries. Antibiotic prophylaxis should also be considered in through-and-through lip laceration, avalusive and degloving scalp laceration, and when the wound involves exposed cartilage of the ear or nose or evidence of devascularization.

    If prophylactic antibiotic therapy is required, then the antibiotic should be selected on the basis of the normal bacterial flora associated with the wound site.

47. **When should scars be revised?***

A scar usually has its worst appearance at 2 weeks to 2 months after suturing. Scar revision should await complete maturation, which may take 4 to 24 months. A good rule of thumb is to undertake no revisions for at least 6 to 12 months after initial repair. The maturation of the wound may be assessed by its degree of discomfort, erythema, and induration.

BIBLIOGRAPHY

Abubaker AO: Use of prophylactic antibiotics in preventing infection of traumatic injuries, *Dent Clin North Am* 53(4): 707–715, 2009. doi: 10.1016/j.cden.2009.08.004. Review.

Amiel GE, Sukhotnik I, Kawar B, et al.: Use of N-butyl-2-cyanoacrylate in elective surgical incisions: long-term outcomes, *J Am Coll Surg* 189:21–25, 1999.

Brown DJ, Jaffe JE, Henson JK: Advanced laceration management, *Emerg Med Clin North Am* 25:83, 2007.

Ernst AA, Gershoff L, Miller P, Tilden E, Weiss SJ: Warmed versus room temperature saline for laceration irrigation: a randomized clinical trial, *South Med J* 96(5):436, 2003.

Farion KJ, Osmond MH, Hartling L, et al.: Tissue adhesives for traumatic lacerations: a systematic review of randomized controlled trials, *Acad Emerg Med* 10:110–118, 2003.

Hollander JE, Richman PB, WerBlud M, et al.: Irrigation in facial and scalp lacerations: does it alter outcome? *Ann Emerg Med* 31:73–77, 1998.

Hollander JE, Singer AJ: Laceration management, *Ann Emerg Med* 34(3):356, 1999.

Horgan MA, Piatt Jr JH: Shaving of the scalp may increase the rate of infection in CSF shunt surgery, *Pediatr Neurosurg* 26(4):180, 1997.

Karounis H, Gouin S, Eisman H, Chalut D, Pelletier H, Williams BA: Randomized, controlled trial comparing long-term cosmetic outcomes of traumatic pediatric lacerations repaired with absorbable plain gut versus nonabsorbable nylon sutures, *Acad Emerg Med* 11(7):730–735, 2004.

Ketch LL: Facial lacerations. In Harken AH, Moore EE, editors: *Abernathy's surgical secrets*, ed 5, Philadelphia, 2005, Mosby.

Lavasani L, Leventhal D, Constantinides M, Krein H: Management of acute soft tissue injury to the auricle, *Facial Plast Surg* 26:445, 2010.

RP L, Flood R, Eyal D, Saludades J, Hayes C, Gaughan J: Cosmetic outcomes of absorbable versus non-absorbable sutures in pediatric facial lacerations, *Pediatr Emerg Care* 24(3):137–142, 2008, http://dx.doi.org/10.1097/PEC.0b013e3181666f87.

Mitchell RB, Nanez G, Wagner JD, et al.: Dog bites of the scalp, face, and neck in children, *Laryngoscope* 113:492–495, 2003.

Nelson CC: Management of eyelid trauma, *Aust N Z J Ophthalmol* 19:357, 1991.

Quinn J, Wells G, Sutcliffe T, et al.: A randomized trial comparing octylcyanoacrylate tissue adhesive and sutures in the management of lacerations, *JAMA* 277:1527–1530, 1997.

Selbst SM, Attia MW: Minor trauma—lacerations. In Fleisher GR, Ludwig S, editors: *Textbook of pediatric emergency medicine*, ed 5, Philadelphia, 2006, Lippincott Williams and Wilkins, p 1571.

Shimoyama T, Kaneko T, Horie N: Initial management of massive oral bleeding after midfacial fracture, *J Trauma* 54(2):332, 2003.

Simon HK, Zempsky WT, Burns TB, et al.: Lacerations against Langer's lines: to glue or suture? *J Emerg Med* 16:185–189, 1998.

Stierman KL, Lloyd KM, De Luca-Pytell DM, et al.: Treatment and outcome of human bites in the head and neck, *Otolaryngol Head Neck Surg* 128:795, 2003.

Sujeeth S, Dindawar S: Parotid duct repair using an epidural catheter, *Int J Oral Maxillofac Surg* 40(7):747–748, July 2011.

---

*Reprinted from Ketch LL: Facial lacerations. In Harken AH, Moore EE, editors: *Abernathy's surgical secrets*, ed 6, Philadelphia, 2009, Mosby.

CHAPTER 35

CRANIOFACIAL SYNDROMES

Michael Jaskolka, Renie Daniel, Lewis Jones

EMBRYOGENESIS/GROWTH/DEVELOPMENT

1. **What are the components of the craniofacial skeleton?**
   The craniofacial skeleton is composed of the neurocranium (cranial vault and cranial base) and the viscerocranium (facial skeleton). The bones of the cranial vault are derived from the paraxial mesoderm and are formed through intramembranous ossification; the formation and expansion of ossification centers are directly within mesenchymal tissue. The bones of the cranial base are formed through endochondral ossification.

2. **Can you describe the rate of growth of the brain cranial vault of a child?**
   The brain is thought to grow in propulsive fashion. Over the first two years of life, the volume of the brain and cranium increase fourfold. Head circumference has reached 86% of its final size by age 1 and 94% by age 5. The maturation age of cranium width is 14 years in females and 15 years in males.

3. **How does the skull form and develop?**
   The cranial vault is formed by intramembraneous ossification, and bone deposition continues at the sutures. Endocranial resorption and ectocranial deposition continue in step with brain growth and expansion of the overlying soft tissue envelope. The three distinct layers of the skull do not develop until 3 to 5 years of life.

4. **What embryologic structures lead to the development of the face?**
   The frontonasal prominence and first pharyngeal arch. At weeks 4 to 5 the stomedial depression is surrounded by primordial structures that develop into facial structures: the frontonasal prominence, paired nasomedial and nasolateral prominences, and paired maxillary and mandibular prominences. The maxillary and mandibular prominences are derived from the first pharyngeal arch with Meckel's cartilage acting as an ossification template for the mandible.

5. **What are the differences among malformation, disruption, and deformation?**
   - **Malformation:** The abnormal formation of tissue as a result of an intrinsic developmental defect. In general, the later the defect occurs in gestation, the less extensive the malformation (e.g., spinal bifida).
   - **Disruption:** This is the breakdown of previously developed tissue causing abnormal morphology due to pressure resulting in amputation or vascular compromise (e.g., amniotic band).
   - **Deformation:** This is changes in morphology caused by external mechanical forces on normal tissue (e.g., oligohydramnios, intrauterine constraint, or abnormal fetal presentation).

6. **What is the functional matrix theory of craniofacial growth?**
   Anatomist Melvin Moss proposed the concept in the 1960s that development of the facial skeleton was directly related to the mechanics and functions of the various units that comprise the facial skeleton. Modern day interpretation has included an intrinsic (genetic) pattern that is altered by extrinsic (epigenetic) factors.

7. **How do remodeling and displacement contribute to craniofacial skeletal harmony?**
   Remodeling occurs as a result of local factors that lead to a change in the size and shape of the facial skeleton. Displacement occurs by the movement of bones away from each other at a suture or articulating surface (e.g., cranial sutures, temporomandibular joints, maxillary sutures). If the processes of remodeling and displacement do not occur in a balanced fashion, a skeletal discrepancy will occur.

8. **Can you name the six functional units that drive craniofacial development?**
   1. Central neurologic system
   2. Optic pathway

3. Speech and swallowing development
4. Airway and pharyngeal development
5. Muscles of facial expression development
6. Tooth development and exfoliation

9. **At what age is the majority of orbital/zygomatic growth completed?**
Approximately 85% of orbitozygomatic growth is completed between 5 and 7 years of age.

DEFORMATIONAL PLAGIOCEPHALY

10. **What is meant by deformational plagiocephaly?**
Deformational plagiocephaly is a nonsynostotic cranial deformity due to external forces. Most commonly, this presents with asymmetric occipital flattening and anterior displacement of the ipsilateral ear and forehead. Severe cases commonly occur in conjunction with torticollis. It is necessary to differentiate between deformational plagiocephaly and lambdoid craniosynostosis, which presents with ridging of the affected suture, severe flattening of the affected occipitoparietal region, ipsilateral retrusion of the forehead, and superior-posterior displacement of the ear (Fig. 35-1).

11. **Why has the incidence of deformational plagiocephaly increased since 1992?**
This is the year that the American Association of Pediatrics (AAP) introduced the "back to sleep" campaign to decrease sudden infant death syndrome (SIDS).

12. **How is deformational plagiocephaly treated?**
In mild cases, observed prone positioning and counterpositioning of the head will support normalization of symmetry over time. In severe cases, families may elect to proceed with the use of a custom molding helmet that is generally worn between the ages of 7 and 14 months of age.

13. **Is there a relationship between deformational plagiocephaly and developmental delay?**
This is a controversial topic that is actively being investigated. A causal relationship has yet to be demonstrated.

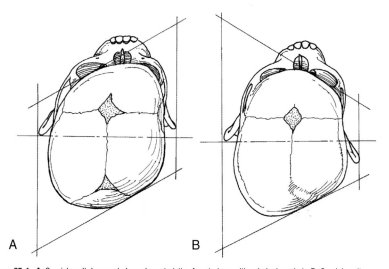

Figure 35-1. A, Cranial vault dysmorphology characteristic of posterior positional plagiocephaly. **B,** Cranial vault dysmorphology characteristic of posterior plagiocephaly secondary to unilateral lambdoid suture craniosynostosis. *(From Caccamese J, Costello BJ, Ruiz RL, Ritter AM: Positional plagiocephaly: evaluation and management,* Oral Maxillofacial Surg Clin North Am *16(4):439–446, 2004.)*

14. **What is torticollis?**

    Torticollis is an abnormal twisting of the head and neck. In children, this is most commonly caused by shortening or contracture of the sternocleidomastoid muscle. Congenital muscular torticollis is present at birth and may be due to intrauterine positioning, birth trauma, neurologic injury/disorder, or tumor, or it may be idiopathic. Acquired torticollis is thought to be a result of supine positioning with prolonged rotation of the head and neck. The clinical appearance is characterized by a rotation and tilting of the head *toward* the affected side with the chin pointing in the contralateral and superior direction. There may be a fibrotic mass depending upon the etiology. Treatment involves physical therapy, observed prone positioning, and counterpositioning of the head. In rare instances, Botox injections or surgical lengthening of the SCM may be required. Delay in treatment or refractory cases may lead to facial and cranial asymmetry and may require management with a cranial orthotic.

NONSYNDROMIC CRANIOSYNOSTOSIS

15. **How many sutures are present in the cranial vault?**

    There are four major cranial vault sutures: metopic, coronal (bilateral), sagittal, and lambdoid (bilateral). There are multiple other minor sutures (Fig. 35-2).

16. **How many fontanelles are present in the developing skull?**

    There are four fontanelles: anterior, posterior, lateral/sphenoid (bilateral), and mastoid (bilateral) (see Fig. 35-2).

17. **What is craniosynostosis?**

    Craniosynostosis is the premature fusion of one or more sutures of the cranial vault. It leads to an arrest of growth along the affected suture(s) that results in compensatory growth at the unaffected sutures leading to characteristic dysmorphology. In general, it occurs as an intrauterine event.

18. **An abnormality in what anatomic structure is thought to lead to craniosynostosis?**

    The dura.

19. **What is Virchow's law?**

    In 1851, Rudolf Virchow described the cessation of growth perpendicular to a fused cranial suture, with compensatory growth occurring at the remaining sutures in a parallel direction. In 1989, Delashaw further expanded this concept with four additional observations to predict the patterns of abnormal cranial morphology in more detail.

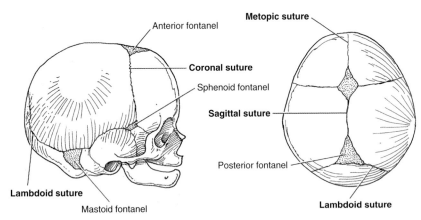

Figure 35-2. Major cranial vault sutures: the metopic, right and left coronal, sagittal, and right and left lambdoid. *(From Ruiz RL, Ritter AM, Turvey TA, Costello BJ, Ricalde P: Nonsyndromic craniosynostosis: diagnosis and contemporary surgical management,* Oral Maxillofacial Surg Clin North Am *16(4):447–463, 2004.)*

Table 35-1. Most Common Forms of Nonsyndromic Craniosynostosis

SUTURE	SHAPE	PREVALENCE	COMMENTS
Sagittal	Scaphocephaly	1:5000	Elongated (length) Narrow (width)
Coronal (unilateral)	Plagiocephaly (anterior)	1:10,000	Shortened orbit, retruded forehead, harlequin eye, contralateral bossing, deviation of the nasal root toward the affected side
Coronal (bilateral)	Brachycephaly (anterior)	Rare	Syndromic Exorbitism
Metopic	Trigonocephaly	1:15,000	Hypotelorism, low incidence of elevated ICP, often associated with other malformations and/or delay
Lambdoid (unilateral)	Plagiocephaly (posterior)	1:150,000	Commonly confused with deformational plagiocephaly
Lambdoid (bilateral)	Brachycephaly (posterior)	Rare	Syndromic

20. **Can you describe the consequences of craniosynostosis?**
    Depending upon the number and type of suture(s) that are involved, craniosynostosis can lead to abnormal morphology of the cranium, orbits, and face.
    In addition, it is thought to be associated with increased intracranial pressure (ICP). In the classic study by Marchac and Renier, approximately 14% of children with untreated single craniosynostosis demonstrated increased ICP. The percentage increased to 42% when two or more sutures were fused. Causality between craniosynostosis and elevated ICP is still debated in the literature.
    Finally, involvement of the coronal suture and ring may result in shortening of the orbit, decreased volume, strabismus, ptosis, abnormal binocular vision, and exorbitism.

21. **What are the clinical findings that may be reported in children with untreated craniosynostosis who develop increased ICP?**
    Headaches, vomiting, sleep disturbance, behavioral changes, and diminished cognitive function have all been reported. Prolonged elevated ICP will produce papilledema, optic nerve atrophy, and eventual vision loss. Signs of elevated ICP in association with single suture craniosynostosis are not usually encountered before 1 year of life.

22. **What are the physical and radiographic signs of craniosynostosis?**
    Absence of the affected suture with an irregular ridge of bone in its place. Abnormal cranial and orbital morphology, depending upon the affected suture(s). Elevated ICP may demonstrate as a scalloped "copper beaten" appearance or thinning and erosion of the inner surface of the skull on CT.

23. **Can you describe the most common forms of nonsyndromic craniosynostosis?**
    See Table 35-1 and Fig. 35-3.

24. **What is the harlequin eye deformity?**
    The harlequin eye deformity is the radiographic appearance of the superior lateral position of the ipsilateral orbit and wing of the sphenoid seen in unilateral coronal craniosynostosis.

25. **At what age does the metopic suture physiologically fuse?**
    The metopic suture has been shown to fuse as early as 3 months of life. When this occurs, there is commonly a nonsynostotic ridge that forms. This can make the diagnosis of metopic craniosynostosis challenging in mild cases.

26. **When should surgical treatment of craniosynostosis take place, and what are the two approaches that are used?**
    See Fig. 35-4. The exact timing depends upon the type of treatment, but surgery generally takes place before 12 months of age.

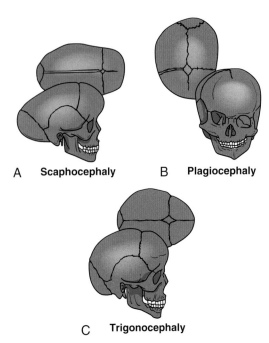

A   Scaphocephaly   B   Plagiocephaly

C   Trigonocephaly

Figure 35-3. Three common forms of nonsyndromic craniosynostosis. *(From Phillips N:* Berry & Kohn's Operating Room Technique, *ed 3, St. Louis, 2013, Mosby.)*

Endoscopic treatment is undertaken at an earlier age, around 3 months of life. It consists of multiple small incisions, suturectomy, and often multiple wedge craniectomies. The use of a postoperative cranial molding helmet is mandatory.

Open treatment is undertaken between 6 and 12 months of life. It consists of a coronal incision, craniectomy, fronto-orbital advancement as indicated, and cranial vault reconstruction. If multiple sutures are involved or the need for treatment is urgent, early surgery may be undertaken with a plan for additional reconstruction.

27. **What is the most important perioperative consideration for patients undergoing correction of craniosynostosis?**
Acute blood loss. Careful attention must be given to volume status. The majority of patients undergoing open treatment require a blood transfusion.

SYNDROMIC CRANIOSYNOSTOSIS

28. **What is the most common location of the genetic mutation found in craniofacial dysostosis syndromes, and how are they transmitted?**
The genetic abnormality is most commonly found on the fibroblast growth factor receptor (FGFR) genes 1, 2, and 3. The most common are the FGFR2-related dysostosis syndromes. They are generally inherited in an autosomal dominant pattern.

29. **What are the general functional considerations in patients with craniofacial dysostosis syndromes?**
- Craniosynostosis may restrict brain growth and be associated with elevated ICP leading to cognitive and behavioral delays as well as optic nerve compression.
- Untreated optic nerve compression will initially cause papilledema and eventually result in optic nerve atrophy and blindness.
- Shallow orbits result in proptosis of the globe that may lead to corneal desiccation/ulcers as well as globe herniation in severe cases. Dystopia and strabismus are also common orbital findings.

A   B   C

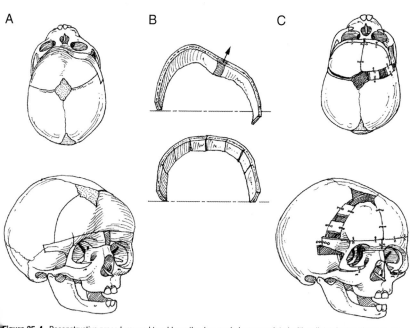

Figure 35-4. Reconstructive procedure used to address the dysmorphology associated with unilateral coronal suture craniosynostosis. **A,** Outline of the bifrontal craniotomy and orbital osteotomies. **B,** The dysmorphic orbital bandeau is removed, and vertical osteomies are used for reshaping. **C,** The reconstructed orbital bandeau is reinserted, and anterior cranial vault reconstruction is performed. *(From Ruiz RL, Ritter AM, Turvey TA, Costello BJ, Ricalde P: Nonsyndromic craniosynostosis: diagnosis and contemporary surgical management,* Oral Maxillofacial Surg Clin North Am *16(4):447–463, 2004.)*

- Hydrocephalus is a concern and is postulated to be secondary to constriction of the cranial base foramina and diminished venous drainage.
- Severe midface hypoplasia may contribute to airway obstruction and sleep apnea. Early evaluation with polysomnogram may be indicated.
- Dental crowding, eruptive abnormalities, and malocclusion are common.

30. **What is Crouzon syndrome?**
    Crouzon syndrome is a form of craniofacial dysostosis that is characterized by bilateral coronal craniosynostosis; other sutures are less often involved. This results in a brachycephalic skull with anterior retrusion, midface hypoplasia and exorbitism. Conductive hearing loss is a common finding. Patients demonstrate a typical IQ.

31. **What is Apert syndrome?**
    Apert syndrome is a form of craniofacial dysostosis that is characterized by bilateral coronal craniosynostosis with a widely patent midline calvarial defect, orbital hypertelorism, ptosis of the upper eyelids and downward slanting lateral canthi, midface hypoplasia, beaked nose, cleft palate (30%), hearing loss (30%), developmental delay, complex syndactyly of fingers and toes, and thick facial skin with increased sebaceous discharge. Macrocephaly and other CNS malformations may be present. Apert syndrome is thought to be associated with advanced paternal age.

32. **What is Pfeiffer syndrome?**
    Pfeiffer syndrome is a form of craniofacial dysostosis that has 3 clinical subtypes with variable penetrance. In general, Pfeiffer syndrome is characterized by craniosynostosis, orbital dystopia, midface hypoplasia, broad and deviated thumbs and toes, and variable syndactyly of the hands and feet. Type 1 is considered the classic form as described above, and patients have a good prognosis. Type 2 is the most severe in presentation and includes the cloverleaf skull deformity, significant

neurologic deficit, and a limited lifespan. Type 3 is similar in severity but does not include the cloverleaf skull deformity. There are a number of other low-frequency limb and organ abnormalities that may occur.

33. **What are the other most common named craniofacial syndromes?**
Carpenter, Saethre-Chotzen, Beare-Stevenson, Jackson-Weiss, and Meunke.

34. **What is the genetic basis for Saethre-Chotzen syndrome?**
Mutation in the TWIST 1 gene and subsequent TWIST 1 protein. A small subset of patients have a chromosomal abnormality in the region of chromosome 7 that contains the TWIST 1 gene.

35. **What is the general sequence of surgical treatment of patients with craniofacial dysostosis syndromes?**
In patients demonstrating increased ICP, early suturectomy and cranial vault expansion are performed. Otherwise, craniectomy and anterior cranial vault reconstruction with fronto-orbital advancement are completed before 12 months of age. Repeat craniofacial expansion may be required during childhood if findings of increased ICP are noted. Residual forehead retrusion, orbital hypertelorism, and midface deficiency can be managed after orbitozygomatic development is largely complete (5 to 7 years of age) by monobloc, facial bipartition, or Le Fort III procedures as indicated by the individual deformity. Final malocclusion is treated with more traditional orthognathic surgical techniques at skeletal maturity.

36. **What are the most common craniofacial conditions that include orbital hypertelorism?**
The craniofacial dysostosis syndromes, (cranio) frontonasal dysplasia, and midline facial clefts.

37. **What are the key features of frontonasal dysplasia?**
The most common presentation includes anterior cranium bifidum, orbital hypertelorism, a widow's peak, wide nasal dorsum with a bifid tip, and a midline cleft of the lip and palate.
    Craniofrontonasal dysplasia is likely a subtype that is inherited in an X-linked dominant pattern and more commonly seen in females. It has similar features, but includes craniosynostosis (most commonly bilateral coronal), thick and wiry hair, and other low-frequency extremity abnormalities.

38. **What are the surgical options for correction of orbital hypertelorism?**
Circumferential orbital osteotomies can be completed through a combined intracranial/extracranial approach. The orbits can be translocated after excision of a portion of the intervening interorbital tissues (frontal and nasal bones, floor of the anterior cranial fossa, ethmoid air cells, and nasal septum). Patients who have severe constriction of the maxilla can be managed with a facial bipartition procedure.

39. **What adjunctive procedures are often necessary at the time of orbital hypertelorism correction?**
Concurrent dorsal nasal augmentation and medial canthopexies.

40. **What is the position of the cribriform plate in patients with orbital hypertelorism, and why is this important?**
The cribriform plate is often inferiorly positioned with prolapse of the frontal lobes. Retraction and elevation are critical for the safe medial translocation of the orbits.

41. **Can you describe the cloverleaf skull deformity?**
Cloverleaf skull, also known as kleeblattschädel, refers to the trilobar skull shape characterized by multiple suture craniosynostosis, towering and bossing of the forehead, flattening of the posterior skull, and expansion or bulging of the temporal regions. The etiology is heterogeneous, and cloverleaf skull anomalies are often seen in conjunction with a spectrum of brain malformations. It can occur in the *absence* of craniosynostosis.

42. **What are the characteristic features of Binder syndrome?**
Variable nasomaxillary hypoplasia that may affect the frontal sinus, nose, upper lip, anterior septum, floor of the nose, and premaxillary-derived tissues. Clinical presentation includes midface deficiency, absence of anterior nasal spine, short nose with limited projection, acute nasolabial angle, and a flat nasofrontal angle. The nostrils appear crescent or semilunar in shape when viewed from below.

BIBLIOGRAPHY

American Academy of Pediatrics Task Force on infant sleep position and sudden infant death syndrome. Changing concepts of sudden infant death syndrome: implications for infant sleeping environment and sleep position, *Pediatrics* 105:650–656, 2000.

Antunes RB, Alonso N, Paula RG: Importance of early diagnosis of Stickler syndrome in newborns, *J Plast Recon Aesthetic Surg* 65:1029–1034, 2012.

Carlson BM: *Human embryology and developmental biology*, ed 5, Philadelphia, 2013, Saunders.

Cohen MM: Craniostenosis and syndromes with craniosynostosis: incidence, genetics, penetrace, variability, and new syndrome updating, *Birth Defects* 15:13–63, 1979.

Cole P, Hollier LH Jr: Craniosynostosis syndromes. In Weisman LE, Firth HV, editors: *UpToDate*, Waltham, MA, UpToDate. http://www.uptodate.com/home/help-manual-citing. Accessed on April 14, 2014.

Costello BJ, Mooney MP, Shand J: Craniomaxillofacial surgery in the pediatric patient: growth and development considerations. In Fonseca RJ, Marciani RD, Turvey TA, editors: *Oral and maxillofacial surgery*, ed 2, St Louis, 2009, Saunders.

Enlow D: *Facial growth*, ed 3, Philadelphia, 1990, Saunders.

Farkas L, Posnick J, Hreczko T: Anthropometric growth study of the head, *Cleft Palate Craniofacial J* 29(4):303–307, 1992.

Farkas L, Posnick J, Hreczko T, Pron G: Growth patterns of the orbital region, *Cleft Palate Craniofacial J* 29(4):315–317, 1992.

Hennekam RC, Beisecker LG, et al.: Elements of morphology: general terms for congenital anomalies, *Am J Genet Part A* 161(11):2726–2733, 2013.

Jones KL: *Smith's recognizable patterns of human malformation*, Philadelphia, 2006, Elsevier.

Kadouch DJM, Mass SM, Dubois L, et al.: Surgical treatment of macroglossia in patients with Beckwith-Wiedemann syndrome: a 20-year experience and review of the literature, *Int J Oral Maxillofac Surg* 41:300–308, 2012.

Kane A, Mitchell L, Craven K, et al.: Observations on a recent increase in plagiocephaly without synostosis, *Pediatrics* 97:877–885, 1996.

Kirshner RE, Kaye AE: Pierre Robin sequence. In Losee J, Kirschner RE, editors: *Comprehensive cleft care*, New York, 2009, McGraw Hill.

Moss M: The functional matrix hypothesis revisited, *Am J Orthodontics* 12(1):8–11, 1997.

Mulliken JB, Kaban LB: Analysis and treatment of hemifacial microsomia in childhood, *Clin Plast Surg* 14(1):91–100, 1987.

Murray JE, Mulliken JB, Kaban LB: Analysis and treatment of hemifacial microsomia, *Plast Reconstr Surg* 74(2):186–199, 1984.

Neville B, Damm D, Allen C, et al.: *Oral and maxillofacial pathology*, Philadelphia, 2002, Saunders.

Posnick J: *Craniofacial and maxillofacial surgery in children and young adults*, Philadelphia, 2000, Saunders.

Ruiz RL, Ritter AM, Turvey TA, et al.: Nonsyndromic craniosynostosis: diagnosis and contemporary surgical management. In Fonseca RJ, Marciani RD, Turvey TA, editors: *Oral and maxillofacial surgery*, ed 2, St Louis, 2009, Saunders.

Ruiz R, et al.: Update in craniofacial surgery, *Oral Max Surg Clin* 16(4):429–605, 2004.

Sulik KK: Orofacial embryogenesis: a framework for understanding clefting sites. In Fonseca RJ, Marciani RD, Turvey TA, editors: *Oral and maxillofacial surgery*, ed 2, St Louis, 2009, Saunders.

Trainor PA, Andrews BT: Facial dysostoses: etiology, pathogenesis and management, *Am J Med Genet Part C Semin Med Genet* 163C:283–294, 2013.

Teichgraeber JF, Ault JK, et al.: Deformational posterior plagiocephaly: diagnosis and treatment, *Cleft Palate Craniofacial J* 39(6):582–586, 2002.

Vargervik K: Classification and management of hemifacial microsomia. In Papel ID, Frodel JL, Holt GR, et al.: *Facial plastic and reconstructive surgery*, ed 3, New York, 2009, Thieme.

Vento AR, LaBrie RA, Mulliken JB: The O.M.E.N.S. classification of hemifacial microsomia, *Cleft Palate Craniofacial J* 28(1):68–77, 1991.

CHAPTER 36

OROMANDIBULAR DYSOSTOSIS

Daniel J. Meara, Renie Daniel, Lewis Jones, Michael Jaskolka

1. **What is the etiology of human facial dysostoses?**
   The human facial dysostoses are felt to result from abnormal migration of neural crest cells to the pharyngeal arches of the face.

2. **Which branchial arches are disturbed in the human facial dysostoses?**
   The first and second branchial arches are affected in these dysostoses. (See Table 36-1.)

3. **How are these groups of conditions subdivided?**
   - Mandibulofacial dysostoses (MFD)
   - Acrofacial dysostoses (AFD)

4. **What differentiates the mandibulofacial from the acrofacial dysostoses?**
   The addition of limb abnormalities results in the designation of acrofacial dysostosis.

5. **What are the common characteristics of oromandibular dysostoses?**
   - Down-slanting palpebral fissures
   - Coloboma of the lower eyelids
   - Hypoplasia of the zygomatic complex
   - Retro-micrognathia
   - Microtia

6. **What is a coloboma?**
   A coloboma is an apparent absence or defect of some ocular tissue, usually due to failure of a part of the fetal fissure to close. Typically, the defect is a skin notch within the lower eyelid that involves the whole thickness of the eyelid, and reconstruction involves all of its layers.

7. **What is the most common and well known of the oromandibulofacial dysostoses?**
   Treacher Collins syndrome. This condition is the result of at least three gene mutations (TCOF1, POLR1D, and POLR1C). It was initially described by British ophthalmologist Dr. Edward Treacher Collins in 1900, and it was more definitively described by Swiss ophthalmologist Dr. Adolphe Franceschetti in 1949.

8. **What is Treacher Collins syndrome?**
   Treacher Collins syndrome, also known as mandibulofacial dysostosis, is inherited in an autosomal dominant fashion and demonstrates variable phenotypic expression. It presents with bilateral abnormalities of the structures of the first and second branchial arches. Incidence is between 1 in 25,000 to 1 in 50,000 live births.

9. **Can you describe the characteristic findings in a patient with Treacher Collins syndrome?**
   Treacher Collins findings typically consist of:
   - Marked underdevelopment of the zygomatic complex
   - Overlying skin and soft tissues are hypoplastic with downward-sloping palpebral fissures and inferiorly positioned lateral canthi.
   - Colobomas of the lower eyelids
   - Varying degrees of microtia may occur as well as conductive hearing loss due to external and middle ear abnormalities.
   - The nose is wide at the bridge with elongation and lacks tip support.
   - The overall facial form is convex due to clockwise rotation of the maxilla-mandibular complex, class II open bite relationship, increased lower facial height, mandibular hypoplasia (especially of the condylar-ramus unit), an obtuse mandibular plane angle, and retrogenia, often resulting in airway impairment and feeding difficulties.
   - The TMJs and musculature are commonly hypoplastic.

Table 36-1. Pharngeal Arch and its Derivatives

PHARYNGEAL ARCH	ARCH ARTERY	CRANIAL NERVE	SKELETAL ELEMENTS	MUSCLES
1	Terminal branch of maxillary arch	Maxillary and mandibular division of trigeminal (V)	Incus, malleus. Upper portion of external ear (auricle), maxilla, zygomatic, squamous portion of temporal bone, mandible	Muscle of mastication, mylohyoid, anterior belly of digastric, tensor tympani, tensor veli palatini
2	Stapedius artery (embryologic) and cortico-tympanic artery (adult)	Facial nerve (VII)	Stapes, styloid process, stylohyoid ligament, lesser horns and upper rim of hyoid. Lower portion of external ear (auricle)	Muscles of facial expression, posterior belly of digastric, mylohyoid stapedius
3	Common carotid artery, most of internal carotid	Glossopharyn-geal (IX)	Lower rim and greater horn of hyoid	Stylopharyngeus
4	Left: Arch of aorta Right: Right subclavian artery	Superior laryn-geal branch of vagus (X)	Laryngeal cartilages	Constrictors of pharynx, crico-hyoid, levator veli palatini
6	Ductus arteriosus; roots of definitive pulmonary arteries	Recurrent laryn-geal branch of vagus (X)	Laryngeal cartilages	Intrinsic muscles of larynx

- Cleft palate may also be present.
- Dental anomalies include missing or hypoplastic teeth.

10. What syndrome is similar in craniofacial presentation to Treacher Collins syndrome, with the addition of extremity abnormalities?

    Nager syndrome, also known as acrofacial dysostosis. Autosomal recessive and dominant causation has been described, and the condition is often sporadic, without familial tendencies.

    The facial features include:
    - Malar hypoplasia
    - Downward-slanting palpebral fissures
    - Mandibular deficiency, often resulting in airway compromise and feeding difficulties
    - Low-set and abnormal ears
    - Conductive hearing loss
    - Cleft palate with significant hypoplasia

    The limb abnormalities may range from hypoplasia to agenesis of the radius and thumbs, with multiple other low-frequency extremity abnormalities.

11. What is craniofacial microsomia (CFM)?

    CFM is a congenital birth defect postulated to be a result of in utero injury to the stapedial artery that leads to variable hypoplasia of the first and second branchial arches, via failed neural crest development and migration.

    Patients commonly clinically demonstrate:
    - Microtia
    - Skin tags
    - Colobomas
    - Facial nerve weakness

Table 36-2. OMENS-Plus Classification

0 (Orbit)	0 – Normal orbit
	1 – Abnormal size
	2 – Abnormal position
	3 – Abnormal size and position
M (Mandible)	0 – Normal mandible
	1 – Hypoplastic mandibular ramus
	2 – Hypoplastic and malformed mandibular ramus
	3 – Absence of ramus, glenoid fossa
E (Ear)	0 – Normal ear
	1 – Auricular hypoplasia
	2 – Absence of external auditory canal
	3 – Absent auricle and malpositioned lobe
N (Facial nerve)	0 – Normal facial nerve
	1 – Upper facial nerve involvement
	2 – Lower facial nerve involvement
	3 – All branches affected
S (Soft tissue structures)	0 – No soft tissue abnormality
	1 – Minimal tissue/muscle deficiency
	2 – Moderate tissue/muscle deficiency
	3 – Severe tissue/muscle deficiency
Plus (Extracranial abnormalities)	Extracraniofacial abnormalities

- Macrostomia
- Underdevelopment of the facial skeleton (including the **characteristic hypoplastic mandible**) and associated muscles, soft tissues, and TMJs
- Congenital heart defects

Other names include hemifacial microsomia, otomandibular dysostosis, and lateral facial dysplasia, and CFM more accurately describes a group of disorders that fall within a spectrum of variable but overlapping clinical findings.

12. **What is oculo-auriculo-vertebral (OAV) spectrum?**
    OAV, often referred to as Goldenhar syndrome, is considered to be a variant within the spectrum of anomalies within CFM.
    Additional clinical findings include:
    - Presence of epibulbar dermoids
    - Vertebral, especially cervical spine, abnormalities
    - Higher incidence of oronasal clefting
    - Pharyngeal and laryngeal abnormalities

13. **How common is CFM?**
    CFM is estimated to occur 1 in 5600 births, and it is the second most common congenital facial anomaly after cleft lip and palate. There is a male predilection as well as right-side predominance. It can occur in a bilateral form; however, the anomaly is unilateral in 80% of cases.

14. **What is the most common classification system for CFM?**
    The OMENS classification assigns a number from 0 to 3 to the primary areas affected: **O**rbital distortion, **M**andibular hypoplasia, **E**ar anomaly, **N**erve involvement, and **S**oft tissue deficiency. A "Plus" designation may also be included to detail any extracraniofacial abnormalities. (See Table 36-2.)

15. **What other classification systems have been developed to describe various aspects of the multiple associated malformations?**
Pruzansky and Kaban, which are often most useful in clinical practice. Pruzansky presented his classification in 1969 as a simple and practical means to define mandibular deficiency or deformity. Kaban modified the classification by adding additional detail and by separating type II deformity into IIA and IIB forms.

16. **What is the Kaban classification of the TMJ, and how is it applied?**
The Kaban classification is used to categorize the anatomy and function of the mandibular ramus-condyle unit, within the TMJ, as well as the need for and timing of surgical reconstruction. This classification is applied to a number of conditions that affect the mandible, temporomandibular joint, and facial musculature, including Treacher Collins syndrome and CFM.
   - **Type I:** All components of the mandible and glenoid fossae are present and mildly hypoplastic. The muscles of mastication are present, and the function of the TMJ is normal.
   - **Type IIA:** All components of the mandible and glenoid fossae are present and moderately hypoplastic. The condyle is displaced anteriorly and medially. The muscles of mastication are hypoplastic, but the TMJ remains functional.
   - **Type IIB:** There is severe hypoplasia of the mandible and glenoid fossae, but a posterior point of contact still remains in an anterior and medial position. The muscles of mastication are severely hypoplastic or partially absent, and the TMJ is abnormal in function.
   - **Type III:** Complete absence of the ramus, the glenoid fossa, the joint structures (disk, capsule, ligaments), and most of the muscles of mastication. The mandible is free floating without a posterior point of contact.

17. **What are the general reconstructive stages for patients with Treacher Collins syndrome and CFM?**
Surgical reconstruction should be considered in an anatomic subunit fashion based upon growth, development, function, and cosmetic/psychosocial considerations.
   - Orbital-zygomatic reconstruction can be undertaken after 5 to 7 years of age; lateral canthopexy is completed concurrently. In type III deformities of the TMJ, glenoid fossa reconstruction should be carried out at the same time.
   - Early mandibular distraction may be considered in cases of airway obstruction. Otherwise the timing of mandibular reconstruction should be based upon the function of the TMJ. Type IIB and III deformities may benefit from distraction or costochondral grafting in the early mixed dentition with attempted management of the maxillary cant by use of an asymmetric acrylic splint. Malocclusion and facial asymmetry are best completed with traditional orthognathic surgical techniques involving the maxilla, mandible, and chin, at skeletal maturity.
   - Microtia reconstruction generally requires multiple procedures. Dr. B. Brent and Dr. S. Nagata have delineated the two most commonly employed sequences using autogenous tissue. Treatment does not usually begin until at least 6 years of age due to costochondral maturity and patient cooperation. When indicated, management of canal atresia and the middle ear are carried out after external ear reconstruction is completed.
   - Soft tissue procedures should be carefully planned after skeletal reconstruction is complete, unless there is a functional indication necessitating early intervention.
   - Orofacial clefting is treated in the typical sequence. Lip repair at 3 to 6 months of life. Cleft palate repair at 8 to 12 months of life, unless airway considerations dictate otherwise.
   - Correction of the macrostomia is typically addressed in the first few months of life, and excision of the skin tags within the first year.

18. **What is Pierre Robin, and what are the pathognomonic clinical findings in Pierre Robin?**
Pierre Robin is a sequence with a primary defect (arrested mandibular development) causing a cascade of secondary anomalies (glossoptosis, cleft palate), which in this sequence leads to airway obstruction.

19. **What is the difference between a sequence and a syndrome?**
A sequence occurs when a single developmental defect results in a chain of secondary defects. A syndrome is a group of anomalies that contain multiple malformations and/or sequences with variable expression.

20. **What are the most important considerations in the care of neonates with Pierre Robin sequence (PRS)?**

   PRS is a clinical entity that is postulated to occur secondary to restricted mandibular growth. It may occur in association with a craniofacial syndrome or be present in isolation. The tongue maintains a posterior position that interferes with the embryonic fusion of the palatal shelves, resulting in a cleft palate.

   PRS is variable in severity of presentation. The most important early considerations are the potential for airway obstruction and feeding difficulties beyond those of a typical child with an isolated cleft palate. Management of the airway is dependent upon the type and location of obstruction and may require prone positioning, nasopharyngeal airway, CPAP, intubation, or surgery. Surgery may include tongue lip adhesion, mandibular distraction, or tracheostomy. Feeding may be complicated by aspiration and reflux and may require the use of medications, a cleft palate feeder, a nasogastric tube, or a g-tube.

21. **What is the most common genetic syndrome associated with PRS?**

   Stickler syndrome.

22. **Can you describe Stickler syndrome?**

   Stickler syndrome is a collagen disorder that is inherited in both autosomal dominant and recessive fashions, depending upon the type. There are five subtypes based upon which collagen (II, IX, XI) gene is involved. In addition to micrognathia and cleft palate, other craniofacial findings may include dorsal nasal and midface hypoplasia. Visual abnormalities are the most concerning as the development of early high myopia and retinal detachment may lead to early blindness if not identified. Varying degrees of sensorineural hearing loss as well as other collagen-based musculoskeletal abnormalities are common.

BIBLIOGRAPHY

Abubaker O, Benson K: *Oral and maxillofacial surgery secrets*, ed 2, Philadelphia, 2007, Elsevier.

American Academy of Pediatrics Task Force on infant sleep position and sudden infant death syndrome. Changing concepts of sudden infant death syndrome: implications for infant sleeping environment and sleep position, *Pediatrics* 105:650–656, 2000.

Antunes RB, Alonso N, Paula RG: Importance of early diagnosis of Stickler syndrome in newborns, *J Plast Reconstr Aesthet Surg* 65:1029–1034, 2012.

Caccamese JF, Costello BJ, Mooney MP: Novel deformity of the mandible in oculo-auriculo-vertebral spectrum: a case report and literature review, *J Oral Maxillofac Surg* 64:1278–1283, 2006.

Carlson BM: *Human embryology and developmental biology*, ed 5, Philadelphia, 2013, Saunders.

Cobb A, Green B, Gill D, et al.: The surgical management of Treacher Collins syndrome, *Brit J Oral Maxillofac Surg* 52:581–589, 2014.

Costello BJ, Mooney MP, Shand J: Craniomaxillofacial surgery in the pediatric patient: growth and development considerations. In Fonseca RJ, Marciani RD, Turvey TA, editors: *Oral and maxillofacial surgery*, ed 2, St Louis, 2009, Saunders.

D'Antonio LL, Rice RD, Fink SC: Evaluation of pharyngeal and laryngeal structure and function in patients with oculo-auriculo-vertebral spectrum, *Cleft Palate-Craniofac J* 35(4):333–341, 1998.

Enlow D: *Facial growth*, ed 3, Philadelphia, 1990, Saunders.

Hennekam RC, Beisecker LG, et al.: Elements of morphology: general terms for congenital anomalies, *Am J Gene A* 161(11):2726–2733, 2013.

Jones KL: *Smith's recognizable patterns of human malformation*, Philadelphia, 2006, Elsevier.

Kirshner RE, Kaye AE: Pierre Robin sequence. In Losee J, Kirshner RE, editors: *Comprehensive cleft care*, New York, 2009, McGraw Hill.

Moss M: The functional matrix hypothesis revisited, *Am J Orthodont* 12(1):8–11, 1997.

Mulliken JB, Kaban LB: Analysis and treatment of hemifacial microsomia in childhood, *Clin Plast Surg* 14(1):91–100, 1987.

Murray JE, Mulliken JB, Kaban LB: Analysis and treatment of hemifacial microsomia, *Plast Reconstr Surg* 74(2):186–199, 1984.

Neville B, Damm D, Allen C, et al.: *Oral and maxillofacial pathology*, Philadelphia, 2002, Saunders.

Posnick J: *Craniofacial and maxillofacial surgery in children and young adults*, Philadelphia, 2000, Saunders.

Posnick J, Ruiz R: Treacher Collins syndrome: current evaluation, treatment, and future directions, *Cleft Palate-Craniofac J* 37(5), 2000.

Ruiz R, et al.: Update in craniofacial surgery, *Oral Maxillofac Surg Clin* 16(4):429–605, 2004.

Schlump J, Stein A, Hehr U, et al.: Treacher Collins syndrome: clinical implications for the paediatrician—a new mutation in a severely affected newborn and comparison with three further patients with the same mutation, and review of the literature, *Euro J Pediatr* 171:1611–1618, 2012.

Sulik KK: Orofacial embryogenesis: a framework for understanding clefting sites. In Fonseca RJ, Marciani RD, Turvey TA, editors: *Oral and maxillofacial surgery*, ed 2, St Louis, 2009, Saunders.

Trainor PA, Andrews BT: Facial dysostoses: etiology, pathogenesis and management, *Am J Med Gene C* 163C:283–294, 2013.

Travieso R, Chang C, Terner J, et al.: A range of condylar hypoplasia exists in Treacher Collins syndrome, *J Oral Maxillofac Surg* 71:393–397, 2013.

Vargervik K: Classification and management of hemifacial microsomia. In Papel ID, Frodel JL, Holt GR, et al.: *Facial plastic and reconstructive surgery*, ed 3, New York, 2009, Thieme.

Vento AR, LaBrie RA, Mulliken JB: The O.M.E.N.S. classification of hemifacial microsomia, *Cleft Palate Craniofac J* 28(1):68–77, 1991.

Weinzweig J: *Plastic surgery secrets plus*, ed 2, Philadelphia, 2010, Mosby Elsevier.

Wieczorek D: Human facial dysostoses, *Clin Gene* 83:499–510, 2013.

CHAPTER 37

SYNDROMES AFFECTING THE OROFACIAL REGION

Dean M. DeLuke, A. Omar Abubaker, Kenneth J. Benson

1. **What is a syndrome?**
   A syndrome is a set of symptoms that occur together. A particular syndrome may have three, four, or 10 manifestations, but a key sequence of symptoms leads to the diagnosis of a particular syndrome.

2. **What is Ellis-van Creveld syndrome?**
   Ellis-van Creveld syndrome is found mostly in the Amish population and includes dwarfism, hidrotic ectodermal dysplasia, and fusion of the mid-upper lip. The syndrome is also called chondroectodermal dysplasia. It is the most common cause of dwarfism among the Amish population.

3. **What are the congenital and acquired causes of macroglossia?**
   Congenital and hereditary conditions causing macroglossia include vascular lesions, such as lymphangioma and hemangioma, hemihypertrophy, cretinism, Beckwith-Wiedemann syndrome, Down syndrome, neurofibromatosis, and multiple endocrine neoplasia (MEN) syndrome type 2B. Acquired causes include long-term edentulous state, amyloidosis, myxedema, acromegaly, angioedema, and tumors of the tongue.

4. **What are the features of achondroplasia?**
   Achondroplasia is a disease with >80% sporadic genetic incidence representing point mutations. The average frequency worldwide is 1 in 25,000 though it occurs more frequently in Latin America. Risk factors for the disease include advanced paternal age at time of conception, and more than 20% are familial, showing autosomal dominant mode of transmission. Systemic features of this syndrome include short limbs, short stubby hands, lordotic lumbar spine, prominent buttocks, protuberant abdomen, and predilection for obesity. The craniomaxillofacial features include macroencephaly (enlarged head), frontal bossing, depression of nasal bridge, midface hypoplasia with relative mandibular prognathism, and otitis media. Otitis media in these patients is common during the first six years of life, which can lead to hearing loss if untreated. Oral features include anterior dental crowding and Class III malocclusion.

5. **What syndromes are associated with mandibular prognathism?**
   Mandibular prognathism may be present in the following syndromes: basal cell nevus syndrome (Gorlin syndrome), Klinefelter syndrome, Marfan syndrome, osteogenesis imperfecta, and Waardenburg syndrome. Down syndrome has been associated with both prognathism and micrognathia.

6. **What common malformation syndromes are associated with midface deficiency?**
   The following syndromes may be associated with midface deficiency: achondroplasia, osteogenesis imperfecta, Apert syndrome, cleidocranial dysplasia, Crouzon syndrome, Marshall syndrome, Pfeiffer syndrome, and Stickler syndrome.

7. **What syndromes are often associated with hyperdontia/hypodontia?**

Syndromes Associated with Hyperdontia	Syndromes Associated with Hypodontia
Cleidocranial dysplasia	Crouzon
Gardner	Down
Hallermann-Streiff	Ectodermal dysplasia
Sturge-Weber	Ehlers-Danlos
Oral-facial-digital, type I	Ellis-van Creveld

Syndromes Associated with Hyperdontia	Syndromes Associated with Hypodontia
Fabry-Anderson	Goldenhar
	Gorlin
	Hallermann-Streiff
	Hurler
	Oral-facial-digital, type I
	Witkop tooth and nail
	Sturge-Weber
	Turner

8. **In what diseases are café au lait spots seen?**
   Café au lait spots are seen in patients with neurofibromatosis (von Recklinghausen disease) and in McCune-Albright syndrome. The spots are described as Coast of California (smooth borders) in neurofibromatosis and Coast of Maine (irregular borders) in Albright syndrome.

9. **What is von Recklinghausen disease?**
   Von Recklinghausen disease is more commonly known as neurofibromatosis in current terminology. Eight forms are recognized, but 85% to 90% are type I (skin related). The disease is autosomal dominant, and occurrence is 1 in 3000 with no sex predilection. The majority of cases exhibit café au lait spots of the skin (melanin pigmentation). The presence of six or more spots that are >1.5 cm in diameter is pathognomonic for the disease. Axillary freckling is called Crow's sign and is often present in this disease. Type I of the disease most frequently involves the skin and oral mucosa. Café au lait spots have smooth borders (coastline of California). The disease is thought to arise from Schwann cells, fibroblasts, and perineural cells. Histologically, proliferation of delicate spindle cells with thin wavy nuclei and myxoid matrix is often seen. There is no curative treatment for the disease. Radiotherapy is ineffective and can be associated with transformation of the lesions into sarcomas.

10. **What is neurilemoma (schwannoma)?**
    Neurilemoma is a slow-growing tumor thought to be derived from Schwann cells. It is an uncommon disease, and 25% to 48% occur in head and neck areas. The tongue is the most common intraoral location. Histologically, the lesions usually show a characteristic palisaded cell pattern (Antoni type A tissue) around central eosinophilic areas known as Verocay bodies. Antoni type B tissue shows a more disorderly arrangement of cells and fibers. The treatment of neurilemoma is surgical excision, and there is a low rate of recurrence.

11. **What is the differential diagnosis of a newborn with a crusty lower lip that wipes off easily, leaving areas of indentation?**
    The differential diagnosis of this condition includes Stevens-Johnson syndrome, herpetic gingivostomatitis, epidermolysis bullosa, dermatitis herpetiforms, herpes zoster, and toxic epidermal necrolysis (Lyell's disease).

12. **What are the clinical features of basal cell nevus syndrome?**
    The syndrome is also known as Gorlin syndrome. It is an autosomal dominant syndrome with very complex and highly variable abnormalities. It has several orofacial and systemic abnormalities, including:
    - Cutaneous anomalies, including basal cell carcinoma, palmar and plantar pitting
    - Dental and osseous anomalies, such as multiple odontogenic keratocysts (OKCs) in 75% of patients, mandibular prognathism, rib anomalies (bifid ribs), vertebral anomalies such as kyphoscoliosis in 50%, and bradymetacarpalism
    - Ophthalmologic and frontal abnormalities, such as ocular hypertelorism (40%), and frontal and temporoparietal bossing
    - Neurologic anomalies in the form of mental retardation, and calcification of falx cerebri
    - Sexual abnormalities in the form of ovarian fibromas and medulloblastomas
    - Oral manifestations, including OKCs, which are indistinguishable from those not associated with the syndrome. The treatment of these cysts is similar to that for other OKCs.

13. **What is Frey syndrome?**

    Frey syndrome (gustatory sweats) is sweating of the temporal cutaneous region upon eating. It usually occurs due to surgical damage to the auriculotemporal nerve during temporomandibular joint (TMJ) or parotid surgery. The damaged nerve regenerates in a misdirected fashion and the parasympathetic salivary nerve supply carried along the auricular region reconnects along sympathetic pathways that innervate the sweat glands. After salivary, gustatory, or psychic stimulation of the parasympathetic fibers, sweating occurs. Confirmation of the diagnosis consists of using Minor's starch iodine test to detect sweating. The treatment for this condition includes topical anticholinergic and local atropine injections, botulinum toxin injections, severing of the auriculo-temporal nerve, or transplantation/interposition of fascia lata graft under the skin in the involved area. This syndrome should be differentiated from a similar condition called crocodile tears, which is a lacrimation that occurs during eating and generally follows Bell's palsy, herpes zoster, or head injury.

14. **What is Ramsay Hunt syndrome?**

    Symptoms of Ramsay Hunt syndrome include facial nerve paralysis, otalgia, and vesicular eruption on the external ear, vertigo, and hearing deficits. It is caused by herpes zoster virus infection of an ipsilateral geniculate ganglion.

15. **What is reactive arthritis (formerly Reiter syndrome)?**

    This syndrome was classically described as a triad of urethritis, conjunctivitis, and arthritis. It usually affects young males (male to female ratio is 9:1). Urethritis or external genital lesions may be present. The joint involvement may include the TMJ, leading to TMJ dysfunction symptoms. The underlying cause is most often either a gastrointestinal or urogenital infection, so it is important to diagnose and treat the underlying condition.

16. **What is Heerfordt syndrome?**

    Heerfordt syndrome also is called uveoparotitis or uveoparotid fever. It is associated with acute sarcoidosis. It is characterized by firm painless enlargement of the parotid gland with uveal inflammation of the tracts of the eyes (conjunctivitis, keratitis) and cranial nerve (CN) involvement (CN VII nerve paralysis in half the cases).

17. **What are the clinical features of Ascher syndrome?**

    There are three features associated with Ascher syndrome:
    - Acquired double lip: seen when lips are tensed, resembling a Cupid's bow
    - Blepharochalasis: drooping of tissue between the eyebrow and edge of upper lid so the tissue hangs loosely over the lid margin
    - Thyroid enlargement, which is not a consistent finding and may not appear until many years after eyelid involvement

18. **What is Melkersson-Rosenthal syndrome?**

    Recurrent attacks of facial paralysis, noninflammatory painless facial edema, cheilitis granulomatosa, and fissured tongue. Facial palsy may begin suddenly in childhood and precede facial edema by many years.

19. **What is the most common human chromosomal abnormality?**

    Down syndrome, also called trisomy 21 syndrome. Clinically, the patient has a flat face, large anterior fontanel, open sutures, fissured tongue, and hypermobility of the joints. It has been associated with both prognathism and micrognathia.

20. **Which syndrome has been referred to as hysterical dysphagia?**

    Plummer-Vinson syndrome, which usually occurs in the fourth and fifth decades of life. Most commonly seen in women, this syndrome is a manifestation of iron deficiency anemia. Symptoms include cracks at commissures, lemon-tinted skin color, red and smooth painful tongue, and dysphagia from esophageal stricture.

21. **What is Papillon-LeFèvre syndrome?**

    This is a syndrome of juvenile periodontitis with associated skin lesions. It is manifest as severe destruction of alveolar bone involving deciduous and permanent teeth, deep periodontal pockets, boggy gingiva, and fetid breath. Skin lesions may be present and include keratotic lesions of palmar and plantar surfaces.

22. **Which syndrome is associated with lower lip pits?**
Lower lip pits are a common manifestation of van der Woude syndrome (lip pit–cleft lip syndrome). Lower lip pits are present in 80% of patients with this syndrome. Patients may also be missing the central and lateral incisors, canines, or bicuspids. In addition, these patients often have a cleft lip, but may or may not have a cleft palate or cleft uvula. Van der Woude syndrome is an autosomal dominant disorder.

23. **What is Horner syndrome?**
Horner syndrome is a combination of ptosis of the upper eyelid, myosis of the pupil, and anhidrosis of the forehead caused by interruption of the cervical sympathetic trunk to the orbit. The ptosis is a result of interruption of the innervation to the superior tarsal muscle, leading to constant ptosis and interference with maintenance of normal elevation of the upper lid. This should be distinguished from the inability to open the eye voluntarily, which usually results from paralysis of the oculomotor nerve, and from the inability to close the lids tightly, which is a result of facial nerve paralysis. The myosis is a result of the unopposed action of the parasympathetic nerves on the ciliary muscles, whereas the anhidrosis is the result of interruption of sympathetic flow to the sweat glands. Isolated Horner syndrome may be caused by trauma to the neck and by tumors involving the carotid artery, or it may even be the first sign of lung cancer.

24. **What is superior orbital fissure syndrome?**
Superior orbital fissure syndrome is a combination of symptoms that result from direct or indirect pressure on the structures passing through the superior orbital fissure. This mostly occurs as a rare complication of orbital fracture, although it can result from neoplastic or inflammatory conditions affecting the superior orbital fissure. The clinical presentation varies in severity, depending on the number of structures involved. The complete presentation of the syndrome includes subconjunctival ecchymosis; proptosis; ptosis; persistent periorbital edema; ophthalmoplegia; loss of corneal, direct, consensual, and accommodation reflexes; and loss of sensation over the forehead extending to the vertex.

25. **What is cherubism?**
Cherubism is a syndrome characterized by bilateral, progressive enlargement of the maxilla and mandible. The onset is often early (between ages two and five). The process may sometimes burn out after puberty. Radiographically, there is a characteristic multilocular or soap bubble appearance of the jawbones. Recontouring procedures may be necessary to reduce bulk and improve esthetics, and this is best done after puberty or when the disease is in a quiescent phase.

26. **What are the four distinguishing features found in patients with osteogenesis imperfecta?**
    1. Brittle bones that are prone to fracture
    2. Blue sclera
    3. Dentinogenesis imperfecta
    4. Maxillary hypoplasia

27. **What are the four distinguishing features found in patients with cleidocranial dysplasia?**
    1. Aplasia of clavicles
    2. Multiple impacted and supernumerary teeth
    3. Short stature
    4. Class III skeletal malocclusion
    5. High-arched palate

28. **What are the four distinguishing features found in patients with Ehlers-Danles syndrome?**
    1. Extreme joint hypermobility (including the TMJ)
    2. Hyperelastic skin that can be stretched readily
    3. Mucosal fragility and early onset of periodontal disease
    4. Hypoplastic enamel and dentin

29. **What are the four distinguishing features found in patients with Gardner Syndrome?**
    1. Intestinal polyposis (with a high risk of malignant transformation)
    2. Multiple supernumerary and impacted teeth
    3. Osteomas of the jawbones
    4. Multiple soft tissue tumors (desmoid tumors, epidermoid cysts)

30. **What is Bechet syndrome?**
Bechet syndrome is a multisystem immune system disorder that may be triggered by viral or bacterial infection. It is characterized by the triad of multiple apthous-like ulcers, uveitis, and genital lesions. In severe cases, treatment with systemic steroids may be indicated.

31. **Describe the distinctions between Stevens-Johnson syndrome (SJS) and toxic epidermal necrolysis (TEN).**
SJS is classically described as a severe form of erythema multiforme with mucosal and skin involvement, along with genital and eye lesions. In TEN, the skin involvement is more progressive and severe, involving skin detachment on more than 30% of skin surfaces. In the majority of cases, a toxic drug reaction is the cause, and a T-cell mediated response is the underlying mechanism.

32. **What is Peutz-Jeghers syndrome?**
Peutz-Jeghers syndrome is characterized by intestinal polyps that often become malignant, and mucocutaneous pigmentation (oral melanosis) that involves intraoral and perioral regions.

33. **What are the multiple endocrine neoplasia (MEN) syndromes?**
MEN encompasses a constellation of syndromes: MEN type 1, type 2A, and type 2B. Common to all are endocrine neoplasias (adrenal, thyroid, pituitary, parathyroid, and pancreas). MEN 2B has associated mucosal neuromas and mandibular prognathism, and patients typically exhibit a marfanoid appearance. The endocrine tumors in type 2B are medullary thyroid carcinoma and pheochromocytoma.

34. **What is the classic triad of symptoms associated with Trotter syndrome, and what is the cause of this syndrome?**
The classic triad of symptoms in Trotter syndrome is hearing loss, soft palate paralysis or deviation, and neuralgia or paresthesia of the third division of the trigeminal nerve (lingual or mandibular branches). Trismus is also a common clinical correlate. The symptoms are all caused by the occurrence and direct extension of a nasopharyngeal carcinoma. The condition is often confused with or misdiagnosed as a temporomandibular disorder.

35. **What is Osler-Rendu-Weber syndrome, and what is its significance for the oral and maxillofacial surgeon?**
Osler-Rendu-Weber syndrome is also known as hereditary hemorrhagic telangiectasia, and it is characterized by multiple arteriovenous malformations. Spontaneous bleeding may occur, and often the presence of multiple areas of telangiectasia on the lips, oral mucosa, and/or perioral lesions may lead to the initial diagnosis.

36. **Give at least three distinguishing features of Papillon-Lefèvre syndrome.**
    1. Early periodontal disease that affects both the primary and permanent dentition
    2. Palmar and plantar keratosis
    3. Calcification of the falx cerebri is a frequent finding.

37. **Give at least three distinguishing features of Prader-Willi syndrome.**
    1. Short stature
    2. Morbid obesity (with an early age of onset) secondary to hypothalamic dysfunction
    3. Small mouth, hands, and feet with dolichocephaly
    4. Tendency to develop diabetes and sleep apnea

38. **Give at least three distinguishing features of Sjogren syndrome.**
    1. Originally described as a triad of dry eyes, dry mouth, and autoimmune disease
    2. Bilateral salivary gland enlargement is a common finding.
    3. Histologically, the diagnosis can be confirmed by biopsy of minor salivary glands in the lip or palate (classic finding is periductal lymphocytic infiltrate).
    4. A predilection to develop lymphoma
        In current terminology, it is also important to distinguish between primary and secondary Sjogren syndrome. Primary Sjogren syndrome refers to involvement of the salivary and lacrimal glands, without evidence of systemic autoimmune disease, while secondary Sjogren syndrome is associated with an autoimmune disease (most often rheumatoid arthritis or systemic lupus erythematosus).

39. **What is the most commonly observed inheritance pattern for syndromes of the head and neck?**
Autosomal dominant.

BIBLIOGRAPHY

Cohen M: Anomalies, syndromes and medical genetics. In *Oral and maxillofacial surgery update*, vol 2, Rosemont, IL, 1998, AAOMS Publications.

DeLuke DM: *Syndromes of the head and neck, an atlas of the oral and maxillofacial clinics of North America*, Philadelphia, 2014, Elsevier.

Goodrich JJ, Hall CD: *Craniofacial anomalies: growth and development from a surgical perspective*, New York, 1995, Thieme Medical.

Hennekam R, Allanson I, Krantz I: *Gorlin's syndromes of the head and neck*, ed 5, New York, 2010, Oxford Press.

Jones KL, Jones MC, del Campo M: *Smith's recognizable patterns of human malformation*, ed 7, Philadelphia, 2013, Saunders.

Neville B, Damm D, Allen C, et al.: *Oral and maxillofacial pathology*, ed 3, Philadelphia, 2008, Saunders.

Salmon AM: *Developmental defects and syndromes*, Aylesbury, England, 1978, HM+M Publications.

CHAPTER 38

CLEFT LIP AND PALATE

Jennifer E. Woerner, A. Omar Abubaker

EMBRYOLOGY

1. **Which processes merge to form the upper lip, anterior maxillary alveolus, the nose, and the mouth?**
   The merger of the maxillary and medial nasal processes forms the upper lip and anterior maxillary alveolus. The merger of maxillary and mandibular processes forms the mouth, whereas the merger of the lateral nasal process forms the ala of the nose.

2. **How does cleft lip develop?**
   Cleft lip develops from failure of fusion of the medial nasal process and the maxillary process.

3. **At what time during gestation do cleft lip and/or palate occur?**
   The upper lip and premaxilla form at approximately 7 weeks' gestation. Disruption around this time results in clefting of the lip and/or alveolus. The palatal shelves fuse at approximately 12 weeks of gestation. Disruption around this time results in clefting of the hard and/or soft palate.

4. **Why are left-sided secondary or palatal clefts more common than right-sided clefts?**
   Up to the seventh week of gestation, the two palatal shelves of the human embryo lie almost vertically. As the neck straightens from its flexed position, the tongue drops posteriorly, and the shelves rotate superiorly to the horizontal position; they fuse from anterior to posterior to form the palate by 12 weeks. In rodents, the right palatal shelf reaches the horizontal position before the left one, leaving the left side susceptible to developmental interruption for a longer period than the right. It is believed that this sequence of changes occurs in humans as well and may account for the higher incidence of left-sided clefts.

ANATOMY

5. **What are the primary and secondary palates?**
   The primary palate comprises the lip, alveolar arch, and palate anterior to the incisive foramen (the premaxilla). The secondary palate comprises the soft palate and hard palate posterior to the incisive foramen. The primary and secondary palates are separated by the incisive foramen (Fig. 38-1).

6. **Which orofacial muscles are anatomically abnormal in cleft lip and palate?**
   In cleft lip, the main muscle involved is the orbicularis oris muscle. In cleft palate, several muscles are usually involved, depending on the extent of the cleft. In *complete* cleft palate, the levator veli palatini, tensor veli palatini, uvular, palatopharyngeus, and palatoglossus muscles are involved (Fig. 38-2).

7. **What is Passavant's ridge?**
   Passavant's ridge is a transverse ridge or a bulge produced by the forceful contraction of the superior pharyngeal constrictor on the posterior pharynx opposite the arch of the atlas. This ridge is observed during gagging and pronunciation of vowels. It is an important mechanism in velopharyngeal closure.

8. **What is the blood supply to the palate?**
   The palate has an abundant blood supply that includes the greater and lesser palatine branches from the descending palatine a. (branch of maxillary a.), palatine branch of the ascending pharyngeal a. (branch of external carotid a.), ascending palatine branch of the facial a., and tonsillar branches of the dorsalis linguae.

EPIDEMIOLOGY

9. **What factors are known to cause cleft deformities?**
   Less than 40% of clefts of lip and palate are of genetic origin, and less than 20% of isolated cleft palates are of genetic origin. Corticosteroids and diazepam taken during the first 8 weeks of pregnancy

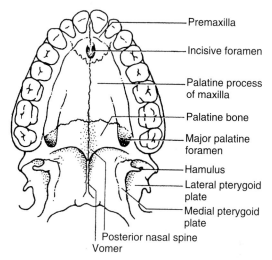

Figure 38-1. Anatomy and divisions of the palate into primary and secondary palates. *(From Randall P, LaRosa D: Cleft palate. In McCarthy JG, editor:* Plastic surgery, *Philadelphia, 1990, Saunders.)*

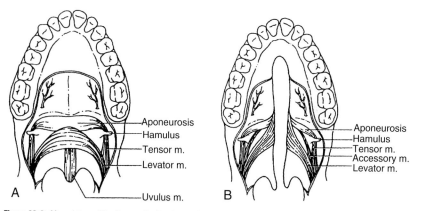

Figure 38-2. Musculature of the **A,** normal soft palate and **B,** cleft soft palate. Note that in the normal musculature, the elevator muscles are oriented transversely and insert in the midpalate. In the cleft palate, the musculature is disrupted and the muscles are oriented more longitudinally, inserting on the posterior edge of the palatal bone and along the bony edges of the cleft. *(From Randall P, LaRosa D: Cleft palate. In McCarthy JG, editor:* Plastic surgery, *Philadelphia, 1990, Saunders.)*

are also believed to be etiologic factors. Viral infections, lack of certain vitamins, and other factors during the first trimester of pregnancy are suspected as well.

10. **What is the incidence of cleft lip with or without cleft palate in the general population? In different ethnic groups?**
   The incidence of cleft lip worldwide is approximately 1 in every 700 to 800 live births. Incidence is highest in the Japanese, about 2.1 to 3.2 in every 1000 births. In Caucasians, incidence is 1.4 in every 1000 births; in Africans, it is 0.3 to 0.43 in every 1000 births.
      The incidence of isolated cleft palate in general is 1:2000.

11. When is a cleft palate associated with a cleft lip?

The most frequent combination is a unilateral cleft of the lip and palate, which is seen more often in boys than girls, and predominantly on the left side. The hereditary incidence in these patients is fairly high. The next most common cleft is isolated cleft palate, which is seen more frequently in girls; the hereditary incidence in these patients is fairly low. Bifid uvula has an incidence of about 2%, but most cases are asymptomatic. However, as many as 20% of patients with bifid uvula have some degree of velopharyngeal incompetence (VPI).

12. What is the familial risk for developing cleft palate?

Family Makeup	Risk of CL/P	Risk of CP
One affected sibling or parent	4%	2.5%
Two affect siblings	9%	1%
One sibling and one parent	16%	15%

13. Is prenatal ultrasound useful in diagnosing cleft deformity?

Successful imaging of the face is usually not possible till approximately 15 weeks' gestation. The lip is most easily visualized in the coronal plane. Identification of isolated cleft palate may be more challenging, but it is easiest to visualize in the axial plane.

14. What is the importance of auditory screening in this population?

The same muscles that elevate the soft palate also help to tense and open the eustachian tube to equalize the middle ear; therefore, children born with cleft palate are at risk for eustachian tube dysfunction and chronic middle ear effusions because these muscles do not function appropriately. It is recommended that all children undergo a newborn hearing screen. If they do not pass, they will have this exam repeated by an audiologist and have a follow-up with an ENT to check for middle ear effusions. It is recommended that this be completed before 6 months of age.

15. What are the currently available feeding aids for cleft patients?

There are multiple specialty feeders for cleft children. The Mead Johnson is a low-cost compressible bottle that allows the caregiver to squeeze the milk into the infant's mouth as he or she is sucking. The Pigeon Nipple has a faster flow and can often be used by older infants on any bottle. The nipple itself is compressed against the hard palate and does not require sucking to dispel milk. The Haberman feeder is a more expensive bottle that is good for children who are small or premature. It contains a one-way valve that keeps milk in a soft chamber and nipple. The chamber can then be pumped to dispel milk into the infant's mouth. The flow can be adjusted by rotating the nipple.

When bottle feeding cleft infants, it is important to remember they swallow more air when sucking than non-cleft infants; therefore, it is important to feed them upright at a 45 degree angle and burp them frequently.

CLASSIFICATION

16. How can clefts be classified?

Clefts can be described as **complete** or **incomplete,** and prepalatal (cleft of the primary palate) or palatal (cleft of the secondary palate). **Prepalatal** can be further divided into unilateral or bilateral; each may be further subdivided into involving one-third, two-thirds, or all (complete cleft) of the lip. Similarly, **palatal** clefts may be described as involving one-third, two-thirds, or all of the soft palate and one-third, two-thirds, or all of the hard palate, extending up to the incisive foramen (Fig. 38-3).

A cleft can also be classified as a submucosal cleft palate or a bifid uvula (see questions 18 and 19).

17. What is the difference between a complete and incomplete cleft of the lip?

A complete cleft lip is a cleft of the entire lip and the underlying premaxilla, or alveolar arch. An incomplete cleft lip involves only the lip.

18. What is a submucous cleft?

A submucous cleft is a deficiency in the musculature of the palate due to failure of the levator muscle fibers to fuse completely in the midline. However, clinically, the palate looks intact because the overlying oral and nasal mucous membranes are present. A submucous cleft is characterized by a bifid uvula, loss of the posterior nasal spine, and a bluish midline streak on the soft palate due to muscular diastases. A notch may be present in the posterior hard palate.

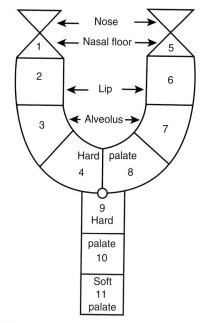

Figure 38-3. Millard's modified classification of Kernahan's and Elsahy's classification of cleft lip and palate. The small circle indicates the incisive foramen. *(Modified from Randall P: Cleft palate. In Smith JW, Aston SJ, editors:* Grabb and Smith's plastic surgery, *ed 4, Boston, 1991, Little, Brown.)*

This type of cleft usually leads to difficulties with speech and to VPI because the muscles of the soft palate are unable to function normally. A congenital absence of the muscularis uvulae may also occur (with or without a bifid uvula) and is often associated with palatal incompetence.

19. What is a bifid uvula?
A bifid uvula is a variation of cleft palate seen in 2% of the normal US population. It may be associated with palatal incompetence, and patients should be followed for possible speech problems.

CLEFT LIP REPAIR

20. What are the criteria for timing of cleft lip repair?
Surgical repair of cleft lip is generally carried out at 10 to 14 weeks of age. However, traditionally, the time of repair of cleft lip often is based on the **Rule of Tens.** According to this rule, cleft lip can be closed when the infant is ≥10 weeks old, the hemoglobin is ≥10 g/dL, and the child's weight is ≥10 lb.

21. What is Simonart's band?
Often defined as the soft tissue band between the margins of the cleft lip, nostril, or alveolar cleft when a complete skeletal cleft of the alveolus is also present. Most of these soft tissue adhesions are located at the base of the nostril. They often help maintain nasal form and decrease the dimensions of the soft tissue cleft and segmental displacement, possibly aiding in primary lip repair.

22. What is the lip adhesion procedure?
Lip adhesion is reserved for very wide clefts in which primary closure may not be possible. It is usually carried out at 3 to 4 months of age with the definitive repair planned for 6 to 12 months of age. Advantages include narrowing of a wide cleft and alignment of the alveolar arches. Disadvantages include an additional anesthetic and possibility of increased scar tissue formation.

23. **What are some of the techniques for cleft lip repair?**
These techniques are the lip adhesion procedure, the Millard rotation advancement flap, the Tennison Randall triangular flap, and the Delaire.

24. **What is the Millard rotation advancement flap?**
The Millard rotation advancement flap is a modified Z-plasty technique placed at the top of the cleft so that the point of greatest tension is placed at the base of the nares. It is the most popular method of cleft lip repair. It is used for complete, incomplete, and wide cleft repairs and is ideal for closing incomplete or narrow clefts. The technique involves downward rotation of the philtrum of the lip as a flap into normal symmetric position, while the lateral lip segment is advanced across the cleft and into the space behind the central lip. The final scar from the suture line closely recreates the philtrum of the lip on the cleft side (Fig. 38-4).

CLEFT PALATE REPAIR

25. **What is the timing for cleft palate repair?**
In most centers, repair of the cleft palate is carried out when the child is 10 to 18 months of age, the age at which articulate speech skills are beginning to develop. In contrast, some centers prefer repair to be delayed until 18 to 24 months of age, after eruption of the first molars. The differences in timing of cleft palate repair are mostly based on different opinions regarding the balance between needs for normal speech versus normal palate growth and occlusion.

26. **What are the goals of successful cleft palate repairs?**
   - Separation of the nasal and oral cavities through closure of both mucosal surfaces
   - Construction of a water-tight velopharyngeal valve
   - Preservation of facial growth
   - Good development of aesthetic dentition and functional occlusion

27. **What are some of the techniques for cleft palate repair?**
These techniques are the von Langenbeck, Furlow palatoplasty, V-Y pushback, and Wardhill-Kilner.

28. **What is the von Langenbeck operation?**
The von Langenbeck operation involves long, relaxing incisions laterally, with elevation of large mucoperiosteal flaps from the hard palate, which is bipedicled anteriorly and posteriorly. The cleft margins of both the hard and soft palates are approximated at the midline. The levator muscles are completely detached from their abnormal bony insertion, and the soft palate musculature is repaired in the midline. A palatal lengthening procedure is not included in this operation (Fig. 38-5).

29. **What is a vomer flap?**
This procedure consists of elevation of a wide, superiorly based flap of nasal mucosa from the vomer to close the hard palate. In bilateral clefts, vomer flaps can be obtained from each side of the vomer. This technique avoids the need for elevating large mucoperiosteal flaps from the hard palate and the potential risk of resultant maxillary growth disturbances.

30. **What are the most common postoperative complications of cleft palate?**
Hypernasal speech is the most common complication following cleft palate repair, occurring in up to 30% of patients. Oral-nasal fistulas are the second most common complication and occur in 10% to 21% of cleft repairs. These fistulas typically occur at either end of the hard palate (i.e., at the anterior alveolus or at the junction of the soft and hard palate).

31. **What are the major sequelae of an unrepaired cleft palate?**
The problems associated with an unrepaired cleft palate are numerous, and they begin at birth and continue for the patient's lifetime:
   - An inability to build up suction and nasal regurgitation
   - Poor eustachian tube function, which may lead to fluid in the middle ear space and inclination toward recurrent otitis media
   - Breathing problems, particularly if the chin is short and the tongue falls backward, causing inspiratory obstruction, as in Pierre Robin sequence
   - Speech problems, including hypernasality with vowel sounds and distortion of the pressure consonants
   - Adjacent teeth angled into the cleft and possibly malformed or absent, if the alveolar ridge is involved
   - Dental caries and severe malocclusion

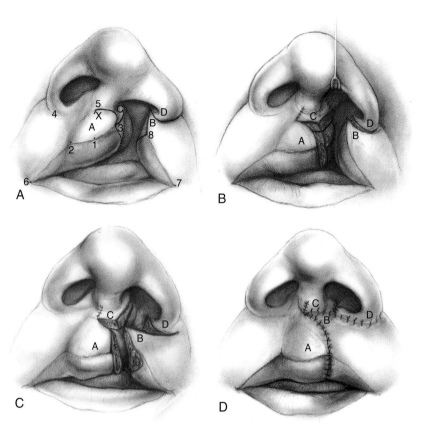

Figure 38-4. Rotation advancement cleft lip repair (Millard, 1958, 1976). **A,** An incision is made at right angles to the vermilion borders into the medial edge of the cleft lip at a point corresponding to the potential height of Cupid's bow on the cleft side *(3)*. From this point superiorly, the cleft-edge vermilion is trimmed. The full-thickness incision is then carried upward following the curvature and position of the philtrum on the normal side until it reaches the base of the columella. The incision is cut to preserve as much muscle as possible on the flap. Without crossing into the normal philtrum, the incision curves under the base of the columella and extends toward the normal side as far as is necessary to rotate Cupid's bow *(flap A)* into a normal horizontal plane. A small back-cut (X) directed obliquely downward facilitates this rotation. **B,** A hook is used to exert upward traction on the cleftside alar rim. This results in a defect at the base of the cleftside columella to be filled with flap C. An incision is made into the membranous septum following the posterior border of flap C. This flap is subsequently undermined and advanced into position to balance the columella. The medial aspect of flap C is tailored and sewn into the superior aspect of the defect created by the downward rotation of flap A. **C,** Flap B is then developed to preserve as much muscle on the flap as possible. The vermilion is trimmed by making an incision at a right angle to the vermilion border at a point *(8)* at which the vermilion becomes attenuated to preserve the length of the lateral element when sutured to the medial element *(flap A)*. The distance between this point *(8)* and the ipsilateral oral commissure *(7)* corresponds to the distance between the apex of Cupid's bow *(2)* and the oral commissure on the non-cleft side *(6)*. The incision is carried up along the vermilion border to include the most superomedial usable lip tissue and then curved laterally around the alar base. Once this is completed, and through an incision in the upper gingivobuccal sulcus, the lateral element is then dissected from the maxilla. At the same time, the cleftside alar base *(flap D)* is released from its pyriform aperture attachment. The orbicularis oris muscle bundles are then carefully dissected, freeing them subcutaneously and submucosally so that when approximated across the cleft, the orientation of their fibers will be changed from a near-vertical direction to the normal horizontal direction. Flap B is then advanced medially and sewn into the defect created by the downward rotation of flap A, and the lip is closed in three layers: muscle, skin, and mucosa. Flap D is then advanced medially to close the nostril floor. A portion of this flap may be deepithelialized and sewn to the base of the nasal septum anteriorly with a permanent suture as a unilateral alar cinch. **D,** The completed repair. (*From Perry RJ, Loré JM Jr: Cleft lip and palate. In Loré JM, Medina JE, editors:* An atlas of head and neck surgery, *ed 4, Philadelphia, 2005, Saunders.*)

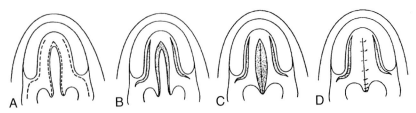

Figure 38-5. The von Langenbeck operation. **A,** Flap design. **B,** The relaxing incisions. **C,** Elevation of the mucoperiosteal flap. **D,** Closure of the nasal mucosa and closure of the oral mucosa. *(From Randall P, LaRosa D: Cleft palate. In McCarthy JG, editor: Plastic surgery, Philadelphia, 1990, Saunders.)*

VELOPHARYNGEAL INSUFFICIENCY

32. What is VPI?

VPI is a confusing term used to describe resonance disorders due to structural abnormalities (velopharyngeal insufficiency), neurologic disorders (velopharyngeal incompetence), or functional issues (velopharyngeal mislearning). During speech production, the velum is elevated and the pharyngeal wall moves to close the nasopharynx off from the oropharynx to produce oral speech sounds. When there is a deficiency in this mechanism, hypernasality, nasal emissions, or compensatory mechanisms can result.

33. How is VPI being diagnosed?

No single technique has been found to be ideal for the diagnosis of VPI. Diagnosis is usually based on a combination of perceptual assessments by a speech language pathologist, visualization of the mechanism during function via direct techniques such as nasopharyngoscopy and videofluoroscopy, and data collected from indirect techniques such a nasometry. This includes a formal speech-language evaluation.

34. Which muscles are the most important in achieving VP closure?

The levator palatini muscles contribute the most to VP closure by pulling the middle third of the soft palate superiorly and posteriorly to produce firm contact with the posterior pharyngeal wall at about the level of the adenoidal pad. Other muscles that contribute to VP closure include the paired palatopharyngeus muscles, which pull the soft palate posteriorly; the muscularis uvulae, which cause the uvula to thicken centrally with contraction; and the superior pharyngeal constrictors, which move the lateral pharyngeal walls medially or the posterior pharyngeal wall anteriorly with contraction.

35. How is VPI managed?

Speech therapy usually begins with parental counseling when the child is 6 months old, and individual child therapy should begin when the child is about age 4 or when the definitive diagnosis is made. Dental prosthesis may also be helpful. About 20% to 25% of VPI cases require surgery. Surgical methods include secondary palatal lengthening, pharyngeal augmentation using soft tissue or implants, and pharyngeal flaps. Such flaps convert the incompetent nasopharynx into two lateral ports and are most successful in patients with good lateral pharyngeal wall motion.

ALVEOLAR CLEFT BONE GRAFTING

36. What are the goals of ACBG?

- Closure of oronasal fistulas
- Give continuity to maxillary arch
- Provide support to ala on cleft side by recreating piriform rim
- Provide bone for eruption of permanent teeth
- Facilitate orthodontic movement of teeth
- Improve lip support
- Create patent nasal airway

37. What is the ideal age for alveolar cleft repair?

Most studies indicate that the bone graft should be placed before the eruption of the permanent canine and when the canine root is one-fourth to one-half or one-half to two-thirds developed. Root resorption and graft failure are common when bone grafts are placed after eruption of the canine. Traditionally, bone grafts are placed at ages 9 to 11, although early grafting at ages 5 to 7 is becoming more popular. Orthodontic treatment to stimulate growth and tooth eruption should be instituted within 3 months before bone graft. Orthodontic expansion of the maxillary arch *after* grafting instead of before grafting, at approximately ages 7 to 12, has also been advocated.

38. **When should the cleft site be orthodontically expanded prior to grafting?**
The maxillary segments should be expanded prior to bone grafting to correct posterior and/or anterior cross-bites. Care should be taken to avoid orthodontic movement or rotation of teeth near the cleft site that may have questionable bony support.

39. **Which is the ideal bone for alveolar cleft repair?**
Particulate bone with cancellous marrow is the best choice for grafting an alveolar cleft because its osteoinduction and osteoconduction qualities are most predictable.

ORTHOGNATHIC SURGERY FOR CLEFT PATIENTS

40. **What are the most common skeletal jaw deformities in the cleft palate patient?**
The skeletal deformities associated with cleft lip and palate vary but generally include one or more of the following: midface deficiency, maxillary transverse deficiency, Class III skeletal and occlusal deformity, and prognathic mandible.

41. **What is the ideal age for cleft orthognathic surgery?**
The ideal age for cleft orthognathic surgery is similar to that of children without cleft lip and palate. Ideally, it should be performed upon completion of facial growth, which is age 14 to 16 in girls and 16 to 18 in boys. Orthognathic surgery can be accomplished earlier for psychosocial considerations, improvement of sleep apnea, or in children with large anterior-posterior deficiencies, with the knowledge that they may require an additional procedure at a later date due to relapse.

42. **What incision modifications should be considered during cleft orthognathic surgery?**
In unilateral cleft lip and palate, a typical Le Fort I, circumvestibular incision can be made during orthognathic surgery. In the bilateral cleft lip and palate patient, it is important to leave the mucosa from canine to canine anteriorly intact to maintain the blood supply to the maxilla. To complete the osteotomy, incisions are made from the distal of the canine to the mesial of the first premolar. Subperiosteal dissection is then completed and the osteotomies are made through these two windows. To use the nasal-septal osteotome, a small stab incision is made in the midline at the height of the vestibule and the osteotome is inserted.

43. **What are generally safe guidelines for maxillary advancement versus distraction osteogenesis?**
Le Fort I advancement can usually be accomplished in patients with cleft palate requiring ≤6 mm of advancement, though up to 10 mm may be indicated in some cases. One must consider the number or previous palatal surgeries and the amount of scarring present. Advancements greater than 6 to 10 mm are generally best treated with distraction osteogenesis.

44. **What are the complications specific to cleft orthognathic surgery?**
When considering either orthognathic surgery or distraction osteogenesis in patients with cleft palate, one must understand the risks of the patient developing VPI. All patients must be informed that the risk of developing hypernasal speech following surgery is common in the cleft population. In most cases, this resolves without intervention in 6 to 12 months, and the speech will return to its preoperative quality. If after 12 months it does not resolve, patients may require a pharyngeal flap to improve their quality of speech.

CLEFT RHINOPLASTY

45. **What are the common features of unilateral cleft nasal deformities?**
- Nasal septum: convex on and deviated toward the cleft side
- Nasal tip: deviated toward the non-cleft side, depressed dome with poor tip support
- Lower lateral cartilage on the cleft side may be weak, smaller, or misshapen; angle between medial and lateral crura is excessively obtuse on the cleft side

- Pyriform aperture: webbing of the soft tissue present on the cleft side
- Nostril: horizontally oriented on the cleft side and may have asymmetry
- Columella may be shorter on the cleft side and commonly deviated toward the non-cleft side
- Nasolabial fistula may be present
- Hypertrophy of the turbinate on the cleft side
- Poor support of the ala on the cleft side due to clefting of alveolus if present

46. **What are the common features of bilateral cleft nasal deformities?**
    - Broad and bifid nasal tip
    - Displacement of alar cartilages inferiorly with hooding of the nostril
    - Wide horizontal nostrils
    - May have shortening of the columella

47. **What is the timing of cleft rhinoplasty?**
    Some of the cleft nasal deformities are addressed at the time of primary cleft lip repair including correction of the flared ala, correction of the nasal-septal deviation, and improvement of nostril symmetry. Some surgeons advocate correction of tip deformities with various techniques at the time of primary lip repair, but this can be controversial due to the possibility of adverse effects on nasal growth. A formal open or closed rhinoplasty is usually reserved for the completion of facial growth, consolidation of the maxillary arch, and correction of maxillary hypoplasia.

48. **What is the traditional sequence of treatment for cleft lip and palate?**
    - At birth, the cleft lip and palate team evaluates the child.
    - At 10 weeks old, the cleft lip is repaired.
    - At age 1 year, the child is reevaluated by the cleft lip and palate team.
    - At 12 to 18 months, the soft and hard palates are repaired.
    - At 5 to 8 years, interceptive orthodontics are used.
    - At 5 to 7 years, the pharyngeal flap (if necessary) is done.
    - At 7 to 8 years, maxillary expansion is done, if needed.
    - At 9 to 11 years, alveolar cleft bone grafting is performed.
    - At 12 to 13 years, comprehensive orthodontics are initiated.
    - At 14 to 16 years, orthognathic surgery and nasal surgery are done, if needed.

BIBLIOGRAPHY

American Cleft Palate-Craniofacial Association: Parameters for evaluation and treatment of patients with cleft lip or palate and other craniofacial anomalies. In Philips BJ, Warren DW, editors: *The cleft palate and craniofacial team*, Chapel Hill, NC, 1993, American Cleft Palate Association.

Grabb WC, Rosenstein SW, Bzoch KR, editors: *Cleft lip and palate: surgical, dental, and speech aspects*, Boston, 1971, Little, Brown.

Hendrick DA: Cleft lip and palate. In Jafek BW, Stark AK, editors: *ENT secrets*, Philadelphia, 1996, Hanley & Belfus.

Johnson MC, Bronsky PT, Millicorsky G: Embryogenesis of cleft lip and palate. In McCarthy JG, editor: *Plastic surgery*, Philadelphia, 1990, Saunders.

Kernahan DA: The striped Y—a symbolic classification for cleft lip and palate, *Plast Reconstr Surg* 47:469–470, 1971.

Millard Jr DR, Latham RA: Improved primary surgical and dental treatment of clefts, *Plast Reconstr Surg* 86:856–871, 1990.

Millard Jr DR: Combining the Von Langenbeck and the Wardill-Kilner operations in certain clefts of the palate, *Cleft Palate J* 29:85–86, 1992.

Millard Jr DR: Cleft lip. In Weinzweig J, editor: *Plastic surgery secrets*, Philadelphia, 1996, Hanley & Belfus.

Natsume N, Kawai T: Incidence of cleft lip and palate in 39,696 Japanese babies born in 1983, *Int J Oral Maxillofac Surg* 15:565–568, 1986.

Randall P, LaRosa D: Cleft palate. In McCarthy JG, editor: *Plastic surgery*, Philadelphia, 1990, Saunders.

Randall P, LaRosa D: Cleft palate. In Weinzweig J, editor: *Plastic surgery secrets*, Philadelphia, 1996, Hanley & Belfus.

Randall P: Cleft palate. In Smith JW, Aston SJ, editors: *Grabb and Smith's plastic surgery*, ed 4, Boston, 1991, Little, Brown.

ORTHOGNATHIC SURGERY

David M. Alfi, Ariel Farahi, A. Omar Abubaker, Bashar M. Rajab

CHAPTER 39

1. **What does the clinical workup of orthognathic surgery consist of?**
   The clinical workup for orthognathic surgery should consist of photographic records, diagnostic casts, interocclusal records, facebow transfer, radiographic examination, and facial measurements. In addition, a thorough medical history and physical examination must be completed. At the minimum, the photographic records should capture the patient's frontal view (with lips relaxed and smiling) and the patient's right profile view in repose. The radiographic examination should include a lateral cephalogram, posterior-anterior (PA) cephalogram, and panoramic radiograph with lips relaxed and teeth in centric relation (CR). The diagnostic casts should be mounted on an anatomic, fully adjustable articulator, and in CR. With the recent availability of cone beam computer tomography (CBCT), its use in orthognathic surgery ranges from generating a lateral cephalogram, PA cephalogram, and panoramic radiograph to being used to assess a posterior airway and, when obtained with a gyroscope, can be used to digitally simulate the surgery.

2. **How is the facial examination of a patient performed?**
   The facial examination of a patient is the most important stage of the surgical planning and is performed with the patient in the natural head position (NHP). The NHP orients the patient's head to a position that is most natural to the observer. In cephalometry, the NHP is approximated by rotating the S–N line down 6 degrees. The facial examination can be divided into three components: the upper third, middle third, and the lower third of the face.

   In evaluating the lower third of the face, the lips are evaluated for static and dynamic symmetry. There is usually a 0.5-5 mm upper tooth show at rest in adults, with females showing more than males and both genders decreasing tooth show with age. In addition, the upper lip length (22 mm) is equal to roughly 30% of the lower third of the face (22 mm + 3 mm + 45 mm) (Fig. 39-1).

3. **How are skeletal age and deceleration of growth determined?**
   Skeletal age is determined by a hand–wrist radiograph. Deceleration of growth is determined by serial cephalometric films.

4. **What is the significance of cervical vertebral maturation in relation to planning orthognathic surgery?**
   Cervical vertebral maturation can be seen on a single lateral cephalometric radiograph. There are six stages of cervical vertebral maturation. The peak of mandibular and craniofacial growth corresponds to the peak in statural height growth, which corresponds to stages three and four of cervical vertebral maturation. As cervical vertebra mature through the six stages, they develop a concavity on the inferior border and assume a more rectangular shape (Fig. 39-2).

5. **What is the role of cephalometric evaluation in pre-surgical treatment planning?**
   The facial skeleton can been quantified and measured by using cephalometric analysis. However, orthognathic treatment planning must depend largely on clinical findings. The use of cephalometrics should support or dispute the clinical impression, similar to the way laboratory blood studies support the medical examination and decision making. Some insurance companies may also base their determinations on cephalometric parameters.

6. **What are the most commonly used analyses and what they are used for?**
   The Steiner, the Downs analysis, and the McNamara analysis are the commonly used bony cephalometric analyses. The Steiner analysis is useful for evaluating the upper and lower incisor position relative to the anterior cranium. The Downs analysis is used to determine the facial angle that describes the relative anteroposterior (AP) relationship of the mandible to the cranium. The McNamara analysis is used to compare the incisor relationship to basal bone.

7. **What are the most common soft tissue facial measurements?**
   1. Facial contour angle
   2. Lower lip length

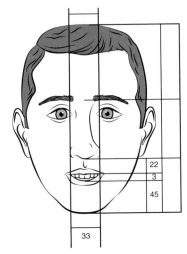

Figure 39-1. Facial evaluation: Ideally, as in this figure, the upper lip length (22 mm) is equal to roughly 30% of the lower third of the face (22 mm + 3 mm + 45 mm).

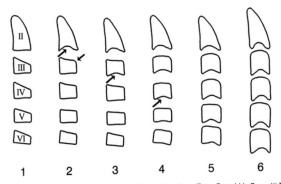

Figure 39-2. The six developmental stages of cervical vertebral maturation. *(From Franchi L, Baccetti T, McNamara JA Jr: Mandibular growth as related to cervical vertebral maturation and body height, Am J Orthodont Dentofac Orthoped 118(3):335–340, 2000.)*

   3. Nasolabial angle
   4. Ricketts E-line
   5. Upper lip length
   6. Upper face height-to-total face height ratio

8. **What is the Holdaway ratio useful for planning?**
   The Holdaway ratio is useful in planning a genioplasty. In this instance, the N-B line should be extended to the inferior border of the mandible and then compare the distances between LI and Pog from this line. In normal Caucasian males, the comparison is 1:1, while in normal Caucasian females, it is 0.5:1.

9. **What is the difference between the goal of nonsurgical orthodontic therapy and the goal of pre-surgical orthodontic therapy?**
   The goals of nonsurgical and pre-surgical orthodontic therapy are essentially opposite. While nonsurgical orthodontics aims to camouflage and mask the patient's true skeletal deformities by attempting to achieve the best occlusion, the purpose of pre-surgical orthodontics is to unmask and

decompensate true skeletal deformities, thereby making the occlusion and the deformity more exaggerated than on initial presentation in a sagittal, transverse, and vertical dimension.

10. **What are the limits of movement in orthodontic-only therapy versus orthognathic surgery?**
The limits of orthodontic-only therapy and orthognathic surgery are believed to fall into an envelope of achievable outcomes as described by Proffit and White. In a growing child, the limits of orthodontic treatment alone are correction of a positive overjet of 8 mm, a negative overjet of 4 mm, and a transverse discrepancy of 3 mm. In an adult, the achievability of orthodontics are even more limited. However, orthognathic surgery can correct up to 25 mm positive overjet and 12 mm negative overjet by surgical intervention in both jaws.

11. **What are the different skeletal discrepancies of growth between with the mandible and maxilla?**
The major discrepancies between the maxilla and the mandible can occur in one or a combination of the following dimensions:
   • Anterior–posterior discrepancy (A–P)
   • Vertical discrepancy
   • Transverse discrepancy

12. **What causes maxillary mandibular A–P discrepancy, and how is it manifested?**
Anterior–posterior maxillary mandibular discrepancy can be the result of normal growth of the maxilla with abnormal growth of the mandible, normal growth of the mandible and abnormal growth of the maxilla, or abnormal growth of both the mandible and maxilla. When the discrepancy is caused by maxillary deficient growth or by excessive growth of the mandible or both, the resulting deformity is Class III skeletal deformity and malocclusion. When the discrepancy is caused by normal growth of the maxilla and deficient growth of the mandible, the resulting deformity is Class II skeletal deformity and Class II malocclusion.

13. **What causes maxillary mandibular transverse discrepancy, and how is it manifested?**
Maxillary mandibular discrepancy is often manifested as a mandibular or maxillary cross-bite, depending on which jaw is affected. Once again this deformity can be caused by a deficient growth in one jaw compared to the opposing jaw or can be caused by extraction of one jaw and advancing the teeth to relieve crowding or in preparation for orthognathic surgery, resulting in a cross-bite.
   Cross-bite can be relative or absolute. Relative cross-bite is what can be observed in the patient's mouth when the patient has a concomitant anterior posterior discrepancy. An absolute cross-bite is when one places the casts of the maxilla and the mandible in Class I canine and still observes a cross-bite.

14. **What is a vertical maxillary mandibular discrepancy?**
Just as with other discrepancies, this deformity often occurs in one jaw independently from the opposite jaw or in combination. Such discrepancies can be manifested as an open bite or deep bite, depending on which jaw they occur.

15. **Can these discrepancies occur in combination?**
Yes. In fact, it is not unusual that the deficient maxillary A–P dimension would be associated with a vertical or transverse deficient leading to not only Class III skeletal deformity but also to decreased vertical height of the maxilla (decrease facial height) or a small maxilla in the transverse dimension leading to a cross-bite.

16. **What are the two types of A–P mandibular deficiencies?**
   1. Low mandibular plane angle type
   2. High mandibular plane angle type
   Each has distinct morphologic and occlusal presentations, but in both types the mandible is small.

17. **What are the features of AP mandibular deficiencies?**
The features of the low mandibular plane angle type **mandibular deficiency** include small mandible, short facial height, curled-over lower lip, and deep labiomental crease. The angles of the mandible and the masseters are usually well developed and well defined, and the maxilla may be vertically deficient. The occlusion shows a curve of Spee, which is generally excessive in both arches. The mandibular

anterior teeth may occlude with the palate, along with an excessively deep bite. Radiographically, the ramus height is usually normal, and the angular and linear cephalometric measurements are usually smaller than normal.

The high mandibular plane angle variety is characterized by normal or excessive face height, a small and retropositioned chin, flattened labiomental fold, and excessive activity of the mentalis muscles. The mandibular ramus is short, the condyles are usually small, and the angles of the mandible are obtuse and hypoplastic. The occlusion is characterized by protrusive maxillary teeth, narrow arch form, constricted mandibular arch, and Class II canine and molar relationships. There may be an open bite, which is indicative of conditions such as rheumatoid arthritis, temporomandibular joint (TMJ) ankylosis, and condylar resorption. If AP mandibular deficiency of the high mandibular plane angle type exists along with vertical maxillary excess, all the features of vertical maxillary excess are present, and the features of mandibular deficiency are exaggerated.

18. **How is mandibular deficiency treated?**

Treatment of isolated mandibular deficiency usually involves mandibular advancement. Bilateral sagittal split osteotomy (BSSO) with rigid fixation is the most frequently performed procedure to accomplish this advancement. Inverted-L osteotomy with rigid fixation and bone grafting is recommended for advancement >1 cm. In general, stability of mandibular advancement is better with smaller amounts of advancements than with large ones. More recently, distraction osteogenesis has become a more popular procedure for treatment of mandibular deficiency and hypoplasia than inverted-L osteotomy with bone graft. Augmentation genioplasty procedures using an alloplastic or osteoplastic technique with and without the BSSO technique occasionally are used to disguise significant mandibular deficiency. Also, mandibular subapical osteotomy may help in leveling the mandibular arch.

19. **What are the features of mandibular prognathism?**

Although isolated mandibular prognathism is a rare condition, mandibular prognathism often is associated with maxillary deficiency. When the two conditions are present together, the appearance of mandibular prognathism is exaggerated. Overclosure of the vertical dimension and centric relation-centric occlusion slides also may coexist and exaggerate such appearance. The chin and lower lip in patients with these conditions are forward relative to the upper lip, often making them the dominant facial feature. The mandibular body and mandibular angle are well defined, often with an obtuse angle. The occlusion is Class III, and often the skeletal discrepancy is greater than the occlusal discrepancy because of the dental compensations. Such compensation is manifested as flared maxillary anterior teeth and upright mandibular anterior teeth.

20. **How is mandibular prognathism treated?**

Sagittal split osteotomy with rigid fixation is the procedure of choice for correction of mandibular prognathism. Transoral vertical ramus osteotomy is advocated by some, especially for large posterior movement and when there is a need for an asymmetric setback. However, problems with control of the proximal segment and adverse postsurgical occlusal changes have been reported with this procedure. Surgery should be undertaken only after dental compensations are eliminated with pre-surgical orthodontics and, preferably, after mandibular growth is completed.

21. **What are the three modifications of BSSO procedure?**

1. **Hunsuck modification**: Extend the cut posteriorly and slightly past the lingula into the retrolingular fossa. This creates an easier procedure and causes less soft tissue trauma.
2. **Dalpont modification**: Make the lateral osteotomy more anterior to the level of the second molar, which increases surface area of contact.
3. **Epker modification**: Dissection is carried out, only as needed, avoiding excessive stripping of the masseter and medial pterygoid muscles. This causes less swelling and postoperative discomfort as well as preservation of blood supply.

22. **What are the possible complications of a BSSO?**

Complications of BSSO are classified as either intraoperative or postoperative. The most common complications of mandibular procedures in general, and BSSO in particular, include unfavorable osteotomy splits (fracture of the proximal or distal segments), nerve injury, vascular injury and bleeding, and proximal segment malpositions. Mandibular dysfunction (including TMJ dysfunction symptoms), relapse, wound infection, and wound dehiscence are some of the postoperative possible complications.

23. What is the incidence of unfavorable split osteotomy during BSSO? How is this complication treated?

An unfavorable split between the proximal and distal segments occurs in 3.1% to 20% of cases. The use of heavy osteotome and twisting technique is believed to be the main cause. An unfavorable split should be treated by completing the osteotomy and using plates and screws to fix the fractured segments.

24. What is the incidence of neurosensory deficits following BSSO?

Neurosensory deficits of the inferior alveolar nerve following BSSO are one of the most significant concerns with this procedure. Complications occur in 20% to 85% of surgeries. However, the incidence is only 9% at 1 year after surgery. This complication is more common in patients older than age 40 and in patients who undergo simultaneous genioplasty.

25. What is the most likely source of profuse bleeding during internal vertical ramus osteotomy (IVRO)?

Masseteric artery: This passes through the sigmoid notch and is approximately 25 mm from the anterior border of the ramus and 8 mm above the sigmoid notch.

Inferior alveolar artery: The mandibular foramen is rarely less than 7 mm away from the posterior border.

Internal maxillary artery: It is found medial to the mandible at the level of the condylar neck.

Retromandibular vein: This is due to excessive retromandibular dissection or accidental damage to this vessel.

26. In which mandibular ramus osteotomy is inferior alveolar nerve (IAN) damage most common?

IAN damage is most common in BSSO, noted in 33% of cases after 20 months of follow-up. On the other hand, IAN injury due to VRO is far less common, with a mean of 9% after 21 months of follow-up. During inverted-L osteotomy, risk of IAN is uncommon and seen far less than in BSSO and VRO, as the osteotomies are performed posterior to the lingula. However, a transcutaneous approach during inverted-L osteotomy may lead to damage to the marginal mandibular nerve.

27. How can tooth damage be prevented in subapical osteotomy?

The horizontal osteotomy should be positioned greater than 5 mm below the root apices to avoid inadvertent tooth injury or devitalization.

28. When is genioplasty indicated?

The genioplasty procedure is used to correct functional as well as cosmetic deformities.

Lower facial height deformities, including excessive length, can contribute to functional problems such as lip incompetence and open mouth posturing. Mental soft tissue strain to compensate for these deficiencies can result in thinning of mandibular alveolar bone. Many cosmetic and functional deformities such as retrognathia, microgenia, asymmetry, and excessive or shallow labiomental fold can be corrected with the osseous genioplasty.

29. What is a consequence of genioplasty due to incorrect suturing?

During genioplasty, closure of the incision must include reconstruction of the mentalis muscles with a **slowly resorbing suture**. The result of incomplete approximation or fast resorbing sutures may be chin ptosis, or a "Witch's Deformity," drooping of the chin below the jawline.

30. What are the different types of genioplasty procedures?

- Horizontal osteotomy with advancement: for correction of pure horizontal microgenia
- Double-sliding horizontal osteotomy: for the correction of significant microgenia
- Horizontal osteotomy with anterior posterior reduction: for correction of an isolated chin excess
- Vertical reduction genioplasty by a horizontal resection: for correction of an isolated vertical excess
- Oblique osteotomy and advancement caudally, or caudally and inferiorly, with placement of interposition graft: for correction of pure vertical deficiency or a combination of vertical and horizontal deficiency
- Alloplastic augmentation

31. How can the angles of the osteotomy influence the movement of the distal segment?

The more parallel the osteotomy line with the occlusal plane and the mandibular plane, the more pure the AP movement. If vertical shortening is desired, the angle of the osteotomy should become more acute compared with the mandibular plane.

32. What are the possible complications of the alloplastic chin augmentation?
    - Infection
    - Bone resorption beneath the implant
    - Extrusion and rejection
    - Less predictable and stable
    - Dehiscence
    - Less versatile
    - Malposition

33. What are the possible complications of osseous genioplasty?
    - Wound dehiscence and infection
    - Soft tissue chin ptosis
    - Hematoma
    - Root exposures
    - Tooth devitalization
    - Asymmetry
    - Neurosensory loss
    - Irregularities and step-type deformities

34. What are the clinical features of vertical maxillary excess (VME)?
    VME is characterized by excessive tooth display at lip repose, excessive gingival exposure on smiling, and lip incompetency. An open bite is almost always present, especially when there are steps in the maxillary occlusal plane. The face height is always long, and the chin is rotated downward and posteriorly. This condition is exaggerated by the presence of a short upper lip or maxillary protrusion. VME can be seen with Class I, II, or III occlusions.

35. How is VME treated?
    VME can be treated with orthodontic intervention early in life (ages 8 to 12) with high-pull head gear or open bite Bionater to control vertical growth of the maxilla. If successful, such treatment may resolve the skeletal abnormalities, and ultimately the soft tissues and other facial structures grow accordingly. However, when an adult presents with this condition, it usually is treated with Le Fort I osteotomy and superior repositioning of the maxilla.

36. Are there any special factors that should be considered when treating VME?
    Yes. Because the vertical growth of the maxilla is the last vector to cease, the excessive vertical development may continue growing later than expected. If significant vertical growth occurs, postsurgical relapse can result. Accordingly, as with most deformities characterized by excessive growth, delaying surgery until growth has slowed or completed is recommended. However, if VME is severe, early surgery may be justified on the basis of psychosocial benefits.

37. What are the causes of posterior VME?
    - When opposing posterior mandibular teeth have been extracted, passive eruption of the maxillary teeth results.
    - Posterior VME also may be caused by excessive maxillary vertical growth, which is usually associated with anterior open bite.

38. What are the clinical and radiographic features of posterior VME?
    A distinct step in the maxillary occlusal plane is usually present. When posterior maxillary vertical excess occurs due to passive eruption of teeth, the condition is usually associated with inadequate inter-arch space, which poses a serious prosthetic challenge. Facial change is not apparent because the passive eruption ceases when the teeth contact the mandibular ridge. When posterior VME occurs in the dentate state, there is an increased facial height with lip incompetency secondary to downward and backward rotation of the mandible. The maxillary incisor-to-lip relationship may be normal, but during animation excessive gingiva shows in the posterior region.
    Radiographic features of both conditions include excessive distance from the palatal plane to the first molar cusp. In the partially edentulous patient, excessive pneumatization of the maxillary sinus may be seen.

39. How is posterior VME treated?
    Treatment of posterior VME involves an interdental osteotomy and superior positioning of the posterior segment. If inadequate space exists between the teeth, orthodontic movement or extraction of a tooth is necessary to avoid damage to adjacent teeth.

In the partially edentulous patient, the anterior occlusion should not change if isolated posterior maxillary osteotomy is performed. In the dentate state, superior repositioning of the posterior maxilla results in closure of the open bite, shortening of the face height, improved lip competency, improved mandibular rotation, and forward projection of the chin.

40. **What are the clinical and cephalometric features of maxillary vertical deficiency?**
    - Maxillary vertical deficiency is often present with other skeletal abnormalities, such as AP or transverse maxillary deficiency or mandibular prognathism.
    - The lower face height is always reduced, and the freeway space is excessive.
    - Often, the maxillary incisors are completely covered by the upper lip at rest, with only a portion of the crowns exposed when smiling, and a proper-sized mandible will appear prognathic because of the over-closed position.
    - The occlusion is typically Class III with differences between centric relation-centric occlusion.
    - Cephalometrically, the palatal plane to first molar distance is always reduced.

41. **How is vertical maxillary deficiency treated?**
    Treatment of vertical maxillary deficiency usually involves Le Fort I osteotomy with down-grafting, often in combination with mandibular osteotomy.

42. **What are the features of maxillary AP deficiency? How is it treated?**
    AP deficiency of the maxilla is typically characterized by paranasal deficiencies, deficiency of the infraorbital region, and lack of zygomatic prominence. The upper lip behind the lower lip is the soft tissue characteristic. The occlusion is Class III with compensatory flaring of the maxillary anterior incisors in the true condition and is overly retracted if premolars have been removed previously to compensate orthodontically for mandibular deficiency. Cephalometrically, the maxillary unit length measurements may confirm the diagnosis. Treatment of maxillary AP deficiency usually consists of Le Fort I advancement with or without bone grafts, depending on the extent of advancement.

43. **What are the clinical characteristics of transverse maxillary deficiency? What is the best radiographic method of diagnosis of this deficiency?**
    The clinical indicators of transverse maxillary deficiency include unilateral or bilateral palatal cross-bite; crowded, rotated, and palatally or buccally displaced teeth; a narrow tapering maxillary arch form; and a narrow, high palatal vault. The soft tissue features are limited to a degree of paranasal hallowing, narrow nasal base, deepened nasolabial folds, and zygomatic hypoplasia. When sagittal and vertical dysplasia exist concomitantly with a maxillary transverse deficiency, they often mask the transverse deficiency. Patients who present with cross-bite should be examined closely to determine whether such finding represents a displacement of the teeth relative to the basal bone or a true skeletal bite due to a wide mandible or narrow maxilla. Generally, if a cross-bite involves more than one or two teeth, the cross-bite is probably skeletal.
    For diagnosis and determination of transverse maxillary deficiency, PA cephalogram has been used for identification and evaluation of transverse skeletal discrepancy. More recently, CBCT can provide more accurate assessment and treatment planning for this deformity.

44. **What are the treatment methods of transverse maxillary deficiency?**
    The method of correction used depends on several factors, including whether the deficiency is skeletal or dental, or both; the patient's skeletal growth; the magnitude of the transverse discrepancy; and the periodontal status of the dentition. The treatment commonly used is either orthopedic maxillary expansion or surgically assisted maxillary expansion (SME). SME is indicated in non-growing patients (skeletal age is 15 years or older) and in failed orthodontic/orthopedic expansion and when the maxillary transverse deficiency is >5 mm, when there is a significant transverse maxillary deficiency associated with a narrow maxilla and wide mandible. It is also indicated if there is extremely thin, delicate gingival tissue, in the presence of significant buccal gingival recession in the maxillary canine–premolar region.
    Sometimes the transverse discrepancy is the result of a mandibular advancement, especially after extraction of the mandibular bicuspid, with a normal maxillary transverse dimension; a midline mandibular osteotomy combined with BSSO and narrowing of the mandible posteriorly can be used to correct such cross-bite.

45. **What are the components of the technique of SME?**
    Although several techniques have been described to accomplish the expansion of the transversely deficient maxilla, most authors agree on the following steps of the technique:
    1. Bilateral osteotomy of the maxilla from the piriform rim to the pterygomaxillary fission
    2. Release of the nasal septum

3. Midline palatal osteotomy
4. Osteotomy of lateral nasal walls
5. Bilateral osteotomy of pterygoid plates from the maxillary tuberosity
6. Activation of the maxillary appliance to a total widening of I.0 to 1.5 mm to assure mobility of both sides of the maxilla
7. Soft tissue closure in a similar fashion to that of Le Fort I osteotomy, preferably using alar cinch and V-Y closure

46. **What are the indications of Le Fort I segmental osteotomy over Le Fort I single-piece osteotomy?**
Le Fort I segmental osteotomy should be utilized in cases of maxillary deformities that include multiple planes of occlusion or steps such as seen in apertognathia that require segmentation to correct. However, use segmental Le Fort I osteotomy to correct transverse maxillary deficiency as seen commonly in Class III malocclusion and VME, but only in cases that require not more than 5 to 7 mm in expansion. It is important to be selective about electing Le Fort I segmental osteotomies as it has a higher risk of necrosis of a dento-osseous segment, periodontal deformities (caused by large steps and gaps in the alveolus), and dental injury.

47. **What are the possible complications of a Le Fort I osteotomy?**
Intraoperative Complications
- Unfavorable osteotomy
- Bleeding
- Improper maxillary repositioning
- Inability to stabilize the maxilla
- False aneurysms
Postoperative Complications
- Relapse
- Ophthalmic injury (rare)
- Bleeding
- Condylar malpositioning (rare)
- Neurologic dysfunction
- Avascular necrosis of segment (rare)
- Unfavorable facial aesthetics
- Infection less than 1% of cases
- Non-union: Few reports are available and the true occurrence is likely understated

48. **Is it necessary to preserve the greater palatine vessels during Le Fort I osteotomy?**
No. Studies have found no change in outcome even when both descending palatine vessels are ligated. This finding is also supported by biologic investigations that determine the blood supply to the maxilla, after the osteotomy, to be provided by the ascending pharyngeal artery, ascending palatal artery, and the adjacent soft tissue pedicles.

49. **What is the incidence of neurosensory dysfunction after Le Fort I osteotomy?**
Injury to cranial nerve V2 is the most common injury, with 25% of patients experiencing reduced nociceptive response to pinpricks. Injury also has been reported to cranial nerve IV and the parasympathetic fibers of the lacrimal gland.

50. **If injured, which artery may cause brisk and serious bleeding during Le Fort I osteotomy?**
The **descending palatine artery,** which passes through the palatine bone to enter the palatal soft tissue at the medial maxillary sinus wall in the posterior hard palate, must be handled carefully to avoid severance. Delayed and serious bleeding can be encountered in the postoperative period as late as several weeks following the procedure. The patient can present with profuse epistaxis >2 weeks after the Le Fort 1 as breakdown of a clot or necrosis of the injured arterial vessels can occur.

51. **What is the most likely source of profuse bleeding following Le Fort I incision but before bony osteotomy?**
The posterior superior alveolar artery, which is located at the posterolateral surface of the maxilla, is often encountered during reflection of the periosteum off the bone before making the bony cut. If these vessels are lacerated, they bleed profusely. This bleeding can easily be controlled with pressure packing.

52. **Is it necessary to preserve the greater palatine vessels during Le Fort I osteotomy?**
No. Studies have found no change in outcome even when both descending palatine vessels are ligated. This finding is also supported by biologic investigations that determine the blood supply to the maxilla, after the osteotomy, to be provided by the ascending pharyngeal artery, ascending palatal artery, and the adjacent soft tissue pedicles.

53. **When is it advised to perform a surgically assisted rapid palatal expansion (SARPE) instead of segmental Le Fort I osteotomy?**
SARPE is indicated in cases that contain in excess of 5 mm of transverse maxillary deficiency at the first molar; in isolated maxillary transverse deficiencies; and in skeletally mature or failed orthodontic expansion. However, complications of SARPE may include periodontal defects if the midline osteotomy does not enter the mid-palatal suture line or when the rate of expansion is greater than biological limits.

54. **Which orthognathic procedure has the highest degree of relapse?**
According to Proffit et al. transverse expansion of the maxilla is the most unstable orthognathic procedure. The greatest relapse is seen in the second molar region, with an average of 50% loss of surgical expansion. After 1 year, inferior maxillary positioning and mandibular setbacks were also found to be less predictable than in other surgical techniques.

55. **What is idiopathic condylar resorption?**
Idiopathic condylar resorption of the mandibular condyle is a progressive dissolution of the condylar head without a history of apparent direct cause. The condition is seen mostly after orthognathic surgery, although it has been reported in patients who are undergoing or who have finished orthodontic treatment.

56. **What are the causes of idiopathic condylar resorption?**
Several clinical and radiographic risk factors have been reported in the literature, but the exact causes and pathogenesis of the condition remain unclear.
Patient-Related Risk Factors
- Age (young)
- High mandibular plane angle
- Gender (female)
- Short posterior height
- Preoperative TMJ dysfunction symptoms
- Small posterior-to-anterior facial height ratio
- Mandibular hypoplasia

Surgery-Related Risk Factors
- Counterclockwise rotation of the proximal and distal segments
- Surgically induced posterior condylar displacement in patients with extremely high mandibular plane angle
- Type of fixation (wire osteosynthesis and intermaxillary fixation; controversial)
- Direction and degree of mandibular movement (severe magnitude mandibular advancement; controversial)
- Condylar displacement after orthognathic surgery (controversial)

57. **What are the clinical manifestations of condylar resorption?**
The clinical signs of occlusal relapse after orthognathic surgery or orthodontic treatment develop before the radiographic sign of condylar resorption. The resorptive process can occur unilaterally or bilaterally and usually starts within the first year after treatment. Clinically, idiopathic condylar resorption is manifested by progressive development of anterior open bite and posterior rotation of the mandible with Class II canine and molar relation. The patient often begins to appear retrognathic and occludes mostly on the posterior teeth. The patient may have pain or changes in range of motion. In some patients, the clinical presentation of condylar resorption is similar to that of rheumatoid arthritis. If pain is present, it usually is mild in proportion to the degree of radiographic changes in the joint.

The radiographic features of condylar resorption include generalized resorption of the condylar head, often bilaterally, with anterior rotation of the condylar stump in the glenoid fossa. The resorption process often continues regardless of treatment until the entire condylar head resorbs. Bone scintigraphy often shows an increased uptake throughout the resorptive process that may not be interrupted by a period of decrease or cessation of uptake.

58. What are the treatment options of condylar resorption?

As with other progressive condylar changes, a critical step in treatment planning for condylar resorption is to determine whether the condition is still progressing or has ceased. A history of recent occlusal changes and scintigraphy is important to determine the stage of the condition. Most authors agree on delaying surgical intervention, especially orthognathic surgery, until the resorptive activity has stopped. During such activity, nonsurgical measures, such as nonsteroidal antiinflammatory drugs (NSAIDs) and splint therapy are recommended. Once the resorptive process ceases, orthognathic surgery or condylar replacement with alloplastic or costochondral graft (the two most common surgical modalities) is performed. Recent reports show higher stability after costochondral graft than with orthognathic surgery alone.

BIBLIOGRAPHY

Abubaker A, Strauss R: Genioplasty: a case for advancement osteotomy, *J Oral Maxillofac Surg* 58:783–787, 2000.
Apinhasmit W, Chompoopong S, Methathrathip D, et al.: Clinical anatomy of the posterior maxilla pertaining to Le Fort I osteotomy in Thais, *Clin Anat* 18:323–329, 2005.
Arnett GW, Tamborello JA: Progressive class II development: female idiopathic condylar resorption, *Oral Maxillofac Surg Clin North Am* 2:699, 1990.
Bailey L, White R, Proffit W, et al.: Segmental Le Fort I osteotomy for management of transverse maxillary deficiency, *J Oral Maxillofac Surg* 55:728–731, 1997.
Bell W: *Modern practice in orthognathic and reconstructive surgery*, Philadelphia, 1992, Saunders.
Bell W, You Z, Finn R, Fields R, et al.: Wound healing after multisegmental Le Fort I osteotomy and transection of the descending palatine vessels, *J Oral Maxillofac Surg* 53:1425–1433, 1995.
Betts N, Dowd K: Soft tissue changes associated with orthognathic surgery, *Atlas Oral Maxillofac Surg Clin North Am* 8:13–38, 2000.
Boye T, Doyle P, Mckeown F, et al.: Total subapical mandibular osteotomy to correct class 2 division 1 dento-facial deformity, *J Cranio-Maxillofac Surg* 40:238–242, 2012.
Cheung L, Chua H, et al.: A meta-analysis of cleft maxillary osteotomy and distraction osteogenesis, *Int J Oral Maxillofac Surg* 35:14–24, 2006.
Cheung L, Fung S, Li T, et al.: Posterior maxillary anatomy: implications for Le Fort I osteotomy, *Int J Oral Maxillofac Surg* 27:346–351, 1998.
Chua H, Hägg M, Cheung L, et al.: Cleft maxillary distraction versus orthognathic surgery—which one is more stable in 5 years? *Oral Surg Med Oral Pathol Oral Radiol Endod* 109:803–814, 2010.
Crawford FG, Stoelinga PJ, Blijchop PA, et al.: Stability after progressive condylar resorption after orthognathic surgery: report of 7 cases, *J Oral Maxillofac Surg* 52:460–466, 1994.
Epker BN, Wolford LM: *Surgical correction of dentofacial deformities*, St Louis, 1980, Mosby.
Franchi L, Baccetti T, McNamara J, et al.: Mandibular growth as related to cervical vertebral maturation and body height, *Am J Orthodont Dentofac Orthop* 118:335–340, 2000.
Fujimura K, Segami N, Kobayashi S, et al.: Anatomical study of the complications of intraoral vertico-sagittal ramus osteotomy, *J Oral Maxillofac Surg* 64:384–389, 2006.
Greer Walker D: Facial development. Lecture presented at Arris and Gale lecture in England, Stoke Mandeville Hospital; Middlesex Hospital; Royal Dental Hospital. In Grubb J, Evans C, et al.: Orthodontic management of dentofacial skeletal deformities. Clinics in plastic surgery , March 28, pp 403–415, 1957.
Guyuron B: *Genioplasty*, Washington, DC, 1993, Library of Congress.
Hoppenreijs TJ, Freihfer M, Stoelinga PJ, et al.: Condylar remodeling and resorption after Le Fort I and bimaxillary osteotomies in patients with anterior open bite. A clinical and radiographic study, *Int J Oral Maxillofac Surg* 27:81–91, 1998.
Huang YL, Pogrel MA, Kaban LB: Diagnosis and management of condylar resorption, *J Oral Maxillofac Surg* 55:114–119, 1997.
Hwang SJ, Haers PE, Zimmermann A, et al.: Surgical risk factors for condylar resorption after orthognathic surgery, *Oral Surg Oral Med Oral Pathol Oral Radiol Endod* 89:542–552, 2000.
Jegal J, Kang S, Kim J, Sun H: The utility of a three-dimensional approach with T-shaped osteotomy in osseous genioplasty, *Arch Plast Surg* 40:433–439, 2013.
Lanigan D, Hey J, West R, et al.: Major vascular complications of orthognathic surgery: false aneurysms and arteriovenous fistulas following orthognathic surgery, *J Oral Maxillofac Surg* 49:571–577, 1991.
Mori Y, Shimizu H, Minami K, Kwon T, Mano T: Development of a simulation system in mandibular orthognathic surgery based on integrated three-dimensional data, *Oral Maxillofac Surg* 15:131–138, 2011.
O'Ryan F: Complications of orthognathic surgery, *Oral Maxillofac Surg Clin North Am* 2:593–613, 1990.
Pereira F, Yaedú R, Sant'ana A, Sant'ana E, et al.: Maxillary aseptic necrosis after Le Fort I osteotomy: a case report and literature review, *J Oral Maxillofac Surg* 68:1402–1407, 2010.
Proffit W, Turvey T, Phillips C, et al.: The hierarchy of stability and predictability in orthognathic surgery with rigid fixation: an update and extension, *Head Face Med* 1–11, 2007.
Proffit W, Turvey TA, Phillips C: Orthognathic surgery: a hierarchy of stability, *Int J Adult Orthodont Orthognath Surg* 11:191–204, 1996.
Reyneke J: *Essentials of orthognathic surgery*, Chicago, 2003, Quintessence Publishers.
Steel B, Cope M, et al.: Unusual and rare complications of orthognathic surgery: a literature review, *J Oral Maxillofac Surg* 1678–1691, 2012.
Tucker M, et al.: Orthognathic surgery versus orthodontic camouflage in the treatment of mandibular deficiency, *J Oral Maxillofac Surg* 53:572–578, 1995.
Turvey TA: Maxillary expansion: a surgical technique based on surgical-orthodontic treatment objectives and anatomical considerations, *J Maxillofac Surg* 13:51–58, 1985.

CHAPTER 40

DISTRACTION OSTEOGENESIS

Din Lam

1. **What is distraction osteogenesis?**
   Distraction osteogenesis is bone formation in the gap between gradually distracted bone ends on each side of a corticotomy. The technique requires the creation of an osteotomy followed by the application of a medical distractor to separate the bone segments at a controlled rate. The process is based on the principle that tension stimulates histogenesis and does not require the use of a bone graft or rigid fixation of the bone segments.

2. **What are the four phases of distraction osteogenesis?**
   Phase I: Osteotomy—creation of bony segments.
   Phase II: Latency—allow soft callus to form. Length of latency depends on patient age. Most protocols ask for 3 to 7 days of latency period, unless the patient is a neonate; in such cases, distraction can start 1 day after osteotomy.
   Phase III: Distraction—0.5 mm twice a day is the most common protocol for distraction.
   Phase IV: Consolidation—allows for hard callus formation. Most protocols recommend a consolidation phase of at least 6 to 8 weeks.

3. **What are the advantages of distraction osteogenesis?**
   - Reduced risk of infection seen in nonvascularized bone grafts
   - Eliminated need for donor site harvesting
   - More predictable bone survival
   - Provides both soft and hard tissue expansion simultaneously

4. **What are the four zones of tissue generation in the intercalary gap?**
   Zone 1: Fibrous central zone
   Zone 2: Transition zone, features osteoid formation along the collagen bundles
   Zone 3: Remodeling zone, osteoclasts work to remodel the newly formed bone
   Zone 4: Zone of mature bone

5. **What are the three types of distraction?**
   1. Unifocal distraction: A single osteotomy is made and distraction forces are applied by a device attached by screws on either side of the osteotomy.
   2. Bifocal distraction: This is one osteotomy with pins on either side of osteotomy and defect and with a single spanning device encompassing the transport system.
   3. Trifocal distraction: Osteotomy is made on both ends of the bony defect. Each end is distracted until the two distracted segments join each other in the center of the intercalary gap.

6. **How are distraction devices categorized?**
   - Internal device versus external device versus semi-buried
   - Unilateral vector versus curvilinear versus multi-vector

7. **What are the vectors of distraction?**
   The vector of distraction is based on the long axis of the distraction device. In the mandible, there are three types of distraction vectors: horizontal, oblique, and vertical. A horizontal vector is 0 degree to 30 degrees, an oblique vector is 30 degrees to 45 degrees, and a vertical vector is greater than 45 degrees. The trajectory of the distracted mandible can be predicted based on the vector of distraction. The horizontal vector is preferred in the patient with mandibular body deficiency. The vertical vector is used in the condyle reconstruction.

8. **How is new bone formed during distraction osteogenesis?**
   Intramembranous ossification.

401

9. **How long does it take the bone in the distraction zone to achieve 90% of normal bony structure?**
Eight months.

10. **What are the etiologies of failure in distraction osteogenesis?**
   - Ischemic fibrogenesis: Inadequate blood supply leads to fibrous formation.
   - Cystic degeneration: Venous congestion leads to a distraction gap filled with cystic cavity.
   - Fibrocartilage nonunion: This is caused by unstable fixation. Cartilage is filled in the distraction gap.
   - Buckling of regenerate is caused by premature removal of distraction device.

11. **What is the primary advantage of an external distraction device versus an internal distraction device?**
Better control of the distraction vector.

12. **How does the stability of moderate (5 to 10 mm) maxillary advancement with distraction osteogenesis compare to that with conventional orthognathic surgery?**
Distraction osteogenesis has not been proven to be superior in stability to conventional orthognathic surgery for moderate maxillary movement. As a result, maxillary distraction is mostly reserved for >10 mm advancement and patients with cleft palate.

13. **Which Kaban subtype of hemifacial microsomia will benefit from distraction osteogenesis?**
Kaban's classification (Class I, IIa, IIb, and III) describes temporomandibular joint defects found in patients with hemifacial microsomia. The type I patient has a mild deficiency that usually does not require surgery, whereas the type III patient has too little bone stock for osteotomy and distractor placement. The type IIa patient can be treated predictably with orthognathic surgery and bone graft. The type IIb patient will benefit the most from distraction osteogenesis.

14. **What is included in the clinical assessment of patients for mandibular distraction?**
Cephalometric analysis, facial nerve function, dental evaluation, photography, and possibly a three-dimensional CT scan.

15. **What incision and osteotomy are used for mandibular distraction?**
Extra-oral skin incision (Risdon incision) with inverted-L osteotomy is by far the most common technique in making mandibular osteotomy and placement of distractor.

16. **What are the possible complications related to mandibular distraction?**
   - Facial scar
   - Loosening of hardware
   - Facial nerve injury
   - Sensory deficits of inferior alveolar nerve
   - Tooth bud injury in young patient
   - Noncompliance

17. **Who are the candidates for neonatal mandibular distraction?**
   - Syndromic patients with poor mandibular growth
   - Beyond 9 months and continued airway compromise secondary to tongue base obstruction
   - Candidates for tracheostomy
   - Failure of nonsurgical management

18. **For neonatal mandibular distraction, what are the physical signs that indicate adequate distraction?**
When the lower alveolar crest is anterior to the maxillary alveolar crest or minimal episodes of oxygen desaturation during close monitoring are good indications of adequate distraction.

19. **For alveolar distraction in the mandible, what is the minimal bone height you need?**
The minimal bone needed for proper placement of a distraction device is 3 to 4 mm. One millimeter of bone will be removed for the osteotomy, and the remaining bone will be needed for screw fixation of the distraction device in the proximal and distal bony segments.

20. **What are the disadvantages of craniofacial distraction?**
Prolonged treatment time, required external device, multiple clinical visits, and close postoperative follow-ups are needed.

21. What is the average age of the patient who needs to undergo midface distraction?

Unless there is a severe upper airway obstruction from midface hypoplasia, midface distraction should not be performed until approximately 3.5 years of age to ensure that there is adequate bone stock to perform the procedure successfully.

22. What orthodontic measures can be practiced during activation and consolidation to achieve the optimal occlusion?

During the activation and consolidation phases, the newly generated bone can be molded and shaped by using guiding elastics to help establish the optimal occlusion. In unilateral mandibular distraction, an intraoral splint can be used to maintain a posterior open bite during the distraction process. The open bite will later close orthodontically by extruding the maxillary dentoalveolus with serial reduction of the bite plate.

23. Where is the area of most bone formation after maxillary distraction?

Most bone formation occurs in the pterygomaxillary region.

CHAPTER 41

SLEEP APNEA AND SNORING

Robert A. Strauss, Kenneth J. Benson, Roman G. Meyliker

1. **How is *snoring* defined?**
   Snoring is a partial airway and pharyngeal flow obstruction that does not cause the individual to have an arousal from sleep. Movement of air through the partially obstructed airway creates vibration and thus the snoring sound.

2. **Does snoring always indicate the presence of obstructive sleep apnea syndrome (OSAS)?**
   No. Although patients who have OSAS are typically loud snorers, and snoring usually indicates some degree of obstructed breathing, not all people who snore have OSAS. In fact, about 25% of adult males snore, and this number increases with age, reaching about 60% at age 60 years. Most snoring is not pathologic and may be reduced or prevented by lifestyle changes. However, with age and weight gain, snoring can eventually degrade into sleep apnea.

3. **Can a snoring patient with excessive daytime somnolence, but without other classic symptoms, have OSAS?**
   Yes. The lack of other classic symptoms of OSAS does not mean the diagnosis of OSAS can be ruled out. Approximately 30% of sleep apnea patients have no other symptoms other than snoring. Because snoring is an indication of partial airway obstruction, understanding the potential of the process to worsen over time is important.

4. **What is the surgical management of snoring?**
   Laser-assisted uvulopalatoplasty (LAUP) and Bovie-assisted uvulopalatoplasty (BAUP) are the most commonly used surgical procedures for the treatment of snoring. Both procedures involve amputation of the uvula and approximately 1 cm of the soft palate. After healing, the soft palate stiffens, reducing its ability to vibrate, and thus reduces snoring. Occasionally the procedure is repeated to resect more tissue without involving the levator muscle and causing velopharyngeal insufficiency. As long as obstructive sleep apnea has been ruled out, the procedure can usually be done under local anesthesia in the office. The advantage of LAUP over BAUP is the prevention of deeper tissue damage and possibility of less postoperative pain, but both procedures are equally effective.

5. **What is obstructive sleep apnea (OSA)?**
   OSA is repetitive, discrete episodes of decreased airflow (hypopnea) or complete cessation of airflow (apnea) for at least a 10 second duration, in association with >2% decrease in oxygen hemoglobin saturation, and that causes an arousal from sleep.

6. **Is there a difference between OSA and OSAS?**
   Yes. These are not the same processes. OSA is an objective lab finding. OSAS involves OSA combined with signs and symptoms of disease.

7. **What are the differences between apnea and hypopnea?**
   Apnea is the cessation of airflow lasting for more than 10 seconds. Hypopnea refers to a greater than two-thirds decrease in tidal volume. Both show a decrease in oxygen saturation of at least 2%.

8. **How many sleep stages are there in normal sleep patterns?**
   There are five sleep stages: one rapid eye movement (REM) stage and four non-REM stages.

9. **During which sleep stages do most obstructive events occur?**
   Stages III and IV and the REM stage, which are the deeper stages of sleep. Pharyngeal wall collapse is more common during these stages because the muscles are most relaxed.

10. **What factors may contribute to OSA events?**
    Anything that effectively causes patient drowsiness or muscle relaxation may contribute to OSA. Alcohol, sedatives, and narcotics are good examples. Weight gain can also potentiate OSA events, as can allergies and upper respiratory infections.

11. What is the primary symptom of OSAS?
    Excessive daytime sleepiness.

12. What other symptoms of OSAS may be present?
    - Loud snoring
    - Morning headache
    - Depression
    - Impotence
    - Restless sleep and frequent arousal at night
    - Hypertension

13. What are the important elements of the physical exam of a patient suspected of having OSA?
    A thorough head and neck exam, including diagnostic nasopharyngoscopy, should be performed in any patient who presents with possible OSA. Exam should include the nose for signs of obstruction or septal deviation, hypertrophic turbinates, and allergic rhinitis. The oral cavity should be examined for large tonsils, redundant soft palate and uvula, redundant lateral pharyngeal walls, macroglossia, and retrognathia. The neck should be evaluated for a thick neck and laryngeal obstruction. The patient should also be screened for signs of hypothyroidism, cor pulmonale, and hypertension.

14. What is the main objective test for diagnosing OSAS?
    Polysomnography is the most commonly performed evaluation for diagnosis of OSAS. It comprises the following tests:
    - Electroencephalography (EEG)
    - Thoracic and abdominal efforts
    - Electrooculography (EOG)
    - Pulse oximetry
    - Chin and leg electromyography (EMG)
    - Electrocardiography (ECG)
    - Nasal and oral airflow

    In some cases, a less formal home sleep study (which can still be very accurate) and multiple sleep latency tests (MSLTs) to confirm daytime sleepiness may also be included.

15. What are the Apnea/Hypopnea Index (AHI) and the Respiratory Disturbance Index (RDI)?
    The AHI represents the number of obstructive respiratory events per hour of sleep. The AHI along with oximetry is the primary clinical indicator in the diagnosis of OSAS. The RDI is the AHI plus any respiratory effort-related arousals (RERA), arousals associated with breathing that do not meet the technical criteria for an apnea or hypopnea (e.g., greater than 10 seconds in duration).

16. How are the AHI and RDI calculated?

    $$AHI = apneas + hypopneas/total\ sleep\ time \times 60$$
    $$RDI = AHI + RERA$$

    An AHI of 5 is the upper limit of normal.

17. What is the modified Muller technique?
    While undergoing fiberoptic nasopharyngoscopy, the patient performs an inspiratory effort against a closed mouth and nose (reverse Valsalva) with the scope first above the soft palate and then secondarily above the base of the tongue. The examiner observes the degree of closure at the oropharyngeal and hypopharyngeal levels.

18. How are lateral cephalograms used in evaluation of patients for OSAS?
    Cephalometric analysis helps confirm physical exam and fiberoptic nasopharyngoscopy exam results. The following are normal measurements of the cephalogram:
    - Posterior nasal spine–tip of palatal uvula (PNS-P): 35 mm or less
    - Mandibular plane–hyoid (MP-H): 15 mm or less
    - Posterior airway space (PAS): 11 mm or greater

19. **What is Fujita's classification of upper airway obstruction?**
    Type I Fujita: upper pharyngeal obstruction including palate, uvula, and tonsils; normal base of tongue
    Type II Fujita: type I obstruction plus base of tongue obstruction
    Type III Fujita: obstruction at tongue base, supraglottis, and hypopharynx; normal palate

20. **What are the classes of sleep apnea?**
    Obstructive, central, and mixed.

21. **What is the difference between OSA and central sleep apnea?**
    With OSA, there is a normal inspiration effort, but upper airway obstruction causes intermittent cessation of airflow. Central sleep apnea is marked by a lack of inspiratory effort secondary to failure of respiratory centers in the central nervous system to provide the phrenic nerve with appropriate afferent information to activate the diaphragm.

22. **What is the prevalence of OSA in the general population in the United States?**
    OSA is present in approximately 6% to 13% of the general US population.

23. **Is there a relationship between the prevalence of OSA and chronic obstructive pulmonary disease (COPD)?**
    According to one study, OSA is highly prevalent in moderate to severe COPD patients. These patients have a greater than expected sleep disordered breathing that can be an important contributory factor to morbidity and mortality of these patients.

24. **Who usually treats central sleep apnea?**
    Neurologists and sleep specialists.

25. **How is OSA classified?**
    The combination of AHI/RDI and lowest oxyhemoglobin desaturation (SaO_2) is a good parameter for scoring OSA severity (Table 41-1).

26. **What are some systemic complications associated with OSAS?**
    - Cor pulmonale
    - Hypertension
    - Daytime somnolence
    - Hypoxia
    - Death
    - Polycythemia vera
    - Depression
    - Stroke

27. **What are the criteria for the cure of OSAS?**
    The surgical cure should have respiratory and sleep results equal to the second night of continuous positive airway pressure (CPAP) titration.
    For patients on CPAP, a nonsurgical treatment, cure is determined as:
    - Although many articles use a postoperative AHI reduction of at least 50% with a maximum of 20 (i.e., an AHI of 26 should be reduced to 13, and an AHI of 80 should be reduced to 20), this can still represent significant OSA. Currently, most experts agree that true cure is only achieved when the AHI is less than 10 regardless of where it began.
    - Postoperative SaO_2 that is normal or with only a few brief falls below 90%
    - Normalization of sleep architecture

Table 41-1. Classification of OSA

	RDI	SAO_2
Mild OSA	10-30	>90%
Moderate OSA	30-50	<85%
Severe OSA	>50	<60%

OSA, obstructive sleep apnea; RDI, respiratory disturbance index.

28. **What are the nonsurgical treatment methods for OSAS?**
    Nasal CPAP is the most effective nonsurgical treatment for OSAS. It usually consists of an airtight mask held over the nose by a strap wrapped around the patient's head. CPAP is maintained by a machine that is similar to a ventilator. Although nasal CPAP is nearly 100% effective in relieving OSAS, it is very poorly tolerated. Even when it is initially successful, many patients (30% to 50%) eventually stop using it because of discomfort or intolerance.

    Mandibular positioning devices are another effective nonsurgical method of treating OSAS. These devices open the airway by holding the mandible, and hence the tongue, forward during sleep. These devices are used with patients with mild to moderate OSA, in patients with lesser degree of oxygen saturation, relatively less daytime sleepiness, low frequency of apnea, and intolerant to CPAP or those who refuse surgery. As with CPAP, discomfort and poor compliance are major problems. Behavioral modifications, such as weight loss and avoidance of alcohol and sedatives, may also reduce OSAS. Again, patient compliance is a major stumbling block.

29. **What are the potential complications of CPAP?**

Mask Related	Pressure/Airflow Related
Skin rash	Rhinorrhea
Conjunctivitis from air leak	Nasal dryness/congestion
	Chest discomfort
	Sinus discomfort
	Tympanic membrane rupture (rare)
	Massive epistaxis (rare)
	Pneumothorax (rare)

30. **What are the surgical options for the management of OSAS?**
    - Tracheotomy
    - Mandibular osteotomy with genioglossus advancement
    - Uvulopalatopharyngoplasty (UPPP) or laser-assisted UPPP (LA-UPPP)
    - Hyoid suspension
    - Robotic base of tongue reduction
    - Maxillary and mandibular advancement (MMA)

31. **What is a "U-triple-P"?**
    UPPP is a surgical procedure performed to enlarge the oropharyngeal airway in an anterior-superior and lateral direction. The tonsils are removed (if they have not been removed previously), along with the posterior edge of the soft palate, including the uvula. The tonsillar pillars are then sewn together, and the mucosa on the nasal side and oral side of the cut edge of the soft palate are sewn together. This was historically the most common surgical procedure performed for treatment of OSAS, although it is actually only moderately effective.

32. **What are the results of UPPP in the treatment of OSAS?**
    UPPP offers promising results to many patients suffering from OSAS, but success rates vary:
    - Elimination of snoring in 80% to 100% of cases
    - Subjective decrease and improvement in excessive daytime somnolence in 80% to 100% of cases
    - Measured RDI decrease by approximately 50% in 50% of patients
    Despite having an approximate 50% reduction in RDI, a patient may still have significant OSA; therefore UPPP may not improve an OSA patient enough to decrease mortality. CPAP and tracheostomy are still the gold standards to decrease OSA mortality rates. However, MMA has now been shown to be highly effective as a surgical cure.

33. **What are the potential complications of UPPP?**
    Bleeding is the most common postoperative complication. Velopharyngeal insufficiency occurs in 5% to 10% of patients but is rarely permanent. Nasopharyngeal stenosis is rare but can be a complication. Other minor complaints include dry mouth, tightness in the throat, and an increased gag reflex.

34. **What is the role of LAUP in OSAS?**
    LAUP is highly effective in the treatment of snoring, with successful results in 85% to 90% of patients. However, the effectiveness of standard LAUP in the treatment of OSAS has been well established to be poor and, in some cases, detrimental. Snoring and OSAS probably represent a continuum of a similar

pathology, but it is still difficult to determine where LAUP is effective and where it is not. Therefore the current recommendation is that all patients should undergo a sleep study before surgery for snoring or OSAS. LAUP should only be used on patients who have no OSA.

35. **What is an appropriate phase I surgical treatment plan for an OSAS patient with a nasooropharyngeal site of obstruction?**
In patients with less severe OSA, phase I or targeted surgical procedures may be attempted. UPPP is excellent for snoring but has only a 40% success rate with OSAS at this obstruction site. Other procedures include nasal surgery and palatal advancement procedures.

36. **What phase I treatment would be appropriate for OSAS in the presence of oropharyngeal and hypopharyngeal obstruction?**
UPPP or nasal surgery and genioglossus advancement with or without hyoid myotomy and suspension are options for this level of obstruction. Newer types of tongue base and hyoid advancements that use sutures around the base of the tongue or hyoid and connected to screws on the inferior border of the mandible may also be effective, especially when used in combination with other phase I procedures.

37. **What is the next step after phase I treatment?**
CPAP treatment is continued for 6 months, at which time the patient is reevaluated with polysomnography. If phase I treatment is unsuccessful, then phase II surgery would be appropriate. Phase II surgery involves orthognathic surgery, which consists of combined MMA. For patients with severe OSA, many surgeons bypass phase I surgery and advance immediately to the more effective phase II surgery (MMA).

38. **What is the most effective surgical management of OSAS?**
Tracheostomy. More recently, MMA has been shown to be highly effective as a surgical treatment with much less morbidity than tracheostomy.

39. **What is the success rate of MMA in the treatment of OSAS?**
Many consider MMA the most promising surgical alternative to tracheostomy. Long-term studies and recent evidence suggest approximately 85% to 95% effectiveness of MMA based on polysomnographic data. Quality of life indicators are also highly correlated. MMA is very effective because it increases the entire airway space.

40. **What are the complications of untreated childhood OSAS?**
    - Failure to thrive
    - Growth impairment
    - Behavior and learning problems
    - Cardiopulmonary complications

41. **What are the signs and symptoms of childhood OSAS?**
    - Snoring
    - Nighttime sweating
    - Restlessness
    - Unusual sleeping positions
    - Chest retraction
    - Paradoxical breathing
    - Use of accessory muscles
    - Paradoxical rib cage motion during inspiration
    - Enuresis
    - Hyponasal speech
    - Nasal obstruction
    - Mouth breathing

42. **What remains the first-line surgical treatment for OSAS in children?**
Adenotonsillectomy has been shown to have high cure rates in healthy children with OSAS.

BIBLIOGRAPHY

Davila DG: Medical considerations in surgery for sleep apnea, *Oral Maxillofac Surg Clin North Am* 7:205–217, 1995.
Hausfeld JN: Snoring and sleep apnea syndrome. In *American Academy of Otolaryngology—Head and Neck Surgery Foundation: common problems of the head and neck*, Philadelphia, 1992, Saunders.

Munoz A: Sleep apnea and snoring. In Jafek BW, Stark AK, editors: *ENT secrets*, Philadelphia, 1996, Hanley & Belfus.

Nelson PB, Riley RW: A surgical protocol for sleep disordered breathing, *Oral Maxillofac Clin North Am* 7:345–356, 1995.

Nimkam Y, Miles P, Waite P: Maxillomandibular advancement surgery in obstructive sleep apnea syndrome patients: long-term stability, *J Oral Maxillofac Surg* 53:1414–1418, 1995.

Prinsell J: Maxillomandibular advancement surgery: a site-specific treatment approach for obstructive sleep apnea in 50 consecutive patients, *Chest* 116:1519–1520, 1999.

Riley R, Troll R, Powell N: Obstructive sleep apnea syndrome: current surgical concepts, *Oral Maxillofac Surg Knowl Update* 2:79–97, 1998.

Riley RW, Powell NB, Guilleminault C: Maxillofacial surgery and obstructive sleep apnea: a review of 80 patients, *Otolaryngol Head Neck Surg* 101:353–361, 1989.

Sher AE: Obstructive sleep apnea syndrome: a complex disorder of the upper airway, *Otolaryngol Clin North Am* 23:593–605, 1990.

Soler X, Gaio E, Powell FL, et al.: High prevalence of obstructive sleep apnea in patients with moderate to severe COPD, *Ann Am Thorac Soc* 12:1219–1225, 2015.

Sterni LM, Tunkel DE: Obstructive sleep apnea syndrome. In Flint PW, editor: *Cummings otolaryngology head and neck surgery*, ed 5, St Louis, 2010, Elsevier.

Tina B, Waite P: Surgical and nonsurgical management of obstructive sleep apnea, *Princ Oral Maxillofac Surg* 3:1531–1547, 1992.

CHAPTER 42

FACIAL PAIN AND MYOFASCIAL DISORDERS

Bhavik S. Desai, Steven G. Gollehon, Gregory M. Ness

1. **How are the treatment modalities to manage temporomandibular joint (TMJ) pain and dysfunction classified?**
   The treatment of TMJ pain and dysfunction is divided into irreversible and reversible modalities. Reversible therapy consists of patient education, medication, physical therapy, and splint therapy. Occlusal adjustments, prosthetic restoration, orthodontic treatment, orthognathic surgery, and TMJ surgery are irreversible therapies that involve permanent changes in the function or morphology of the masticatory system.

2. **What is the most common form of pain and discomfort associated with TMJ disorders?**
   Masticatory myalgia or myofascial pain.

3. **How is the etiology of muscle pain categorized?**
   - Muscle hyperactivity (functional and dysfunctional)
   - Muscle inflammation (myositis) secondary to injury or infection
   - Myalgia associated with muscle hyperactivity

   In contrast to episodic myofascial pain, myofascial pain dysfunction (MPD) syndrome is chronic and self-perpetuating. Sustained muscular hyperactivity results in increased loading of the articular surfaces, and microtrauma leads to inflammation, arthralgia, reflex muscle splinting, and continued myospasm.

4. **What is a differential diagnosis of conditions that can cause pain of non-odontogenic origin in the head and neck region?**
   - Temporomandibular joint disorders including capsular, bony, and disc pathologies
   - Myofascial pain to muscles of mastication
   - Referred pain from maxillary sinus
   - Pain of traumatic origin (including iatrogenic trauma)
   - Trigeminal neuralgia
   - Neurovascular pain such as migraines and tension headaches
   - Trigeminal autonomic cephalgias such as cluster headaches, paroxysmal hemcrania, and SUNCT (Short-lasting, Unilateral Neuralgiform-headache attack with Conjunctival injection and Tearing)
   - Pain secondary to salivary gland pathology such as infections and neoplasms
   - Persistent idiopathic facial pain (atypical facial pain)
   - Burning mouth syndrome (stomatodynia/glossodynia)

5. **What are the hallmarks of trigeminal neuralgia?**
   Trigeminal neuralgia, briefly, is characterized by recurring episodes of severe, sharp, stabbing, lancinating or electric shock-like pain along the V1, V2, or V3 branches of the trigeminal nerve. Symptoms are typically unilateral, and the highest incidence of the condition is in middle-aged adults with a female predilection. Pain is episodic, lasts seconds to a few minutes, and may occur multiple times a day with refractory periods between pain episodes. It may occur spontaneously or may be triggered by touching the face, exposure to wind, or by intraoral stimuli, such as tooth brushing and flossing. A small percentage of cases are associated with central tumors. A patient with symptoms of trigeminal neuralgia under age 40 should be evaluated for multiple sclerosis. It is recommended to obtain an MRI of the brain in suspected cases of trigeminal neuralgia. Medical management includes use of anticonvulsant and neuropathic medications.

6. **What are some salient features of migraine headaches an oral surgeon or dentist should be aware of?**

Migraines are a group of episodic, recurring headache disorders of neurovascular origin. They have a mean age of incidence in the second to fourth decades of life and are more common in females than males. A migraine episode is typically characterized by severe, throbbing unilateral pain supraorbital or localized in the periorbital region that could radiate to the frontalis and temples. Some patients can identify triggering factors, such as alcohol, caffeine, food products, noises, etc., that may precipitate a migraine attack. An episode of migraine may accompany gastric discomfort or nausea, and some patients report prodromal symptoms prior to the onset of pain. An episode of migraines can last for a few hours to days and is followed by a recovery phase. Medical management of migraines includes use of medications such as triptans, neuropathic and anticonvulsant medications, and painkillers along with avoidance of triggering factors when possible. It is pertinent for an oral surgeon or dental provider to include migraines, especially those on the midface and temples, in the differential diagnosis of temporomandibular joint disorders, myofascial pain, and trigeminal neuralgia.

7. **What are cluster headaches?**

Cluster headaches are a well-characterized group of recurring headaches within the neurovascular group of trigeminal autonomic cephalgias that also includes paroxysmal hemicrania and SUNCT. It is characterized by intense, stabbing pain episodes in the ocular region and frontal/temporal region lasting minutes to a few hours and accompanied by autonomic signs on the ipsilateral side such as conjunctival tearing and rhinorrhea. It is more common in male patients than female, and peak incidence is during the second and third decades of life. Its medical management is very similar to that of migraines.

8. **What is the relationship between TMJ disc displacement and clinical symptoms of pain and discomfort?**

Despite the clinical evidence supporting the existence of TMJ disc derangement, many questions remain unanswered, raising doubts about its clinical significance. Because pain is usually aggravated by functional and parafunctional movements, it would appear that pain originates from pressure and traction on the disc attachments. However, many, and perhaps the majority of, patients with displaced discs have no pain, whereas some have severe pain. Studies by Kircos et al. (1987) and Westesson et al. (1989) show a 30% incidence of disc displacement in asymptomatic patients with normal TMJ exams and an 88% incidence of disc displacement in the contralateral asymptomatic joint in patients with unilateral pain and discomfort, respectively. These findings make it clear that disc displacement is not necessarily related to pain.

9. **Does preemptive analgesia reduce postsurgical pain and chronic pain following surgery in patients with TMJ disorders?**

Recent studies have demonstrated that dynamic processing by neurons in the affected pathway may facilitate nociception. The old view that nociceptive pathways are merely static conductors of signals generated by noxious stimuli appears to be invalid. As a result, preemptive analgesic techniques may reduce postsurgical pain and, perhaps, reduce the possibility of chronic pain in the operated patient.

10. **What is the main goal in the postoperative management of patients with TMJ dysfunction?**

Chronic pain and restricted jaw movement are the most common complaints of multiply operated TMJ dysfunction patients. Typically, pain restricts the patient's ability to comply with postsurgical physical therapy, contributing to a gradual decline in jaw mobility. Therefore the major management objective should be adequate pain control coupled with effective physical therapy to maintain jaw function.

11. **What are the management strategies used to treat pain and discomfort in the multiply operated patient with TMJ dysfunction?**

Strategies include pharmacologic approaches, behavioral modification techniques, psychiatric counseling, and physical therapy. Obviously, the success of any approach will depend on an accurate assessment of the patient's physical and emotional status. Furthermore, combination therapies (provided by a coordinated, multidisciplinary team of qualified health care providers) are often required to optimize the patient's condition. Further surgery is ineffective at reducing pain in the multiply operated patient and is not indicated unless a specific mechanical obstruction to function is identifiable and amenable to surgical correction (e.g., ankylosis). In such cases, the patient must understand that improvements in range of motion and function are not likely to be accompanied by pain reduction.

12. **What is peripheral sensitization? What is its role in hyperalgesia in facial pain?**
According to Hargreaves and Wardle, small-diameter group III and IV afferent nerve fibers innervate joints and muscles and respond to stimuli that can be perceived as noxious, such as pressure, algesic chemicals, and inflammatory agents. Ischemia also is an effective stimulus if present for significant amounts of time and is associated with muscle contractions. These nociceptors may be excited by a variety of stimuli, and their sensitivity may be increased following mild, persistent injury. As a result, this peripheral sensitization is thought to be a major factor in the production of hyperalgesia. In conjunction with central sensitization, peripheral sensitization explains the persistent, chronic nature of myofascial pain and the pain of TMJ disorders.

13. **How is the subnucleus of the trigeminal tract related to reception and processing as a second-order sensory neuron in the modulation of facial and TMJ-derived pain?**
Electrophysiologic data acquired in the past two decades generally support the view that subnucleus caudalis of the cranial verve five (CN V) spinal tract nucleus is an essential V brainstem relay for orofacial pain. Neurons responsive to noxious mechanical stimuli or to algesic chemicals applied to articular and muscular tissues predominate in the superficial and deep laminae of the subnucleus caudalis, where anatomic studies indicate projections of deep afferent inputs terminate. Evidence is emerging that the role of the subnucleus caudalis in pain is related primarily to processing of nociceptive information from facial skin and deep tissues, whereas the more rostral components, such as the subnucleus oralis, may be more involved in intraoral and perioral pain mechanisms.

14. **What are the main types of neurons that perceive and transmit nociceptive stimuli from the orofacial region?**
Second-order nociceptive-specific and wide dynamic range neurons in the nucleus caudalis of V receive nociceptive input from peripheral nociceptors in skin and deep muscle tissues. The transmission, interaction, and feedback mechanisms at the level of higher order sensory neurons in the thalamus and somatosensory cortex remain unknown and are an intense area of research.

15. **What is the rationale behind the use of conservative therapy for Temporomandibular Disorders (TMD)?**
Over 90% of patients with TMD can be managed conservatively without surgical intervention. Early diagnosis and adequate medical management can potentially minimize the chances of a patient with TMD needing surgical treatment and account for more successful therapeutic outcomes. Conservative therapy for TMD includes use of nonsteroidal antiinflammatory agents and muscle relaxant medications, physical therapy to muscles of mastication, home exercises, occlusal orthotic appliances against bruxism, clenching cessation, avoidance of foods that are difficult or time-consuming to chew, and chewing gum cessation, among others.

16. **Which comorbidities are found in association with TMD/myofascial pain?**
Chronic head and neck pain including myofascial pain to muscles of mastication and TMDs simultaneously exist with comorbid conditions such as migraines, tension headaches, fibromyalgia, sleep disorders, irritable bowel syndrome, cervical pain, and arthralgia on other joints in the body.

17. **How is a diagnosis of atypical facial pain made?**
Atypical facial pain, also referred to as persistent idiopathic facial pain, is defined as pain in the maxillofacial region lasting at least a few hours a day and is not attributable to any other source of pain. It is an example of a chronic neuropathy that is diagnosed by excluding all other sources of pain in this region such as odontogenic pain, temporomandibular joint and myofascial disorders, trigeminal neuralgia, migraines, trigeminal autonomic cephalgias, and referred pain from the sinuses, neck, and head. It is typically associated with no positive pathologic or abnormal findings on clinical examination or imaging. Local anesthetic injection in the area of pain may elucidate an equivocal response without achieving complete anesthesia of the region. Atypical facial pain is managed largely by neuropathic, anticonvulsant, analgesic, and antidepressant medication along with psychological or behavioral support.

18. **What are the salient features of burning mouth syndrome, and how is it managed?**
Burning mouth syndrome, or glossodynia, is a chronic neuropathy characterized by chronic burning sensation inside the mouth, with no visible mucosal pathology to explain the symptoms. Symptoms are most commonly found on the tongue, palate, and lips. This disorder may also manifest with symptoms of altered taste or a raw feeling on the dorsal tongue. Diagnosis is usually made by excluding

systemic causes of oral burning such as xerostomia, deficiencies of vitamin B12, folate, and iron, hypothyroidism, and undetected diabetes mellitus and by ruling out local causes of oral burning such as mucosal disease, candidiasis, dental or prosthetic irritation, and parafunctional tongue habits. Management involves correction of underlying source of oral burning, where applicable, and medication with neuropathic drugs or sialogogues.

BIBLIOGRAPHY

Charleston 4th L: Burning mouth syndrome: a review of recent literature, *Curr Pain Headache Rep* 17(6):336, June 2013.

Dolwick MF: Temporomandibular joint disk displacement: clinical perspectives. In Sessle BJ, Bryant PS, Dionne RA, editors: *Temporomandibular disorders and related pain conditions: progress in pain research and management*, ed 4, Seattle, 1995, IASP Press.

Hargreaves AS, Wardle JJ: The use of physiotherapy in the treatment of temporomandibular disorders, *Br Dent J* 155:121–124, 1983.

Hoffmann KD: Differential diagnosis and characteristics of TMJ disease and disorders, *Oral Maxillofac Surg Knowl Update* 1:43, 1994.

Kircos LT, Ortendahl DA, Mark AS, et al.: Magnetic resonance imaging of the TMJ disc in asymptomatic volunteers, *J Oral Maxillofac Surg* 45:852–854, 1987.

Kopp S: Degenerative and inflammatory temporomandibular joint disorders: clinical perspectives. In Sessle BJ, Bryant PS, Dionne RA, editors: *Temporomandibular disorders and related pain conditions: progress in pain research and management*, ed 4, Seattle, 1995, IASP Press.

Lambert GM: Degenerative and inflammatory temporomandibular joint disorders: basic science perspectives. In Sessle BJ, Bryant PS, Dionne RA, editors: *Temporomandibular disorders and related pain conditions: progress in pain research and management*, ed 4, Seattle, 1995, IASP Press.

Milam SB: Nonsurgical management of the multiply operated TMD patient, *Selected Readings Oral Maxillofac Surg* 6:4, 1999.

Milam SB: Articular disk displacements and degenerative temporomandibular joint disease. In Sessle BJ, Bryant PS, Dionne RA, editors: *Temporomandibular disorders and related pain conditions: progress in pain research and management*, ed 4, Seattle, 1995, IASP Press.

Milam SB, Zardeneta G: Oxidative stress and degenerative temporomandibular joint disease: a proposed hypothesis, *J Oral Maxillofac Surg* 56:214–223, 1998.

National Institutes of Health: *Management of temporomandibular disorders: National Institutes of Health Technology Assessment conference statement*, Bethesda, MD, 1996, NIH.

Sessle BJ: Masticatory muscle disorders: basic science perspectives. In Sessle BJ, Bryant PS, Dionne RA, editors: *Temporomandibular disorders and related pain conditions: progress in pain research and management*, ed 4, Seattle, 1995, IASP Press.

Stohler CS: Clinical perspectives on masticatory and related muscle disorders. In Sessle BJ, Bryant PS, Dionne RA, editors: *Temporomandibular disorders and related pain conditions: progress in pain research and management*, ed 4, Seattle, 1995, IASP Press.

Westesson PL, Eriksson L, Kurita K: Reliability of a negative clinical temporomandibular joint examination: prevalence of disk displacement in asymptomatic temporomandibular joints, *Oral Surg Oral Med Oral Pathol* 68:551–554, 1989.

Zakrzewska JM: Differential diagnosis of facial pain and guidelines for management, *Br J Anaesth* 111(1):95–104, 2013.

CHAPTER 43

TEMPOROMANDIBULAR JOINT PATHOPHYSIOLOGY AND SURGICAL TREATMENT

David W. Lui, Renato Mazzonetto, Steven G. Gollehon, Daniel B. Spagnoli, Gregory M. Ness

1. **What is the main function of cartilage?**

   Cartilage is aneural, avascular, and alymphatic. Its main function is to withstand compressional forces during frictional joint loading. The articular cartilage functions to resist forces of compression and joint friction between the condyle and fossa. Chondrocytes within the cartilage also secrete important biochemicals for joint function, such as lubricin, which acts to maintain joint integrity and reduce functional wear.

2. **What is the difference between temporomandibular joint (TMJ) articular cartilage and cartilage of other synovial joints?**

   Most synovial joints have hyaline cartilage on their articular surface; however, a number of joints, such as the sternoclavicular, acromioclavicular, and TMJs, are associated with bones that develop from intramembranous ossification. These have fibrocartilage articular surfaces.

3. **What are the unique properties of the TMJ and its articular disc?**

   The articular disc is tightly attached to the lateral and medial poles of the condyle. Therefore, during mouth opening, the condyle-articular disc complex moves in a sliding movement relative to the temporal bone to or beyond the apex of the articular eminence, whereas the condyle rotates underneath the disc. Because the TMJ has characteristics of both a hinge joint (ginglymus) and a gliding joint (articulatio plana), it is classified as a ginglymoarthrodial joint. A unique feature of the TMJ is that it is rigidly connected to both the dentition and the contralateral TMJ.

4. **What are the main protective and functional responsibilities of the articular disc of the TMJ?**

   The main functions of the disc are to absorb shock and to resist stretching and compressional forces by transforming them into tension stresses in the collagen fibers. These stresses are dispersed throughout the collagen network and consequently reduced. Another function of the articular disc is to establish joint stability while translatory movements of the condyle occur.

5. **What is synovium?**

   Synovium is the thin epithelioid tissue lining nonarticular surfaces of diarthrodial joints. In the healthy TMJ, the anterior and posterior recesses of both the superior and inferior joint spaces are lined with synovium. The synovium contains specialized cell types A and B. Type A cells are derived from the monocyte/macrophage lineage and are phagocytic, filling an important role in the catabolic metabolism of articular cartilage. Type B cells are more fibroblastic in nature and secrete hyaluronic acid and proteoglycans, components of synovial fluid. Synovial fluid is a dialysate of blood plasma containing hyaluronate and proteoglycans, and it is important for joint surface nutrition, oxygenation, and lubrication.

6. **What are the external causes of internal derangements of the TMJ?**

   External causes of internal derangements are classified as macrotrauma or microtrauma. External factors such as clenching, grinding, bruxing, nail biting, and other parafunctional habits can cause excessive joint loading and lack of motion. These actions lead to inflammatory biochemical alterations in the joint that promote degradation, synovial inflammation, and formation of adhesions.

7. **What clinical sign is pathognomonic for the first stage of internal derangement of the articular disc?**

   Reciprocal clicking is considered pathognomonic for the first stage of disc displacement. In the first stage of internal derangement, clicking begins suddenly and spontaneously or after an injury. The noise is often loud and may be audible to others, but it is rarely associated with severe pain. The patient may be aware of a feeling of obstruction within the joint during movement until the click occurs. The mandible frequently deviates toward the affected side until the click occurs and then returns to the midline after the click.

8. **What are the hallmarks of the second stage of internal derangement?**
The second stage of disc derangement is reciprocal clicking with intermittent locking. The typical patient complains that the jaw becomes locked, and there is usually, but not always, severe pain over the affected joint. Patients may describe a feeling of obstruction to opening within the joint. Patients may be able to manipulate the joint to restore function. In some cases, the jaw may unlock spontaneously. In nearly all cases, there is a prior history of clicking of the affected joint.

9. **How does stage 3 of internal derangements of the articular disc differ?**
The third stage of disc derangement is associated with limited opening and has been termed *closed lock*. A limited opening of <27 mm and severe pain over the affected joint are characteristic findings. A deviation of the mandible on opening is also seen. Again, the patient often describes a feeling of fullness or obstruction. In contrast to stage 2, few patients are able to unlock or relocate their closed lock and restore normal function.

10. **Why is the fourth stage of internal derangement less painful when compared with earlier stages of disc derangement?**
The fourth and final stage in the classification of internal derangement involving the articular disc is characterized by an increase in opening and crepitus occurring within the joint during movement due to degenerative changes in the disc and articular surfaces. This stage appears to be less painful than previous stages because the neurovascular tissue is no longer impinged between the condyle and the glenoid fossa.

11. **What is the relationship between osteoarthritis and TMJ disc displacement?**
The relationship between osteoarthritis and disc displacement is a subject of debate. Disc displacement may be a sign, as well as a cause, of TMJ osteoarthritis. However, it often is a concomitant phenomenon, with an initial disturbance of molecular and cellular processes leading to osteoarthritis in cartilaginous tissues. The concomitant manifestation of both osteoarthritis and disc displacement comprises a substantial portion of all TMJ disorders, although both conditions may manifest separately and may be mutually independent. Currently, osteoarthritis, alone or in combination with disc displacement, is one of the most prevalent TMJ disorders.

12. **How do external factors lead to anatomic alterations in the TMJ?**
Acute macrotrauma to the joint, such as direct or coup-contrecoup injuries, may result in displacement, contusion, hemorrhage, and irreversible deformation of the joint tissues with the potential for intracapsular interferences, restrictive fibrosis, and inflammation.
Functional overload, or microtrauma, is another frequent cause of internal derangements. Chronic microtrauma is associated with parafunctional activities such as chronic clenching habits, grinding, nail biting, and gum chewing that alter the lubricating properties of the joint; introduce friction between the disc and the condyle, causing degenerative changes; and result in gradual anterior displacement and eventual perforation of the disc.

13. **What is the sensitive balance between anabolism and catabolism that exists in the TMJ synovium and articular disc?**
Because the articular cartilage is avascular and alymphatic, nutrition and elimination of waste products are dependent on diffusion through the cartilage matrix from and to the synovial fluid. Joint loading significantly stimulates disc diffusion and is essential to chondrocyte nutrition. Because cartilage is avascular, chondrocytes have to function under almost anaerobic conditions. Consequently, they have relatively low metabolic activity, which renders them vulnerable to toxic influences. Chondrocytes are unable to regenerate after major trauma, but they have considerable recuperative abilities. Although once thought of as an inert tissue, articular cartilage is now recognized as a dynamic system that is capable of remodeling under functional demands and turnover of extracellular matrix components. As long as the environment of the TMJ synovium and articular cartilage exists in a balance between net breakdown and net build-up, most destructive processes in the TMJ remain subclinical. It is when the net catabolism (breakdown) exceeds the anabolic build-up (reparative processes) that most chronic inflammatory conditions begin to become symptomatic.

14. **What is synovitis, and how does it occur?**
Synovitis is an inflammatory disorder of the synovial membrane that is characterized by hyperemia, edema, and capillary proliferation in the synovial membrane. Synovitis occurs when the level of

cellular debris and the concentration of biochemical mediators of inflammation and pain produce levels that the synovial membrane is unable to ingest, absorb, or process.

15. **Biochemically, what compounds have been linked to the pathogenic pathway in TMJ osteoarthritis?**

    In osteoarthritic cartilage, which is characterized by tissue degradation, an imbalance between protease and protease inhibitor levels or activities has been postulated as a possible pathogenic pathway in osteoarthritis. In support of this, high levels of active metalloproteases, in particular MMP-2, MMP-9, and MMP-3, were found in lavage fluids of affected TMJs.

16. **What is weeping lubrication? What is its origin and function in maintaining TMJ homeostasis?**

    Loading of cartilage during joint movement results in an increase of the internal hydrostatic pressure. If the hydrostatic pressure exceeds the osmotic pressure exerted by the proteoglycans, water is squeezed out of the extracellular matrix, contributing to the lubrication of the joint surfaces during joint movement. This so-called weeping lubrication occurs particularly under high loads. Under low loads, the so-called boundary lubrication functions through a lubricating glycoprotein, lubricin. The proteoglycans, in collaboration with the collagen network, determine the viscoelastic properties of the cartilage and provide it with its resilience, elasticity, shear strength, and self-lubrication. In addition, proteoglycans can function as internal membrane receptors.

17. **What are the goals of nonsurgical management of TMJ disorders?**

    Some patients with TMJ disorders can be managed successfully without surgery. Between 2% and 5% of all patients treated for TMJ disorders undergo surgery. Physical therapy, occlusal splint therapy, pharmacologic therapy, occlusal adjustments, and patient counseling can treat joint pain and limitation in mouth opening. The goals are:

    • To eliminate pain or at least decrease it to a level that the patient can manage
    • To decrease or eliminate jaw dysfunction and to increase masticatory ability
    • To restore jaw movement to a normal range of motion
    • To counsel the patient about habits that tend to decrease TMJ function

18. **What are the indications to proceed with TMJ surgery?**

    Patients with pain and dysfunction whose signs and symptoms do not respond satisfactorily to nonsurgical therapy within a period of 3 months may be candidates for surgery, particularly if they are diagnosed with advanced internal derangement caused by ankylosis, rheumatoid arthritis, or severe degenerative osteoarthritis. Patients with no improvement in range of motion and mouth opening despite conservative treatment are also candidates for surgical therapy. Some clinicians recommend earlier (within days or weeks) invasive management by arthrocentesis of conditions such as acute closed lock.

19. **When is TMJ arthrocentesis indicated?**

    Arthrocentesis is used to manage TMJ problems in patients who do not respond well to nonsurgical therapy. The major indications for its use are (1) acute or chronic limitation of motion because of an anterior displaced disc without reduction and (2) hypomobility resulting from restriction of condylar translation in the upper joint space. Patients with normal range of motion despite an anterior disc displacement with reduction, who nonetheless have chronic pain, also respond favorably to arthrocentesis. Arthrocentesis also may be used to manage pain and dysfunction in patients who have undergone previous invasive procedures that have failed to relieve pain with limitation of function. The alteration of the biochemical environment within the intracapsular space by arthrocentesis to relieve various vasoactive pain mediators is also another strong indication for treatment. Arthrocentesis may bridge the gap between nonsurgical therapy or nonsurgical and pharmacologic therapy and invasive TMJ surgery.

20. **What are the major advantages of TMJ arthroscopic surgery over open joint surgery?**

    A minimally invasive surgical procedure, arthroscopy allows direct visualization of the anatomic structures of the TMJ, biopsy of pathologic tissue, and removal of osteoarthritic fibrillation tissue, as well as direct injection of steroid into inflamed synovial tissues and correlation of clinical findings with the actual joint pathology or previous imaging studies. Patients experience decreased morbidity, faster recovery time, and less intraarticular inflammation and destruction than with open joint procedures.

21. **When is arthroscopic surgery contraindicated?**

    Contraindications to arthroscopy are similar to those for other elective procedures, such as any medical condition that places the patient at an increased risk from general anesthesia or the surgical procedure itself. Local contraindications include skin or ear infections and severe or advanced fibrous ankylosis resulting in severe limitations and movement of the condyle. Emotional instability, obesity that prevents the joints from being palpated adequately, and other circumstances unique to the patient are also considerations.

22. **Why is preservation of the synovial membrane, articular cartilage, and disc important during TMJ surgery?**
    The synovial membrane must be maintained to provide joint lubrication. Excessive removal of synovial tissue with shavers, cautery, or laser should be avoided to prevent scar formation and the subsequent formation of dense connective tissue. Articular cartilage should be preserved when possible to maintain resiliency and compressibility of the joint; moreover, only the fibrillated osteoarthritic tissue should be removed conservatively during arthroscopy. Disc preservation is important because it gives the joint a biochemical advantage by facilitating intracapsular boundaries and hydrostatic weeping lubrication. Many surgeons achieve favorable results using arthroscopic lysis and lavage alone, removing no tissues at all.

23. **What role does disc repositioning play in achieving successful TMJ surgery outcomes?**
    There is debate over this question among surgeons. Most would advocate preservation of as much normal joint structure and architecture as possible for the reasons listed previously. Patients who undergo disc removal develop radiographic changes, such as condylar flattening and osteophyte formation, similar to those seen in advanced osteoarthritis, although these postsurgical changes are often asymptomatic. On the other hand, procedures such as meniscectomy have high clinical success rates, and disc repositioning has been found to be temporary in many cases following arthroscopy or meniscoplasty procedures, suggesting that the clinical benefit is not dependent on restoring a reduced disc position.

24. **Do lasers have advantages over conventional rotary instruments in arthroscopic procedures?**
    Yes. The effectiveness of joint surgery has improved greatly with the application of laser technology. Diseased tissues can be removed without mechanical contact, thus minimizing trauma to the articular cartilage and surrounding synovial surfaces. Coagulation of bleeding occurs instantly without thermal damage. Bone spurs are easily removed, minimizing the use of larger mechanical instruments in narrow places, which further reduces local tissue insult.

25. **What are the indications for alloplastic total joint reconstruction?**
    - Severe arthritic conditions: osteoarthritis, traumatic arthritis, rheumatoid arthritis
    - Ankylosis including, but not limited to, recurrent ankylosis with excessive heterotopic bone formation
    - Revision procedures where other treatments have failed (e.g., alloplastic reconstruction, autogenous grafts)
    - Avascular necrosis
    - Multiply operated joints
    - Large benign neoplasms
    - Malignancy (e.g., post-tumor excision)
    - Severe condylar resorption
    - Developmental condylar agenesis

26. **What are the contraindications for alloplastic total joint reconstruction?**
    - Active or chronic infection
    - When there is insufficient quantity or quality of bone to support the components
    - Systemic disease with increased susceptibility to infection
    - Partial TMJ joint reconstruction is not recommended because the natural condyle can resorb when functioning against a metal fossa, and a metal condyle will erode through the natural fossa
    - Known allergic reaction to any materials used in the components
      Note: Patients with known or suspected nickel sensitivity should not have Co-Cr-Mo devices implanted because this material contains nickel.
    - Patients with mental or neurological conditions who are unwilling or unable to follow postoperative care instructions

- Skeletally immature patients
- Patients with a foreign body reaction due to previous implants

27. **What are the stages of osteoarthritis?**
    1. Initial stage
    2. Repair stage
    3. Degradation stage
       - Early
       - Progressive
    4. Late stage

28. **What occurs during the initial and repair stages of osteoarthritis?**
    If a primary insult, whether biochemical, biomechanical, inflammatory, or immunologic, disturbs the chondrocyte control balance between synthesis and degradation of extracellular matrix components in normal tissue turnover, cartilage degradation ensues. Initially, cartilage degradation caused by increased proteolytic activity will be counteracted by attempts at repair. In the repair stage, an increased degradation of extracellular matrix components by protease is counteracted by an increased anabolic cytokine-mediated synthesis of these components by chondrocytes. This results in a new balance between increased degradation and increased synthesis of extracellular matrix components. Histologically, the repair stage is characterized by the proliferation of chondrocytes. Clinically, the cartilage changes in the repair stage of osteoarthritis may remain asymptomatic for many years. In general, osteoarthritis is progressive and ultimately manifests clinically. However, what causes the established balance to tip, resulting initially in a focal net degradation of extracellular matrix components, still is not known.

29. **How does the early degradation stage of osteoarthritis differ from the initial and repair stages?**
    In the early stages of osteoarthritis, the degradation caused by the increased synthesis and activity of protease exceeds the increases of extracellular matrix components by the chondrocytes. This results in an initial focal degradation and loss of articular cartilage. The key feature of disease progression is the enzymatic breakdown of the cartilage. Consequently, the content of several extracellular matrix components is reduced focally, whereas the composition and distribution of the other extracellular matrix components are altered. The collagen network shows signs of electron-microscopic disorganization. The fibrils, of the articular surface in particular, appear disoriented and separated more widely than normal. In addition, the histochemical stains for proteoglycans show uneven staining with focally increased affinity, especially in areas of swelling and focal loss of metachromasia. Also, the chondrocytes may produce free radicals that will cause cleavage of extracellular matrix molecules. The content of proteolytic enzymes, including acid phosphatase, serine protease, and metalloprotease such as collagenase and stromelysin-1, is increased in early osteoarthritic cartilage proportional to the severity of the disease process.

30. **What role does synovial clearance play in the initial clinical manifestations of osteoarthritis?**
    The degradation products of the extracellular matrix components are further degraded by the chondrocytes or diffused into synovial fluid, where they are removed by the circulation or are phagocytosed by synovial A lining cells. This latter phenomenon is called *synovial clearance* and frequently induces a secondary synovitis. Often, the osteoarthritic process becomes manifest only when a secondary synovitis develops, causing joint pain and, frequently, a limitation of joint movement. Moreover, the involvement of the synovial tissues in the osteoarthritic process initiates a cascade of secondary events, creating a vicious circle that leads to further cartilage damage by the synthesis of inflammatory and pain mediators.

31. **What is the clinical importance of interleukin-1 and prostaglandins in the early breakdown stages of osteoarthritis?**
    Interleukin-1 induces increased synthesis of prostaglandins, prostaglandin E2 (PGE2) in particular, by synoviocytes. This increase in prostaglandins may be responsible for several of the symptoms observed in this stage of osteoarthritis. Prostaglandins and leukotrienes are mediators of inflammation. In response to inflammatory changes, nonmyelinated sensory neurons in the synovial tissues may release substance P and other pain mediators. Among other effects, substance P may enhance the synthesis of collagenase and PGE2 by the synovial lining cells, thereby perpetuating the catabolic process.

32. **What molecular events may contribute to degenerative disease in the TMJ?**
The inflammatory, catabolic changes that lead to osteoarthritis of the TMJ may be provoked by oxidative stress triggered by several possible mechanisms. A variety of potentially injurious cytokines, neuropeptides, cartilage matrix degrading enzymes, and arachidonic acid metabolites have been identified in the synovial fluid of diseased TMJs. Oxidative stress is the accumulation of reactive free radical molecules that may then injure tissues both directly and indirectly by stimulating the production of these molecules. The free radical formation may be initiated (1) by direct mechanical stress to cartilage, erythrocytes, or other tissues, (2) by cyclic hypoxia-reperfusion injury to tissues within the joint, or (3) as a direct result of neurogenic inflammation, in which free radicals may modulate cytokine production.

33. **What role does estrogen play in the female predilection for TMJ dysfunction?**
In general, women tend to report more pain and exhibit a higher incidence of joint noise and mandibular deflection with movement than do men. Functional estrogen receptors have been identified in the female TMJ but not in the male TMJ. Estrogen may also promote degenerative changes in the TMJ by increasing the synthesis of specific cytokines, whereas testosterone may inhibit these cytokines. It is likely that sex hormones profoundly influence several cell activities that may be associated with remodeling or degenerative processes in the human TMJ.

34. **What is the incidence of TMJ dysfunction and pain in patients with rheumatoid arthritis?**
The occurrence of TMJ pain caused by rheumatoid arthritis depends on the severity of the systemic disease. According to several clinical investigations, about one-third to one-half of patients with rheumatoid arthritis will experience pain in this joint at some time, with nearly 60% of patients suffering from bilateral joint dysfunction. For more than one-third of patients, temporomandibular dysfunction symptoms begin within 1 year after the onset of general disease. Fifteen percent to 16% of these patients will develop great functional disability.

35. **What occurs during progression of rheumatoid arthritis in the TMJ?**
The target tissue of rheumatoid arthritis is the synovial membrane. Progression in the TMJ follows a general scheme with exudation, cellular infiltration, and pannus formation. The articular surfaces of the temporal and condylar components are destroyed, the disc becomes grossly perforated, and the subchondral bone is resorbed. Complete ankylosis of the joint seldom occurs, although most persons have reduced mandibular mobility and loss of posterior height, resulting in apertognathia. The progression of rheumatoid arthritis is slow in most people, although a few experience severe joint destruction within a few months. The presence of a high erythrocyte sedimentation rate is a negative prognostic factor.

36. **How is chondromalacia defined as it applies to the TMJ?**
Chondromalacia is a term used rather loosely by the medical profession to describe a clinically distinctive posttraumatic softening of the articular cartilage of the patella in young people. The term is now also applied to the TMJ and mimics lesions of early osteoarthritis. Osteoarthritis starts focally in a joint; clinical symptoms occur when it is present to a certain degree or when a certain area is affected.
The grading of chondromalacia is as follows:
- Grade I: softening of cartilage
- Grade II: furrowing
- Grade III: fibrillation and ulceration
- Grade IV: crater formation and subchondral bone exposure

37. **How do primary and secondary osteoarthritis differ as they apply to the TMJ?**
Primary osteoarthritis will result in degenerative changes, disc displacement, and finally changes in joint morphology. All signs and symptoms seem to be the result of this primary idiopathic process. Secondary osteoarthritis shows degenerative changes due to joint afflictions, such as rheumatoid arthritis, but also may be due to disc displacement. Osteoarthritis of the TMJ deals with synovial joint pathology, primarily with a connective tissue disease.

38. **What occurs during the progressive degradation stage of osteoarthritis?**
In this stage, the anabolic process has become increasingly defective relative to catabolic effects. The synthesis of extracellular matrix components fails or, as the synthesis and activity of protease remain increased, results in a progressive degradation, erosion, and loss of articular cartilage. Histologically,

the progressive degradation stage of osteoarthritis is characterized by fibrillation, detachments, and thinning of the cartilage from mechanical wear. Irregularities and reduplication of the tide mark have been observed, although less often in the TMJ than in other osteoarthritic synovial joints.

39. **What are the hallmark arthroscopic features of the progressive degradation stages of osteoarthritis?**
Arthroscopically, the articular cartilage of the TMJ may appear fibrillated or eroded. Fibrillation of the cartilage of the articular eminence may be focal or extensive. Articular disc displacement, either reducing or nonreducing, is frequently seen. Angiogenesis in the cartilage of the articular eminence may be observed, whereas creeping synovitis may be seen on the posterior wall of the glenoid fossa and the articular disc. The synovial tissues may appear hypervascularized and redundant or may show fibrotic changes in local areas. In addition, adhesion formation may result in a reduction of the anterior and posterior joint recesses.

40. **What occurs during the late stages of osteoarthritis?**
The content of several extracellular matrix components, including water, proteoglycans, and collagen, is further reduced. The synthesis and activity of protease may remain increased or may be finally reduced when the articular cartilage is nearly destroyed, resulting in so-called residual osteoarthritis. Histologically, the late stage of osteoarthritis is characterized by an extensive fibrillation of the cartilage, eventually resulting in severe thinning of the articular cartilage layer or even denudation of the subchondral bone. Chondrocyte necrosis often occurs. The collagen network is severely disorganized and disintegrated, whereas histochemical stains for proteoglycans show severe depletion of proteoglycans. Biochemically, the late stage of osteoarthritis is characterized by continuous increased syntheses of protease or by decreased synthesis of protease in the case of residual osteoarthritis. The content of several extracellular matrix components is further reduced to levels in residual osteoarthritis.

41. **What arthroscopic findings are seen in the late stage of osteoarthritis?**
Cartilage may appear severely fibrillated and eroded. Denudation of subcondylar bone is seen, and angiogenesis of the cartilage of the articular eminence may be present. Disc displacement or disc perforation may have developed. The synovial tissues may appear hypervascularized and redundant or may have become fibrotic. In the latter stages of this disease, adhesion formation with opposing surfaces frequently results in limited joint recesses.

42. **What are the clinical manifestations of the late stages of osteoarthritis?**
- Clinically, the late stages of osteoarthritis may be manifest by joint pain and limitation of joint movement.
- Joint noises may be present if the disc displacement or proliferation has developed or may be caused by articular cartilage surface irregularities.

In the case of residual osteoarthritis of the TMJ, clinical signs and symptoms may have ceased.

43. **Can you describe the classifications of TMJ ankylosis?**
See Table 43-1.

44. **What is the treatment protocol for pediatric TMJ ankylosis?**
1. Aggressive excision of fibrous and/or bony mass via gap arthroplasty
2. Ipsilateral coronoidectomy
3. Contralateral coronoidectomy if maximal incisal opening is less than 35 mm or no contralateral TMJ dislocation
4. Lining of joint with temporalis fascia or native disc, if salvageable
5. Reconstruction of ramus-condyle unit with either distraction osteogenesis (DO) or costochondral graft (CCG) and rigid fixation
6. If DO, early mobilization of mandible starting day of surgery
7. If CCG, early mobilization with minimal maxillomandibular fixation for no more than 10 days
8. Aggressive postoperative physical therapy

45. **What serious complications may arise from arthroplasty for TMJ bony ankylosis?**
Injury to the middle ear with loss of hearing, damage to the facial nerve (specifically the temporal or zygomatic branches), and severe intraoperative bleeding, usually from the internal maxillary artery, are significant risks of this operation.

Table 43-1. Classifications of TMJ Ankylosis

TOPAZIAN (1964)	SAWHNEY (1986)	HE ET AL. (2011)
Stage I: Ankylotic bone limited to condylar process Stage II: Ankylotic bone extending to sigmoid notch Stage III: Ankylotic bone extending to coronoid process	Type 1: Extensive fibrous adhesions around joint, condyle present Type 2: Bony fusion, especially at lateral articular surface, no fusion in the medial joint space Type 3: Bony bridge between ascending ramus of mandible and temporal bone/zygomatic arch Type 4: Joint is replaced by a mass of bone between ramus and skull base	A1: Fibrous ankylosis without bony fusion A2: Bony ankylosis in lateral joint, residual condyle fragment is larger than 50% of contralateral normal condyle A3: Similar to A2, residual condyle is smaller than 50% of contralateral normal condyle A4: Complete bony ankylosis

BIBLIOGRAPHY

Buckley MJ, Merrill RG, Braun TW: Surgical management of internal derangement of the temporomandibular joint, *JOMS* 51(Suppl 1):20–27, 1993.

Dijkgraaf LC, Milam SB: Osteoarthritis: histopathology and biochemistry of the TMJ, *Oral Maxillofac Surg Knowl Update* 3:1–20, 2000.

Dijkgraaf CL, Spijkervet FK, de Bont LG: Arthroscopic findings in osteoarthritic temporomandibular joints, *J Oral Maxillofac Surg* 57:255–268, 1999.

Frost DE, Kendell BD: The use of arthrocentesis for treatment of temporomandibular joint disorders, *J Oral Maxillofac Surg* 57:583–587, 1999.

Giannakopolous HE, Sinn DP, Quinn PD: Biomet microfixation temporomandibular joint replacement system: a 3-year follow-up study of patients treated during 1995 to 2005, *JOMS* 70:787–794, 2012.

Hall DH: The role of discectomy for treating internal derangements of the temporomandibular joint, *Oral Maxillofac Surg Clin North Am* 6:287–296, 1994.

He D, Yang C, Chen M, et al.: Traumatic temporomandibular joint ankylosis: our classification and treatment experience, *JOMS* 69:1600–1607, 2011.

Hoffmann KD: Differential diagnosis and characteristics of TMJ disease and disorders, *Oral Maxillofac Surg Knowl Update* 1:43–66, 1994.

Israel HA: The use of arthroscopic surgery for treatment of temporomandibular joint disorders, *J Oral Maxillofac Surg* 57:579–582, 1999.

Kaban LB, Bouchard C, Troulis MJ: A protocol for management of temporomandibular joint ankylosis in children, *JOMS* 67:1966–1978, 2009.

Laskin DM: Etiology and pathogenesis of internal derangements of the temporomandibular joint, *Oral Maxillofac Surg Clin North Am* 6:217–229, 1994.

Mercuri LG: Alloplastic temporomandibular joint replacement: rationale for the use of custom devices, *IJOMS* 41:1033–1040, 2012.

Quinn JH: Arthroscopic histopathology, *Oral Maxillofac Surg Knowl Update* 1:115–132, 1994.

Sanders B: Arthroscopic management of internal derangements of the temporomandibular joint, *Oral Maxillofac Surg Clin North Am* 6:259–269, 1994.

Sawhney CP: Bony ankylosis of the temporomandibular joint: follow-up of 70 patients treated with arthroplasty and acrylic spacer interposition, *Plast Reconstr Surg* 77:29–38, 1986.

Spagnoli DB: Anatomy of the TMJ, *Oral Maxillofac Surg Knowl Update* 1:1–41, 1994.

Topazian RG: Etiology of ankylosis of the temporomandibular joint: analysis of 44 cases, *J Oral Surg* 22:227–233, 1964.

Wilkes CH: Internal derangements of the temporomandibular joint. Pathological variations, *Arch Otolaryngol Head Neck Surg* 115:469–477, 1989.

CHAPTER 44

ORAL AND MAXILLOFACIAL CYSTS AND TUMORS

David Webb

1. **What is the most common odontogenic cyst and tumor?**

   The most common odontogenic cyst is the periapical cyst (with an inflammatory etiology). The most common developmental odontogenic cyst is the dentigerous cyst, which is usually diagnosed between ages 10 and 30 years. The dentigerous cyst represents a pathologic expansion of the dental follicle: a sac-like structure surrounding the crown of an unerupted tooth.

   The most common odontogenic tumor is the odontoma, with prevalence exceeding that of all other odontogenic tumors combined. The odontoma is a hamartoma and is classified as complex or compound. The second most common odontogenic tumor is the ameloblastoma (excluding the KCOT), with much greater morbidity and mortality than the odontoma.

2. **What is the differential diagnosis for a mixed density (radiopaque/radiolucent) lesion in the posterior mandible above the mandibular canal?**

   The two most prevalent categories are odontogenic and fibro-osseous. Odontogenic etiology includes odontoma (mixed density if still forming), ameloblastic fibro-odontoma (usually in children), adenomatoid odontogenic tumor (usually in teenagers), osteoblastoma (younger patients), cementoblastoma (attached to tooth root), calcifying epithelial odontogenic tumor, calcifying odontogenic cyst, and developing tooth. Fibro-osseous etiology includes cement-osseous dysplasia, fibrous dysplasia (disease **of** bone = indistinct lesion margins), and ossifying fibroma (disease **in** bone = distinct lesion margins). If the radiographic border of the lesion is poorly demarcated, consider osteomyelitis, metastatic carcinoma, osteosarcoma/osteochondroma.

3. **What if the same lesion crosses the mandibular midline?**

   Cement-osseous dysplasia, osteomyelitis, metastatic carcinoma, osteosarcoma.

4. **What is the differential diagnosis for a multilocular radiolucency in the posterior mandible above the mandibular canal?**

   Keratocystic odontogenic tumor, ameloblastoma, myxoma (stepladder appearance with perpendicular trabeculae), idiopathic bone cavity (traumatic bone cyst is an incorrect term as there is no cyst lining), and cherubism (bilateral).

5. **Define the following terms: *enucleation, curettage, peripheral ostectomy, linear margins,* and *anatomic margins.***

   - *Enucleation*: removal of the soft tissue lining and cyst/tumor produced by the lesion from its bony cavity
   - *Curettage*: using a curette to scrape or scoop the soft tissue and some hard tissue produced by the lesion from its bony cavity
   - *Peripheral ostectomy*: removal of a layer of hard tissue from a bony cavity (usually with a rotary handpiece and bur) after removal of all visible soft tissue
   - *Linear margin*: bony radiographic margin that is measured from the extent of the resected lesion
   - *Anatomic margin*: a distinct tissue layer or vital structure sacrificed or preserved during an ablative procedure

   Both linear and anatomic margins are planned based upon the diagnosis of the lesion. For example, ablative principles for a solid ameloblastoma of the mandible would call for 1 cm linear margins (determined radiographically) and one uninvolved anatomic barrier (i.e., a supraperiosteal dissection in the setting of cortical plate perforation).

6. **What is the incidence of development of cystic lesions around retained, asymptomatic, impacted mandibular third molars?**

   According to various literature reports, it ranges from 0.3% to 37%.

7. **Is it necessary to remove teeth that are in close association with a cyst?**
   Appropriate imaging techniques should be obtained to ascertain that teeth are indeed involved by the lesion. Usually teeth with displaced but intact roots can be treated endodontically and preserved. Teeth showing root resorption should be extracted. The removal of teeth associated with odontogenic keratocysts is appropriate to prevent recurrence.

8. **What is the accepted diameter required to radiographically diagnose a nasopalatine duct cyst?**
   The nasopalatine duct cyst (NPDC) is the most common nonodontogenic cyst in the maxilla. Radiolucencies >6 mm in the area of the incisive foramen are considered pathologic. 28% of NPDCs contain respiratory epithelium on histologic analysis.

9. **How can chronic inflammation affect the prognosis of an untreated odontogenic cyst?**
   Malignant transformation is one concern when tissue is exposed to chronic inflammation. Primary intraosseous squamous cell carcinoma ex-odontogenic cyst is most commonly associated with radicular cyst, dentigerous cyst, and keratocystic odontogenic tumor. Clinical features of pain, swelling, perforation of the buccal and lingual cortical plates, and adherence of the cyst lining to the bony cavity are all suspicious for malignancy. The estimated incidence of malignant change in cysts is between 0.31% and 3%.

10. **Why was the odontogenic keratocyst (OKC) redesignated as the keratocystic odontogenic tumor (KCOT)?**
    Redesignation of the OKC as the KCOT by the World Health Organization in 2005 was due to behavior, histology, and genetics. Abnormal function of the tumor suppressor gene PTCH occurs in both nevoid basal cell carcinoma syndrome and sporadic KCOTs.

11. **How are odontogenic keratocysts treated?**
    Evidence suggests that these cysts can be managed effectively by a conservative approach. Good results have been achieved with decompression or marsupialization with or without later cystectomy, enucleation combined with excision of overlying mucosa and Carnoy solution application to the bony defect, and enucleation combined with liquid nitrogen application to the osseous cavity. It appears that although odontogenic keratocysts are notorious for their capricious nature relative to their tendency to recur, block resection of these lesions is hardly justifiable.

12. **What is the difference among a Partsch I, Partsch II, and decompression procedure?**
    A Partsch I procedure is synonymous with marsupialization. In this one-step procedure, the cystic cavity is converted into a pouch by creating a bony window over the cyst and suturing the cut edges of the cyst lining to the surrounding oral mucosa. A Partsch II procedure is enucleation of the lesion followed by primary closure. Decompression is distinguished from marsupialization by making a smaller window into the lesion and securing a tube for daily irrigation. A second surgery is necessary for definitive enucleation when using the decompression method.

13. **What are the three possible reasons for persistence of a keratocystic odontogenic tumor?**
    First, incomplete removal: KCOTs are difficult to enucleate as the epithelial lining is thin (five to eight cell layers) and friable. Multilocular lesions further complicate complete removal. Second, some authors believe daughter or satellite tumors persist within the bone beyond the perceived margin. This may explain the high recurrence rate or rather persistence for marsupialization or enucleation alone as definitive treatment. Last, epithelial remnants from the dental lamina may reside within the attached alveolar mucosa overlying the primary lesion. These harboring remnants can potentially develop into new lesions. For this reason, some authors recommended excision of the overlying mucosa in addition to the lesion.

14. **Name the five types of ameloblastomas and treatment of each.**
    See Table 44-1.

15. **What are the six histologic patterns of solid/multi-cystic ameloblastoma?**
    Follicular (most common), plexiform, acanthomatous, granular cell, desmoplastic, and basal cell (least common). The desmoplastic pattern is unique as it may present as a mixed density lesion radiographically.

Table 44-1. Types of Ameloblastomas and Treatment

AMELOBLASTOMA TYPE	DESCRIPTION	TREATMENT
Peripheral ameloblastoma	Firm, exophytic, non-ulcerative, painless gingival mass	Excision with 2 to 3 mm margins (include one uninvolved layer)
Unicystic ameloblastoma	Well-circumscribed radiolucency (90% unilocular, 10% multilocular) usually posterior mandible, associated with impacted tooth in 20 yo. **Three histologic patterns: intraluminal, luminal, and mural**	Intraluminal, luminal are enucleated (+/− curettage). Mural must be resected. Be wary of enucleate/curettage after incisional biopsy yields intraluminal or luminal as mural ameloblastoma may exist elsewhere in the cyst lining
Solid (multi-cystic) ameloblastoma	Multilocular radiolucency, posterior mandible, painless expansion in 20 to 60 yo. Desmoplastic variant can appear radiographically as mixed density lesion	Resect all **six histologic patterns** with 1 to 1.5 cm linear margins and one uninvolved anatomic layer
Malignant ameloblastoma	A **benign** ameloblastoma with **metastatic potential** whose metastatic foci will also be benign	Resection/excision of primary and metastatic tumors (see solid)
Ameloblastoma carcinoma	A **malignant** ameloblastoma with **metastatic potential** whose metastatic foci will also be malignant	Radical resection, +/− chemotherapy, +/− XRT

16. Are all unilocular radiolucent ameloblastomas unicystic?
    No. While ~90% of unilocular radiolucent ameloblastomas are unicystic, ~10% are multi-cystic. Conversely, ~10% of multilocular radiolucent ameloblastomas are unicystic.

17. What is the doubling time of ameloblastoma vs. oral cavity squamous cell carcinoma (OCSCC), and when does each most often recur?
    Doubling time of ameloblastoma is 2 to 5 years versus OCSCC ~1 month. Average recurrence of ameloblastoma is ~5 years vs. OCSSC within first year.

18. What is the recommended length of follow-up for recurrent odontogenic tumors such as ameloblastoma, myxoma, calcifying epithelial odontogenic tumor, and keratocystic odontogenic tumor?
    These lesions can recur after decades with no prior evidence of disease. Accordingly, indefinite follow-up with imaging annually for the first 5 years and biannually thereafter is prudent.

19. Why is the adenomatoid odontogenic tumor (AOT) referred to as the *lesion of two-thirds*?
    The AOT occurs during the second decade of life in two-thirds of cases, maxilla:mandible is 2:1, and F:M is 2:1. This tumor is commonly associated with an unerupted maxillary canine and can often be distinguished from a dentigerous cyst by radiolucency surrounding the apex, not just crown, of the involved tooth. The circumscribed unilocular radiolucency occasionally contains snowflake radiopacities, further differentiating the AOT from a dentigerous cyst. The thick capsule facilitates easy enucleation with almost no recurrence.

20. What histologic features are present in the calcifying epithelial odontogenic tumor (CEOT)?
    The CEOT is a slow-growing tumor of odontogenic origin. Most common between ages of 30 to 50, usually a painless, slow expansion of the posterior mandible paired with radiographic findings of a uni- or multilocular radiolucency. Radiopaque calcifications may be present. The histopathologic features are unique and may include sheets of polyhedral cells, amyloid deposits, and multiple

calcifications (Leisegang rings). After staining with Congo red, the amyloid exhibits apple-green birefringence under polarized light. Treatment involves resection with 1.0 to 1.5 cm margins.

21. **What common anatomic structures share histologic features with the odonto-genic myxoma?**
The developing dental papilla and hyper-plastic tooth follicle are strikingly similar to the myxoma microscopically. If located in the maxillary sinus, nasal polyps can also resemble myxoma. It is important to distinguish these structures using clinical and radiographic correlation. Treatment of myxoma includes surgical resection with 1.0 to 1.5 cm bony margins and one uninvolved anatomic barrier.

22. **What histologic features are present in the calcifying odontogenic cyst (COC)?**
Like the ameloblastoma, the COC is an uncommon lesion that can have cystic, solid, and peripheral variants, with the solid variant being the most aggressive. The lesion is considered by many to be a neoplasm rather than a cyst. Intraosseous lesions can be cystic or solid (neoplastic) with a very small number of solid types known to be malignant (odontogenic ghost cell carcinoma). Diagnostic histologic findings include ghost cells. 10% to 20% of COCs are involved with an odontoma.

23. **What are the two variants of ameloblastic fibroma?**
Literature suggests the ameloblastic fibroma can be categorized into neoplastic and hamartomatous variants based on clinical and radiographic features. Lesions in patients over the age of 22 are considered true neoplasms, while those in younger patients may be either true neoplasms or odontomas in early stages of development. Histologic analysis of the two are indistinguishable. Asymptomatic small unilocular lesions with no or minimal bone expansion are likely developing odontomas, while large expansile lesions with extensive bone destruction are neoplasms.

24. **Which jaw lesions include histology containing multinucleated giant cells?**
Central giant cell lesion, giant cell tumor, brown tumor of hyperparathyroidism, cherubism, and aneurysmal bone cyst

25. **Compare and contrast the aneurysmal bone cyst (ABC) with the idiopathic bone cavity (IBC).**
Both the ABC and SBC share a peak incidence in the second decade of life. Both lesions lack an epithelial lining and are not true cysts. Both have an unknown etiology, though the ABC is believed to be reactive, resulting either as a primary entity stemming from trauma or secondary to a dilated vascular bed in a preexisting bony lesion. Clinical features of both include swelling, mild painful symptoms, and vital teeth with or without tooth displacement. The IBC is located almost exclusively in the mandible, with a tendency for the body of the mandible. The ABC has predominance in the posterior mandible with more uniform distribution in the maxilla. Surgical exploration into the IBC reveals either an empty cavity or cavity filled with serosanguineous fluid. Surgically the ABC appears as a blood-soaked sponge, usually without marked hemorrhage, and is known to have a high recurrence rate.

26. **Which genetic diseases are central giant cell lesions associated with?**
The brown tumor of hyperparathyroidism associated with neurofibromatosis-1 (NFM-1), cherubism, and Noonan syndrome all are characterized by central giant cell lesions, often multifocally. For this reason, parathormone levels may be indicated with a histologic diagnosis of central giant cell lesion, as well as genetic testing to rule in/out Noonan syndrome. Noonan syndrome is an uncommon disorder characterized by short stature, short neck with webbing, deformity of the sternum, cardiac anomalies, and cryptorchidism. Craniofacial features include dysmorphism, hypertelorism, downward eye slant, ptosis, and low-set posteriorly rotated ears. Cherubism is an autosomal dominant disease process that ceases after puberty. In the absence of severe functional disturbance, treatment is usually deferred until disease stabilization and/or regression.

27. **How does one treat giant cell lesions?**
Central giant cell lesions can be aggressive or nonaggressive but share the same benign histology. Aggressive lesions tend to recur, are large, can erode teeth, and can be associated with pain. As such, nonaggressive lesions can be definitively treated with enucleation while aggressive lesions may require en bloc resection. Generally speaking, surgery and chemotherapy are indicated if patients are ≤10 years old. For patients >10 years old, only surgery is required. Adjunctive chemotherapy options include intranasal or subcutaneous calcitonin, intralesional glucocorticoids, and antiangiogenic therapy with interferon alpha.

28. What types of chemotherapy regimens are used to treat giant cell lesions?
    - *Interferon alpha*: 3 million units/m^2 SQ daily. Side effects can include fatigue, fever, headache, and hair loss. Favorable response has been reported, especially in patients <10 years old.
    - *Systemic calcitonin*: 50 IU SQ QD until tolerated, then advance to 50 IU SQ BID until tolerated, then advance to 100 IU SQ QD for 6 to 9 months (until lesion resolves radiographically). The downside to calcitonin is decreased serum Ca^{2+} levels and peptic ulcer disease.
    - *Intralesional steroids*: Weekly injections of 30 mg triamcinolone (often combined with local anesthetic) for 6 weeks. GCLs are very vascular lesions so one drawback for intralesional steroid use includes systemic absorption potentially resulting in a cushingoid response.

29. How should fibrous dysplasia be treated?
    Re-contouring is usually performed in cases in which aesthetic and functional improvement is required, but it is more effective when the dysplastic site has undergone maturation. Although complete resection of fibrous dysplasia has been decried in the past, current refined instrumentation and craniofacial surgical techniques allow a more aggressive, non-disabling approach, particularly when vital anatomic structures are affected by the lesion.

30. What surgery is indicated for osteosarcoma of the mandible?
    Wide surgical resection (2.0 to 3.0 cm margins). Adjuvant therapy has been shown to be beneficial in cases when surgical margins are positive or uncertain.

31. What are the workup and treatment for a diagnosis of solitary plasmacytoma of bone?
    A solitary plasmacytoma is a unifocal, monoclonal, neoplastic proliferation of plasma cells occurring most often within bone but may be found within soft tissue. The disease mostly affects men over the age of 50. It is rarely found in the jaws, with mandible more common than maxilla. Plasmacytosis must be ruled out with a complete radiographic survey and a bone marrow biopsy. Urine and serum electrophoresis demonstrate a monoclonal immunoglobulin M spike in up to 25% of cases. 70% of patients with solitary lesions develop multiple myeloma. Treatment of solitary plasmacytoma includes radiation therapy.

CHAPTER 45

CANCER OF THE ORAL CAVITY

David L. Hirsch, Lauren G. Bourell, Ray Cheng

1. **What is the typical presentation of oral cancer?**
   Oral cancer may present as an irregular color change or thickening in the mucosa. It may be a mass that is exophytic or endophytic, ulcerated or non-ulcerated. When larger, it is typically indurated. It may be friable and bleed and is usually, although not always, painful.

2. **What is the prevalence of oral cancer?**
   Worldwide, oral cancer is the twelfth most common cancer; all head and neck cancers combined rank fifth overall. In the US, there are about 45,000 new head and neck cancer cases per year, of which about 12,000 are oral cavity cancers. Oral cancer is more common in males by a ratio of 2:1 and most common in the fifth to sixth decades of life.

3. **What is the most common location in the oral cavity for cancer to present?**
   The most common sub-site is tongue, followed by floor of mouth. Buccal mucosa and retromolar trigone areas are next in frequency.

4. **What does TNM stand for, and what is the TNM system in reference to oral cancer?**
   Tumor Node Metastases (TNM) is a staging system for cancer of the oral cavity. TNM staging can be different in different head and neck sub-sites. (See Table 45-1.)

5. **How is oral cancer staged? What is the average 5-year survival for each stage?**
   See Table 45-2.

6. **What is the difference between clinical staging and pathologic staging?**
   Clinical staging depends on clinical examination of tumor size, palpable lymph nodes, and radiologic evidence of cervical lymph nodes and distant metastasis. Pathologic staging is determined by the size of tumor and evidence of cervical lymph nodes based on final pathology.

7. **What are the common risk factors for oral cancer?**
   Tobacco and alcohol use (which has a synergistic effect when combined with tobacco) are two of the most common risk factors for oral cancer. In parts of the world were paan or betel quid (arica nut) products are used, this is also a risk factor. Diets low in fresh fruits and vegetables are associated with an increased cancer risk as well.

8. **What is the role of HPV (human papillomavirus) in oral cancer?**
   Particular strains of the HPV, especially HPV-16, are independent risk factors for oropharyngeal squamous cell carcinoma. For oral squamous cell carcinoma, the rate of HPV+ in oral cavity cancer is significantly lower, and its association with oral cavity cancer is controversial.

9. **Which oral lesions are considered premalignant?**
   Potentially malignant lesions of the oral cavity include leukoplakia, erythroplakia, lichen planus, lichenoid reaction, submucous fibrosis, discoid lupus erythematosus, actinic keratosis, and epithelial dysplasia.

10. **What is the risk of progression to oral cancer for these premalignant lesions?**
    For leukoplakias without dysplasia and for lichen planus and lichenoid reactions, the risk of malignant transformation is <1%. Erythroplakia has a much higher rate of malignant transformation of 23.4%, while leukoplakias with dysplasia have the highest rate of transformation at 36.4%.

11. **What is the management of these premalignant lesions?**
    Smoking and alcohol cessation should be encouraged for all patients with leukoplakia. Various forms of surgical treatment, including scalpel excision, NdYAG laser or CO_2 laser-assisted excision, or photodynamic therapy, have been advocated as treatment for leukoplakia with or without evidence of dysplasia.

Table 45-1. Oral Cavity Squamous Cell Carcinoma TNM Description

PRIMARY TUMOR (T)		REGIONAL LYMPH NODES (N)		DISTANT METASTASIS (M)	
T_X	Primary tumor cannot be assessed	N_X	Regional lymph nodes cannot be assessed	M_0	No distant metastasis
T_0	No evidence of primary tumor	N_0	No regional lymph node metastasis	M_1	Distant metastasis
T_{is}	Carcinoma in situ	N_1	Met in single ipsilateral lymph node less than 3 cm		
T_1	Tumor size 2 cm or less	N_2			
T_2	Tumor size between 2 and 4 cm	N_{2a}	Met in single ipsilateral lymph node greater than 3 cm less than 6 cm		
T_3	Tumor size greater than 4 cm	N_{2b}	Multiple ipsilateral lymph nodes, none greater than 6 cm		
T_{4a}	Tumor invades adjacent structures only (cortical bone, deep extrinsic muscle of tongue, maxillary sinus, skin of face)	N_{2c}	Bilateral or contralateral lymph nodes, all less than 6 cm		
T_{4b}	Tumor invades masticator space, pterygoid plates, or skull base and/or encases internal carotid artery	N_3	Mets in lymph node greater than 6 cm in size		

From Edge SB, Byrd DR, Compton CC, et al., editors: AJCC cancer staging manual, ed 7, New York, 2010, Springer.

Table 45-2. Oral Cavity Squamous Cell Carcinoma TNM Staging

Stage	T	N	M	5-Year Survival
0	T_{is}	N_0	M_0	
I	T_1	N_0	M_0	91%
II	T_2	N_0	M_0	77%
III	T_1	N_1	M_0	61%
	T_2	N_1	M_0	
	T_3	N_1	M_0	
IVA	T_{4a}	N_0	M_0	32%
	T_{4a}	N_1	M_0	
	T_1	N_2	M_0	
	T_2	N_2	M_0	
	T_3	N_2	M_0	
	T_{4a}	N_2	M_0	
IVB	Any T	N_3	M_0	25%
	T_{4b}	Any N	M_0	
IVC	Any T	Any N	M_1	4%

From Edge SB, Byrd DR, Compton CC, et al., editors: AJCC *cancer staging manual,* ed 7, New York, 2010, Springer.

Erythroplakia and lesions demonstrating dysplasia should be treated more seriously as they carry a higher risk of malignancy. Patients with lichen planus require an initial biopsy and periodic follow-up.

12. **What is PVL (proliferative verrucous leukoplakia), and what is its premalignant potential?**
PVL is a corrugated-appearing, papillomatous lesion of the oral cavity, more common in elderly women who had leukoplakia for many years, with no etiologic factors proven to date. There is an approximately 74% rate of malignant transformation to squamous cell carcinoma or verrucous carcinoma, recurrences after treatment in 86.7% of cases, new lesions during follow-up in 83.3%, and oral cancer eventually in 63.3% with high incidence on the gingival.

13. **How does depth of invasion of cancer of the oral tongue affect prognosis?**
Tumors with greater thickness and greater depth of invasion into underlying structures represent later stage disease. Tumors with depth of invasion <4 mm have increased locoregional control and better disease-specific and overall survival compared to tumors with depth of invasion ≥4 mm, which have worse locoregional control and decreased survival. There is also an increased risk of neck metastasis with >4 mm depth of invasion. According to Shah et al. there is also an increased risk of neck recurrence in patients with low-risk T1-2 tongue cancer with >4 mm thickness who underwent partial glossectomy and ipsilateral elective neck dissection without postoperative radiation.

14. **What is the current staging system for oral cancer?**
The TNM staging system is shown in Tables 45-3 to 45-5.
Some inherent inadequacies of this system have prompted the proposal of certain modifications and revisions in an effort to enhance its prognostic significance.

15. **Which levels are commonly associated with regional metastasis from oral cavity SCC?**
Levels I-III are the most commonly involved sites in neck metastasis. Level IV only represents a very small subgroup of patients. Level IV lymph node may be at a higher risk when the presence of metastasis in levels I-III is found. Level V is an uncommon finding in oral cavity SCC but significant in other head and neck cancer sites.

Table 45-3. Tumor Classification of Cancer of the Oral Cavity

CLASS	TUMOR SIZE
T_1	≤2 cm at greatest dimension
T_2	>2 cm but ≤4 cm at greatest dimension
T_3	>4 cm at greatest dimension
T_4	Tumor invades adjacent structures

From Edge SB, Byrd DR, Compton CC, et al., editors: AJCC *cancer staging manual,* ed 7, New York, 2010, Springer.

Table 45-4. Node Classification of Cancer of the Oral Cavity

CLASS	DESCRIPTION
N_X	Regional lymph nodes cannot be assessed
N_0	No regional lymph node metastasis
N_1	Metastasis in a single ipsilateral lymph node, ≤3 cm at greatest dimension
N_2	Metastasis in a single ipsilateral lymph node, more than 3 cm but not more than 6 cm at greatest dimension *or* Multiple ipsilateral lymph nodes, none more than 6 cm at greatest dimension *or* Bilateral or contralateral lymph nodes, none more than 6 cm at greatest dimension
N_{2a}	Metastasis in a single ipsilateral lymph node, >3 cm but ≤6 cm at greatest dimension
N_{2b}	Metastasis in multiple ipsilateral lymph nodes, none >6 cm at greatest dimension
N_{2c}	Metastasis in bilateral or contralateral lymph nodes, none >6 cm at greatest dimension
N_3	Metastasis >6 cm at greatest dimension in a lymph node

From Edge SB, Byrd DR, Compton CC, et al., editors: AJCC *cancer staging manual,* ed 7, New York, 2010, Springer.

Table 45-5. Metastasis Classification of Cancer of the Oral Cavity

CLASS	DESCRIPTION
M_X	Distant metastasis cannot be assessed
M_0	No distant metastasis
M_1	Distant metastasis

From Edge SB, Byrd DR, Compton CC, et al., editors: AJCC *cancer staging manual,* ed 7, New York, 2010, Springer.

16. **What is meant by the term *neck dissection* in reference to surgical treatment of oral cancer?**
    A neck dissection is a lymphadenectomy, or removal of lymph nodes, from the cervical region of the neck extending below the mandible to just above the clavicle and posteriorly to the trapezius muscle. Depending on the type of neck dissection, the sternocleidomastoid muscle, internal jugular vein, and/or spinal accessory nerve may also be included in the neck dissection specimen. Neck dissection is a therapeutic, diagnostic, and staging procedure for the oral cancer patient.

17. **What are the types of neck dissections?**
    There are various systems for classifying neck dissections. The most aggressive approach is called a radical neck dissection. This refers to removal of all lymph nodes in the neck from levels I-V along with the SCM (sternocleidomastoid), the internal jugular, and the spinal accessory nerve. The modified radical neck dissection is a version of the radical neck that removes all lymph nodes from levels I-V but spares one (or more) of the named structures. A type I modified radical neck dissection spares the spinal accessory, type II spares the spinal accessory and the internal jugular, and type III

spares all three: spinal accessory, internal jugular, and SCM. There is also a selective neck dissection that includes removal of selected lymph nodes only, from levels of the neck most likely to be involved with a particular tumor (as an example, a selective neck dissection for an oral cavity cancer would usually include levels I–III—sometimes also referred to as a supraomohyoid neck dissection).

18. **Which patients are indicated for a neck dissection?**
Patients with clinical evidence of cervical lymph node metastasis, either a neck mass on physical exam or a positive lymph node on diagnostic imaging (>15 mm in size, central lucency, ring enhancement), are indicated for neck dissection. Patients with T2 and larger tumors usually receive an ipsilateral neck dissection, with consideration for a contralateral neck dissection if the tumor crosses the midline or if they have contralateral neck disease.

19. **What is an SLNB (sentinel lymph node biopsy) in reference to oral cancer?**
The sentinel lymph node is the first lymph node in a chain or group of lymph nodes to receive the lymphatic drainage from a tumor. This sentinel node can be identified and examined for the presence of metastatic cancer cells—the presence or absence of cancer cells in the sentinel node is taken as evidence of the likelihood that cancer has spread to the remainder of the lymph node chain. The benefit of identifying and removing the sentinel node (a sentinel node biopsy) is that for negative sentinel nodes, the patient can be spared a more invasive neck dissection procedure.

20. **Which patients benefit from this technique (SLNB)?**
SLNB does not replace traditional neck dissection and is not indicated for patients in whom a neck dissection is indicated. SLNB is best for patients with small lesions (T1, some T2) and N0 necks. Patients should be informed that, in the case of a positive SLNB, they will require a formal neck dissection.
The sensitivity of SLNB was 87.5% and 77.8% for permanent and frozen sections, respectively. The specificity was 100% for permanent and frozen sections, respectively.

21. **What are the types of imaging that may be used in the work-up of an oral cancer patient?**
Panoramic or plain radiography, CT (computed tomography), and MRI (magnetic resonance imaging) may all be used in the work-up of a patient with known or suspected oral cancer. Imaging of the chest with plain film or CT scan should also be done initially to rule out metastatic or second primary disease.
Panoramic radiography has good specificity for bony invasion but poor sensitivity and is useful for imaging the dentition and for periapical/periodontal infections that may be missed by traditional CT.
CT scan has 100% specificity for bony invasion. Intravenous contrast is needed to assess nodal metastasis in the neck. Dental restoration can adversely affect the quality of imaging.
MRI also has 100% specificity for bony invasion and is slightly more sensitive than traditional CT scan. MRI may be degraded by motion artifact, and MRI may overestimate bony involvement if edema is present. MRI is suitable for soft tissue imaging of the primary tumor and cervical lymph nodes (with contrast).

22. **What are the primary treatment modalities of oral cancer?**
The preferred treatment for oral cancer is surgical resection, followed by radiation or radiation plus chemotherapy as needed for high-risk patients. Radiation as a primary treatment for oral cancer has a small role, although cancers of the oropharynx, larynx, and hypopharynx are more often treated with radiation as the primary modality.
Randomized controlled trials comparing surgery to radiation for treatment of oral cancer (T2+ lesions) were terminated early due to markedly poorer outcomes in the radiation treatment arm; in general, the overall survival and disease-free survival of patients receiving primary radiation therapy for oral cancer is roughly half that of those receiving surgery as their primary modality of treatment.

23. **What is the accepted margin of normal (uninvolved) tissue surrounding a tumor that a surgeon proposes to take during surgical resection of an oral cancer?**
A margin of 1 to 1.5 cm circumferentially around a tumor is the goal during resection of oral cancer. In reality, this margin may not be achievable due to proximity of vital structures. Furthermore, there is a considerable specimen shrinkage after resection and fixation of tissue that can vary in surgical site. Mistry et al. found mean shrinkage of tumor margins for tongue and buccal specimen were 23.5% and 21%, respectively. Less shrinkage is appreciated in higher stage T3/T4 than for lower stage T1/T2 tumors.

24. What is meant by the terms *adjuvant* and *neo-adjuvant* treatment in reference to oral cancer treatment?

    Adjuvant treatment includes radiation or radiation plus chemotherapy that is given after surgery. Neo-adjuvant treatment for oral cancer refers to chemotherapy alone given prior to planned surgery. The use of RT before surgery in head and neck cancer has been abandoned due to poor treatment outcome as found in RTOG 73-03.

25. What types of adjuvant treatments are available for oral cancer?

    Radiation is the main adjuvant treatment that is recommended to patients. Chemotherapy is sometimes given concurrently with adjuvant radiation (positive postoperative margin and extra-capsular spread in metastatic lymph node). It is currently recommended that radiation therapy commence within 6 weeks after surgery and that the entire radiation treatment be completed within 100 days. This recommendation is based on data demonstrating worse locoregional control and poorer outcomes when radiation therapy was delayed or the treatment course prolonged.

26. Which types of patients are typically recommended to receive adjunctive radiation therapy or chemotherapy?

    Patients are candidates for adjuvant radiation if they have perineural invasion, cervical lymph node metastasis, and late-stage and bulky tumors (stages III-IV). Adjuvant radiation improves locoregional control of oral cancer and increases overall survival. According to results from RTOG 9501 and EROTC 22931 studies, patients with extra-capsular extension of disease or microscopic evidence of tumor at the resection margins are candidate to receive concomitant chemotherapy and radiation.

27. What are some of the key differences between traditional radiotherapy and IMRT (intensity modulated radiotherapy) as it relates to oral cancer?

    IMRT uses three-dimensional CT-based mapping of the tumor site to design a radiation treatment plan that attempts to spare vital structures such as major salivary glands while still delivering the total treatment dose to critical areas such as the tumor bed. The appeal of IMRT is the promise of equal efficacy as conventional radiation therapy with fewer side effects such as hyposalivation and trismus. Studies have generally shown good efficacy, although data is mixed about benefits of IMRT regarding side effects. The cost of IMRT is more than traditional radiotherapy.

28. Which chemotherapeutic agents are most commonly given?

    Commonly given agents include the platinum agents such as cisplatin and carboplatin (radiation sensitizers). 5-fluorouracil and docetaxel are the other commonly used agents. The biological agent cetuximab (brand name Erbitux) is also used in head and neck cancer. Cetuximab is an EGFR (epidermal growth factor receptor) inhibitor. Currently, it is used together with cisplatin or radiation therapy for non-resectable or recurrent disease.

29. What is the most important prognostic factor regarding survival in oral cancer?

    The most important prognostic factor is the presence or absence of cervical lymph node metastasis. The presence of cervical lymph node metastasis decreases 5-year survival by 50%. Extracapsular extension is the second most important prognostic factor since it significantly lowers 5-year survival by decreasing regional control and requires addition of chemotherapy to treatment regimen.

30. What is the average survival time after diagnosis of distant metastasis in oral squamous cancers?

    Survival time after the discovery of distant metastasis is typically less than 6 months.

31. What is the follow-up schedule for patients after they have finished active treatment (surgery/radiation/etc.) for oral cancer?

    Oral cancer patients require close follow-up after they have completed treatment for their malignancy. This follow-up should include regular head and neck exams, supplemented by FDL (fiberoptic direct laryngoscopy) or DL (direct laryngoscopy) as indicated, and appropriate imaging studies. Patients should have follow-up with any specialists necessary for their ongoing care, particularly speech and swallow pathologists, radiation oncologists, medical oncologists, and their primary care providers both medical and dental. Typical follow-up protocol calls for monthly follow-up for the first 2 years, with increasing intervals through 5 years.

32. **What is the role of PET/CT in post-cancer surveillance?**

PET/CT has a role in helping to detect early recurrence in head and neck cancer patients. Traditional CT may be difficult to interpret in these patients due to anatomic changes that occur post-surgically and post-radiotherapy—the addition of PET can aid in distinguishing new lesions of concern. PET scan is based on the fundamental principal of higher metabolic activity of tumor cells compared to that in normal tissue. An area with increased glucose uptake is correlated with the presence of cancer cells.

BIBLIOGRAPHY

Ang KK, Trotti A, Brown BW, et al.: Randomized trial addressing risk features and time factors of surgery plus radiotherapy in advanced head-and-neck cancer, *Int J Radiat Oncol Biol Phys* 51:571–578, 2001.

Bagan J, Scully C, Jimenez Y, Martorell M: Proliferative verrucous leukoplakia: a concise update, *Oral Dis* 16:328–332, 2010.

Centers for Disease Control and Prevention (CDC): Human papillomavirus–associated cancers—United States, 2004-2008, *MMWR* 61(15):258–261, 2012.

Ganly I, Goldstein D, Carlson DL, et al.: Long-term regional control and survival in patients with "low-risk," early stage oral tongue cancer managed by partial glossectomy and neck dissection without postoperative radiation. The importance of tumor thickness, *Cancer* 119:1168–1176, 2013.

Glenny AM, Furness S, Worthington HV, et al.: The CSROC Expert Panel. Interventions for the treatment of oral cavity and oropharyngeal cancer: radiotherapy, *Cochrane Database of Sys Rev*, 2010. Issue 12, Art. No.: CD006387.

Kademani D, Dierks E: Management of locoregional recurrence in oral squamous cell carcinoma, *Oral Maxillofac Surg Clin N Am* 18:615–625, 2006.

Lingen MW, Xiao W, Schmitt A, et al.: Low etiologic fraction for high-risk human papillomavirus in oral cavity squamous cell carcinomas, *Oral Oncol* 49:1–8, 2013.

Morris LG, Sikora AG, Patel SG, et al.: Second primary cancers after an index head and neck cancer: subsite-specific trends in the era of human papillomavirus-associated oropharyngeal cancer, *J Clin Oncol* 29(6):739–744, February 2011.

National Comprehensive Cancer Network (NCCN). NCCN clinical practice guidelines in oncology. http://www.nccn.org/professionals/physician_gls/f_guidelines.asp (accessed on April 01, 2014).

Parsons JT, Mendenhall WM, Stringer SP, et al.: An analysis of factors influencing the outcome of postoperative irradiation for squamous cell carcinoma of the oral cavity, *Int J Radiat Oncol Biol Phys* 39(1):137–148, 1997.

Schiff PB, Harrison LB, Strong EW, et al.: Impact of the time interval between surgery and postoperative radiation therapy on locoregional control in advanced head and neck cancer, *J Surg Oncol* 43:203–208, 1990.

Silverman S, Gorsky M, Lozada F: Oral leukoplakia and malignant transformation, a follow-up study of 257 patients, *Cancer* 53:563–568, 1984.

Weinstock YE, Alava I, Dierks EJ: Pitfalls in determining head and neck surgical margins, *Oral Maxillofacial Surg Clin N Am* 26:151–162, 2014.

Weiss MH, Harrison LB, Isaacs RS: Use of decision analysis in planning a management strategy for the stage N0 neck, *Arch Otolaryngol Head Neck Surg* 12:699–702, 1994.

CHAPTER 46

SALIVARY GLAND DISEASES

Christos A. Skouteris

1. **What are the appropriate diagnostic methods in evaluating salivary obstruction?**
   Clinical Exam
   - Palpation of the gland
   - Bimanual palpation along the course of the duct
   - Visual confirmation of diminished or absent salivary flow
   - Assessment of the type of any ductal discharge
   Sialoendoscopy (used for diagnosis and treatment of sialolithiasis)
   Imaging Techniques
   - Plain films: occlusal, frontal, lateral, lateral oblique, and panoramic views
   - Sialography: contraindicated in the presence of acute sialadenitis and when sialoliths have been positively identified on clinical exam and plain films
   - Ultrasonography
   - Computed tomography (CT): useful in identifying parenchymal or extraparenchymal masses that can cause obstruction by pressure or ductal invasion
   - Radionuclide scanning: evaluates the effect of the obstruction on glandular dynamics and function

2. **Can peripheral facial nerve paralysis be a sign of nonmalignant conditions affecting the parotid gland?**
   Yes. It has been reported that peripheral facial nerve paralysis can be associated with acute suppurative parotitis, nonspecific parotitis with inflammatory pseudotumor, amyloidosis, and sarcoidosis of the parotid.

3. **Is fine-needle aspiration biopsy (FNAB) efficacious in the diagnosis of salivary gland pathology? Would it change the course of management?**
   Refinements in sampling techniques and specimen preparation, as well as improvements in cytologic interpretation, have considerably increased the diagnostic value of FNAB in the evaluation of salivary pathology. The specificity of the procedure ranges from 96% to 100%, and the sensitivity is 85% to 99%.
   FNAB changed the clinical approach in 35% of patients in a study by Heller et al. It aided in avoiding surgical resection of lymphomas and inflammatory masses, in adopting a more conservative approach for benign tumors in elderly and high surgical risk patients, and in better preoperative counseling of patients regarding the nature of the tumor, the likely extent of the resection, the management of the facial nerve, and the possible need for a neck dissection.

4. **Is incisional biopsy indicated for the diagnosis of pathologic conditions of the parotid gland?**
   Yes, it is indicated for the diagnosis of suspected systemic disease with parotid involvement, particularly when FNAB findings are inconclusive. Systemic conditions in which incisional parotid biopsy can be of great diagnostic value include sarcoidosis, Sjögren's syndrome, lymphoma, and sialosis.

5. **What are the clinical manifestations of a tumor involving the deep lobe of the parotid?**
   Tumors of the deep parotid lobe can grow undetected until they are large and clinically evident. In cases in which the tumor has grown into the lateral pharyngeal space, a bulging in the lateral pharyngeal wall can be seen. Extensive tumors in this anatomic location can displace the soft palate and uvula, with resultant difficulties in speech, breathing, and deglutition.

6. **What are the contemporary imaging modalities for visualizing tumors of the major salivary glands?**
   - CT
   - MR sialography
   - CT sialography
   - Positron emission tomography (PET)

- Magnetic resonance imaging (MRI)
- Ultrasound

7. **Are sialoliths always visible on radiographs?**
No. Sialoliths in the early stage of development are quite small and not adequately mineralized to be visible radiographically. It has also been reported in the literature that 30% to 50% of parotid and 10% to 20% of submandibular sialoliths are radiolucent. These radiolucent sialoliths can be visualized indirectly by the imaging defect that they produce on sialography, or directly through sialoendoscopy.

8. **What methods are used for the treatment of sialolithiasis?**
Transoral removal of palpable sialoliths should be considered as the treatment of choice in patients suffering from submandibular stones located within either the floor of the mouth or the perihilar region of the gland. Methods include:
- Stone removal through sialoendoscopy
- Extracorporeal shockwave lithotripsy
- Intracorporeal shockwave lithotripsy (endoscopically controlled, stone fragmentation via laser or pneumoballistic energy)
- Fluoroscopically guided basket retrieval
- Laser surgery for sialolithiasis (sialolithectomy with CO_2 laser)

There is increasing evidence to show that the submandibular gland regains function after stone removal, and sialoadenectomy may not be the treatment of choice for proximal calculi. In cases of severely impacted hilar calculi or intraparenchymal calculi that are associated with frequent recurrent episodes of sialadenitis, excision of the submandibular gland or superficial parotidectomy is warranted. Submandibular sialoadenectomy can be accomplished through the conventional cervical approach or, more recently, by intraoral or extraoral endoscopic excision.

9. **What is considered an effective method for the treatment of salivary duct stenosis?**
Strictures of the submandibular or parotid duct can be treated by balloon dilatation of the duct under fluoroscopic guidance (per oral balloon sialoplasty).

10. **What types of lesions can result from mucous escape?**
Mucoceles and ranulae.

11. **What are the different types of clinical presentation of a ranula?**
A ranula can present as a floor-of-the-mouth swelling, as a plunging ranula with an intraoral and a cervical component, and as a purely cervical ranula without an intraoral component. An extreme case of ranula is the thoracic ranula, which can originate in the submandibular area and extend into the subcutaneous tissue planes of the anterior chest wall.

12. **What are the treatment modalities for the different types of ranulae?**
Intraoral ranula:
- Excision (for small lesions) ± excision of sublingual salivary gland
- Marsupialization (for larger lesions) ± excision of the sublingual salivary gland
- Cryotherapy
- Laser ablation (CO_2) or laser excision (diode)
- Hydrodissection
- Intracystic injection of the streptococcal preparation OK-432

Excision, wherever feasible, or marsupialization with excision of the sublingual salivary gland is the preferred method for the treatment of floor of the mouth ranulae, especially in recurrent cases.
Plunging ranula:
- Intraoral marsupialization with excision of the sublingual gland (preferred method)
- Extraoral removal of lesion with excision of the sublingual gland
- Intraoral fenestration and continuous pressure
- Intralesional injection of OK-432

Cervical ranula: excision of lesion and sublingual salivary gland through a cervical approach

13. **How can you differentiate between viral and bacterial parotitis?**
Viral parotitis infection is bilateral and is preceded by prodromal signs and symptoms of 1 to 2 days' duration, including fever, malaise, loss of appetite, chills, headache, sore throat, and preauricular tenderness. Purulent discharge from Stensen's duct is rare but, if present, might be the result of the development of secondary bacterial sialadenitis. Lab investigations reveal elevated serum titers for mumps or influenza virus, leukopenia, relative lymphocytosis, and high levels of serum amylase.

14. **How is acute bacterial parotitis diagnosed?**
    - History, with emphasis on diabetes, dehydration, malnutrition, immunosuppressive therapy, antisialic drugs, debilitating systemic disease, and recent surgery
    - Physical exam, including palpation and observation for purulent ductal discharge
    - Imaging, including ultrasound and CT
    - Culture of purulent discharge and antibiotic sensitivity testing

15. **What are the most common causes of xerostomia?**
    Xerostomia can be idiopathic, drug-induced, radiation-induced, or the principal manifestation of primary and secondary Sjögren's syndrome.

16. **Is there an association between salivary disease and AIDS?**
    Yes. Conditions affecting the salivary glands in AIDS patients include parotid lymphoepithelial lesions, cysts, lymphadenopathy, Kaposi's sarcoma, AIDS-related intraglandular lymphoma, salmonella and cytomegalovirus parotitis, and a Sjögren's syndrome-like condition with xerostomia.

17. **What syndromes can affect the salivary glands?**
    Primary Sjögren's syndrome is usually characterized by parotid and lacrimal gland enlargement, xerostomia, and xerophthalmia. Secondary Sjögren's syndrome involves autoimmune parotitis that occurs with rheumatoid arthritis, lupus, systemic sclerosis, thyroiditis, primary biliary cirrhosis, and mixed collagen disease. Sarcoidosis may involve the parotid gland. Sarcoidosis of the parotid gland, along with fever, lacrimal adenitis, uveitis, and facial nerve paralysis, is called Heerfordt's syndrome. Recently, a sicca syndrome-like condition has been recognized in HIV-positive children. This condition presents with parotid gland enlargement, xerostomia, and lymphadenopathy.

18. **What are the signs and symptoms of salivary gland malignancy?**
    Rapid tumor growth or a sudden growth acceleration in a long-standing salivary mass, pain, peripheral facial nerve paralysis, skin involvement, nodal metastasis, and history of cutaneous cancer (scalp, face, ear, lids).

19. **Can ultrasonography, CT, MRI, and PET scanning distinguish between benign and malignant salivary gland tumors?**
    Ultrasonography can be useful in differentiating between benign and malignant tumors. Recent evidence suggests that malignant tumors (with the exception of lymphomas) are characterized sonographically by attenuation of posterior echoes, whereas benign tumors exhibit distal echo enhancement. CT can effectively differentiate among benign, malignant, and inflammatory lesions in approximately 75% of cases. MRI appears to be the most suitable for evaluation of salivary gland tumors, especially malignant tumors. However, PET scanning is not able to distinguish between benign and malignant tumors. Recently, new MR technologies such as dynamic contrast-enhanced MRI (DCE-MRI), diffusion-weighted MRI (DW-MRI), and proton MR spectroscopy (MRS) have shown promising results in the differentiation between benign and malignant salivary gland tumors. Malignant salivary gland tumors can be differentiated from pleomorphic adenomas but not from Wharthin's tumors using DCE-MRI at a time of peak enhancement of 120 seconds. A washout ratio of 30% enabled the additional differentiation between malignant and Wharthin's tumors. Using time-signal intensity curves on the basis of time to peak enhancement of 120 seconds and a washout ratio of 30% had high sensitivity (91%) and specificity (91%) in the differentiation between benign and malignant tumors.

20. **What is the role of radionuclide imaging in the diagnosis of salivary gland pathology?**
    In addition to assessing salivary function, salivary scintigraphy can be useful in the diagnosis of acute and chronic sialadenitis of specific or nonspecific etiology, abscesses, lymphomas, and tumors. In salivary neoplasia, radionuclide imaging can identify glandular masses >1 cm in diameter, distinguish between certain tumor types based on their specific uptake characteristics, and, in some instances, differentiate benign from malignant disease.

21. **What is the most common benign tumor of minor and major salivary glands?**
    Pleomorphic adenoma.

22. **What are the most important histologic features associated with the incidence of recurrence of pleomorphic adenoma?**
    Hypocellular pleomorphic adenomas often have a thin capsule and constitute the most frequently encountered histologic type in recurrence. Pseudopodia—fingerlike tumor extensions outside the pseudocapsule—are considered to be an additional factor in recurrence.

23. **What is the incidence of tumors affecting the sublingual salivary glands?**
Sublingual salivary gland tumors comprise <1% of all salivary gland neoplasms. These tumors are predominantly malignant (>80%) and are usually adenoid cystic or mucoepidermoid carcinomas.

24. **What are the most common malignant tumors of minor and major salivary glands?**
    • Mucoepidermoid carcinoma in the parotid gland
    • Adenoid cystic carcinoma in the submandibular, sublingual, and minor salivary glands

25. **What is the incidence of metastatic neck disease in patients with malignant salivary tumors?**
In a large series of patients with malignant tumors of the parotid, submandibular, sublingual, and minor salivary glands, the reported overall incidence of metastatic cervical lymphadenopathy was 15.3%. Parotid cancer is associated with metastatic lymph node involvement in 18% to 25% of cases.

26. **Is it possible to determine accurately the actual clinical extent of an adenoid cystic carcinoma? Why?**
No. Adenoid cystic carcinoma tends to spread perineurally. Therefore, it can extend well beyond its primary location. The terms *perineural invasion* (PNI), *neurotropism,* and *perineural spread* (PNS) are used to describe perineural tumor growth. An important distinction has been made in the literature between PNI, which is a microscopic finding of tumor cells infiltrating or associated with small nerves (which cannot be radiologically imaged) and PNS, which describes the presence of gross tumor spread along a nerve, at least in part distinct from the main tumor mass. Adenoid cystic carcinoma has less of a tendency for PNI and more of PNS, whereas polymorphous low-grade adenocarcinoma (PLGA) and salivary duct carcinoma (SDC) have a tendency for PNI rather than PNS.

27. **Are there central (intraosseous) salivary tumors?**
Yes. Although rare, salivary tumors arising in the maxilla and mandible have been reported. These tumors are thought to derive from heterotopic salivary gland inclusions and are mostly mucoepidermoid carcinomas. However, other salivary malignancies, such as acinic cell carcinoma, clear cell carcinoma, and myoepithelial carcinoma in pleomorphic adenoma, have also been reported to occur centrally within the jaws.

28. **What types of surgical procedures can be used for the management of benign and malignant tumors of the parotid?**
    • Extracapsular excision or lumpectomy—tumor removal with a safety margin without facial nerve dissection
    • Partial superficial parotidectomy—tumor removal with adequate cuff of normal parotid tissue. No need for dissection of the full facial nerve or excision of the entire superficial lobe. Indicated for small, localized, benign tumors of the parotid (usually tail)
    • Superficial parotidectomy—with preservation of the facial nerve. Indicated for large benign tumors of the superficial lobe
    • Deep lobe parotidectomy—with facial nerve preservation. Indicated for benign deep lobe tumors
    • Total parotidectomy—indicated for tumors extending to the deep lobe and for malignant tumors
    • Extended parotidectomy—indicated in cases of malignant tumors with invasion of skin, ear and temporal bone, mandible, parapharyngeal space, and infratemporal fossa
Total or extended parotidectomy for malignancies can be combined with selective or radical neck dissection. When the facial nerve is involved or is in close proximity to the tumor, its sacrifice is inevitable, and nerve repair may be followed by immediate or late nerve grafting.

29. **Which are the surgical approaches for parotidectomy?**
    1. Preauricular transcervical incision
    2. Rytidectomy (face lift) incision

30. **What are the most reliable anatomic landmarks in locating the main trunk of the facial nerve during parotid surgery?**
Recent studies have shown that the tympanomastoid fissure is the most reliable landmark in locating the main trunk of the facial nerve. An almost equally dependable anatomic landmark is the tragal cartilage pointer. Main trunk distance from anatomic landmarks:
Posterior belly of digastric muscle: 5.5 ± 2.1 mm
The tragal pointer: 6.9 ± 1.8 mm

The junction between the bony and cartilaginous ear canal: 10.9 ± 1.7 mm

The tympanomastoid fissure: 2.5 ± 0.4 mm

In general, the facial nerve will be found running deep to the tissue between the pointer and the mastoid attachment of the posterior belly of the digastric muscle. The nerve also lies superficial to the retromandibular vein and the stylomastoid artery lies superficial to the nerve as it enters the gland.

If great difficulty is encountered in locating the main trunk of the facial nerve, retrograde dissection of peripheral branches is a viable option.

31. **Are there any imaging techniques for visualization of the facial nerve?**
High-resolution MRI using a three-dimensional Fourier transform gradient-echo sequence is able to visualize the facial nerve in its course from the stylomastoid foramen to the level of the retromandibular vein. However, this technique, as well as others, has not been successful in visualizing the intraparotid divisions and course of the nerve, which are of great clinical importance. Another recently introduced modality for preoperative visualization of the facial nerve is diffusion tensor (DT) tractography that may be useful for assessing facial nerve course and displacement.

32. **Is there a role for intraoperative frozen-section evaluation of tumors of the major salivary glands?**
Yes. When FNA biopsy is inconclusive and because open biopsy is not indicated, intraoperative frozen sections might provide information that can modify the treatment plan. Frozen section is more accurate in the evaluation of benign tumors, whereas its sensitivity for malignancy is 61.5% and its specificity is 98%.

33. **What is Frey's syndrome?**
A late complication of parotidectomy. The syndrome of gustatory sweating was first described by Łucja Frey-Gottesman, a Polish neurologist, in 1923. Its incidence varies considerably in the literature, ranging from 1.7% to 97.6%. More recent studies report an incidence of 23%. The pathophysiology of the syndrome is related to the aberrant cross-reinnervation between the postganglionic secretomotor parasympathetic fibers to the parotid gland by the auriculotemporal nerve and the postganglionic sympathetic fibers supplying the sweat glands, subdermal vascular plexus, and piloerector muscles of the skin.

34. **What is the role of radiation and chemotherapy in the management of malignant salivary gland tumors?**
Postoperative radiation therapy should be administered when the tumor is high stage or high grade, the adequacy of resection is in question, or the tumor has ominous pathologic features. Neutron beam therapy shows promise in controlling locoregional disease but requires further study. Currently, chemotherapy is clearly indicated only for palliation in patients with recurrent or unresectable disease.

35. **What are the most common nonneoplastic salivary gland pathology in children?**
   - Acute viral sialadenitis
   - Sialolithiasis
   - Acute bacterial sialadenitis
   - Mucoceles

36. **Which are the most common salivary neoplasms in children?**
Hemangiomas and lymphangiomas of the salivary glands, followed by pleomorphic adenomas, are the most common benign tumors. Malignant neoplasms are very rare, but the rate of malignancy in children is much higher than in adults. The most common malignant salivary tumor is mucoepidermoid carcinoma, followed by acinic cell carcinoma.

BIBLIOGRAPHY

Carlson ER: The comprehensive management of salivary gland pathology. In *Oral and maxillofacial clinics of North America*, vol 7. Philadelphia, PA, 1995, Saunders.

Carvalho MB, Soares JM, et al.: Perioperative frozen section examination in parotid gland tumors, *Sao Paolo Med J* 117:233, 1999.

Iizuka K, Ishikawa K: Surgical techniques for benign parotid tumors: segmental resection vs extracapsular lumpectomy, *Acta Otolaryngol Suppl* 537:75, 1998.

Shintani S, Matsuura H: Fine needle aspiration of salivary gland tumors, *Int J Oral Maxillofac Surg* 26:284, 1997.

Spiro RH: Treating tumors of the sublingual glands, including a useful technique for repair of the floor of the mouth after resection, *Am J Surg* 170:457, 1995.

Spiro RH: Management of malignant tumors of the salivary glands, *Oncology* 12:671, 1998.

Witt RL: Facial nerve function after partial superficial parotidectomy, *Otolaryngol Head Neck Surg* 121:210, 1999.

CHAPTER 47

VASCULAR ANOMALIES

Shelly Abramowicz, Arin K. Greene

1. **What is the difference between an infantile hemangioma and a vascular malformation?**
   Infantile hemangioma is a benign vascular tumor that rapidly grows during the first few months of age and then regresses after infancy. Vascular malformations occur as result of abnormal embryonic development—they are present at birth, slowly progress over the life of the patient, and never regress.

2. **Which children have highest incidence of hemangioma?**
   Caucasian, premature (less than 1200 g), female.

3. **How many infants have multiple hemangiomas? Where are they located?**
   Approximately 20% have more than 1 skin lesion. Infants with more than 5 cutaneous hemangiomas have a 16% risk of having a hepatic hemangioma.

4. **How are vascular malformations categorized?**
   Based on the primary type of vessel that is affected: capillary malformation, lymphatic malformation, venous malformation, or arteriovenous malformation.

5. **Can you describe the life cycle of infantile hemangioma?**
   - Proliferating phase (2 weeks of age to 9 months)
   - Involuting phase (12 months to 4 years)
   - Involuted phase (>4 years of age)

6. **What is Kasabach-Merritt phenomenon?**
   - Profound thrombocytopenia (<10,000 mm^3)
   - Petechiae
   - Bleeding
   - Affects 50% of infants with kaposiform hemangioendothelioma (it is not associated with infantile hemangioma)

7. **What is PHACE association?**
   Plaque-like hemangioma in a segmental/trigeminal dermatomal distribution of the face with at least one of the following: **P**osterior fossa brain malformation, **H**emangioma, **A**rterial cerebrovascular anomalies, **C**oarctation of aorta and cardiac defects, **E**ye/**E**ndocrine abnormalities. Affects approximately 2% of patients with hemangiomas.

8. **What are congenital hemangiomas? What are the two types?**
   These are fully grown at birth and do not enlarge postnatally. Unlike infantile hemangioma, they are more likely to be located on the trunk or extremities. They are purpler than infantile hemangioma and often have a peripheral pale halo.
   There are two types: RICH and NICH.
   - Rapidly involuting congenital hemangioma (RICH) involutes immediately after birth and is completely regressed by 14 months of age.
   - Non-involuting congenial hemangioma (NICH) remains unchanged over the patient's life and does not regress.

9. **How are hemangiomas managed nonsurgically?**
   - Ninety percent of lesions are simply observed as they enlarge and then regress because most are small, localized, and do not involve aesthetically or functionally important areas.
   - Ulcerated lesions are managed with local wound care (e.g., hydrated petroleum, topical antibiotic ointment, and dressing changes).
   - Small, localized problematic lesions at risk for causing a significant deformity or obstructing a vital structure are managed by intralesional corticosteroid injection (triamcinolone <3 mg/kg). Patients may require additional injections every 4 to 6 weeks during the rapid growth phase.

- Problematic infantile hemangiomas that are too large to be treated with a corticosteroid injection are managed with either oral prednisolone (initiated at 3 mg/kg/day) or propranolol (2 mg/kg/day). Pharmacotherapy is discontinued at approximately 10 months of age when the hemangioma is no longer proliferating.

10. **How are infantile hemangiomas managed surgically?**
Resection is rarely indicated during the proliferative phase because the lesion is very vascular. Indications include a problematic lesion that has failed pharmacotherapy.

 Ideally, operative intervention for infantile hemangiomas is reserved for a residual deformity after the tumor has finished involuting between 3 and 4 years of age. At this time, the lesion is much less vascular, and the procedure is safer. Approximately 50% of hemangiomas leave behind a permanent deformity following involution (e.g., scarred skin, fibrofatty tissue, anetoderma, or damaged structures).

11. **What are potential local/systemic complications associated with vascular malformations?**
 - Local complications: destruction of anatomic structures, infection, obstruction, pain, thrombosis, ulceration, disfigurement
 - Systemic complications: disseminated intravascular coagulation, pulmonary embolism, thrombocytopenia, congestive heart failure

12. **What is capillary malformation (CM)?**
A capillary malformation (also known as port-wine stain) is present at birth and persists throughout life. It appears as a macular pink stain that blanches with pressure and can occur anywhere on the body. Over time, the lesion darkens to deep purple, the skin thickens, and multiple nodular fibrovascular lesions appear.

13. **What is Sturge-Weber syndrome?**
CM in ophthalmic and/or maxillary trigeminal nerve distribution associated with leptomeningeal capillary and venous anomalies and vascular lesions of ocular choroid. Potential for refractory seizures, hemiplegia, and variable delayed motor and cognitive development.

14. **What oral/dental manifestations are associated with facial CM?**
Possible overgrowth of facial soft tissues and skeleton in area of stain. Intraorally, there is potential for gingival overgrowth and pyogenic granulomas. Good oral hygiene and regular dental cleanings are most important in preventing complications.

15. **What special precautions are necessary for oral procedures in areas associated with facial CM?**
None. Procedures such as gingivectomy, extraction, and/or osteotomies can be done without concern for excessive bleeding.

16. **What is management of facial CM?**
Pulsed-dye laser (multiple treatments), contour resection of labial ptosis, and/or orthognathic surgery depending on extent of soft tissue and skeletal involvement/hypertrophy.

17. **What is the etiology of lymphatic malformation (LM)?**
LM results from an error in the embryonic development of the lymphatic system. Lymphatics may become separated from primitive lymph sacs or from the main lymphatic channels. Lymphatic tissue also may form in an abnormal location.

18. **What can cause sudden increase in size of LM?**
Viral/bacterial infection anywhere in the body.

19. **What complications can occur with LM?**
 - Intralesional bleeding (spontaneous or because of local trauma)
 - Infection

20. **What is the management of LM?**
 - Observation (small/asymptomatic lesions)
 - Prophylactic antibiotics for patients with more than three infections/year
 - CO_2 laser or radiofrequency ablation to treat intraoral vesicles that are bleeding or leaking
 - Sclerotherapy for macrocystic LMs, which involves aspiration of the cyst(s) followed by injection of an inflammatory sclerosant that causes shrinkage and scarring of the lesion. Sclerosants that are commonly used include ethanol, sodium tetradecyl sulfate, doxycycline, and OK-432.

- Resection is generally reserved for symptomatic macrocystic lesions that can no longer be sclerosed or for microcystic LMs that are not amenable to sclerotherapy.

21. **What is a venous malformation (VM)?**
Developmental abnormality of veins composed of thin-walled, dilated, abnormal channels of variable size and mural thickness. Normal endothelial lining and deficient smooth muscle. They grow proportionately to the child and can expand during puberty. They are easily compressible and enlarge when the affected area is dependent.

22. **How can craniofacial structures be affected by VM?**
Can progressively distort facial features by causing skeletal changes and hypertrophy with/without intraosseous involvement. Oral VMs can cause malocclusion, cross-bite, and/or open bite deformity because of mass effect.

23. **How are VMs managed?**
- Asymptomatic lesions can be observed.
- First-line therapy for symptomatic lesions is sclerotherapy (usually 1% sodium tetradecyl sulfate) that causes cellular destruction, thrombosis, and inflammation; resulting scarring shrinks the lesion.
- Small, localized lesions can be treated without image guidance.
- Large VMs require fluoroscopy and treatment by an interventional radiologist. VMs usually require multiple treatments because recanalization causes re-expansion.
- Resection is generally reserved for symptomatic lesions that no longer can be treated with sclerotherapy.

24. **What can cause enlargement of VMs?**
Intralesional clotting, trauma, puberty, pregnancy.

25. **What is an arteriovenous malformation (AVM)?**
AVM results from an error in vascular development during embryogenesis. It is composed of abnormal communications between arteries and veins without normal intervening capillary bed.

26. **What is the Schobinger system?**
Clinical staging system for AVMs. Four stages: quiescence, expansion, destruction, and decompensation.

27. **What does each stage of the Schobinger system consist of?**
Stage I (quiescence): pink-bluish stain, warmth, arteriovenous shunting by Doppler
Stage II (expansion): same as above with enlargement, pulsations, thrill, bruit, tortuous/tense veins
Stage III (destruction): same as above with dystrophic skin changes, ulceration, bleeding, persistent pain, or tissue necrosis
Stage IV (decompensation): same as above, plus cardiac failure

28. **How are AVMs managed?**
- Nonoperative: This includes compression garments for extremity lesions, hydrated petroleum to prevent desiccation/ulceration.
- Embolization of the nidus is generally first-line therapy for a symptomatic AVM.
- Operative management is reserved for symptomatic lesions that have failed embolization. Because AVM is often diffuse and involves multiple tissue planes and vital structures, resection is typically not curative. Preoperative embolization is performed to reduce intraoperative blood loss during the resection.

29. **What is the treatment for asymptomatic AVM?**
None. Embolization or incomplete excision of an asymptomatic lesion may stimulate it to enlarge and become problematic.

30. **If tooth extraction is planned in the site of an AVM, what needs to be done preoperatively?**
Preoperative embolization, with tooth extraction 48 to 72 hours later before recanalization and angiogenesis restore blood to lesion.

31. **What is Rendu-Osler-Weber disease?**
Also known as hereditary hemorrhagic telangiectasia. The first vascular anomaly to be understood at a genetic level with two causative genes on chromosome 9q. Lesion begins in capillary beds, and tiny capillary-venous shunts appear in skin, mucous membranes, lungs, liver, and brain.

32. What is blue rubber bleb nevus syndrome?

Rare, sporadic disorder composed of cutaneous and gastrointestinal VMs. Skin lesions can occur anywhere in body but have predilection for trunk, palms, and/or soles of feet. VMs are soft, blue, and increase in size and number with age. Gastrointestinal lesions are most common in small bowel and can cause bleeding, intussusception and volvulus.

33. What is Klippel-Trenaunay syndrome?

A sporadic capillary-lymphatic-venous malformation (CLVM) associated with soft tissue/skeletal hypertrophy of a limb.

BIBLIOGRAPHY

Abramowicz S, Padwa BL: Vascular anomalies in children, *Oral MaxillofacSurg Clin North Am* 24:443–455, 2012.

Chen MT, Yeong EK, Horng SY: Intralesional corticosteroid therapy in proliferating head and neck hemangiomas: a review of 155 cases, *J Pediatr Surg* 35:420–423, 2000.

Greene AG: Management of hemangiomas and other vascular tumors, *Clin Plast Surg* 38:45–63, 2011.

Greene AK, Orbach DB: Management of arteriovenous malformations, *Clin Plast Surg* 38:96–106, 2011.

Greene AK, Taber SF, Ball KL, et al.: Sturge-Weber syndrome: frequency and morbidity of facial overgrowth, *J Craniofac Surg* 20:617–621, 2009.

Hogeling M, Adams S, Wargon O: A randomized controlled trial of propranolol for infantile hemangiomas, *Pediatrics* 128:e259–e266, 2011.

Kaban LB, Mulliken JB: Vascular anomalies of the maxillofacial region, *J Oral Maxillofac Surg* 44:203–213, 1986.

Marler JJ, Mulliken JB: Current management of hemangiomas and vascular malformations, *Clin Plast Surg* 32:99–116, 2005.

Mulliken JB, Fishman SJ, Burrows PE: Vascular anomalies, *Curr Probl Surg* 37:517–584, 2000.

Mulliken JB, Glowacki J: Hemangiomas and vascular malformations in infants and children: a classification based on endothelial characteristics, *Plast Reconstr Surg* 69:412–422, 1982.

Padwa BL, Mulliken JB: Vascular anomalies of the oral and maxillofacial region. In Fonseca RJ, Marciani RD, Turvey T, editors: *Oral and maxillofacial surgery*, vol 2. St Louis, MO, 2008, Saunders, pp 577–591.

Sloan GM, Renisch JF, Nichter LS, et al.: Intralesional corticosteroid therapy for infantile hemangiomas, *Plast Reconstr Surg* 83:459–467, 1989.

CHAPTER 48

OSTEORADIONECROSIS/ OSTEONECROSIS OF THE JAWS

Regina Landesberg, Lisa Marie Di Pasquale

1. **What is ORN?**
   Radiation plays a key role in the treatment of head and neck cancer. Due to the location of the tumor or lymph node metastases, the salivary glands, oral cavity, and jaws are often included in the treatment radiation fields. As a result, these tissues often undergo changes secondary to radiation damage. Osteoradionecrosis (ORN) is often defined as an area of exposed bone that persists for at least 3 months in bone that has been irradiated. This definition may be insufficient, as ORN can present radiographically as a pathologic fracture with intact mucosa or skin.

2. **What are the risk factors for ORN?**
   Multiple risk factors predispose to the development of ORN. Treatment-dependent factors include cumulative radiotherapy doses to the bone, particularly those that exceed 5000 cGy. This is particularly true of the molar region of the mandible. Other important predisposing factors include the anatomic site of the primary tumor, tumor stage, proximity of the tumor to bone, external beam versus internal radiation therapy, extent of surgery, and concomitant chemotherapy. Host factors that increase the likelihood of developing ORN include the nutritional status of the patient, existing dental disease, oral hygiene, and continued tobacco or alcohol use (Table 48-1).

3. **What is the incidence of ORN?**
   The incidence of ORN ranges from 2% upward. The mandible is the most common site of radiation-induced tissue damage following treatment of head and neck cancers.
   ORN can occur anywhere from a few months up to 30 years after irradiation. It may be related to traumatic injuries such as pre- or post-radiation extractions, denture trauma, and other iatrogenic contributions. Additionally, ORN may occur spontaneously due to the progression of existing dental disease.

4. **Why is the mandible a more common location for ORN than the maxilla?**
   In contrast to the relatively well-vascularized maxilla, the mandible consists primarily of cortical bone that is essentially supported by a single arterial blood supply (inferior alveolar artery), thus making it at increased risk of ischemic radionecrosis.

5. **Does the mode of radiation delivery affect ORN incidence?**
   The different forms of radiation do not produce the same biologic effects. The initial delivered dose of radiation becomes an effective dose with a biologic effect under the influence of three main parameters: radiation type (type of atomic origin, level of energy), tissue type, and radiation schedule (fractionation, dose per fraction, total cumulative dose). It has been shown that external beam radiation is more positively correlated with ORN incidence than internal implant radiation therapy. Total radiation doses associated with increased risk of ORN are those higher than 5000 cGy, particularly 6000 to 7000 cGy.

6. **What is the pathophysiology of ORN?**
   Four hypotheses have been described for the development of ORN. First described was a series of local injury and infection following radiation exposure. Later, the "Triple H" hypothesis (hypocellular, hypoxic, and hypovascular) was described where ORN was thought to occur as a result of microvascular damage resulting in a damaged blood supply. A more recent proposal implicates radiation-induced suppression of osteoclast-mediated bone turnover in the pathogenesis of ORN. Finally, a fourth hypothesis is based on the histopathological features seen in ORN-proposed fibroatrophic bone changes called radiation-induced fibrosis (RIF). The sum of these four hypotheses indicates that irradiated bone has reduced cellular viability, obliteration of vessels, and compromised bone turnover compared to healthy bone.

Table 48-1. Risk Factors for Osteoradionecrosis

PATIENT-RELATED FACTORS	TUMOR-RELATED FACTORS	TREATMENT-RELATED FACTORS
Active dental disease	Anatomic location of the tumor	Field of radiation
Oral hygiene	Clinical state of the tumor	Total radiation dose
Pre-radiation oral care	Presence of lymph node	Dose rate/day
Alcohol and tobacco use	Metastasis	Mode of radiation delivery
		Tumor surgery

Table 48-2. Classification of Osteoradionecrosis and Recommended Therapy

1	< 2.5 cm length of bone affected (damaged or exposed); asymptomatic
	Medical treatment only
2	> 2.5 cm length of bone; asymptomatic, including pathologic fracture or involvement of the inferior alveolar nerve or both
	Medical treatment only unless there is dental sepsis or obvious loose, necrotic bone
3	> 2.5 cm length of bone; symptomatic, but with no other features despite medical treatment
	Consider debridement of loose or necrotic bone, and local pedicled flap
4	> 2.5 cm length of bone; pathologic fracture, involvement of the inferior alveolar nerve, orocutaneous fistula or a combination
	Reconstruction with free flap if patient's overall condition allows

From Lyons A, Osher J, Warner E et al., Osteoradionecrosis-A review of current concepts in defining the extent of the disease and a new classification proposal, *Br J Oral Maxillofac Surg* 52:392-395, 2014.

7. What are the clinical and radiographic features of ORN?
   Diagnosis of ORN is primarily based on clinical findings and patient history. The clinical manifestations of ORN may present several years after irradiation. By definition, ORN occurs in patients with a history of radiation and include one or several of the following that have failed to heal in at least 3 months:
   - Nonhealing ulcer
   - Exposed bone
   - Pain/dysesthesia/anesthesia
   - Orocutaneous fistula
   - Pathologic fracture
   Recently, Lyons et al. (Table 48-2) developed a new classification and recommendations for treatment of ORN based on the extent of the condition.

8. What is included in radiographic criteria?
   - Increased density
   - Periosteal thickening
   - Diffuse radiolucency
   - Mottled areas of osteoporosis
   - Sclerosis
   - Sequestration
   - CT scan or bone scintigraphy can also be used to evaluate the extent of the ORN.

9. What are the preventive methods of management of ORN?
   The decision to extract symptomatic and asymptomatic teeth before radiation therapy has traditionally been based on empirically designed protocols and not on "evidence-based" dentistry. Consideration is given to the preexisting condition of the teeth in the radiation field and to teeth that might cause post-irradiation complications if left in place. Pre-radiation extraction is indicated for teeth with advanced or symptomatic periodontal disease, advanced carious decay, pulpal involvement, mobility with root furcation, periapical pathology, and residual root tips

not covered by alveolar bone. Critical to the decision-making process is the patient's previous history of good oral hygiene and commitment to routine and ongoing professional dental visits. For optimum healing after extractions, 3 weeks prior to the initiation of radiotherapy is desirable; however, in most situations this is not feasible. An atraumatic approach should be employed in the pre-radiation extraction procedure with care taken to remove all sharp bony edges. If possible, an attempt to achieve primary closure is made. Patients undergoing radiation therapy ideally should be treated with a fluoride regimen of 1.1% NaF (5000 parts per million) gel and fluoride trays. Frequent surveillance and care by dental providers is essential both during and after radiation therapy.

10. **What are the conservative methods of management of ORN?**
    In the early stages of ORN, there is typically only a small nonhealing lesion present. Conservation management, commonly pain relief, and antibiotic therapy can be considered. Superficial debridement, or sequestrectomy, has been shown to promote soft tissue coverage. Irrigation and excellent oral hygiene are essential. Over half of these early stage lesions can be cured in this manner. Hyperbaric oxygen therapy has also been used in conservative management of ORN. Early study (Phase II), based on the hypothesis of radiation-induced fibrosis, has shown promising results with a cocktail regimen of pentoxifylline-tocopherol-clodronate (PENTOCLO).

11. **What is hyperbaric oxygen (HBO) therapy? What are the uses of HBO in ORN?**
    HBO therapy is another nonsurgical treatment modality for ORN. The use of HBO therapy is based on the Triple H theory (previously described). HBO is thought to increase the blood-tissue oxygen gradient, improving the diffusion of oxygen in hypoxic tissues, which promotes angiogenesis by increasing growth factors such as vascular endothelial growth factor (VEGF), as well as stimulating osteogenesis.
    HBO has been used therapeutically to treat ORN or prophylactically in irradiated bone prior to surgical intervention. Additionally, HBO is used in treatment of necrotizing skin infections, gas gangrene, and refractory osteomyelitis.

12. **What is the HBO protocol?**
    Therapeutic HBO treatment consists of 30 HBO dives to 2.4 atm for 90 minutes. If the wound shows definitive clinical improvement, additional dives may be added. Dives are typically once a day, 5 days a week.
    Although surgery is contraindicated in heavily irradiated fields, when it cannot be avoided HBO has been used in an attempt to avoid the development of ORN. Patients usually receive 20 dives preoperatively, followed by 10 dives postoperatively.
    Although HBO therapy seemed to be effective in early investigations using animal models, more recent studies have failed to conclusively show its benefit. A recent systematic review of the literature by Fitz et al. failed to identify any reliable evidence to support or refute the efficacy of HBO in the prevention of postextraction ORN in irradiated patients.

13. **What are surgical treatment options for ORN?**
    In the more advanced stages of ORN and in cases where conservative measures failed, surgical treatment, with or without HBO, is required. First, a possible local recurrence of a malignancy should be excluded via biopsy. As previously described in Table 48-1, management may be medical and/or surgical depending on the extent of the lesion.

14. **What is osteonecrosis of the jaws (ONJ)?**
    Osteonecrosis of the jaws (ONJ), also known as medication-related osteonecrosis of the jaws (MRONJ) and antiresorptive osteonecrosis of the jaws (ARONJ), is a clinical entity with the diagnostic characteristics defined by a number of medical and dental professional societies (AAOMS, ASBMR, ADA). Although there are slight differences in the various definitions of ONJ, a breach in the oral mucosa leading to exposed bone that fails to heal in 6 to 8 weeks is a mandatory element in the diagnosis of this condition. Additionally, patients must have a history of receiving antiresorptive therapy and no previous head and neck radiation. While the occurrence rate of ONJ in oncology patients ranges from 1.5% to 15%, patients treated for benign conditions (most commonly osteoporosis) appear to have a much lower incidence of ONJ (1/10,000 to 1/100,000).

15. **What causes ONJ?**
    While many questions regarding the incidence, pathoetiology, and natural history of this condition still need to be answered, it appears this disorder is multifactorial in nature. There seems to be a strong association between antiresorptive therapy (bisphosphonates, anti-RANK ligand) and ONJ;

Table 48-3. Antiresorptives

BENIGN			MALIGNANT		
	Antiresorptive	Route		Antiresorptive	Route
Bisphosphonate			**Bisphosphonate**		
	Alendronate (Fosamax)	PO		Pamidronate (Aredia)	IV
	Risedronate (Actonel)	PO			
	Ibandronate (Boniva)	PO			
	Zoledronate (Reclast)	IV		Zometa (Reclast)	IV
Monoclonal antibody	Denosumab (Prolia)	SQ	**Monoclonal antibody**	Denosumab (Xgeva)	SQ

however, a definitive cause-and-effect relationship between the two has not been established. Development of ONJ is often preceded by a traumatic event, most commonly an extraction. The fact that many of ONJ are immunosuppressed by medications (steroids, chemotherapy) or disease (diabetes, rheumatoid arthritis, cancer) suggests that an alteration in wound healing may play a significant role in the development of ONJ. Furthermore, the unique microbial environment and the high susceptibility of the oral cavity to frequent traumatic events may explain why ONJ lesions show a preference for the craniofacial region.

16. What are bisphosphonates?
    Bisphosphonates (BPs) are a widely used class of drugs indicated for the prevention and treatment of postmenopausal and steroid-induced osteoporosis, Paget's disease of bone, hypercalcemia of malignancy, multiple myeloma, and bone metastases associated with breast, prostate, lung, and other soft tissue tumors (Table 48-3).

17. What is denosumab?
    Denosumab (Dmab), a receptor activator of NF-kappa Bligand (RANKL) inhibitor, has recently been approved for similar indications to BPs, and it has also been strongly associated with ONJ (see Table 48-3).

18. What is the staging system for ONJ?
    The ONJ staging system, originally described in 2009 by a special committee of the AAOMS, has been largely accepted by both the medical and dental professions. This system has essentially remained unchanged in the most recent AAOMS 2014 update on MRONJ. The stage of disease is based on the severity of clinical symptoms as well as radiographic findings. Of note is the inclusion of a Stage 0 category where only nonspecific radiographic findings are identified in a patient receiving antiresorptive therapy (Table 48-4).

19. How is ONJ treated?
    Several studies have shown that patients who have a screening examination and appropriate treatment of dental disease prior to the initiation of antiresorptive therapy have a significant decrease in the risk of developing ONJ. The present recommendations by both the ADA and AAOMS do not include a drug holiday or CTX (C-terminal telopeptide) testing in patients requiring oral surgical procedures who are on antiresorptive therapy for benign conditions. In contrast, surgical procedures in individuals who have cancer and are receiving antiresorptive therapy should be avoided if at all possible. Nonsurgical therapies, such as endodontic treatment, are preferred in these patients.
    The management of patients with ONJ has traditionally been conservative, with the recommendation that surgical intervention only be performed in the most severe cases (Stage 3) where the patients have significant symptomatology. See Table 4. It should be noted, however, that Carlson as well as others have recently reported success rates of greater than 90% when using aggressive surgical resections to treat ONJ.

Table 48-4. ONJ Staging System

STAGING	TREATMENT
At-risk category: No apparent necrotic bone in patients who have been treated with either oral or IV bisphosphonates	• No treatment indicated • Patient education
Stage 0: No clinical evidence of necrotic bone, but nonspecific clinical findings, radiographic changes, and symptoms	• Systemic management, including the use of pain medication and antibiotics
Stage 1: Exposed and necrotic bone, or fistulae that probe to bone, in patients who are asymptomatic and have no evidence of infection	• Antibacterial mouth rinse • Clinical follow-up on a quarterly basis • Patient education and review of indications for continued bisphosphonate therapy
Stage 2: Exposed and necrotic bone, or fistulae that probe to bone, associated with infection as evidenced by pain and erythema in the region of the exposed bone with or without purulent drainage	• Symptomatic treatment with oral antibiotics • Oral antibacterial mouth rinse • Pain control • Debridement to relieve soft tissue irritation and infection control
Stage 3: Exposed and necrotic bone or a fistula that probes to bone in patients with pain, infection, and one or more of the following: exposed and necrotic bone extending beyond the region of alveolar bone (i.e., inferior border and ramus in the mandible, maxillary sinus and zygoma in the maxilla) resulting in pathologic fracture, extraoral fistula, oroantral and oronasal communication, or osteolysis extending to the inferior border of the mandible or sinus floor	• Antibacterial mouth rinse • Antibiotic therapy and pain control • Surgical debridement/resection for longer term palliation of infection and pain

From Ruggiero SL, Dodson TB, Fantasia J, et al.: American Association of Oral and Maxillofacial Surgeons Position Paper on Medication-Related Osteonecrosis of the Jaw-2014 Update. *J Oral Maxillofac Surg*, 72(10): 1938–1965, 2014.

BIBLIOGRAPHY

Assael LA: New foundations in understanding osteonecrosis of the jaws, *J Oral Maxillofac Surg* 62(2):125–126, 2004.

Carlson ER: Management of antiresorptive osteonecrosis of the jaws with primary surgical resection, *J Oral Maxillofac Surg* 72(4):655–657, 2014.

Delanian S, Chatel C, Porcher R, Depondt J, Lefaix JL: Complete restoration of refractory mandibular osteoradionecrosis by prolonged treatment with a pentoxifylline-tocopherol-clodronate combination (PENTOCLO): a phase II trial, *Int J Radiat Oncol Biol Phys* 80(3):832–839, 2011.

Dimopoulos MA, Kastritis E, Bamia C, Melakopoulos I, Gika D, Roussou M, Migkou M, Eleftherakis-Papaiakovou E, Christoulas D, Terpos E, Bamias A: Reduction of osteonecrosis of the jaw (ONJ) after implementation of preventive measures in patients with multiple myeloma treated with zoledronic acid, *Ann Oncol* 20(1):117–120, 2009.

Edwards BJ, Hellstein JW, Jacobsen PL, et al., and the American Dental Association Council on Scientific Affairs Expert Panel on Bisphosphonate-Associated Osteonecrosis: Updated recommendations for managing the care of patients receiving oral bisphosphonate therapy: an advisory statement from the American Dental Association Council on Scientific Affairs, *J Am Dent Assoc* 139(12):1674–1677, 2008.

Fritz GW, Gunsolley JC, Abubaker O, Laskin DM: Efficacy of pre- and postirradiation hyperbaric oxygen therapy in the prevention of postextraction osteoradionecrosis: a systematic review, *J Oral Maxillofac Surg* 68(11):2653–2660, 2010.

Hellstein JW, Adler RA, Edwards B, et al., and the American Dental Association Council on Scientific Affairs Expert Panel on Antiresorptive Agents: Managing the care of patients receiving antiresorptive therapy for prevention and treatment of osteoporosis: executive summary of recommendations from the American Dental Association Council on Scientific Affairs, *J Am Dent Assoc* 142(11):1243–1251, 2011.

Khosla S, Burr D, Cauley J, et al.: American Society for, and R. Mineral, Bisphosphonate-associated osteonecrosis of the jaw: report of a task force of the American Society for Bone and Mineral Research, *J Bone Miner Res* 22(10):1479–1491, 2007.

Landesberg R, Woo V, Cremers S, et al.: Potential pathophysiological mechanisms in osteonecrosis of the jaw, *Ann N Y Acad Sci* 1218:62–79, 2011.

Lyons A, Osher J, Warner E, et al.: Osteoradionecrosis–a review of current concepts in defining the extent of the disease and a new classification proposal, *Br J Oral Maxillofac Surg* 52(5):392–395, 2014.

Marx RE: A new concept in the treatment of osteoradionecrosis, *J Oral Maxillofac Surg* 41(6):351–357, 1983.

Marx RE, Tursun R: Suppurative osteomyelitis, bisphosphonate induced osteonecrosis, osteoradionecrosis: a blinded histopathologic comparison and its implications for the mechanism of each disease, *Int J Oral Maxillofac Surg* 41(3):283–289, 2012.

McCaul JA: Pharmacologic modalities in the treatment of osteoradionecrosis of the jaw, *Oral Maxillofac Surg Clin North Am* 26(2):247–252, 2014.

Oh HK, Chambers MS, Garden AS, Wong PF, Martin JW: Risk of osteoradionecrosis after extraction of impacted third molars in irradiated head and neck cancer patients, *J Oral Maxillofac Surg* 62(2):139–144, 2004.

Ripamonti CI, Maniezzo M, Campa T et al.: Decreased occurrence of osteonecrosis of the jaw after implementation of dental preventive measures in solid tumour patients with bone metastases treated with bisphosphonates. The experience of the National Cancer Institute of Milan, *Ann Oncol* 20(1):137–145, 2009.

Ruggiero SL, Dodson TB, Assael LA et al.: Task Force on Bisphosphonate-Related Osteonecrosis of the Jaws, American Association of Oral and Maxillofacial Surgeons position paper on bisphosphonate-related osteonecrosis of the jaw - 2009 update, *Aust Endod J* 35(3):119–130, 2009.

Ruggiero SL, Dodson TB, Fantasia J, et al.: American Association of Oral and Maxillofacial Surgeons Position Paper on Medication-Related Osteonecrosis of the Jaw-2014 Update, *J Oral Maxillofac Surg* 72(10):1938–1956, 2014.

Sulaiman F, Huryn JM, Zlotolow IM: Dental extractions in the irradiated head and neck patient: a retrospective analysis of Memorial Sloan-Kettering Cancer Center protocols, criteria, and end results, *J Oral Maxillofac Surg* 61(10):1123–1131, 2003.

CHAPTER 49

NECK MASS

HuiShan Ong, Tong Ji, Chen Ping Zhang

1. What are the main categories of neck masses?
   Congenital, infectious/inflammatory, and neoplastic (benign/malignant)

2. What can the age of a patient tell you?
   The patient's age should be a prime consideration in differential diagnosis. Three main age groups are taken into consideration: pediatric (≤15 years), young adult (16 to 40 years), and adult (>40 years). See Table 49-1.

3. How do you establish a differential diagnosis based on the average duration of the patient's symptoms?
   Rule of 7:
   - Swelling from **inflammation** will have existed for **7 days.**
   - Swelling from **neoplasm** will have existed for **7 months.**
   - Swelling from **congenital deformity** will have existed for **7 years.**

4. How do you establish differential diagnoses for a neck mass in an adult?
   Rule of 80s after age of 40:
   - **80%** of all **nonthyroid** neck masses will be **neoplastic**.
   - **80%** of neoplastic masses are **malignant**.
   - **80%** of malignant mass are **metastatic**.
   - **80%** of metastases are from primary sites above the level of the clavicle.
   - **80%** of metastatic lymph nodes (LNs) in adults are **SCC**.

5. How do you diagnose a neck mass?
   A diagnosis can develop from patient's chief complaint, patient's age, location, onset and duration, size, pain, drainage/exudates, characteristics and progression of a neck mass, and past medical history including previous head neck surgery.

6. What are the clinical investigations in evaluating the cervical mass?
   - Ultrasound
   - Contrast-enhanced CT
   - Fine needle aspiration cytology (FNAC)
   - PET-CT
   - MRI
   - Clinical palpation

7. What is a normal LN?
   Clinically palpable normal LN is about 1 cm in size (at a range of 0.5 to 2 cm), relatively soft in consistency, and mobile. Tender upon palpation does not differentiate between normal and cancerous. But the size of the LN can be various among different age groups. See Table 49-2.
   Therefore, any node greater than 2 cm beyond these normal hyperplastic zones shall be evaluated with caution.

8. In what circumstances should you be particularly concerned about a neck mass?
   - **Hard** or **fixed** mass
   - Obstructive airway/breathing difficulty
   - **Elderly** patient
   - Medically compromised patient
   - Presence of **oropharyngeal mass** when simple pharyngitis or dental infection has been ruled out
   - Signs of **cachexia**
   - A history of persistent **hoarseness of voice** or complaining of **dysphagia**

Table 49-1. Patient's Age and How It Relates to Differential Diagnosis

Pediatric:	Inflammatory > congenital > malignant > benign
Young adult:	Inflammatory > congenital > benign > malignant
Adult:	Malignant > benign > inflammatory > congenital

Table 49-2. Size of LN According to Different Age Groups

Infant:	Small palpable LNs are more readily palpated in the posterior cervical region.
Pediatric:	Small palpable LNs are palpable over the submandibular region > anterior cervical chain > posterior cervical region.

9. **How does a contrast-enhanced CT compare to MRI in evaluation of neck mass?**
   CT images can significantly manifest an enhanced rim with center liquefaction lymph node to indicate a regional metastasis. Signal intensity on MRI with intravenous gadolinium administration is still ineffective in demonstrating a metastatic lymph node; MRI lymph node assessment relies more on analysis of enhancement kinetics (peak and washout timing slope) after bolus administration of gadolinium chelate agents that are technically dependent. Furthermore, an MRI cannot identify an intranodal calcification, which is a particular concern for metastatic prediction in papillary carcinoma of the thyroid gland.

10. **How do you evaluate a neck mass with a minimally invasive approach?**
    FNAC. It is a cytological study of aspirated cells.

11. **What are the limitations in FNAC?**
    It does not allow evaluation of cellular morphology. Sometimes, accurate diagnosis cannot be established due to sampling error, handling, and processing errors or reading errors. A repeated aspiration or an excisional biopsy should be considered if the cytology result did not correspond to clinical presentation.

12. **How can aspirated content help to provide diagnostic information?**
    Fluid content aspiration. Detection of fluid content can aid in primitive diagnosis establishment. Color and consistency of fluid content:
    - **Plugging ranula**: **Clear** fluid, **viscous fluid** enriched with amylase and total protein content
    - **Cystic hygroma**: Clear to yellowish fluid, **serous fluid**
    - **Vascular malformation**: Hemorrhagic content (**blood**) when blood vessel was **not** being punctured
    - **Dermoid/epidermoid cyst**: **Clear content** fluid with some **debris**, **serous** fluid. Occasionally, no fluid can be aspirated as the entire content was filled with debris (cheesy and semisolid).

13. **What is the most common congenital mass in the lateral neck?**
    Branchial cleft cyst.

14. **What is a branchial cleft cyst?**
    It is a congenital mass frequently found in children or young adults. It is manifested as a developing mass or draining tract anywhere between the preauricular region and supraclavicular fossa within the anterior triangle depending on branchial arch origin (Table 49-3). The etiology of the cyst is related to incomplete involution of branchial cleft during development.

15. **What is the treatment option for a branchial cleft cyst?**
    Surgical excision is the primary management for branchial cleft cyst. An infected cyst needs to be treated with an antibiotic before definitive management. A fistula, sinus tract, or previous dissected plane/path might harbor an epithelial remnant; thereby they shall be completely resected together with the underlying cyst.

16. **What is a thyroglossal duct cyst (TGDC)?**
    It is the most common congenital mass found in the midline of the neck. It can present anywhere between the base of the tongue and the superior aspect of the thyroid gland. It moves in a vertical plane, especially during swallowing and tongue protrusion. It is typically painless, but it can also cause exacerbated pain when infected.

Table 49-3. Comparison of different types of branchial cleft cyst

BRANCHIAL ARCH REMNANT	ASSOCIATED LOCATION	SINUS TRACT	PRECAUTION
First	Preauricular region	External auditory canal	Facial nerve
Second	Superior one-third and beneath to SCM, part of the lesion extended anteriorly to SCM	Extended superior medially running between Internal Carotid Artery (ICA) and External Carotid Artery ECA and running superiomedially beneath the posterior belly of digastric muscle to enter tonsil fossa	Marginal mandibular nerve, spinal accessory nerve, and hypoglossal nerve Carotid sheath superior laryngeal nerve
Third and Fourth	Middle one-third to mediastinal	Piriform fossa	Recurrent laryngeal nerve

ICA, Internal Carotid Artery; ECA, External Carotid Artery

17. **How do you manage a TGDC?**
First, ensure the presence of a functioning orthotopic thyroid gland prior to surgical resection. TGDC requires a Sistrunk procedure during surgical excision, as the hyoid bone (arises from the second branchial arch) starts to develop after the descent of the thyroid gland, which results in the thyroglossal duct located posteriorly to hyoid bone. Fusion of the second branchial arch at midline will cause an entrapment of the thyroglossal duct over the hyoid bone. Therefore, Sistrunk resection requires a removal of the middle third of hyoid bone. A center cuff of muscles (mylohyoid raphe, part of genioglossus and hyoglossus muscle) around the tract is circumcised at a 45° angle posterosuperiorly up to the foramen cecum. The overlying tongue base mucosal can be kept intact or violated. Lastly, passing a 3-0 suture in a "figure 8" to ensure a watertight closure and prevent postoperative seepage or surgical site infection.

18. **Why should you suspect a neck mass in an adult might be a malignancy instead of a second branchial cleft cyst?**
Both of them share the same anatomic region. The second branchial cleft cyst is more commonly found in children than adults; radioimages are important to support a differential diagnosis. Branchial cleft cysts typically appear as a well-defined and homogeneous nonenhancing mass of fluid attenuation at the characteristic location [second branchial cleft cyst: immediately anterior or beneath upper one-third of sternocleidomastoid muscle (SCM)]. On the other hand, a radiopaque-enhanced rim with central necrosis. Intralesional solid components or irregular outer border shall prompt a diagnosis of metastatic cancer.

19. **Why do cervical lymph nodes need to be assessed?**
Evaluation of nodal status and the staging of lymph nodes is essential for determining an appropriate therapeutic option (surgical resection with neck dissection and postoperative radiation, chemotherapy, and prognosis prediction).

BIBLIOGRAPHY

Cianchetti M, Mancuso AA, Amdur RJ, Werning JW, Kirwan J, Morris CG, Mendenhall WM: Diagnostic evaluation of squamous cell carcinoma metastatic to cervical lymph nodes from an unknown head and neck primary site, *Laryngoscope* 119:2348–2354, 2009.

Cohen SM, Burkey BB, Netterville JL: Surgical management of parapharyngeal space masses, *Head Neck* 27:669–675, 2005.

Cummings CW, Flint PW, Harker LA, et al.: Overview of diagnostic imaging of the head and neck. In *Otolaryngology—head and neck surgery*, ed 4, Philadelphia, 2005, Elsevier Mosby, pp 25–92.

Edwards SP: Pediatric malignant tumors of the head and neck. In Bagheri SC, Bell RB, Khan HA, editors: *Current therapy in oral and maxillofacial surgery*, ed 1, Saunders, 2011, pp 820–827.

Ferrer R: Lymphadenopathy: differential diagnosis and evaluation, *Am Fam Physician* 58(6):1313–1320, 1998.

Goffart Y, Hamoir M, Deron P, et al.: Management of neck masses in adults, *B-ENT* 1:133–142, 2005.

Lin S, Tseng FY, Hsu CJ, et al.: Thyroglossal duct cyst: a comparison between children and adults, *Am J Otolaryngol* 29:83–87, 2008.

Meier JD, Grimmer JF: Evaluation and management of neck masses in children, *Am Fam Physician* 89:353–358, 2014.

Myers EN, Suen JY, Myers JN, et al.: Lymphomas presenting in the head and neck: current issues in diagnosis and management. In *Cancer of the head and neck*, ed 4, Philadelphia, 2003, Saunders, pp 601–610.

Rosa PA, Hirsh DL, Dierks EJ: Congenital neck masses, *Oral Maxillofac Surg Clin North Am* 20:339–352, 2008.

CHAPTER 50

BONE GRAFTING TO FACILITATE DENTAL IMPLANT PLACEMENT

George R. Deeb, Fahad M. Alsaad

1. **Which branchial arch are the maxilla and mandible derived from, and what type of ossification do they undergo?**
   Both the maxilla and the mandible are derived from the first branchial arch, which is derived from the neural crest ectomesenchyme. Craniofacial bone development is preceded by formation of cartilaginous and membranous precursors that give rise to the neurocranium and viscerocranium. The maxilla and mandible form by intramembranous ossification of the membranous viscerocranium. Maxillary ossification begins at the infraorbital foramen, and mandibular ossification begins at the mental foramen.

2. **What is the basic histology of bone tissue and the cells within it?**
   Osteoprogenitor cells are the precursor to the bone matrix forming osteoblasts. They are located on the endosteal surface of trabecular bone and periosteal surface of cortical bone. Once mature, osteoblasts secrete type I collagen as well as other matrix proteins forming immature bone known as *osteoid*, which subsequently mineralizes up to two-thirds of the bone matrix. These osteoblasts are called *osteocytes*. As they become trapped with the matrix they form and are considered to be at the terminus of their differentiation. They communicate with each other and the surface with an extensive canalicular network.
   Osteoclasts are responsible for bone resorption and are derived from bone marrow monocyte-macrophage precursor cells. The resorption process forms Howship's lacunae where the osteoclasts are housed.

3. **Can you describe the difference between cortical and trabecular bone?**
   Cortical bone is made of dense, compact bone containing a series of osteons known as the Haversian system, which is the functional unit of compact bone. Haversian canals lie within the osteons and contain vasculature. Biochemical communication between osteons occurs via Volkmann's canals.
   The functional unit of trabecular bone is the trabecular packets, which like the Haversian system is formed of concentric lamellae of bone matrix. Turnover of trabecular bone is much higher than cortical bone, and it is involved in mineral metabolism.

4. **Can you describe primary bone healing?**
   Primary bone healing implies direct bone contact or a gap of less than 1 mm. Healing occurs in the same process of bone turnover, by direct remodeling of the Haversian system. Osteoclasts work to create a cutting cone, resorbing edges of the fracture, and osteoblasts follow and secrete osteoid for future mineralization.

5. **What are the three phases of secondary bone healing?**
   The primary phases of secondary bone healing are:
   1. Inflammatory phase: Bleeding at the fracture edges forms a hematoma, which turns into granulation tissue.
   2. Repair phase: Inflammatory cells and fibroblasts invade the tissue. These cells cause the recruitment of osteoblasts and provide a scaffold for vascular ingrowth. Osteoblasts lay down osteoid and form a soft callus that eventually ossifies, forming woven bone.
   3. Remodeling phase: This phase occurs over the next months to a year and restores bone to its original shape and strength, by converting the woven bone to lamellar bone.

6. **How do cortical bone grafts heal?**
   Block bone grafts heal by creeping substitution, a process similar to primary bone healing.

7. **Do cortical bone grafts undergo complete resorption and replacement?**
   No, cortical block grafts are never completely resorbed and replaced by new bone. The nonvascularized cortical bone block remains as necrotic centers with the newly formed bone.

About 17% of resorption of the mandibular block autograft when combined with particulate auto- and xenografts was noted on human studies, and an average of 5.0mm of vertical height was gained in ridge augmentation procedures. Maintenance of the vitality of autografts is achieved by revascularization, which protects against graft infection and necrosis.

8. **Can you describe the healing of autogenous cancellous bone grafts?**
Autogenous marrow contains both osteocompetent marrow stem cells as well as osteoblasts. These cells remain viable through plasmatic diffusion. During the first week of healing, platelets release an array of growth factors that promote angiogenesis and regeneration. During weeks 2 through 8, the graft is revascularized by capillary ingrowth, and the osteoblasts begin to synthesize osteoid. Remodeling is initiated by osteoclasts, which are stimulated by growth factors released during osteoid formation. After 6 months of healing, 90% of the graft is matured.

9. **What are the bone density categories and locations in the maxilla and mandible?**
   - D1: Dense cortical bone in the anterior mandible and in the posterior mandible
   - D2: Dense to porous cortical bone in the anterior mandible and surrounding; dense trabecular bone in the posterior mandible and anterior maxilla
   - D3: Thin porous cortical bone in the anterior maxilla surrounding; fine trabecular bone and posterior maxilla
   - D4: Fine trabecular bone in posterior maxilla

10. **How are alveolar ridge deficiencies classified according to Seibert's nomenclature?**
   - Class 1: Horizontal tissue loss with normal ridge height
   - Class 2: Vertical tissue loss with normal ridge height.
   - Class 3: Combined horizontal and vertical bone loss.

11. **Which type of defect (vertical or horizontal) is more challenging to reconstruct?**
Vertical alveolar bone loss is more challenging to reconstruct than horizontal bone loss.

12. **What is another classification scheme for describing alveolar defects?**
Defect classification can be described by the number of walls remaining. For example, an intact extraction socket has five walls. When the buccal plate is missing, a defect has four walls remaining. The more walls missing, the more difficult is the reconstruction. Total vertical bone loss has only one wall remaining, which is the apical wall, and therefore is the most challenging to reconstruct.

13. **What is an osteogenic graft?**
A graft that transfers osteocompetent cells to begin the bone-forming process. These cells along with the osteocompetent cells at the defect site form new bone. Autogenous bone grafts are the only osteogenic grafts and considered the gold standard in bone grafting.

14. **What is an osteoinductive graft?**
Osteoinductive grafts begin bone formation by stimulating host mesenchymal cells to differentiate. This process occurs through the transfer of proteins in the graft. These proteins begin a signaling cascade for the host to form bone.

15. **What is an osteoconductive graft?**
Osteoconductive grafts provide scaffolding for the host to form bone. These grafts do not contain proteins or cells and therefore do not biologically influence the host.

16. **What are the classifications of bone grafts based upon their source?**

Autograft	Graft taken from the same host
Allograft	Graft taken from a genetically similar donor, as in cadaveric graft
Xenograft	Graft taken from a genetically dissimilar donor, most commonly bovine or porcine source
Synthetic graft	Graft not taken from a living donor No cellular or protein products in this graft

17. **What are the most common bone graft materials based on their source?**

Autograft	Cadaver cortical/cancellous bone, FDBA (freeze-dried bone allograft), DFDBA (decalcified freeze-dried bone allograft)

| Xenograft | Bio-Oss, Endobon, coralline HA, red algae |
| Alloplast (synthetic) | Calcium sulfate, calcium phosphate, bioactive glass, hydroxyapatite, porous nickel titanium |

18. **What are the most common bone grafts based upon their osseous induction potential?**

Osteogenic	Autograft
Osteoinductive	BMP (bone morphogenic protein), DFDBA (decalcified freeze-dried bone allograft), DBM (demineralized bone matrix)
Osteoconductive	Bio-Oss, Endobon, calcium phosphate, calcium sulfate, collagen, FDBA, glass ionomers, HA (hydroxyapatite), (NiTi) porous nickel titanium

19. **What are the most common factor-based materials?**
Platelet-rich plasma (PRP), bone morphogenic proteins (BMPs), platelet-derived growth factor (PDGF).

20. **What are the most common sites for harvesting regional bone autografts?**
- Mandibular symphysis
- Mandibular ramus and body
- Mandibular coronoid process
- Zygomatic buttress

21. **What is the harvest of a mandibular symphysis graft?**
Either a sulcular of vestibular incision is made. Sulcular incisions will result in recession in some patients with a thin periodontium, or in the presence of crown and bridge work. Distal oblique releases are made distal to the second premolar. The vestibular incision is similar to that for a genioplasty. The vestibular incision will bleed more due to the mentalis and gives slightly less access than the sulcular. The vestibular incision should be closed in two layers to avoid chin ptosis. The vestibular incision is associated with wound dehiscence, scar band formation, and pain more often. The sulcular incision is closed in an interrupted fashion through the papilla.

The superior osteotomy line should be 5 mm below the root apices. All portions of the osteotomy should completely penetrate the labial plate. The osteotomy is completed using round or fissure burs, and thin chisels. The dimensions of the corticocancellous blocks are usually adequate for reconstructing the width of three teeth, or up to 6 mm in horizontal and vertical dimensions.

22. **What is the harvest of a mandibular ramus graft?**
The incision to access the mandibular ramus for grafting begins on the edentulous crest distal to the teeth and includes mesial and distal oblique releases as necessary for access. The superior osteotomy is made 5 mm medial to the external oblique ridge. The vertical osteotomies are made mesially and distally according to bone grafting needs and 10 to 12 mm in vertical height. The inferior osteotomy scores the lateral cortex at the height desired. Using a thin chisel, the bone is outfractured. In 10% to 12% of patients the inferior alveolar nerve will be visible. The wound is closed in a running or interrupted fashion.

23. **Can you describe the harvest of mandibular coronoid bone?**
An incision over the ascending ramus should be made beginning at the level of the occlusal table of the mandibular molar and extended to the midpoint of the ramus. Complete striping of the temporalis is required. The coronoid is grasped with a forceps and a reciprocating saw used to amputate it inferiorly to the forceps. The lingula is located 10 mm below the sigmoid notch, so the osteotomy should not be made more than 5 mm inferior to the notch. The coronoid process has sufficient bone to augment one or two teeth width and 3 to 4 mm in a horizontal or vertical direction. The wound is closed in a running or interrupted fashion.

24. **What is the procedure for harvesting bone from the zygomatic buttress?**
Access to the zygomatic buttress is gained by making a vestibular incision from the canine distally to the first molar area. Superolateral dissection is carried out. Four osteotomies, two vertical and two horizontal, are outlined and completed with a fissure bur. The bone is removed with a chisel. The limiting anatomic barriers are the sinus inferiorly and the infraorbital nerve superiorly. The wound is closed in a running or interrupted fashion.

25. Can you describe the bone resorption in an alveolus after extraction?

The thin cortical buccal plate of an extraction socket is predisposed to a more rapid post-extraction resorption when compared to other walls of the socket. This explains the decrease in ridge width compared to height. Up to 50% of the buccal ridge width and 20% of the ridge height may resorb within the first 6 months after extraction.

26. What are some of the surgical requirements and principals necessary for block graft success?

For a more predictable successful outcome in block grafts, it is critical to insure stability and contact with the host recipient bed. Stabilization may be achieved with fixation screws or immediate placement of the dental implant into the graft. Other techniques that can improve success rate are recipient bed preparation, i.e., decorticating holes to expose the cancellous marrow and improve revascularization of the graft and subsequently its integration. Corticocancellous grafts are favored over cortical block grafts due to their faster revascularization. Graft resorption can be minimized with the use of barrier membranes.

27. What procedure will help minimize bone resorption after extraction?

Socket preservation. Most studies support the concept of grafting an extraction site to minimize bone resorption. Nonetheless it is an additional procedure that adds more cost and a potential for complications. Therefore the clinician should be selective of when to graft, as it has been shown in animal and human studies that ungrafted extraction sites with completely intact bony walls heal without significant defects on their own.

Sites where the buccal cortical bone is thin and resorption is anticipated, such as the anterior maxilla, socket grafting is recommended. The use of a barrier membrane is also advocated to prevent fibrous encapsulation of the graft.

28. What are guided bone regeneration (GBR) and guided tissue regeneration (GTR)?

GBR refers to the formation of bone alone, while GTR refers to the regeneration of the supporting apparatus including cementum, periodontal ligament, and alveolar bone. GTR and GBR use barrier membranes for space maintenance over a defect promoting ingrowth of osteogenic cells and preventing ingrowth of overlying soft tissues into the wound.

29. How much vertical ridge height can be augmented with the use of a barrier membrane?

Studies have shown that up to 4.0 mm of bone can be grafted vertically, without the use of grafting materials, using titanium-reinforced membranes. Additional vertical height can be achieved using grafting materials. Studies have shown an implant success rate of 97.5% in vertically grafted bone, which is comparable to implant success placed in native or horizontal bone.

30. Describe some of the nonresorbable membrane options for bone grafting.

Expanded polytetrafluoroethylene (ePTFE) is the most common type of nonresorbable membrane used. Subtypes of it include porous ePTFE, which allows tissue adherence to the membrane for stabilization, high-density ePTFE that prevents tissue ingrowth, and titanium reinforced for better space maintenance in larger defects. Plain titanium has also been used for ridge augmentation procedures.

31. What are the advantages of use of titanium mesh in bone grafting in preparation for implant placement?

The rigidity of titanium mesh helps maintain the space where bone proliferation is intended and prevents collapse of the soft tissue envelope.

32. What are the types of bioabsorbable barriers available for intraoral bone grafting?

There are two main types of bioabsorbable membranes, which are natural or synthetic. Natural membranes are mostly derived from collagen of an animal origin, and they resorb by enzymatic digestion. Synthetic membranes are polymer products such as polylactic and polyglycolic acid. Those degrade by hydrolysis process.

33. What are the approaches to sinus augmentation?

There are two main techniques to consider when the maxillary sinus requires an augmentation. A conservative approach is performed through a crestal osteotomy using the sequenced implant drills, leaving a thin interface of bone at the sinus floor that will tap into the sinus cavity with osteotomes designed for that purpose, while care is taken to avoid tears to the schneiderian sinus membrane. Particulate bone graft material may be packed into the prepped site. About 3 to 5 mm of sinus floor elevation is gained with this method.

When more sinus elevation is desired, a more invasive approach may be considered. This involves a modification of the Caldwell-Luc procedure, where a window at the lateral sinus wall is made, without perforation into the schneiderian membrane, creating a trapdoor access. The membrane is carefully dissected and lifted from the floor. The bony segment of the sinus window is tucked in as part of the graft, and the reminder of the space between the sinus and its membrane is filled with a graft material. Resorbable membrane is placed to cover the lateral window, and the tissue flap is closed primarily.

The choice between one method over the other depends on the length of the implant, amount of preoperative crestal bone, and the timing of implant placement, whether at the time of sinus augmentation or as a secondary stage.

34. **What materials are used for sinus bone grafting?**
There are numerous grafting materials that can be used in sinus augmentation, all of which show high success rates. These materials include autogenous grafts, xenografts, hydroxyapatite, particulate allografts, and BMP-2. In other studies, tenting of the maxillary sinus membrane with the implant fixture without placement of a graft resulted in bone formation and similar success. It is recommended to place a resorbable barrier membrane over the sinus window to protect and contain the graft.

35. **Are there any contraindications to sinus floor augmentation?**
Clinical or radiographic evidence of sinusitis or any other sinus pathology warrants a referral to an otolaryngologist evaluation and management before considering augmentation procedure at the maxillary sinus.

36. **What is a ridge-splitting procedure? What is a two-stage ridge-splitting procedure?**
A ridge-splitting procedure involves making a longitudinal crestal osteotomy using chisels or a piezotome to separate the buccal and lingual cortices, thus widening the ridge and gaining horizontal width. An interpositional graft may be placed at the intercortical gap to provide stability, along with primary closure.

A modification to this technique involves a two-stage procedure. The initial surgery is aimed toward making a horizontal apical and two vertical osteotomies on the buccal cortex after a full thickness mucoperiosteal flap. The osteotomies outline the buccal segment to be split in stage two. One month later, the second surgery is performed where a split thickness flap is reflected to maintain blood supply to the previously osteotomized segment, which can now be split to widen the ridge. At this stage implants may be placed or an interpositional graft. The rationale for the two-staged approach is to have predictable buccal segment size and prevent unfavorable fractures.

37. **Can you describe the tunneling technique used for horizontal lateral ridge augmentation?**
Alveolar ridges with thin crestal bone usually have a wider base and are indicated for this tunneling technique. A vertical incision is made anterior to the site to be augmented. While being cognizant of the mental nerve in mandibular grafts, a subperiosteal pocket is made. Soft tissue is only reflected from the thin portion to receive the graft, where the wider basal bone will act as a shelf to hold the particulate graft, which is packed into the pocket. Finally the incision is closed primarily with sutures.

38. **What are the different methods of managing a vertically deficient posterior mandibular ridge?**
   - Inferior alveolar nerve lateralization
   - GBR and onlay grafts
   - Use of short implants
   - Interpositional grafts

39. **Can you describe the vertical ridge augmentation technique with an interpositional graft?**
After local anesthesia is administered, a horizontal vestibular incision is made about 15 mm apical to the crest, while being cognizant of the mental nerve. Then a vertical release incision is made in the interdental space one tooth anterior to the planned osteotomy. A buccal flap may be reflected while

preserving the crestal and lingual periosteal attachment to the crestal alveolus to maintain its blood supply. A piezotome is used to complete horizontal and vertical osteotomies, carefully avoiding perforating the lingual soft tissue. Vertical osteotomies must be slightly diverging at the crest to prevent undercut locking of the segment. Next, the segment is mobilized vertically to the extent allowed by the lingual tissue and fixated with small bone plate. Finally a particulate bone graft material is packed into the created gap. The flap then is closed without tension.

40. **How much vertical bone height may be gained from an interpositional graft technique?**
The lingual tissue attachment allows about 4 to 5 mm of crestal segment elevation. In severely deficient ridges where the osteotomized crestal segment is close to the floor of the mouth, the laxity of the lingual tissue may allow for up to 7 to 8 mm of elevation.

BIBLIOGRAPHY

Block M: *Color atlas of dental implant surgery*, ed 3, St Louis, MO, 2010, Saunders, p 80.
Clarke B: Normal bone anatomy and physiology, *Clin J Am Soc Nephrol* 3(Suppl 3):S131–S139, November 2008.
Fonseca R, Marciani R, Turvey T: *Oral and maxillofacial surgery*, ed 2, vol 2. St Louis, MO, 2008, Saunders. 144–147.
Horowitz R, Holtzclaw D, Rosen P: A review on alveolar ridge preservation following tooth extraction, *J Evidence Based Dent Pract* 12(Suppl 3):149–160, 2012.
Irinakis T: Rationale for socket preservation after extraction of a single-rooted tooth when planning for future implant placement, *J Can Dent Assoc* 72(10):917–922, 2006.
Kao S, Scott D: A review of bone substitutes, *Oral Maxillofac Surg Clin N Am* 19(4):513–521, 2007.
Lundgren S, Cricchio G, Palma VC, Salata L, Sennerby L: Sinus membrane elevation and simultaneous insertion of dental implants: a new surgical technique in maxillary sinus floor augmentation, *Periodontology 2000* 47(1):193–205, 2008.
McAllister B, Haghighat K: Bone augmentation techniques, *J Periodontol* 78(3):377–396, 2007.
Misch C: *Contemporary implant dentistry*, ed 3, St Louis, MO, 2007, Mosby.
Peterson L: *Peterson's principles of oral and maxillofacial surgery*, ed 2, Hamilton, Ontario, 2004, BC Decker. eBook, p 1055.
Proussaefs P, Lozada J: The use of intraorally harvested autogenous block grafts for vertical alveolar ridge augmentation: a human study, *Int J Periodont Restorat Dent* 25(4):351–363, 2005.
Rachana CN, Sridhar, Rangan AV, Rajani V: Horizontal ridge augmentation using a combination approach, *J Ind Soc Periodontol* 16(3):446–450, 2012.
Roden D: Principles of bone grafting, *Oral Maxillofac Surg Clin N Am* 22(3):295–300, 2010.
Sadler TW: *Langman's medical embryology*, ed 12, Baltimore, MD, 2012, Lippincott Williams & Wilkins. eBook, p 264.
Seibert JS: Reconstruction of deformed partially edentulous ridges, using full thickness onlay grafts. part I. technique and wound healing, *Comp Contin Educ Dent* 4:437–453, 1983.
Shimono K, Oshima M, Arakawa H, Kimura A, Nawachi K, Kuboki T: The effect of growth factors for bone augmentation to enable dental implant placement: a systematic review, *Jpn Dent Sci Rev* 46(1):43–53, 2010.
Sittitavornwong S, Gutta R: Bone graft harvesting from regional sites, *Oral Maxillofac Surg Clin N Am* 22(3):317–330, 2010.
Stavropoulos F, Nale J, Ruskin J: Guided bone regeneration, *Oral Maxillofac Surg Clin N Am* 14(1):15–27, 2002.
Van der Weijden F, Dell'Acqua F, Else Slot D: Alveolar bone dimensional changes of post-extraction sockets in humans: a systematic review, *J Clin Periodontol* 36:1048–1058, 2009.
Villar C, Cochran D: Regeneration of periodontal tissues: guided tissue regeneration, *Dent Clin N Am* 54(1):73–92, 2010.
Zhang Y, Zhang X, Shi B, Miron RJ: Membranes for guided tissue and bone regeneration, *Ann Oral Maxillofac Surg* 1(1):10, February 01, 2013.

CHAPTER 51

LOCAL AND REGIONAL FLAPS

Din Lam

1. **What is the principle of the reconstructive ladder?**
   Mathes and Nahai originally introduced the concept of the reconstructive ladder in 1982 to provide a systematic way of thinking about wound closure. The "ladder" included primary closure at the bottom rung and ascended through increasingly complex reconstructive means such as skin grafts or local flaps toward microvascular free tissue transfer at the top. It is an important concept designed to improve predictability of wound coverage. In the head and neck reconstruction, however, rungs of the ladder are often skipped to achieve more ideal restoration of form and function. For instance, a composite mandibular defect may be closed using a regional flap such as the pectoralis major that would be lower on the reconstructive ladder than a free flap. However, given the widely recognized predictability of free flaps, an osteocutaneous free tissue transfer may be selected as a more ideal reconstruction.

2. **How does a skin graft heal?**
   Skin graft healing require three phrases. During the first 48 hours, the process of plasmatic imbibition allows the graft to survive the immediate post-graft period before circulation is established. Imbibition is a process that allows nutritive materials to diffuse from the host bed to the skin graft. After 48 hours, anastomotic connections are established between host and graft vessels (inosculation). At the same time, angiogenesis occurs in the skin graft.

3. **What is the difference between full-thickness skin grafts (FTSGs) and split-thickness skin grafts (STSGs)?**
   STSGs are 0.30 to 0.45 mm thick. The skin is sectioned below the papillary dermis, so it will only contain epidermis and a portion of the upper reticular dermis. Because the skin adnexa (hair follicles and associated sebaceous glands, eccrine and apocrine sweat glands) originate in the midreticular dermis or in the subcutaneous fat layer, they are generally not included in STSGs.

   In FTSGs, the dermis is not split. The plane of cleavage is designed to separate the subcutaneous fat from the dermis. The actual thickness of an FTSG is extremely variable and depends on the location on the donor site and the sex, age, and health of the patient.

   The eyelid and supraclavicular and postauricular skin are the thinnest on the body, whereas the palms, soles, and trunk are the thickest. Women have thinner skin. The dermis is very thin in children; it increases until age 50, and then it atrophies. Conditions such as malnutrition, chronic steroid therapy, and insulin-dependent diabetes mellitus also affect dermal thickness.

4. **What are primary and secondary contractions?**
   Primary contraction refers to the immediate elastic recoil of the graft as it is harvested. Secondary contraction occurs during the healing process of the graft and is clinically more significant. The less dermis, the more the graft will contract secondarily.

5. **What percentage of contraction can be expected from STSG and FTSG?**
   A full-thickness graft loses about 40% of its original area, and a thin, split-thickness graft contracts by approximately 10%. In contrast, STSG has significantly more secondary contraction.

6. **When are meshed grafts used?**
   Meshed grafts are useful when insufficient donor skin is available, when a highly convoluted area must be covered, when the recipient bed is less than optimal, or when moderate drainage is anticipated. Graft meshing is usually performed in 1:1.5 or 1:2 ratios.

7. **What are the best types of dressings for a donor site?**
   Donor site dressing for skin grafts can be categorized into four types: open, semiopen, semiocclusive, and occlusive. Open technique is associated with prolonged healing time and increased pain. Semiopen technique utilizes Xeroform gauze to be place over the harvesting site and secured with regular wound dressing. Semiocclusive dressing, such as Op-site and Tegaderm, are bacteria- and

liquid-impermeable but permeable to moisture. They promote faster and less painful healing but are more labor intensive. Fluid or exudates tend to collect under the dressings and need to be drained frequently. Occlusive dressing, such as Duoderm, enhances the rate of epithelialization and collagen synthesis and reduces the bacteria count by decreasing the pH of the exudate. Furthermore, because it does not adhere to the bed, it does not cause irritation or pain.

8. What are the advantages of using local flaps in the head and neck?
   - Similar color and texture of the skin for the site of the defect.
   - Donor sites frequently can be closed directly.
   - Little or minimal scar contracture.

9. What factors most affect aesthetics and function following reconstruction with local flaps?
   Using physical characteristics of tissue can lead to better functional and aesthetic results after reconstruction with local flaps. Such characteristics include integration of relaxed skin tension lines, taking into consideration the cosmetic units of the face, and better use of the physical properties of the skin.

10. Can you describe the various types of local flaps?
    - Random flap: Blood supply is from subdermal plexus.
    - Axial flap: Blood supply is from a segmental artery that runs the length of the flap.
    - Advancement flap: The skin adjacent to the defect is undermined and advanced.
    - Rotation flap: A flap is rotated along an arc into the defect.
    - Transposition flap: A flap is passed over an incomplete bridge of skin.
    - Interpolated flap: A flap is passed over or under a complete bridge of skin, which separates the flap from the defect (paramedian flap).

11. What is stress relaxation?
    As a constant load is applied to the skin causing it to stretch, the load required to maintain this stretch will decrease.

12. What is tissue creep?
    As a sudden load is applied to the skin and kept constant, the amount of extension of the skin will increase as more time is applied.

13. Where should incision lines for local flaps and donor area fall?
    Lines of minimal relaxed tension. The skin tension is at right angles to these lines.

14. In the design of a Z-plasty, what angles yield what percentage of gain in length?
    - 30° will yield 25% gain in length.
    - 45° will yield 50%.
    - 60° will yield 75%.

15. What are the indications for a Z-plasty?
    - To realign scars within the resting skin tension lines
    - To adjust contours by reorienting the tissue
    - To lengthen any linear scar contractures
    - To disperse scars for cosmetic adjustments

16. What are Burrow's triangles?
    This is excess skin that one will find at the base of an advancement flap. This skin needs to be excised to complete the flap.

17. In a rotation flap, what is the typical shape should the defect be excised? And where is the line of greatest tension?
    A triangle with the base as the shortest side is the typical defect repaired with a rotation flap. The line of greatest tension extends from the pivot point of the flap to the edge of the defect nearest to where the flap previously lay.

18. What are the causes of local flap failures in the head and neck?
    - A small flap designed to fill a large defect
    - Hematoma
    - Compromised blood supply

- Tension during closure
- Unfavorable flap design (length:width ratio > 3:1)

19. **What are the most common regional flaps with their vascular supply?**
See Table 51-1.

20. **What is the most common complication related to a temporalis flap? And how can it be prevented?**
Temporal hollowing is commonly noticeable when the donor site is not properly reconstructed. A temporalis flap can be divided into two pedicles: anterior and posterior pedicles. Most defects can be repaired with only the anterior pedicle, where the posterior pedicle can be advanced anteriorly to prevent temporal hollowing. Alternatively, an alloplastic implant can also be used to restore the donor site defect.

21. **How can one prevent vessel injury when harvesting a submental island flap?**
To ensure safety of the submental island flap, a portion of anterior digastric muscle should be harvested with the vascular paddle. Further precaution can be taken if incorporating a portion of mylohyoid muscle with the vascular paddle. This modification helps to sandwich the vessel between two muscle tissues.

22. **Can a submental island flap be used in reconstructing an ablative defect from malignant pathology?**
The major concern of using a submental island flap in a malignant patient is related to incomplete removal of lymphatic tissue in the Level IA region. Although Hayden et al. have reported a series of reconstructive cases with submental island flap on patients with squamous cell carcinoma, the utility of this flap in this patient population remains controversial. This flap, however, will be a great option for the surgeon in treating malignant pathologies that carry a low metastatic rate to the neck, such as adenoid cystic carcinoma and sarcoma.

Table 51-1. The Most Common Regional Flaps with Their Vascular Supply

FLAP	DOMINANT BLOOD SUPPLY
Pectoralis major myocutaneous	Thoracoacromial artery Superior and lateral thoracic arteries contribute
Deltopectoral skin	Perforators from internal mammary artery
Temporalis muscle	Anterior and posterior deep temporal arteries
Temporoparietal fascia	Superficial temporal artery
Paramedian flap	Supratrochlear artery
Nasolabial flap	Random flap or axial flap based on angular artery
Submental island flap	Submental artery
Facial arterial myomucosal flap	Branch of facial artery
Tongue flap	Most common tongue flap is random flap. Axial flap design is based on dorsal-lingual branch of lingual artery
Palatal island flap	Greater palatine artery
Platysma myocutaneous	Submental branch of facial artery
Trapezius myocutaneous	Transverse cervical artery
Latissimus dorsi myocutaneous	Thoracodorsal artery
Sternocleidomastoid myocutaneous	Branches of occipital and superior thyroid arteries
Trapezius flap	Dorsal scapular artery
Supraclavicular flap	Supraclavicular artery

23. When harvesting a pectoralis major myocutaneous flap, how much skin paddle off the muscle can one incorporate?

Size and location of skin paddle depends on reconstructive needs. Typical skin paddle is harvested at the infero-medial border of the pectoralis major muscle. The sixth costal cartilage serves as a landmark for the inferior border of the muscle. Skin overlying any portion of the muscle can be utilized, and the larger the skin paddle, the more likehood the skin will survive due to the increased number of myocutaneous perforators. Additional 3–5 cm length can be harvested beyond the inferior edge of the pectoralis muscle as a random pattern flap.

24. When reconstructing a head and neck defect with a pedicled latissimus dorsi myocutaneous (LDM) flap, how does one transfer this flap to the recipient site?

A pedicled LDM flap is not commonly used in head and neck reconstruction since the increasing popularity of free flap. However, it remains an important flap for the reconstructive surgeon, especially in the case of a patient with depleted neck vessels. A pedicled LDM flap is easy to harvest and provides a large volume of tissue. Once the flap is raised, the pedicled LDM flap will be delivered to the recipient site by creating a subcutaneous tunnel around the deltopectoral region or between the pectoralis major and minor muscles.

25. For a palatal island flap, is it possible to harvest the entire palatal tissue based on a single artery?

Yes. A rich anatomic network, called the trilaminar macronet, exists within the mucosa, submucosa, and periosteum between the right and left greater palatine arteries. This dense network allows the entire palatal tissue to be harvested based on single greater palatine artery.

26. What are the two variations of a facial arterial myomucosal (FAMM) flap?

A FAMM flap can be either a superiorly or inferiorly based flap, depending on the location of the defect. A superiorly based FAMM flap is based on the retrograde flow of the facial artery and is used to reconstruct a soft tissue defect found in the maxilla, palate, or floor of the nose. An inferiorly based FAMM flap is based on the antegrade flow of the facial artery and is used to reconstruct a soft tissue defect found in the floor of the mouth and lower jaw.

27. When performing a tongue flap, what determines whether it should be an anteriorly or posteriorly based flap?

The location of the defect determines where a tongue flap is based. For defects of the soft palate, retromolar region, and posterior buccal mucosa, a posteriorly based flap is used. Anterior-based flaps are used for hard palate defects, defects of the anterior buccal mucosa, and anterior floor of the mouth or lips.

28. How long before you can safely divide the pedicle when using a tongue flap to repair oronasal communication?

Most tongue flaps used for oral cavity reconstruction require a two-stage procedure. The first stage is to harvest and to insert the flap to the recipient sites. At this stage, the flap remains attached to the donor site for its blood. After 10 to 14 days, a new blood supply to the recipient site is established, and attachment to the donor site can be safely divided.

BIBLIOGRAPHY

Baker SR, Swanson NA: *Local flaps in facial reconstruction*, ed 2, St Louis, 1995, Mosby. Print.

Chim H, Salgado C, Seselgyte R, Wei Fu-C, Mardini S: Principles of head and neck reconstruction: an algorithm to guide flap selection, *Semin Plast Surg* 24(2):148–154, 2010. Print.

Chu EA, Byrne PJ: Local flaps I: bilobed, rhombic, and cervicofacial, *Fac Plast Surg Clin North Am* 17(3):349–360, 2009. Print.

Tschoi M, Hoy EA, Granick MS: Skin flaps, *Surg Clin North Am* 89(3):643–658, 2009. Print.

Neligan PC: Head and neck reconstruction, *Plast Reconstr Surg* 131(2):260e–269e, 2013. Print.

Patel KG, Sykes JM: Concepts in local flap design and classification, *Oper Tech Otolaryngol-Head Neck Surg* 22(1):13–23, 2011. Print.

Urken ML: *Atlas of regional and free flaps for head and neck reconstruction: flap harvest and insetting*, ed 2, Philadelphia, 2012, Wolters Kluwer Health/Lippincott Williams & Wilkins. Print.

Ward BB: The palatal flap, *Oral Maxillofac Surg Clin North Am* 15(4):467–473, 2003. Print.

Ward BB: Temporalis system in maxillary reconstruction: temporalis muscle and temporoparietal galea flaps, *Atlas Oral Maxillofac Surg Clin* 15(1):33–42, 2007. Print.

Wei Fu-C, Mardini S: *Flaps and reconstructive surgery*, ed 1, Philadelphia, 2009, Saunders/Elsevier. Print.

CHAPTER 52

RECONSTRUCTION OF THE FACIAL SUBUNITS

Melvyn S. Yeoh, Andrew T. Meram

1. **What are the principles related to closing large forehead defects?**
   - When encompassing more than half of the forehead, reconstruction of the entire forehead as a single aesthetic unit should be considered.
   - If the defect includes a portion of one eyebrow, consideration should be given to preserving the intact eyebrow while reconstructing the affected eyebrow.

2. **What area of the forehead has the thinnest and most pliable skin?**
   The glabella region.

3. **Local blockade of which nerves can provide adequate anesthesia to the forehead?**
   Supraorbital and supratrochlear nerves.

4. **Where are the resting skin tension lines on the forehead?**
   Transversely in the forehead and vertically in the glabella region.

5. **What are some of the options available for forehead reconstruction?**
   - Primary closure
   - Closure by secondary intention
   - Skin grafting
   - Local rotational flaps
   - Distant pedicled flaps
   - Skin expansion
   - Microvascular composite tissue transplantation
   - Flap prefabrication

6. **How must primary closure best be obtained, and what type of defect is best suited for primary closure?**
   Most suitable for elliptical defects transversely oriented in anterior portion of forehead parallel to lines of resting skin tension. Transverse dimension can be as long as the full width of the forehead but must have limited vertical height.

7. **How might one obtain additional length for flaps of the forehead and/or scalp?**
   Galeal scoring spaced 0.5 to 1 cm apart.

8. **What are common types of forehead local flaps?**
   Rhomboid, dual rhomboid, banner, bilobed flaps, Worthen flap, shutter flap.

9. **How is the eyebrow best reconstructed?**
   Hair follicular transplantation.

10. **What are options for total eyebrow reconstruction?**
    - Hair plug transplants
    - Hair strip grafts
    - Pedicled scalp flaps

11. What are some options for lower eyelid reconstruction?
    - Direct closure: It can be used in full-thickness defects of up to 30% of the lower eyelid in a young patient and up to 45% in an elderly patient.
    - Tenzel semicircular rotational flap: It can be used for defects of up to 60% of the lid.
    - Hughes tarsoconjunctival flap: It can be used for defects of more than 50% of the lower lid. This upper lid to lower lid sharing technique requires a secondary stage to separate the flap.
    - Mustardé cheek flap: It can be used for very large defects up to the entire lower lid.

12. What are some options for upper eyelid reconstruction?
    - Direct closure: It can be used in full-thickness defects of up to 33% of the lower eyelid in a young patient and up to 40% in an elderly patient.
    - Tenzel semicircular rotational flap: It can be used for defects of up to 60% of the lid.
    - Sliding tarsoconjunctival flap: It can be used on defects of the upper lid that are too large for direct closure by horizontally sliding a section of tarsus from the remaining lid to close the defect and placing a skin graft.
    - Cutler-Beard (bridge) flap: It can be used to repair full-thickness upper lid defects of more than 60% up to defects of the entire upper lid. This procedure requires a secondary stage and an inset ear cartilage graft to reconstruct the tarsus.

13. What are the nasal subunits?
    Dorsum, tip, columella, paired sidewalls, alae, and soft triangles.

14. Can you describe skin quality on the different nasal subunits?
    Skin quality differs from one region to the other. Skin of the nasal dorsum and sidewalls is thin, smooth, and pliable. Skin of the tip and alar subunits is thick, stiff, and pitted with sebaceous glands.

15. How do split-thickness skin grafts heal on the nose?
    They always appear thin and shiny after transfer secondary to the temporary ischemia associated with revascularization.

16. How does a full-thickness skin graft on the nose differ depending on the location?
    It will blend well in the smooth-skinned zones of the dorsum or sidewalls. In contrast, a thin, shiny skin graft will appear as a patch if placed within the normally thick, pitted tip or ala. These regions are better suited for local or regional flap reconstruction.

17. What are potential donor sites for skin grafting of the nose?
    Superficial defects of the upper two-thirds of the nose in the zone of smooth skin can be grafted with full-thickness skin grafts with good results. Preauricular skin provides an ideal match. Postauricular skin may also be harvested, but it tends to heal with a red hue. Supraclavicular skin is another choice to resurface the entire nose, although color match is less satisfactory as it tends to heal with a brownish hue. Split-thickness skin grafts are generally not used in nasal reconstruction.

18. What are the indications for local flap reconstruction of the nose?
    - Small nasal defects less than 1.5 cm in diameter with no cartilage grafts needed
    - To reconstruct defects in the thin, mobile skin of the upper nose

19. What are some types of nasal local flaps?
    Bilobed flap, nasolabial flap, paramedian forehead flap, rhomboid flap, single-lobed flap.

20. What are options for large defects?
    As there is not enough nasal skin to redistribute over the nose to cover large defects, a forehead or nasolabial flap is required for defects greater than 1.5 cm in diameter or those requiring reconstruction of a cartilage framework.

21. What is the blood supply to the nasolabial flap?
    Based on the perforators from the facial and angular arteries that pass through the underlying levator labii and zygomatic muscles to the skin.

22. **What types of forehead flaps can be performed to reconstruct nasal defects, and what are their blood supplies?**
    - New's sickle flap (unilateral superficial temporal artery)
    - Converse's scalping flap (contralateral superficial temporal artery)
    - Median forehead flap (bilateral supraorbital vascular arteries)
    - Paramedian forehead flap (unilateral supratrochlear artery)

23. **Can you describe the paramedian forehead flap?**
    The flap can be designed on either the right or left supratrochlear vessel, but the reach of the flap is easier when it is based on the same side of the lateral defect. A template of the required missing forehead skin should be placed at the hairline and designed with a 1.5-cm pedicle above the supratroch-lear vessels. If the arc of rotation is short, an additional 1.5 cm can be added by extending the flap tip into hair-bearing scalp. The flap should be designed vertically to maintain its axial blood supply.

24. **When is a paramedian forehead flap divided?**
    The paramedian forehead flap can be divided as early as 2 weeks, but most advocate 3 weeks. Often a contouring procedure is done at this time by elevating the flap at an intermediate operation, creating a bipedicle flap that extends from the brow to the columellar inset. The flap can be defatted and thinned and repositioned on the nose with peripheral and quilting sutures. The pedicle is not transected. Three weeks later, the pedicle can be divided.

25. **How and why are primary bone and cartilage grafts used in nasal reconstruction?**
    For nasal reconstruction, bone and cartilage create the framework for the soft tissue. A composite defect will require reconstruction of both the covering soft tissue and the underlying framework.

26. **What donor tissues are available for nasal support?**
    Septal cartilage is the first choice for most nasal grafts. Auricular cartilage is a good choice for ala and tip support. Rib cartilage, cranial bone, and temporoparietal fascia mixed with diced cartilage can be used for nasal dorsum support.

27. **What is the normal size of the adult ear?**
    Height between 5.5 and 6.5 cm and width generally 66% of height in children and 55% of height in adults.

28. **What are general guidelines for proper aesthetic ear reconstruction?**
    - The ear should lie one ear length posterior to the lateral orbital rim.
    - The lateral protrusion of the helix from the scalp is between 1.5 and 2.0 cm.
    - The mean inclination of the ear from the vertical is 20° posterior.

29. **Can an amputated ear be replanted?**
    Yes, by microanastomosis of the posterior auricular artery and a posterior auricular vein to donor vessels.

30. **In case of total ear avulsion, microvascular replantation is not possible; what other options are available?**
    Mladick's two stages pocket technique is a possible option. In this technique, skin of the avulsed ear is removed, and the remaining cartilage is stored in the retroauricular area. This cartilage is retrieved at a later time for construction of auricular framework. Alternatively, this denuded cartilage can be reattached to its proper location and covered with temporoparietal fascia and a split-thickness skin graft. Unlike Mladick's procedure, this is a one-stage procedure.

31. **When total auricular reconstruction is needed, which costal cartilages are harvested?**
    The costal cartilages from ribs 6 to 9 are most commonly used.

32. **What are the goals of lip reconstruction?**
    - Maintain oral sphincter competence.
    - Restore anatomic landmarks.

- Provide adequate stomal opening for speech and eating.
- Preserve sensation.
- Restore aesthetic appearance.

33. **Restoration of what structure is critical in commissure reconstruction?**
The orbicularis oris muscle.

34. **What discrepancy in vermilion border can be noticeable and at what distance?**
1-mm discrepancy is noticeable at 3 ft.

35. **How much tissue loss still permits satisfactory closure of the lips?**
Up to 25% of the upper lip and 33% of the lower lip.

36. **Why is the lower lip a more suitable donor for reconstruction than the upper lip?**
- It has no distinguishing features such as Cupid's bow, philtrum, or tubercle.
- It may sustain greater tissue loss.
- It can donate tissue for upper lip reconstruction.

37. **What are options for repair of localized mucosal or vermilion defects?**
Notch or saddle deformities of the lower lip involving the vermilion can be managed by excision and Z-plasty, V-Y mucomuscular advancement flap, or the lateral mucomuscular advancement flap.

38. **What are the indications for an Abbe flap?**
- A moderate-sized defect of the lower lip that is off-center and spares the commissure
- A defect of the philtrum of the upper lip
- Restoration of symmetry to an overly small lower lip

39. **What is the Abbe flap?**
It is a V-shaped lower lip flap based on the inferior labial artery and designed opposite the area of defect for the central upper lip region. It is raised, transposed 180 degrees, and inset. The donor site is closed primarily. Second stage division of the pedicle and final inset are performed 14 days later.

40. **What are the indications for an Estlander flap, and what is its major disadvantage?**
Most useful in medium-sized lateral defects of the upper or lower lip that includes the commissure. It produces a rounded commissure that may result in a smaller oral aperture, possibly requiring secondary revisions.

41. **Can you describe the Estlander flap?**
A triangular flap based on the superior labial artery and designed for reconstruction of the lateral lower lip defects involving the commissure. The flap is transposed 180 degrees from the upper lip to the lower lip.

42. **What is the Karapandzic flap?**
It is a technique that maintains the neurovascular pedicle in the soft tissue while rotating and restoring sphincter continuity. Central defects of up to 80% can be reconstructed.

43. **What is the Gillies fan flap?**
Fan-shaped rotational advancement flap based on the superior labial artery and designed for large defects involving greater than 50% of the lower lip. It is made lateral to the defect around the nasolabial fold with a 1 cm back cut.

44. **What is a disadvantage of the Gillies fan flap?**
It may result in decreased oral aperture.

45. **Can you describe the McGregor flap?**
Rectangular-shaped flap modified from the Gillies fan flap and based on the superior labial artery. It is rotated around the commissure without altering the size of the oral aperture. The width of the flap

equals the vertical height of the defect, while the length of the flap equals the width of the defect plus the width of the flap.

46. **What is a drawback to the McGregor flap?**
A mucosal advancement flap is required to reconstruct the lip mucosa.

47. **What structures must be accounted for in malar reconstruction to prevent a poor esthetic outcome?**
The lower eyelid and canthal areas.

48. **How might one prevent lower lid ectropion?**
By suturing the advancing flap to the periosteum of the zygoma.

49. **What are the common reconstruction techniques for repairing cheek defect?**
- Small: Primary closure and local flap
- Moderate defect: Nasolabial flap
- Large defect: Cervicofacial rotational flap or submental island flap
- Through-and-through defect: Anterolateral thigh (ALT) free tissue flap

50. **What are the critical elements of the cervicofacial flap?**
- Extensive undermining of the cervical cheek, retroauricular area, and chin
- Rotation is in a superomedial direction.
- Superior dissection lateral to the eye must be performed to prevent ectropion.
- Dissection into the mucosa can allow closure of intraoral and through-and-through defects.

BIBLIOGRAPHY

Bauer BS, Bauer EM: Ear reconstruction. In *Plastic surgery secrets plus*, ed 2, Philadelphia, 2010, Mosby Elsevier, pp 395–400.
Carlson ER, Guerra A: Lip cancer – ablative and reconstructive surgery. In *Current therapy in oral and maxillofacial surgery*, St Louis, MO, 2012, Saunders Elsevier, pp 516–526.
Ghali GE, Herford AS: Local and regional flaps. In *Peterson's principles of oral & maxillofacial surgery*, Shelton, CT, 2012, People's Medical Publishing House, pp 877–892.
Hebda PA: Wound healing of the skin. In *Essential tissue healing of the face and neck*, Shelton, CT, 2009, People's Medical Publishing House, pp 1–15.
Holmes JD: The temporalis system of flaps in head and neck reconstruction: temporoparietal fascia and temporalis muscle flaps. In *Current therapy in oral and maxillofacial surgery*, St Louis, MO, 2012, Saunders Elsevier, pp 527–532.
Hong RW, Menick F: Nasal reconstruction. In *Plastic surgery secrets plus*, ed 2, Philadelphia, 2010, Mosby Elsevier, pp 381–387.
Mankani MH, Mathes SJ: Forehead reconstruction. In *Plastic surgery secrets plus*, ed 2, Philadelphia, 2010, Mosby Elsevier, pp 373–380.
McClure SA, Best SP: Ear reconstruction. In *Current therapy in oral and maxillofacial surgery*, St Louis, MO, 2012, Saunders Elsevier, pp 558–565.
McConnell MP, Evans GRD: Local flaps of the head and neck. In *Plastic surgery secrets plus*, ed 2, Philadelphia, 2010, Mosby Elsevier, pp 363–372.
Perciaccante VJ, Jelic SJ: Oral and maxillofacial reconstruction. In *Oral and maxillofacial secrets*, ed 2, St Louis, MO, 2007, Mosby Elsevier, pp 389–403.
Salama AR: Flap classification and principles of flap design for head and neck reconstruction. In *Current therapy in oral and maxillofacial surgery*, St Louis, MO, 2012, Saunders Elsevier, pp 11–18.
Seki JT: Lip reconstruction. In *Plastic surgery secrets plus*, ed 2, Philadelphia, 2010, Mosby Elsevier, pp 401–408.
Shetty V, Bertolami CN: Wound healing. In *Peterson's principles of oral & maxillofacial surgery*, Shelton, CT, 2012, People's Medical Publishing House, pp 3–16.

CHAPTER 53

MICROVASCULAR SURGERY

Srinivasa Chandra, Rui Fernandes, Jacob Yetzer

1. What is microvascular surgery?

Microsurgery is simply any surgery performed using a microscope for magnification. *Microvascular surgery* refers to microsurgery that includes repair and anastomosis of small blood vessels (generally < 3 mm). This term is often used interchangeably with the term *microvascular reconstruction*. This technique is important in head and neck reconstruction because it allows for tissue to be transferred from a distant site to the defect site with its own blood supply intact. The tissue donor tissue is harvested with the vascular pedicle (supplying artery and vein) and anastomosed or connected to corresponding recipient site vessels.

2. How are flaps classified?

Free flaps can are most commonly classified on a basis of their *tissue composition* and their *blood supply*. Flaps can be composed of skin alone, skin and fascia, skin and muscle, bone alone, or skin muscle and bone together. The nomenclature for these flaps includes cutaneous, fasciocutaneous, myocutaneous, osseous, and osteomusculofasciocutaneous flaps.

Numerous classifications based on blood supply have been published. Probably the most commonly referenced is the Mathes and Nahai classification of muscular flaps listed in Table 53-1.

Cormack and Lamberty and Nakajima also contributed named classifications for cutaneous and fasciocutaneous flaps. The common feature these share is a description of the course of the supplying perforator vessel. For practical purposes, perforator vessels can all be described as "direct," meaning they travel directly from the main vascular pedicle through a fascial plane to supply the skin, or "indirect," meaning they pass through other tissue (usually muscle) before reaching the skin.

3. What is a perforator vessel?

These are identifiable, but unnamed vessels arising from a named source vessel and directly or indirectly supplying a portion of the skin. So-called perforator flaps allow for significant flexibility and creativity in flap harvest.

4. What is an angiosome?

The concept of the angiosome was introduced by Taylor and Palmer in 1987. They divided each half of the body into 40 territories based on the source artery providing the vascular supply. Each anatomic territory can be further divided based on perforators originating from the source vessel. Of clinical importance is the fact that each angiosome is connected to adjacent angiosomes by anastomotic vessels referred to as *choke vessels*. Because of the presence of choke vessels a flap can have a clinical territory somewhat larger than the anatomic territory of the feeding vessel.

5. What is a chimeric flap?

A chimeric flap is a flap that includes multiple tissue paddles that are physically independent from one another, each with a blood supply that originates from a single vascular pedicle. An example would be a scapula flap based on the circumflex scapular artery that includes latissimus dorsi as a separate paddle fed by the thoracodorsal artery. Both the circumflex scapular and thoracodorsal arteries originate from the subscapular artery.

6. When is microvascular reconstruction indicated?

- Posttraumatic defects
- Oncologic resections
- Post-radiation areas with vascular, chronic infection, functional, or structural complications
- Congenital and acquired malformations

Table 53-1. The Mathes and Nahai Classification of Muscular Flaps

FLAP TYPE	VASCULAR SUPPLY	EXAMPLES
Type I	One dominant vascular pedicle	Gastrocnemius, rectus femoris, tensor fascia lata
Type II	Dominant vascular pedicle and minor pedicle	Gracilis, peroneus longus, platysma, soleus, sternocleidomastoid, temporalis, trapezius, vastus lateralis
Type III	Two dominant pedicles	Gluteus maximus, rectus abdominis, serratus anterior
Type IV	Multiple segmental pedicles	Extensor digitorum longus, extensor hallucis longus, sartorius, tibialis anterior
Type V	One dominant pedicle and secondary segmental pedicles	Pectoralis major, latissimus dorsi

7. What are the goals of microvascular reconstruction?
Essentially, this is an autotransplant with its own vascular pedicle. Flaps may be inclusive of skin, fascia, muscle, and bone to an area deficient of structure, vascularity, and function. In general, the goal is to achieve restoration of form and function by replacing "like with like"—that is, soft tissue with soft tissue, bone with bone, and so forth. When insufficient local tissue is unavailable or geometrically insufficient for reconstruction, a soft tissue flap is a solution. Osseous free flaps are useful in reconstructing long bony defects (> 5 to 6 cm) or in those sites where the recipient bed is poorly vascularized or irradiated. Finally, composite defects, where multiple tissue types are needed to be replaced, are readily reconstructed by a composite free flap that suits the needs of the defect.

8. What are contraindications to microvascular reconstruction?
There are few absolute contraindications to microvascular reconstruction. Relative contraindications include a hypercoagulable state, ongoing infection at the recipient or donor site, a patient unable to tolerate a prolonged surgery due to medical comorbidities, poor nutritional status, and inadequate recipient vessels. Also, there are donor site-specific contraindications to consider. For instance, history of upper arm trauma or cephalic vein harvest would be a contraindication for a forearm flap. Likewise, a lower extremity flap would be contraindicated in the setting of peripheral vascular disease. Each flap has its own donor site morbidities to consider that also bear weight in the decision to use a flap.

9. What is the success rate of microvascular free flap transfer?
Success rate is around 95% to 98%.

10. In which order are the artery and vein anastomosed?
The decision should be based on intraoperative anatomy. If repair of the artery will result in poor exposure of the veins, venous repair should be done first. The reverse is also true.

11. What are the microvascular anastomotic techniques for diameter discrepancies?
Diameter of vessel mismatch can be resolved by proportional suturing, differential dilation. and bevelling. Thickness discrepancy can be matched with radial proportional suturing the outer wall while matching the inner diameter.

12. What are the commonly used soft tissue free flaps for craniomaxillofacial reconstruction?
Radial forearm fasciocutaneous, lateral arm fasciocutaneous, latissimus dorsi myocutaneous, anterolateral thigh fasciocutaneous, rectus abdominis myocutaneous.

13. What are the bone flaps commonly used for craniomaxillofacial reconstruction?
Fibula osseous or osteocutaneous, iliac crest osseous or osteocutaneous, scapula osseous or osteocutaneous, radial forearm osteocutaneous.

14. **What is the arterial and venous supply to each of the flaps listed in question 13?**
    - Radial forearm: radial artery, vena comitantes, and cephalic vein (dual outflow)
    - Lateral arm: perforators of the posterior radial collateral artery, vena comitantes, cephalic vein (dual outflow)
    - Latissimus dorsi: thoracodorsal artery and vein
    - Anterolateral thigh: perforators from the descending branch of the lateral circumflex femoral artery and vena comitantes
    - Rectus abdominis: deep inferior epigastric artery and vein
    - Fibula: peroneal artery and vein
    - Iliac crest: deep circumflex iliac artery and vein
    - Scapula: circumflex scapular artery and vein

15. **What is unique about the scapula flap?**
    The scapula flap is based on the circumflex scapular artery, which is a branch of the subscapular system. Branches of the subscapular system not only provide blood supply to the latissimus dorsi, but the circumflex scapular artery has multiple distinct cutaneous and osseous branches. This means that multiple areas of skin and tissue types can be harvested based on one vascular pedicle as a chimeric flap. This allows flaps of the subscapular system to reconstruct geometrically complex defects. Also, unlike the other osseous flaps often used in head and neck reconstruction, the scapula flap will not interfere with postoperative ambulation.

16. **Which recipient site vessels are commonly utilized in the head and neck?**
    Generally, one of several branches of the external carotid artery is selected for anastomosis. The most commonly used are the ipsilateral facial artery, superior thyroid artery, and superficial temporal artery (for upper facial reconstruction). If these are unavailable, other vessels may be selected, the contralateral neck can be used, and vein grafting or vessel transposition are options for the vessel-depleted neck.

17. **What should be included in the workup prior to microvascular reconstruction?**
    In addition to planning the reconstruction on a basis of the anticipated defect, the history and physical should focus on prior surgeries or trauma to the recipient site. If there has been prior surgery, obtaining the operative report can be helpful in elucidating which recipient vessels may still be available. If this is still in question, a computed tomography angiography (CTA) and magnetic resonance angiography (MRA) of the neck may be helpful. If bony reconstruction is planned, consideration ought to be given to obtaining a stereolithographic model to aid in planning and plate contouring. Virtual surgical planning can also be very helpful in this setting.
    Similar considerations should be given to the anticipated donor site. Again prior surgery or trauma will affect the availability of local tissue or vascular pedicle. The particular morbidities of any given flap should be considered in light of the patient's overall status. For instance, a patient with known peripheral vascular disease may be a poor candidate for a fibula flap.

18. **When should imaging of the lower extremity be performed prior to harvesting the fibula flap?**
    When planning a lower extremity flap such as the fibula flap, collateral blood supply to the distal extremity must be confirmed or the patient may suffer disastrous outcomes such as loss of a foot. Normally, the anterior and posterior tibial arteries as well as the peroneal artery supply the lower extremity. When the fibula flap is harvested, the peroneal vessel is eliminated, and the patient loses some of this vascular redundancy. Imaging such as CTA or MRA should be obtained if there is any concern for peripheral vascular disease to confirm three-vessel runoff.
    Be alert for risk factors such as smoking, hypertension, hypercholesterolemia, and history of coronary or cerebrovascular disease. Also, claudication, cold extremities, hair loss, and absent pulses are clinical indicators of peripheral vascular disease.

19. **What is the Allen's test?**
    This is a clinical test used to confirm collateral flow to the hand. This is important when planning a radial forearm flap, which eliminates the radial artery as a nourishing vessel to the hand. The patient raises his hand and makes a tight fist to exsanguinate the hand. The physician then occludes both the radial and ulnar vessels by compressing them. The patient then opens his hand. When the

surgeon releases the ulnar artery alone, blood flow in the form of blush should return to the hand in less than 5 to 6 seconds. This indicates that the deep and superficial palmar arches are present and communicate, thus assuring that the radial and ulnar vasculature share collateral flow. In a smaller percentage of patients, this may not be the case—this is an absolute contraindication for a radial artery flap.

20. **Which of the flaps discussed above poses a risk of postoperative ileus or hernia?**
    The iliac crest and rectus abdominis free flaps both present a risk for ileus and hernia as dissection of the abdominal fascia and retraction of the abdominal contents are unavoidable during harvest of these flaps. Watertight closure of the fascia and gentle retraction during harvest will help avoid these complications. However, patients should be monitored postoperatively for signs including abdominal distention, nausea, vomiting, frequent belching, and lack of flatus or bowel movement.

21. **What is the best way to monitor a free flap postoperatively?**
    Clinical examination. Hourly clinical exam of the flap during the first 24 hours after surgery includes the following:
    - Color: A white flap indicates arterial insufficiency; a cyanotic or blue flap indicates venous congestion.
    - Temperature: The temperature should be the same as surrounding tissue. A cool flap can indicate either an arterial or venous problem. Note: This can be misinterpreted inside the oral cavity.
    - Turgor: Decreased turgor may indicate arterial occlusion; increased turgor indicates venous congestion.
    - Capillary refill: A slow or absent refill indicates arterial occlusion; a brisk refill indicates venous congestion.
    - Pinprick: No bleeding may represent arterial occlusion, while brisk, dark block may be due to venous congestion. Note: The pinprick test is not done regularly.

22. **What are adjuncts to the clinical exam when monitoring a flap?**
    External, handheld Doppler monitoring is the most commonly used adjunct followed by implantable Doppler. Other modalities include laser Doppler monitoring, oxygen probe, and near infrared spectroscopy.

23. **Can you list the potential causes for flap failure?**
    - Thrombosis: This may be caused by vessel trauma during surgery, a hypercoagulable state, or reperfusion injury.
    - Mechanical problems: These may be kinking or compression of the pedicle due to patient position, tight surrounding tissue or hematoma, or inadequate vessel match or size.
    - Physiological: It may be caused by factors such as hypotension or hypovolemia.

24. **Which is more common, arterial or venous occlusion?**
    Venous occlusion is the most common cause of flap failure.

25. **What are postoperative considerations to treat or prevent flap congestion?**
    Topical nitric oxide paste can be applied to the flap, which acts on vascular smooth muscle to vasodilate local vessels. Warm compresses over the flap will have a similar effect. Leech therapy is another consideration, which both increases outflow and has an antithrombotic effect due to the *hirudin* in the leech's saliva. If leech therapy is used, prophylactic coverage of *Aeromonas hydrophila* is required as there is a risk of transmission.

26. **What is meant by the term *ischemia-reperfusion* injury?**
    In any free tissue transfer there is an ischemic episode created when the flap is divided from its vascular supply. This leads to anaerobic metabolism. With time, membrane transporters fail and intracellular calcium accumulates, leading to an inflammatory cascade and production of free radicals. The injury is compounded when the blood supply is re-established (reperfusion). The inflammatory process, which has already begun, is continued by the influx of neutrophils and further production of reactive oxygen species. This process leads to cell death in the form of apoptosis and necrosis, which can lead to flap failure. The surgeon must be expeditious with flap harvest to minimize ischemia time and maintain meticulous tissue handling during anastomosis to prevent secondary ischemia due to

vaso-occlusive episodes. In essence, consideration is needed to eliminate Virchow's triad of stasis, hypercoagulability, and vessel injury as the key to increase flap survival.

27. What methods can be used to minimize ischemia?

Meticulous planning is the most important factor to minimize the effects of ischemia. All recipient vessels should be selected before donor vessels are ligated. In general, muscle does not tolerate warm ischemia well for more than 2 hours. Skin and fasciocutaneous flaps can tolerate longer ischemia times (4 to 6 hours).

28. What is the no-reflow phenomenon?

After performing a patent anastomosis, the flap still fails to reperfuse. This no-reflow phenomenon appears to be related to an obstruction in the microcirculation secondary to endothelial injury, reperfusion injury, or platelet aggregation.

29. How long does it take for new endothelium to cover the anastomosis site?

Pseudointima is formed within the first 5 days of healing. New endothelium starts to cover the anastomosis site after 1 to 2 weeks.

BIBLIOGRAPHY

Budd M, Evans G: Postoperative care. In *Wei and Mardini flaps and reconstructive surgery*, London, 2009, pp 137–142.
Foster RD, Anthony JP, Sharma A, Pogrel MA: Vascularized bone flaps versus nonvascularized bone grafts for mandibular reconstruction: an outcome analysis of primary bony union and endosseous implant success, *Head and Neck* 21(1):66–71, 1999.
Hidalgo DA: Fibula free flap: a new method of mandible reconstruction, *Plast Reconstr Surg* 84:71–79, 1989.
Mathes SJ, Nahai F: Classification of the vascular anatomy of muscles: experimental and clinical correlation, *Plast Reconstr Surg* 67:177–187, 1981.
Pratt GF, Rozen WM, Westwood A, et al.: Technology-assisted and sutureless microvascular anastomoses: evidence for current techniques, *Microsurgery* 32:68–76, 2012.
Song YG, Chen GZ, Song YL: The free thigh flap: a new free flap concept based on the septocutaneous artery, *Br J Plast Surg* 37:149–159, 1984.
Taylor GI, Palmer JH: The vascular territories (angiosomes) of the body: experimental study and clinical applications, *Br J Plast Surg* 40:113–141, 1987. Accessed February 26, 2014.
Urken ML: *Atlas of regional and free flaps for head and neck reconstruction*, New York, 1995, Raven.
Van den Heuvel MG, Buurman WA, Bast A, van der Hulst RR: Review: Ischaemia-reperfusion injury in flap surgery, *J Plast Reconstr Aesthet Surg* 62:721–726, 2009.
Wei FC, Jain V, Celik N: Have we found an ideal soft-tissue flap? An experience with 672 anterolateral thigh flaps, *Plast Reconstr Surg* 109:2219–2226, 2002. discussion 27–30.
Yap LH, Butler CE, *Principles of microsurgery, Grabb and Smith's plastic surgery,* ed 6, edited by C. Thorne. Philadelphia, 2007, Lippincott Williams & Wilkins, pp 66–72.

CHAPTER 54

EVALUATION OF THE AGING FACE

Faisal A. Quereshy, Sarah Naghibi

1. **Can you identify the key elements in the evaluation of the aging face?**
   The cornerstone to the evaluation of the aging face is the physical assessment. Key elements included in this assessment are skin quality and bony structures. These are further divided into the evaluation of the facial thirds: upper, middle, and lower and neck. Although aesthetic surgery will often involve the soft tissue, the underlying bony structures will serve as a critical factor both in the approach and final outcome.

2. **What elements of the skin should be evaluated?**
   The initial evaluation should begin with an analysis of the individual's skin. Aspects of the aging skin that warrant attention are skin laxity, skin phototyping, presence or absence of rhytides, persistency of rhytides against tension, and rhytides from mechanical contraction and gravity.

3. **Can you describe skin phototyping and the Fitzpatrick scale?**
   Skin phototyping is quantified by the Fitzpatrick scale and represents a significant prognostic predictor in aesthetic facial surgery. The scale classifies the skin's varying response to UV light in the setting of aesthetic procedures. The practitioner can deduce from the scale an individual's response to specific procedures such as resurfacing and chemical peels. Fitzpatrick I and II patients have lighter skin and heal better; therefore they are more ideal candidates for laser resurfacing, chemical peels, dermabrasion, and microdermabrasion. Fitzpatrick I, II, and III have a lower risk for complications such as discolorations, burning, and scarring. However, these types tend to have deeper tension lines, and thus they are less suitable for resurfacing. Types IV to VI encompass darker skin patients who are not suitable for resurfacing, although they do not have deep dynamic lines like the former. They are also at a much higher risk for complication.

4. **What is Glogau's classification, and how does treatment strategy change for each group?**
   Glogau's classification of photoaging divides patients into four groups based on the degree of actinic keratosis, wrinkling, acne scarring, and the amount of makeup worn by the patient. This classification helps to assess and quantify the degree of sun damage in patients.

5. **What is Dedo classification, and how does it help with treatment planning?**
   Dedo classification helps to categorize cervical deformity based on the deepest tissue later involved in each: Class I is a normal patient, Class II is related to skin, Class III is fat, Class IV is platysma muscle, and Class V and VI are related to hyoid bone. Based on the etiology of the defect, treatment will be different from one group to the other. Submental liposuction alone will be ideal for Class III patients, whereas Class IV patients will benefit from surgical management of platysma muscle. Class V patients will require mandibular osteotomy or genioplasty. Class VI patients have low hyoid bone positioning, which limits the effectiveness of submental surgery.

6. **How do you evaluate skin laxity?**
   The pinch test is used to differentiate between superficial and deep skin laxity. Pinch test interpretation is as follows: easy lateral and shallow movement of skin is superficial. This superficial laxity manifests itself as rhytides. The physical exam will identify superficial laxity, while photographic analysis based on regions of the face will help identify laxity in the upper, middle, and lower and neck thirds. Specific areas of laxity across the facial thirds include the eyelid fold, nasojugal fold, melolabial fold, jowls, and platysma bands. Each laxity region is then quantified by severity from Class 0 to 5, 0 being devoid of laxity and 5 being the most severe laxity.

7. **What are the common signs found in the aging face?**
   - Ptotic and wrinkled brow
   - Glabellar laxity
   - Ptotic eyelid

- Droopy nasal tip
- Laxity of the cheeks
- Ptotic earlobes
- Perioral wrinkling
- Jowls
- Platysma bands
- Laxity of cervical skin

8. **What signs of facial aging are reversible by aesthetic surgery?**
   - Skin laxity in the cheek and neck region
   - Prominence of nasolabial folds
   - Jowling
   - Rhytides

9. **What are the common complaints found in patients with aging upper third of the face?**
   A frequent complaint of patients in regard to the aging face in this region is the appearance of a sustained tired or angry expression that is inconsistent with their actual disposition. When considering the forehead, aging leads to eyebrow or eyelid ptosis, which results in compensatory contraction of the frontalis muscle. The end result is forehead wrinkles.

10. **How does one evaluate frontalis compensation?**
    There are two ways to evaluate frontalis compensation: one is with the patient smiling, which eliminates the compensation. A second is closing eyes tightly and then slowly opening until sight is first established—compensation appears when eyes are fully open. The depth of existing forehead wrinkles will determine the surgical method—deep lines benefit from a subcutaneous approach, whereas laser resurfacing and endoscopic approaches favor finer wrinkles.

11. **How does glabellar angle change with age?**
    The glabellar angle of the forehead is formed by the intersection of the glabella-nasion and nasion-pronasale. The normal angle is 132 degrees with a 15 degree variation in either direction. Therefore, this angle can be assessed as excessive, normal, or deficient. Excessive angle indicates frontal bossing, whereas aging causes the normally round and projected glabellar to appear flat or depressed.

12. **What changes occur in the eyebrows with age?**
    Gravity is the primary force in brow position changes with age. The ideal female brow at the medial aspect coincides with a vertical plane from alar base to the medial canthus, and the lateral end parallels a line from the alar base to the lateral canthus. In females, the medial and lateral aspects of the brow should lie on the same horizontal plane, and the superior arch of the brow should be at its greatest height above the lateral limbus, with a 1 cm extension above the supraorbital rim. The male brow rests similarly but at a more level plane than the female arch. Brow correction from aging includes Botox, which can lift the brow, or surgical lifting involving endoscopic approach or transblepharoplasty.

13. **What changes occur in the upper eyelids with age?**
    The upper eyelid is usually the first feature of the upper face that exhibits signs of aging. These aging signs are due to skin quality, skin excess, and soft tissue changes. Attention must be given to the aesthetic areas in the upper eyelid: the lid sulcus, orbital palpebral fold, supratarsal fold, pretarsal crease, lacrimal gland, pretarsal skin, upper eyelid margin, and orbital fat. Skin laxity can be examined by gently grabbing pretarsal skin and pulling to create lagophthalmos. Excess skin laxity may result in the inability to fully close the eye. Redundant orbital fat can be evaluated in a similar fashion, and excess represents a consequence of aging and indication for correction. Skin laxity and excess can also lead to the obliteration of the superior palpebral fold in addition to its surrounding anatomy. Thus, the major goal of blepharoplasty is to reestablish this fold. Furthermore, excision of excess skin, which diminishes the eyelid's natural concavity, can restore a more youthful appearance.

14. **What are the important factors in evaluating lower eyelid aesthetic surgery?**
    The lower eyelid differs in its evaluation and surgical approach, depending on the etiology of the changes. Lower eyelids must be evaluated for lid laxity, fat pseudoherniation, and history of dry eyes. Ideally, the lower lid is slightly superior to the lower limbus. The lower lid position moves inferiorly with age, most commonly due to skin laxity and gravity. Excess sclera may be visible. As part of the physical exam, a snap test should be performed to assess for lid laxity. This entails

grasping the lower lid and gently pulling inferiorly and laterally. A normal response would be an instantaneous recoil. Delayed return to its original position signifies increased laxity and tissue redundancy, which may be an indication for lateral canthal tightening with or without lower blepharoplasty.

15. **Can you describe evaluation of the middle third of the face?**

The middle third of the face is punctuated by malar convexity, the depiction of youthful facial features. This convexity is supported by the zygoma and its associated soft tissue. With aging comes the descent of the soft tissue due to gravity and atrophy of the supporting subcutaneous tissue resulting in loss of the youthful convexity. The inferior movement of the cheek results in distinct aging characteristics: a deepening of the nasolabial fold and nasojugal groove and inferior displacement of the buccal fat pads. This can further result in effacement of the jawline with the now excess displaced tissue.

16. **What are the major causes of aging in the lower third of the face?**

Aging of the lower third of the face is predominantly caused by maxillary and mandibular bony resorption, increased skin laxity, and thinning of the subcutaneous fat.

17. **Can you describe the changes with age in the perioral region?**

In general, the upper lip tends to thin out more than the lower lip. Gravity contributes to ptosis of the superficial musculoponeurotic system (SMAS) and fat, both of which are necessary to create a tight, smooth lower facial appearance. The ptosis causes jowls to develop, which creates a widened lower facial width. Aging of the lower face can further be evaluated by locating a horizontal line connecting the oral commissures. This line should be parallel to a corresponding horizontal line between the canthi in young patients. Aging patients will demonstrate a posterior tilt of the oral commissure line.

18. **What are the changes that are found in the aging neck?**

The aging cervical region is largely dependent on bony structures. Specifically, hyoid position, chin prominence, and midface vector should all be thoroughly evaluated in the aging patient. The cervicomental angle is formed by the horizontal submandibular plane and vertically by the neck. An angle between 90 and 100 degrees is considered a youthful aesthetic. Wider angles are often due to a low and anteriorly positioned hyoid bone. Cervicomental angle is also influenced by chin position. Retrognathia can increase the angle. This creates a dulled transition between face and neck. Furthermore, the appearance of the neck becomes heavier and blunted.

The aging patient can be evaluated for tissue redundancy in the neck, which will obscure youthful landmarks and contours. During the physical exam, the practitioner can pull the redundant tissue upward, just inferior and anterior to the ear, which will cause those landmarks to reappear. If the tissue is easily displaced it is considered redundant. During this maneuver, the underlying residual fullness and lipomatosis can be better visualized. The pinch test can also be used to differentiate between redundant tissue and fat—the redundant being easily pinched. To evaluate skin laxity, the patient can protrude the mandible forcefully while the clinician assesses for skin laxity.

Evaluate the platysma and its associated lipomatosis via palpation during contraction to observe midline crossing patterns, which occur at various levels relative to the location of lipomatosis in the neck. In the aging patient, lipomatosis is commonly found deep to the platysma and midline. This maneuver also helps the surgeon quantify the amount of subcutaneous fat in addition to its location relative to the platysma.

19. **What differences are noted between men and women in evaluating patients for aesthetic surgery?**
    - Position of the eyebrows is different
    - Different patterns of hair growth in the scalp
    - Presence of a beard in men, which causes an increase the thickness and blood supply in the region
    - Psychological differences

BIBLIOGRAPHY

Guyuron B, Eriksson E, Persing JA, et al.: *Plastic surgery: indications and practice*, St Louis, MO, 2008, Saunders.
Kaminer MS, Arndt KA, Dover JS, et al.: *Atlas of cosmetic surgery*, ed 2, St Louis, MO, 2009, Saunders, pp 37–43.

1. **Can you describe the motor and sensory innervation of the eyeball, eyelids, and associated structures?**
   - The superior oblique muscle has motor innervation from the trochlear nerve (cranial nerve IV).
   - The lateral rectus muscle has motor innervation from the abducens nerve (cranial nerve VI).
   - The remainder of the extraocular muscles receive motor innervation from the oculomotor nerve (cranial nerve III).
   - Sensory innervation of the eye is from the trigeminal nerve (cranial nerve 5, V1 branch, mainly through the ciliary nerve).
   - Visual sensory is from the optic nerve (cranial nerve).
   - Lid opening is from the levator palpebrae superioris, which is innervated by the oculomotor nerve (cranial nerve III).
   - Lid closing is a result of the orbicularis oculi contraction, which is innervated by the facial nerve (frontal and zygomatic branches of cranial nerve VII).
   - Mueller's muscle is innervated by the autonomic nervous system and contributes to the last several mm of eye opening.

2. **What are the common anatomic structures in the upper and lower eyelids?**
   - The upper eyelid has two preaponeurotic fat pads, one medial (also called nasal) and one central. The medial and central fat pads are separated by the superior oblique muscle. The lacrimal gland lies in the superior lateral orbit and has been mistaken for fat and inadvertently removed. This obviously is a significant complication.
   - The lower eyelids have three fat pads: the medial (nasal), central, and lateral (also called temporal). The medial and central pads are separated by the inferior oblique muscle, and the central and lateral fat pads are separated by the arcuate expansion of the inferior oblique muscle.

3. **Can you name the anatomic tissue and tissue planes involved with routine cosmetic upper eyelid blepharoplasty?***
   - The skin is the most outer layer.
   - The orbicularis oculi muscle is the next layer encountered in cosmetic blepharoplasty.
   - The orbital septum is the next layer progressing deeper.
   - The periorbital fat pads (preaponeurotic fat) are the next layer encountered in routine cosmetic upper blepharoplasty.
   - The next layer involves the levator palpebrae superioris muscle, and the levator aponeurosis is the base layer seen when the fat pads are reduced. The levator is not generally addressed in cosmetic upper lid blepharoplasty, but it may be addressed if simultaneous ptosis surgery was to be performed.

4. **What are the common aging changes seen in the periorbital region?†**
   - There is a descent of the forehead, the eyebrows, and the upper eyelid skin.
   - The eyelid skin on both lids becomes atrophic, sun damaged, pigmented, and crinkly. This is known as *dermatochalasis*.
   - The orbital septum becomes lax, and fat protrusion can occur in both eyelids. This is manifested by "sausages" of protuberant fat that makes patients look older and tired.
   - The nasojugal groove (tear trough) becomes accentuated. This groove deepens and represents soft tissue changes over the inferior orbital rim. The soft tissue atrophy and descent changes in the midface also contribute to the "tear trough" deformity.
   - The lateral canthal skin develops horizontal lines called "crow's feet."

---

*Niamtu J: Cosmetic blepharoplasty. In Niamtu J, editor: Cosmetic facial surgery, St Louis, 2011a, Mosby Elsevier, pp 129–174.
†Niamtu J: Contemporary blepharoplasty: less can be more, Expert Rev Dermatol 5(4):489–490, 2010a.

5. **How can true dermatochalazia be differentiated from pseudodermatochalazia?**
   Pseudodermatochalazia occurs when brow ptosis contributes to an appearance of dermatochalazia. Specific measurements are used to identify the brow location. A female brow should be elevated above the supraorbital rim 0 to 2 mm medially, 10 mm at the apex, and taper at the tail. A male brow should lie at the supraorbital rim. If these measurements are not found on the patient, a brow lift may be indicated.

6. **How do you correctly measure lid ptosis?**
   The palpebral fissure should measure 10 mm. The margin reflex distance-1 (MRD-1) can also be used, which is the distance between the light reflex in the cornea and the center of the upper lid margin. The normal MRD-1 is 5 mm. The MRD-2 will measure lower lid ptosis, and it is also 5 mm. The anatomic points for MRD-2 are also from the light reflex in the cornea down to the center of the lower lid margin.

7. **What is the snap test?**
   This is used to measure lower lid laxity prior to blepharoplasty. The lower lid is pulled away and allowed to "snap" back. This test can predict postoperative ectropion with moderate to severe lid laxity during the snap test.

8. **What is the Schirmer test?**
   The test evaluates dry eyes. Once the lower fornix is dried, a Schirmer strip is placed into the lateral aspect and left in place for 5 minutes. Fifteen mm of wetness at 5 minutes is normal. An abnormal test is not an indicator for surgical treatment.

9. **What are common surgical modalities used to remove excess upper eyelid skin, muscle, and fat?**
   - Cold steel (scalpel or scissors)
   - Microneedle cautery or radio wave surgery
   - CO_2 laser
   - Battery "hot wire" cautery (uncommon)
   - Electrosurgery, radiosurgery, or CO_2 laser are preferable as they provide a bloodless surgical field, which reduces complications, lessens bruising and pain, and promotes faster healing.

10. **What are the common surgical approaches to the lower eyelid blepharoplasty?**
    Subciliary and transconjunctival lower blepharoplasty.

11. **Can you describe the advantages and disadvantages of the most common surgical approaches to the lower eyelid for cosmetic blepharoplasty and their respective advantages or disadvantages?[‡]**
    - The subciliary approach is the oldest surgical approach for lower eyelid blepharoplasty. This technique involves making an incision several mm below the lash line that has a downward limb at the lateral canthus. This incision includes skin and orbicularis oculi muscle, and dissection proceeds over the orbital septum. The orbital septum is then incised, and the three lower fat pads are visualized and reduced or recontoured. After the fat is addressed, a controlled amount of eyelid skin and orbicularis oculi muscle is removed to deal with the dermatochalasis and lower lid skin excess. Advantages of this technique include that it is a direct vision procedure with easy access to all tissues. Disadvantages include that this approach violates the orbital septum (middle lamella), and postoperative septal contraction can result in lower lid malposition where the lower eyelid is retracted and shows excess sclera at the inferior limbus of the iris. Making the skin incision at the ciliary margin and making the orbicularis incision several mm lower leaves a small amount of pretarsal orbicularis, which may aid in preserving normal eyelid position. In the past decade the subciliary approach has fallen out of favor and is less commonly utilized due to the associated lid position problems. More contemporary surgeons prefer the transconjunctival approach.
    - Transconjunctival lower blepharoplasty has become the favored approach for accessing the lower eyelid fat pads. An incision is made from the lacrimal punctum to the lateral canthus through the

[‡]Niamtu J. Blepharoplasty incisional modalities: 4.0 Radiosurgery vs. CO_2 Laser In Pearls and Pitfalls in Cosmetic Oculo-plastic Surgery. Hartstein ME, Holds JB, Massry GG, (eds.) Springer: NY, 2009,

conjunctiva and lower eyelid retractors (capsulopalpabral fascia). This incision is made approximately 4 mm inferior to the lower tarsal margin or 9 mm inferior to the ciliary margin. Scalpel, electrosurgery, radio wave microneedle, or laser are the most common incision modalities. An advantage of this approach is that it is a retroseptal approach and does not disturb the lower lid orbital septum (middle lamella) and therefore does not significantly affect lower lid malposition. Disadvantages of this approach include that the excess skin is not addressed, and the visibility of the fat pads is harder to access and learn. When using the transconjunctival approach to lower eyelid blepharoplasty, the lower eyelid skin is addressed by laser skin resurfacing, chemical peel, skin pinch, or subciliary skin removal with septal preservations.

12. **What causes dark circles on the lower eyelids?**
Dark circles are multifactorial and can include shadowing from protruding lower lid fat pads, actual pigmentation in the skin (which can be significant in some racial groups such as people from eastern Asia). They can also result from underlying blood vessels that show through the thin eyelid skin and from hemosiderin pigment that extravasates from blood vessels.

13. **What are common treatments for dark circles on the lower eyelids?**
Treatments include bleaching creams such as hydroquinone 40% to bleach the skin, laser or chemical peel skin resurfacing to remove the epithelium and create new skin, and direct skin excision.[4]

14. **What minimally invasive procedures are used for nonsurgical periorbital rejuvenation?**
Numerous modalities are used to address nonsurgical periorbital rejuvenation. Neurotoxins are used to treat lateral canthal wrinkles, and injectable fillers can be used to treat the same wrinkles and are also used to fill the tear trough (nasojugal groove) to mitigate the severe depression seen over the inferior orbital rim. Latisse (Bimatoprost) is a topical prostaglandin analogue that stimulates the lash follicles to produce thicker, darker, and longer lashes.[5]

15. **How is the tear trough deformity treated?**
The tear trough can be injected with fillers or autologous fat. This area is vascular, so careful placement with small-gauge needles and low-pressure injection is essential to avoid intravascular injection, which can lead to tissue necrosis and blindness. Hyaluronic acid fillers are favored because they are safe, predictable, and can be reversed with hyaluronidase if necessary. The fillers are not injected in the subcutaneous plane because they can produce a Tyndall effect, which is a blue tinge or hue visible through the skin. Instead they are injected at the periosteal plane and more superficially, but still under the orbicularis oculi muscle. The filler, once injected, can be "walked" across the tear trough from central to medial to fill the area that otherwise may be difficult or more dangerous to inject. Blunt injection cannulas can also be used in lieu of needles.[6,7]

16. **Can tear trough filler be reversed if the patient does not like result?**
The hyaluronic acid fillers (Juvederm, Restylane, Perlane, Voluma, Belotero) can be reversed with hyaluronidase. This enzyme will hydrolyze the hyaluronic acid and degrade it in a matter of hours. Generally 50 to 80 units of hyaluronidase injected into the same plane as the unwanted filler will remove the filler. Nonhyaluronic acid fillers such as Radiesse, silicone oil, Sculptra, Artefil, and autologous fat cannot be reversed with hyaluronidase or any other substance.

17. **Can you name some of the common complications associated with cosmetic blepharoplasty?**
   - Edema
   - Corneal abrasion
   - Lagophthalmos (inability to close the eyes)
   - Asymmetry
   - Subconjunctival ecchymosis (blood over the white sclera)
   - Chemosis (conjunctival edema)
   - Ecchymosis of periorbital region
   - Retrobulbar hematoma (emergent complication)
   - Suture line "cysts" (upper lids)

18. **What is retrobulbar hematoma?**

    Retrobulbar hematoma (RBH) is a potentially severe complication that can cause blindness. It is a result of bleeding behind the globe, and since the blood cannot escape, an expanding phenomenon occurs that can compress the retinal artery and result in permanent vision loss. Any bleeding during blepharoplasty must be taken seriously for the fear of RBH. RBH can be a result of intraoperative or postoperative bleeding. After cosmetic blepharoplasty, patients must refrain from any strenuous activity that may increase blood pressure and produce bleeding in or behind the eye. This includes bending, lifting, straining during bowel movement, or anything that can produce a Valsalva maneuver or cause bleeding. Cold compresses are applied immediately after surgery and for 48 hours after surgery. Preoperatively, patients must refrain from any drug or supplement that may affect coagulation. This includes aspirin, aspirin-containing medications, megadoses of certain vitamins, and certain supplements such as gingko, ginseng, and fish oil. Any of these products must be discontinued 2 weeks before surgery.

19. **What is the purpose of brow and forehead lifting?**

    As inane as that sounds, the answer is important in that the reason to do a brow lift is to lift the brow. Many patients develop ptotic brows with aging. This produces an older and tired look and adds to upper eyelid hooding, which is the condition where the lateral eyelid skin becomes ptotic and redundant. An additional reason to perform brow and forehead lifting is to improve the vertical and horizontal forehead wrinkles. Not all patients need a brow and forehead lift as many people never have elevated or arched brows, and their brows remain in the same position all their life.

20. **Why is the option of brow and forehead lifting important?**

    Contemporary cosmetic surgeons realize the importance in brow and forehead rejuvenation in comprehensive upper one-third facial rejuvenation. It is not uncommon to see surgeons who are not skilled in this procedure, and they do not perform brow and forehead lifting. Instead they perform aggressive upper eyelid blepharoplasty to remove redundant lid skin. Although this benefits the patient, it does not address the root of the problem if the brows are ptotic. In addition, if the patient is interested in a brow lift in the future, it may be impossible if excess upper lid skin has been removed because lifting the brows and forehead will cause lagophthalmos (inability to close the eyelids). Unfortunately, some patients are never able to have a rejuvenating brow and forehead lift because they don't have adequate upper lid skin because they were treated with blepharoplasty instead of brow lift. Finally, performing aggressive upper eyelid blepharoplasty on a patient with ptotic brows can actually pull down drooping brows even further.[8]

21. **Can blepharoplasty and brow and forehead lift be performed simultaneously?**

    Yes, if the patient has sufficient brow ptosis and excess upper lid skin. By performing conservative blepharoplasty with a brow and forehead lift, the surgeon can improve results with the synergistic effects. The blepharoplasty can complement the brow lift by making a more sculpted and crisp upper eyelid complex. The caveat is that when performed in combination, it is critical to be conservative enough with each procedure to allow normal eyelid closure.

22. **What is the function of the musculi frontalis, and what muscles oppose its function?**

    The major function of the frontalis is elevating eyebrows. Corrugator supercilii, procerus, and orbicularis oculi muscles are responsible in opposing the brow-lifting activity of the frontalis muscle.

23. **What are the main sensory and motor nerves associated with the brow and forehead lifting procedures?**

    - The supratrochlear nerve is a bilateral sensory nerve that resides 17 mm lateral to the glabellar midline and innervates the anterior medial forehead and scalp.
    - The supraorbital nerve is a bilateral sensory nerve that resides 27 mm lateral to the glabellar midline and innervates the anterior and posterior scalp.
    - The temporal branch of the facial nerve lies bilaterally between the lateral brow and the temporal hair tuft and provides motor innervation for the frontalis muscle.

24. **What systematic approach should be used to evaluate the contour and position of the eyebrow?**

    The ideal location of the brow for a female is approximately 1 cm above the supraorbital rim; whereas it is only slightly above the rim for a male patient. The contour of the brow is evaluated in thirds: medial, central, and lateral. The medial and lateral ends of the eyebrow lie at approximately the same horizontal level. The apex of the brow lies directly above the lateral limbus of the eye.

25. What are the approaches for brow and forehead lift?
Coronal, anterior hairline, trichophytic, direct brow, and endoscopic approaches.

26. What are the advantages and disadvantages for using a coronal approach?
"Old school" brow and forehead lifting was commonly performed using a coronal approach similar to trauma coronal flaps. The positive effect of this approach is unparalleled vision of the surgical site and access to numerous tissue planes and anatomic units. The flap was raised and dissection over the superior orbital rims was performed. The approach over the forehead is subperiosteal. The periosteum on the soft tissue side of the flap is cross-hatched to provide flap elasticity, and the brow depressors could be transected to enhance effect and longevity. Numerous problems exist with the approach including:
- Extremely aggressive surgery when more conservative approaches are now available
- Large surgical scar that can be visible, especially in patients with unstable hairlines
- Hair loss on the scar
- Sensory nerve dysfunction due to aggressive treatment that includes pain, itching, and numbness
- Increased recovery

27. Why is direct brow lift no longer a popular approach in elevating brow position?
Direct brow-lifting techniques have also been performed and have largely fallen out of common use. These techniques involve removing an ellipse of forehead skin just above the brows on the mid-forehead. By removing skin above the brow, the brow is elevated when the defect is closed. The negative aspect is the fact the scars are visible, and there is little control of the total brow and forehead complex.

28. Why is a trichophytic incision a more preferable approach compared to an anterior hairline incision? What is the indication for using these approaches?
Anterior hairline brow-lifting approaches have remained popular as they are effective in addressing the entire brow and forehead lift, are less aggressive than coronal approaches, and are direct vision procedures that do not require specialized surgical equipment. Also, they do not elevate the hairline. This approach can utilize a pre-trichophillic incision (in front of the hairline), but this author never performs that approach as it is visible, unnatural, and frequently hypopigments, which makes it noticeable.

The trichophytic or transfollicular approach is favored by the author as the incision is made about 5 mm posterior to the hairline with an extreme bevel. The bevel transects some hair shafts but does not cut through the follicle. This allows the transected shafts to grow through the surgical scar and helps hide it. This is an open surgical approach and allows excellent access to the brow and forehead. The author performs this as a subcutaneous dissection that is between the dermis and frontalis. Approximately 20 mm of skin is received across the forehead and makes this a stable and long-lasting procedure. Being transcutaneous, the vertical and horizontal rhytides are more effectively addressed than with subperiosteal approaches. Due to the incision design, the hairline is not elevated with the anterior hairline approaches.

29. What are the major operative principles of an endoscopic forehead lift?
The endoscopic brow and forehead lift is a contemporary technique that became popular in the mid-1990s and is a minimally invasive incision approach to elevating the upper face. The endoscopic technique is more conservative in terms of incisions when compared to open techniques, but it is more aggressive in terms of tissue dissection. It is subperiosteal in the central skull and involves deeper soft tissue planes in the lateral skull.

The basic premise of an endoscopic brow and forehead lift is to make hidden hairline incisions and access the subperiosteal plane over the calvarium and frontal region. As stated, the temporal access involves the staying in the plane immediately superior to the deep temporal fascia. The frontal nerve travels in the superficial fascia or the temporoparietal fascia, and this plane is avoided to protect the nerve. Once the various tissue planes are elevated, the brow depressors are frequently addressed with myotomy or myectomy to reduce postoperative downward pull on the elevated brow. The periosteum is incised just above the supraorbital rims, and the scalp is elevated. The elevation is fixated by numerous methods with suture suspension. The suspension sutures are fixed to the frontal skull by various methods including bone tunnels, titanium screws, resorbable screws, bone plates, and resorbable barbed devices.

30. **What are the disadvantages of an endoscopic forehead lift?**
    There is learning curve for a new surgeon and also the initial cost for surgical instruments. Deep wrinkles of the forehead and glabellar area cannot be completely eradicated.

31. **What are common complications seen with brow and forehead lifting?**
    Regardless of the technique utilized, complications can result from brow and forehead lift. Overcorrection is a significant problem as it can affect the ability to close the eyes, which can cause cornea damage. Some patients may appear overcorrected initially but look normal when the edema subsides. Under-correction can also be seen but can be revised. Hair loss around incisions and hypertrophic or hypotrophic scarring can be seen. Frontal nerve damage is a possible complication, although it can be transient. Sensory nerve damage of the supratrochlear and supraorbital nerves can be seen, which results in paresthesia or dysaesthesia of the distribution of the nerves including the forehead and posterior scalp. Hardware infection is a possibility, as is asymmetry.

BIBLIOGRAPHY

Niamtu J: *Cosmetic blepharoplasty.* In Naimtu J, editor: *Cosmetic facial surgery*, St Louis, 2011a, Mosby Elsevier, pp 129–174.
Niamtu J: Contemporary blepharoplasty: less can be more, *Expert Rev Dermatol* 5(4):489–490, 2010a.
Niamtu J: Blepharoplasty incisional modalities: 4.0 radiosurgery vs. CO2 laser. In Hartstein ME, Holds JB, Massry GG, editors: *Pearls and pitfalls in cosmetic oculoplastic surgery*, New York, 2009a, Springer.
Niamtu J: Contemporary laser resurfacing. In Eremias, editor: *Office-based cosmetic procedures and techniques*, New York, 2010b, Cambridge, pp 212–214.
Niamtu J: Neurotoxins in cosmetic facial surgery. In Niamtu J, editor: *Cosmetic facial surgery*, St Louis, 2011b, Mosby Elsevier,
    pp 604–639.
Niamtu J: Filler injection with micro-cannula instead of needles, *Dermatol Surg* 35(12):2005–2008, December 2009b.
Niamtu J: Adjunctive facial aesthetic procedures. In Milaro M, Ghali GE, Parsen P, Waite P, editors: *Peterson's principles of oral and maxillofacial surgery*, ed 3, Shelton, CT, 2012, Peoples Medical Publishing House, pp 1609–1620.
Niamtu J: *Brow and forehead lifting.* In Niamtu J: *Cosmetic facial surgery*, St Louis, 2011c, Mosby Elsevier, pp 90–128.

CHAPTER 56

RHYTIDECTOMY

Tirbod Fattahi

1. **What is a rhytidectomy?**
   A rhytidectomy is also commonly known as a "facelift." The goals of the surgery are to eliminate facial rhytides and skin laxity through the re-suspension and fixation of the superficial fascia, muscles, and subcutaneous tissue of the face.

2. **What are the indications for rhytidectomy?**
   Rhytidectomy has the potential to correct wrinkling in only the lower thirds of the face and neckline. It also helps to redefine the lower jaw line, platysma banding, and elimination of jowls.

3. **What are jowls?**
   Ovoid masses of fibrofatty subcutaneous tissue immediately adjacent and lateral to the inferior extremity of the nasolabial creases.

4. **Can you define the superficial musculoaponeurotic system (SMAS)?**
   The SMAS is the inferior extension of the temporoparietal fascia and superior extension of the platysma. It is a fibrous dissectible layer that can be used to provide traction on facial tissues during rhytidectomy.

5. **Why is the SMAS structurally important to a rhytidectomy?**
   The SMAS is connected to the facial skin by a layer of fibrous septa that can be dissected away during rhytidectomy, allowing the skin to be re-suspended to reduce the wrinkled appearance of the face. Because it is superficial to most of the sensory and motor nerves of the face, the surgeon can apply traction to the SMAS to tighten the facial skin.

6. **For a conventional rhytidectomy, what are the three components in the incision design?**
   - Preauricular incision
   - Postauricular incision
   - Occipital hairline incision

7. **What are the acceptable incisions for the preauricular incisions?**
   - The contoured pretragal incision is a good choice for a smoker, male patient, and patient with visible pretragal wrinkle.
   - Tragal edge incision is a good choice for a youthful female without visible pretragal wrinkle.
   - Retrotragal incision has a similar indication as the tragal edge incision; however, it carries a higher risk for tragal deformity.

8. **Where is the ideal location to place incision in the postauricular skin?**
   - The vertical postauricular incision should be made in the junction of the postauricular skin and the posterior ear skin.
   - The incision should turn horizontally across the scalp at a point at least two-thirds of the distance from the lobular sulcus to the superior extremity of the concha. The angle should be close to 90 degrees.

9. **What determines how far posterior along the hairline the facelift incision is made?**
   The extent of submental fullness and redundancy; the more redundant tissue, the farther back along the hairline the incision must be.

10. **Why is the facelift skin flap elevated with 4 to 5 mm of fat on its deep side?**
    To preserve the subdermal vascular plexus.

11. What is the main axial blood supply to a facelift flap?
Perforator branch of the transverse facial artery and perforator branch of the submental artery.

12. The SMAS flap during the facelift is elevated in which plane? And how is it commonly being managed?
Deep to skin and superficial to parotid gland capsule (parotideomasseteric fascia). Once the SMAS flap is elevated, it can be either plicated (folded) or imbricated (excised). Plication carries less risk in facial nerve injury, but preserved redundant SMAS tissue can look bulky in the preauricular region.

13. What are the different types of facelift procedures?
• Skin only
• Skin and SMAS-platysma
• Skin and SMAS-platysma and mid-face suspension
• Deep-plane rhytidectomy

14. How do you select the appropriate type of facelift for the patient?
A skin-only facelift is recommended if the defect is found only with skin laxity and rhytides of the face and neck but does not have platysmal banding, jowls, marionette lines, submalar concavity, and other features of deep facial tissue relaxation due to aging. Skin and SMAS lift should be recommended if deep-tissue ptosis is suspected. Deep-plane rhytidectomy is recommended for the patient who needs significant improvement in the nasolabial folds.

15. Can you describe the anatomy of the nasolabial fold?
The nasolabial fold is formed by the insertion of muscles originating on the zygoma and the insertion of the thinned SMAS. This fold arises above the nasal ala and descends toward the mandible lateral to the parasymphysis. Of clinical significance, dissection anterior to the fold produces little change in the contour of the nasolabial fold. It is important to address this possibility preoperatively to the patient who will be undergoing a rhytidectomy procedure to prevent unrealistic expectations.

16. What are the osteocutaneous retaining ligaments in the face?
These are areas where the skin is attached to the underlying bone or fascia directly. The areas of the bony ligaments are the zygoma and mandible at the parasymphysis. The ligaments to the fascia are to the platysma, the platysma-auricular ligament, and the parotid and masseter area. The significance of these ligaments is that they must be released to adequately re-drape the skin.

17. What are the complications that are associated with rhytidectomy?
• Facial nerve injury (1% to 2%)
• Greater auricular nerve injury (5%)
• Hematomas and seromas (4% to 5%)
• Skin slough near the auricular incision (3% to 4%)
• Alopecia near the hairline incision (<2%)

18. Which nerve is most commonly injured in a rhytidectomy?
The greater auricular nerve, which supplies sensation to the skin of the ear and nearby skin, is the most commonly injured. The nerve lies deep to the SMAS about 6.5 cm inferior to the external auditory canal. After emerging from the posterior border of the sternocleidomastoid muscle (Erb's point), it lies on the surface of this muscle with close proximity to the external jugular vein.

19. What are the common telltale signs of facelift surgery?
• Visible scars
• Over-lifting of the temporal hairline
• Stepped occipital hairline
• Distorted tragus
• Distorted earlobes (i.e., pixie ear)

20. How is a pixie ear deformity avoided?
Passive placement of earlobe over the skin flap and judicious trimming of skin flap around the lobe.

21. **What is the treatment for expanding hematoma?**
A small expanding hematoma can be treated with suction-aspiration. Manual pressure to ensure all hematoma is evacuated. A large expanding hematoma may require removal of suture and exploring the surgical site to control the bleeding.

22. **Which patients are more at risk for flap ischemia?**
Smokers, diabetics, and hypertensive patients.

23. **What do you recommend for the prevention of facelift flap ischemia?**
Smoking cessation should start 3 weeks before surgery and 10 days after surgery. Slow-acting niacin (250 mg 3 times a day for 3 weeks before surgery) may be helpful in counteracting the effects of smoking on the small vessels. If smoking cannot be discontinued, the flap should be raised with both skin and SMAS to ensure adequate blood supply to the skin.

24. **What organisms are the most prevalent in facelift infection?**
Staphylococcus aureus, gram-negative bacilli, streptococci, and *Candida albicans*.

25. **What is the main concern regarding simultaneous facelift and laser resurfacing?**
Possible damage to subdermal plexus and skin flap necrosis.

26. **What is the ideal time to see a facelift patient following surgery?**
Within 24 hours, in case a hematoma or seroma needs to be evacuated.

27. **What is the main indication for performing an isolated platysmaplasty?**
Platysmal redundancy or banding, submental fullness but no jowling.

28. **Can you discuss the variation and significance of the platysma muscle anatomy in the midline?**
Platysma in the anterior midline has three different variations with respect to the decussation of its fibers. In general, fibers cross at the level of the thyroid cartilage, submentally, or at the mentum. Platysma banding is caused by a laxity in the platysma that does not decussate across the midline.

29. **How much fat can typically be harvested during a submental liposuction?**
10 to 15 cc from supraplatysmal fat compartment.

30. **What is the ideal patient for isolated submental liposuction?**
Young patient with mild submental fullness with good skin tone and elasticity.

31. **What vessels may be encountered during the subplatysmal dissection in the central neck area?**
Anterior jugular veins.

BIBLIOGRAPHY

Baker DC, Conley J: Avoiding facial nerve injuries in rhytidectomy. Anatomical variations and pitfalls, *Plast Reconstr Surg* 64(6):781–795, December 1979.

Baker DC: Minimal incision rhytidectomy (short scar facelift) with lateral SMASectomy: evolution and application, *Aesthet Surg J* 1426, January/February 2001.

Fattahi T: Submental liposuction versus formal cervicoplasty: which one to choose? *J Oral Maxillofac Surg* 70(12): 2854–2858, December 2012.

Hamara ST: *Composite rhytidectomy*, St Louis, 1993, Quality Publishing.

Millard Jr DR, Garst WP, Beck RL, Thompson ID: Submental and submandibular lipectomy in conjunction with a face life in the male or female, *Plast Reconstr Surg* 49:385, 1992.

Mitz V, Peyronie M: The superficial musculoponeurotic system (SMAS) in the parotid and cheek area, *Plast Reconstr Surg* 34:598, 1964.

Niamtu J: Expanding hematoma in face-lift surgery: literature review, case presentations and caveats, *Dermatol Surg* 31:1134–1144, 2005.

Peterson RA: Facelift: inconspicuous scars about the ears, *Clin Plast Surg* 19:425–431, 1992.

Ramirez O: The subperiosteal approach for the correction of the deep nasolabial fold and the central third of the face, *Clin Plast Surg* 22:341–356, 1995.

Webster RC, Smith RC, Papsidero MJ, Karolow WW, Smith KF: Comparison of SMAS plication with SMAS imbrication in face lifting, *Laryngoscope* 92(8 Pt 1):901, August 1982.

RHINOPLASTY

Shahrokh Bagheri, Behnam Bohluli

CHAPTER 57

1. **What are the routine steps in the preoperative nose examination?**
   Clinical examination is usually the first step after a comprehensive interview. The nose is palpated to find out the quality and thickness of skin. A slight pressure on the nasal tip may indicate tip support. Nasal bones are palpated to grossly measure the size of nasal bones.[1-3]

   Functional evaluation is a determinant part of clinical examinations. External and internal nasal valves are carefully assessed, and adequate illumination and the use of a speculum allow detecting any intranasal deformities.[4]

2. **How can we evaluate and document the external nasal airway patency in preoperative work-ups?**
   The forced inspiration test is a known method to evaluate the external nasal valves. In this test, the patient is asked to deeply breathe, and his or her nostril walls are carefully observed; partial or total collapse of lateral nasal valve shows partial or total valve incompetency. This test may be documented by standard basal photography made during the test. The same test may be performed and documented in selected postoperative intervals.[5]

3. **How can we evaluate and document the internal nasal airway patency in preoperative work-ups?**
   Rhinomanometry and acoustic rhinometry are standard methods in evaluating the internal nasal valves. These methods measure the airway's resistance and patency.[4] They need special instruments and are somewhat technique-sensitive, so alternatively the Cottle test may be applied. In this simple test, the patient is asked to deeply breathe. Then breathing is repeated while a cotton applicator is inserted into the nose, and a gentle lateral pressure is applied. A marked improvement of breathing shows that there are some problems in the internal nasal valves (valve incompetency), while subtle improvement or no change in airflow shows competent nasal valves (Fig. 57-1).[4,6,7]

4. **What is a boxy tip?**
   A broad and wide nasal tip with quadrangular contour is sometimes named a *boxy tip*. A boxy tip usually indicates wide, strong lower lateral cartilages that are divergent from each other. There are some treatment options to treat this condition: suturing techniques, cephalic resection of lower lateral cartilages, dome dividing, and new dome formation are some of the known techniques.[8,9]

5. **What is a tension nose?**
   A tension nose is a relatively common nasal deformity in which there is an overgrowth of septal cartilage and a prominent cartilaginous hump. The nasal tip is usually pushed anteriorly and inferiorly. Treatment of this deformity is based on reducing the height of septum and conservative trimming of the upper lateral cartilages. Tip grafts are sometimes applied for harmony between the tip and the dorsum and to prevent over-resection of the prominent dorsal hump.

6. **What is a crooked nose?**
   Crooked or twisted nose means that there are asymmetries, curves, or bends in the long axis of the nose. These deformities pose a challenge in rhinoplasty. The first step in treating these noses is usually to find the etiology. Traumatic noses have better prognosis, while developmental deformities and those combined with facial asymmetries have the worst prognosis. The surgical plan may be a combination of several rhinoplasty techniques. Two-level osteotomy, asymmetrical hump resection, and camouflage grafts are some common maneuvers employed in these types of deformities.[10,11]

7. **What underlying anatomic structures are associated with the proximal, middle, and distal thirds of the nose?**
   - Proximal one-third: nasal bones
   - Middle one-third: upper lateral cartilages
   - Distal one-third: lower lateral cartilages

487

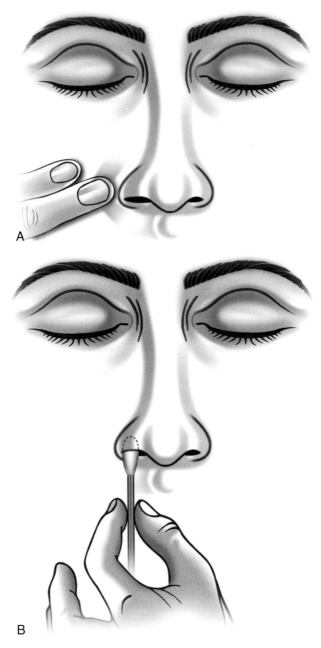

Figure 57-1. Cottle test is a known way to evaluate internal nasal valve.

8. **What are tip support mechanisms?**
   Tip support mechanisms are generally divided into major and minor tip supports. Three major tip supports include:[12]
   1. Size, shape, strength, and resilience of lower lateral cartilages
   2. Attachment of medial crura to the caudal border of the septum
   3. Attachment of lower lateral cartilages to upper lateral cartilages
   And six minor tip supports may include:[12]
   1. Ligamentous sling that covers the domes of the alar cartilages
   2. Dorsal portion of the cartilaginous septum
   3. Membranous nasal septum
   4. Sesamoid cartilages
   5. Attachment of the lower lateral cartilages to the overlying skin and musculature
   6. Nasal spine

9. **What is the tripod concept?**
   The tripod concept is a simplified description of nasal tip cartilages. In this concept, alar cartilages are compared to a tripod, in which two lateral legs of lower lateral cartilages make lateral limbs, and two medial cruras make the third limb of this tripod. This simple description of Anderson has helped to describe the dynamic of each tip plasty and predict the effects of each technique.[13,14]

10. **What are the major steps in a primary aesthetic nose surgery?**
    After precise injection of local anesthesia (lidocaine + epinephrine), incisions are made first, and skeletonization is performed. Then hump resection and basic tip plasty techniques such as cephalic trim are done. Septoplasty and graft harvesting are the next steps. The procedure is followed by lateral and medial osteotomy. At this stage, advanced dorsal surgery techniques such as radix augmentation and spreader fixation[15,16] are applied. Final tip plasty techniques such as tip suture and tip grafts are the next procedures. In the end, internal splints and external splints are used.[1-3,17]

11. **Is the open rhinoplasty technique superior to the closed?**
    The open approach has brought a new era in rhinoplasty. This approach provides a direct access to the cartilaginous framework of the nose so that all the deformities and asymmetries are clearly evaluated. Furthermore, versatile tip grafting techniques and different tip suturing methods can be easily performed in open approach rhinoplasty.[18]
    On the other hand, many surgeons prefer closed approach, and they preserve the open approach for their complex cases such as cleft and secondary rhinoplasty. They believe that the closed approach leads to less trauma and edema and that the possibility of columellar scar is totally eliminated.[19,20]

12. **What are the routine incisions in rhinoplasty?**
    Marginal incision: In this incision, a double hook is used to retract the lateral wall of the nostril. Then a finger press is applied so that the caudal edges of the lateral crural cartilages are visible inside the nose. A No. 15 blade is used to incise the skin. It is important to note that this incision must be exactly caudal to the alar cartilage borders (Fig. 57-2).[1,2]
    Intercartilaginous incision: This is a curvilinear incision that is done in the internal nasal valves where the upper and lower lateral cartilages contact each other. This incision is an integral part of the closed approach, though it may be applied in some open cases as well (Fig. 57-3).[1,2]
    Columellar incision: In this incision, an inverted V or a stair-step incision is made on the columellar skin. The incision is connected to the rim incisions on both sides, and it provides a wide access in the open approach rhinoplasty (Fig. 57-4).[1-3]

13. **What are the main maneuvers to refine nasal tip?**
    Tip plasty is generally composed of some reductive and additive techniques. In a reductive session, a small strip of the cephalic part of lowered lateral cartilages is marked, cut, dissected, and resected to provide a more delicate cartilaginous framework. Divisions of cartilages in dome, medial crura, and lateral crura are some other reductive maneuvers that are frequently performed in tip plasty.[21]
    These reductive techniques may be followed or replaced by additive or augmentation techniques to provide stabler and more reproducible results. Suture tip plasty and tip grafts are the main augmentation methods that are frequently used in modern rhinoplasty.[1-4]

14. **What are the possible consequences of respective tip techniques?**
    Breathing problems: Resection or division of lower lateral cartilages in any part may potentially weaken the nose; nasal valves may be directly affected, and nasal valve incompetency is a common sequence of reductive rhinoplasty.[3,4]

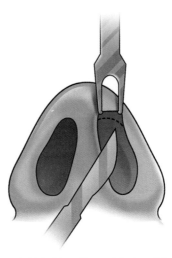

Figure 57-2. To do marginal incision, a double hook is used to retract the alar wall; finger pressure helps the surgeon to see the borders of lower lateral cartilage and make marginal incision.

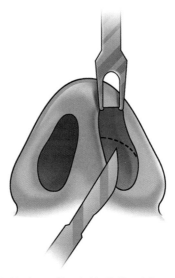

Figure 57-3. An intercartilaginous incision is a curvilinear incision that is made in connection of upper and lower lateral cartilages.

Instability of the nose: Reductive procedures impair nasal stability, so nasolabial angle may change gradually, and tip projection may be reduced.[22] Pinch deformity and asymmetries are the other possible consequences of reductive rhinoplasty.[3,4]

15. **How can suturing techniques help us to make a smaller tip?**
   Suture tip plasty is composed of numerous techniques that are aimed to change the architecture of the lower lateral cartilages.[20,23,24]

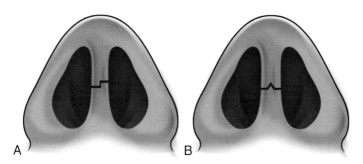

Figure 57-4. Stairstep (A) and inverted V (B) are two common ways to make columellar incisions.

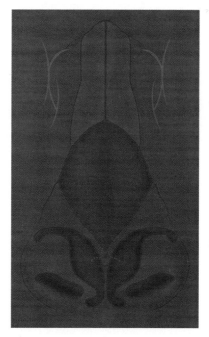

Figure 57-5. An interdomal suture is used to approximate wide interdomal space and to change the angle between two domes.

An interdomal suture is applied to approximate two domes. This technique is especially useful in wide nasal tips with strong cartilages, boxy tips, and grooved nasal tips. Reduction of the interdomal space will lead to a more refined tip (Fig. 57-5).[20,23,24]

An intradomal suture (tip-spanning suture) is a mattress suture that is passed through the dome. This suture will modify the angle between lateral and medial crura so a better contour of the nose will form (Fig. 57-6).[20,23,24]

An intercrural suture is used to approximate medial cruras. This technique helps to narrow and refine a wide columella.[20,23,24]

A foot-plate suture is a mattress suture that is passed from the base of columella in one nostril to the other nostril and is turned back into its first place. This suture is aimed to approximate wide foot plates.[23,24]

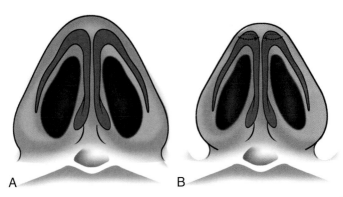

Figure 57-6. An intradomal or tip spanning suture is a mattress suture that is used to change the anatomy of domes.

16. **What are the possible side effects of suture tip plasty?**
   Tip sutures seek to improve the architecture of lower lateral cartilages, whereas overtightening of sutures or deep cartilage bites may distort the cartilages. Pinch deformity, tip asymmetry, and pointed tip are some common sequelae of these seemingly conservative techniques.[3,4]

17. **What are the approaches to the nasal septum?**
   The nasal septum may be accessed by two main approaches:
   1. The dorsal approach is usually used in open rhinoplasty. In this approach, after wide skeletonization, upper lateral cartilages are separated from the septum on both sides. Then subperichondrial dissection is completed until total access to the septum is obtained. This approach provides the best visualization, and dorsal deviations are easily managed.
   2. Transfixion is also a common approach after a semitransfixion or full transfixion incision, which is a common step when closed rhinoplasty, unilateral, or bilateral subpericondral dissection is done, and the septum is accessed by making subperichondrial tunnels.[4]

18. **How much of the nasal septum may be safely extracted during septoplasty or graft harvesting?**
   It is generally accepted that septal support should not be disturbed during septoplasty or cartilage graft harvesting; so a strong L-strut (in which dorsal cartilage is the long arm, and caudal of the septum is the short arm) would be mandatory. It is sometimes said that each limb should be at least 10 mm in width.[4]

19. **How can we prevent external nasal valve damages during a rhinoplasty?**
   Any reductive surgical maneuver on the lower lateral cartilages such as cephalic trimming or cartilage splitting may weaken the nasal valve. So it is usually recommended to select conservative approaches and try to preserve the integrity of the lower lateral cartilages as much as possible. Meanwhile, if due to any reason a weak lower lateral cartilage is encountered during an aesthetic nose surgery, an appropriate augmentation technique might be combined with reductive techniques to preserve external nasal competency or even restore preoperative deficiencies.[1-4]
   A lateral crural transposition flap is a reinforcing technique; here, excessive parts of lateral cartilages, which are planned to be trimmed, are elevated from their underlying skin and folded beneath the remaining cartilages. In this way, cephalic trimming is done while strength of the cartilage is preserved.[25]

20. **How can we reinforce external nasal valves?**
   Cartilage grafts are the mainstay in reinforcing external nasal valves.
   In a lateral crural transposition flap, the excessive parts of lower lateral cartilages, which are usually trimmed and excised in routine rhinoplasty, are marked. These segments are gently dissected away from their underlying skin until they have only a small connection to the dome. Then the cartilage is turned down and fixed underneath the remaining strip of lateral crural cartilages.[25]
   In a lateral crural strut graft, after adequate injection of local anesthesia, lateral crural cartilage is completely stripped off from its underlying skin until the dome genus is accessed. A rectangular

piece of cartilage, which has been previously harvested from the septum or concha, is fixed under the lateral crus. Then the reinforced cartilage is turned back into its initial place.

Alar contouring graft is a narrow strip of cartilage that is inserted in a pocket, which is prepared in the soft tissue of alar rim.[4]

21. **How can we prevent internal nasal valve damage during rhinoplasty?**
    Internal nasal valves made by the upper lateral cartilages (as lateral limbs), septal cartilage, and floor of the nose. Dorsal hump reduction and lateral osteotomy are two main steps that may damage the function of internal nasal valves.[26] There are some key points to avoid causing breathing problems in rhinoplasty.

    Dorsal septal cartilage and upper lateral cartilages that make two limbs of this triangle might be trimmed conservatively. Integrity of underlying mucosa is a crucial factor in the proper function of the internal nasal valve in small hump resections. Intact mucosa will work like a spreader and will prevent the collapse of the valve.[4,26]

22. **What are the indications of a lateral osteotomy?**
    A lateral osteotomy is usually done to narrow a wide, bony pyramid, though this step may also be beneficial in widening a narrow, bony vault, to close an open roof of the nose after hump removal, or help in straightening a crooked nose.[26]

23. **What are the indications for medial osteotomy?**
    Medial osteotomy is sometimes done to complete the desired effects of lateral osteotomy. It is usually indicated in extremely wide noses, asymmetrical bony vaults, and in cases where, based on intraoperative evaluations, bony medicalization is not adequate, and further steps might be taken to gain the optimal bony contour.[26]

24. **What is the importance of preserving Webster's triangle in lateral osteotomy?**
    A deep lateral osteotomy may potentially impair the internal nasal valve area, so it is recommended to leave a small bony pyramid on each side of the pyriform aperture (Webster's triangle) and not to involve it in the osteotomy plan. It is believed that these pyramids will not move during the mobilization of the osteotomy segment; rather they will preserve the nasal valve area (Fig. 57-7).[4,26]

25. **Modern rhinoplasty is based on different types of grafts. What are the main donor sites?**
    Septal cartilage is still the material of choice in rhinoplasty. It may be easily harvested from the septum and used as block, diced, or crushed grafts.

    Conchal cartilage has an inherent anatomic curvature that makes it an ideal material for reconstructing lower lateral cartilages. Rib graft and temporalis fascia are some common autologous grafts that may be used in their specific indications.[4]

26. **What may be done when intraoperative bleeding occurs?**
    A hypotensive anesthesia will definitely help to control the hemorrhage. Proper injection of local anesthesia with epinephrine, atraumatic surgical approach, and dissection in the correct surgical plane are the other dominant factors that may be emphasized in otherwise healthy rhinoplasty patients.[1,2]

27. **What may be done if septal collapse is encountered during septoplasty?**
    Like many other complications, the best protocol is to avoid this event. A strong remaining L-strut and conservative manipulation of the nose after septoplasty are the mainstays to prevent this problem.

    Though in case it happens, the nasal septum should be carefully reduced to its proper place; then it is fixed with several sutures to the nasal bones and upper lateral cartilages.[4,26]

28. **What may be done if an excessive amount of dorsum is excised inadvertently?**
    The best time to restore an over-resected hump is immediately after hump excision. The resected hump is carefully evaluated to find out the amount of excessive resections. Then it is trimmed, tailored, and reinserted in its place. This procedure may be repeated several times to achieve the best profile of the nose. Then this segment is fixed to the nose by suture. In case the resected hump does not provide an acceptable graft, other sources such as nasal septum and temporalis fascia might be considered.[4,26]

29. **What may be done if septal collapse is encountered during septoplasty?**
    Like many other complications, the best protocol is to avoid this event. A strong remaining L-strut and conservative manipulation of the nose after septoplasty are the mainstays to prevent this problem. In case it happens, however, the nasal septum should be carefully reduced to its proper place; then it is fixed with several sutures to the nasal bones and upper lateral cartilages.[4,26]

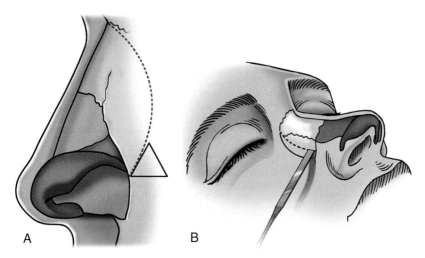

Figure 57-7. Lateral osteotomy is designed in a way that two small triangles of bone are preserved in the base of the pyriform aperture; these pyramids may prevent collapse of internal nasal valves.

30. **What is rocker deformity, and how can it be avoided?**
Rocker deformity is a bony spicule that appears after lateral osteotomy. The presence of this deformity means that osteotomy lines have entered the thick bony parts of the nasal radix and that medicalization of bony segments has caused protrusion of the bones into the radix. This deformity may be easily avoided by limiting the osteotomy lines up to the medial canthus on both sides. Further extensions may lead to severe complications without any considerable gain. It might be emphasized that these deformities will not be resolved by time and are best addressed intraoperatively.[4,26]

31. **What logic supports the use of internal nasal splints after surgery?**
Nasal splints may control postoperative intranasal swelling. In cases that internal incisions are used, synechia may be prevented. Intranasal splints are claimed to be useful in complex septoplasty procedures. These splints will preclude hematoma formation, and they will hold the septal cartilages during the first days of the healing phase.[1-4]

32. **When may internal splints be removed postoperatively?**
Internal splints may be removed 5 to 7 days after surgery, but in the case of aggressive septoplasty procedures such as extracorporeal septoplasty or inadvertent septal collapse, these splints may remain for 1 month to provide better support during the healing phase.[1-4]

33. **What is the importance of taping and extranasal splints after rhinoplasty?**
Taping will help the skeletonized nasal tissue to re-drape over the newly formed nasal framework. Proper taping may eliminate dead spaces so granulation tissue formation will be minimized. A hard external splint holds the bones in their new positions. In addition, it may control postoperative edema and help to provide better recovery and healing.[1-4]

34. **What is best time to revise minor postoperative deformities?**
Major revisions are best postponed for 6 months to 1 year post operation. This period of time is usually necessary for the edema to subside, to see the final results of the surgery, and to plan for a more accurate revision rhinoplasty. Some minor revisions such as alar base surgeries may be performed a few weeks after the surgery.[4]

REFERENCES
1. Bagheri SC: Primary cosmetic rhinoplasty, *Oral Maxillofac Surg Clin North Am* 24(1):39–48, 2012.
2. Bagheri SC, Khan HA, Cuzalina A: Rhinoplasty: current therapy, *Oral Maxillofac Surg Clin North Am* 24ix–x, 2012.
3. Bagheri SC, Khan HA, Jahangirnia A, et al.: An analysis of 101 primary cosmetic rhinoplasties, *J Oral Maxillofac Surg* 70(4):902–909, 2012.

4. Bohluli B, Bagheri SC: *Revision rhinoplasty. Current therapy in oral and maxillofacial surgery*, 2012. Pages 901–910.

5. Constantian MB: The incompetent external nasal valve: pathophysiology and treatment in primary and secondary rhinoplasty, *Plast Reconstr Surg* 93(5):919–931, 1994; discussion 932– 933.

6. Tikanto J, Pirilä T: Effects of the Cottle's maneuver on the nasal valve as assessed by acoustic rhinometry, *Am J Rhinol* 21(4):456–459, 2007.

7. Murrell GL: Components of the nasal examination, *Aesthet Surg J* 33(1):38–42, 2013.

8. Constantian MB: The boxy nasal tip, the ball tip, and alar cartilage malposition: variations on a theme–a study in 200 consecutive primary and secondary rhinoplasty patients, *Plast Reconstr Surg* 116(1):268, 2005.

9. Rohrich RJ, Adams Jr WP: The boxy nasal tip: classification and management based on alar cartilage suturing techniques, *Plast Reconstr Surg* 107(7):1849–1863, 2001; discussion 1864–1868.

10. Potter JK: Correction of the crooked nose, *Oral Maxillofac Surg Clin North Am.* 24(1):95–107, 2012.

11. Cerkes N: The crooked nose: principles of treatment, *Aesthet Surg J* 31(2):241–257, 2011.

12. Dyer 2nd WK: Nasal tip support and its surgical modification, *Facial Plast Surg Clin North Am* 12(1):1–13, 2004.

13. Larrabee Jr WF: The tripod concept, *Arch Otolaryngol Head Neck Surg* 115(10):1168–1169, 1989.

14. Swartout B, Toriumi DM: Rhinoplasty, *Curr Opin Otolaryngol Head Neck Surg* 15(4):219–227, 2007.

15. Byrd HS, Meade RA, Gonyon Jr DL: Using the autospreader flap in primary rhinoplasty, *Plast Reconstr Surg* 119(6):1897–1902, 2007.

16. Sheen JH: Spreader graft: a method of reconstructing the roof of the middle nasal vault following rhinoplasty, *Plast Reconstr Surg* 73(2):230–239, 1984.

17. Krause CJ: Steps in primary rhinoplasty, *Aesthetic Plast Surg* 26(Suppl 1):S14, 2002.

18. Koento T: Versatile grafting at the nasal tip, *Facial Plast Surg* 28(2):152–157, 2012.

19. Tebbetts JB: Open and closed rhinoplasty (minus the "versus"): analyzing processes, *Aesthet Surg J* 26(4):456–459, 2006.

20. Daniel RK: Rhinoplasty: open tip suture techniques: a 25-year experience, *Facial Plast Surg* 27(2):213–224, 2011.

21. Quatela VC, Kolstad CK: Creating elegance and refinement at the nasal tip, *Facial Plast Surg* 28(2):166–170, 2012.

22. Bohluli B, Bgheri SC, Behkish B, et al.: Immediate effects of different steps of rhinoplasty on nasolabial angle and tip projection, *Rashad J Craniofac Surg* 25(5):e404–e406, 2014.

23. Behmand RA, Ghavami A, Guyuron B: Nasal tip sutures part I: the evolution, *Plast Reconstr Surg* 112(4):1125–1129, 2003; discussion 1146–1149.

24. Guyuron B, Behmand RA: Nasal tip sutures part II: the interplays, *Plast Reconstr Surg* 112(4):1130–1145, 2003; discussion 1146–1149.

25. Ashtiani AK, Bohluli B, Bateni H, et al.: Lateral crural transposition flap in tip correction: Tehran retrospective rhinoplasty experience, *Ann Plast Surg* 71(1):50–53, 2013.

26. Bohluli B, Moharamnejad N, Bayat M: Dorsal hump surgery and lateral osteotomy, *Oral Maxillofac Surg Clin North Am.* 24(1):75–86, 2012.

CHAPTER 58

MINIMAL-INVASIVE COSMETIC SURGERY

Alia Koch

1. **What considerations are important in the evaluation of soft tissue prior to facial cosmetic surgery?**
   Initially, the overall health of the skin needs to be evaluated. Lesions should be evaluated prior to surgery. Skin laxity, quality, and extent of any prior damage are important indicators and may dictate operative procedure and healing expectations. Facial animation is important to evaluate for overactive muscles of facial expression.

2. **What is the Fitzpatrick Classification?**
   This system is used to determine the effects of UV radiation on skin. It is commonly used as a means to determine postoperative pigmentation problems after laser resurfacing. See Table 58-1.

3. **What is the benefit of laser resurfacing over chemical peels?**
   Laser resurfacing allows for a precise depth of peel.

4. **What is the Glogau Classification?**
   This system measures the amount of actinic damage the skin has received. It is used when patients are considering peels to address their facial wrinkles. The deeper the underlying pathology, the worse the actinic damage. See Table 58-2.

5. **Which patient is ideal when considering a chemical peel?**
   Fitzpatrick types 1, 2, and 3.

6. **What is chemical peeling?**
   Chemical peeling is the application of exfoliating agents to the skin, which leads to destruction of epidermis and possibly underlying dermis. This process will subsequently lead to regeneration of new epidermal and dermal tissues. Chemical peel can be categorized based on the depth of chemical penetration. Superficial peeling penetrates to the stratum granulosome-papillary dermis layer, medium-depth peeling reaches the upper reticular dermis, and deep-depth peeling can reach the mid-reticular dermis.

7. **What are different agents used for facial chemical peels?**
   See Table 58-3.

8. **What are the indications for chemical peeling?**
   Chemical peeling may be used for photoaging (actinic keratosis, solar elastosis, solar lentigo, and rhytides), pigmentary disturbances (melasma), superficial scarring, acne vulgaris, rosacea, and milia.

9. **How is the skin prepared for a chemical peel?**
   Topical tretinoin is used for 4 to 6 weeks prior to the peel. This decreases the stratum corneum, allowing for more uniform penetration. Prophylactic antivirals are also used preoperatively to prevent herpetic outbreaks. In those patients for whom postinflammatory hyperpigmentation might be a problem, preoperative hydroquinone is indicated as well.

10. **Can peeling be done simultaneously with surgery?**
    Yes; however, peeling should be done conservatively in an area where skin has been surgically altered. Due to disruption of the underlying blood supply, aggressive peeling can lead to skin necrosis.

Table 58-1. The Fitzpatrick Classification

1	Always burns, never tans
2	Always burns, sometimes tans
3	Sometimes burns, tans easily
4	Never burns, always tans
5	Moderately pigmented skin
6	Black skin

Table 58-2. The Glogau Classification

1	Minimal wrinkles and mild pigmentary changes
2	Wrinkles with motion
3	Wrinkles at rest with dyschromias and telangiectasias
4	Heavy wrinkling

Table 58-3. Types of Chemical Peels

PEEL AGENT	DEPTH
Alpha hydroxy acid	Superficial
Jessner's solution	Superficial
Trichloroacetic acid	Superficial to medium depth
Phenol*	Deep peel

*Hepatic and renal toxic, may cause cardiac arrhythmias

11. If both surgery and peeling will be planned, but not at the same time, which one should be done first? And how long should one wait before commencing the next procedure?
The sequence of the procedure should be based on the total timing of the treatment and primary concern of the patient. Surgery should be the primary treatment if sagging of the face is the primary concern, whereas eliminating lines of the face can be easily addressed with chemical peeling. Usually, a 2 to 3 months' wait is needed before chemical peeling if surgery is planned first. A longer waiting period is needed if peeling is performed first.

12. What are the complications that may be encountered after peeling?
    - Skin pigmentation
    - Prolonged erythema (>3 months)
    - Hypertrophic scarring
    - Systemic effects such as hepatic, renal, or cardiac abnormalities associated with phenol

13. What is Botox cosmetic?
Botulinum toxin type A, which is an exotoxin produced by *Clostridium botulinum*. The exotoxin is an A-B neurotoxin, which binds at the presynaptic neuron and inhibits acetylcholine release, causing flaccid paralysis. The use in facial surgery is aimed at reducing or eliminating furrows caused by active muscle movement.

14. Which muscles are treated with Botox cosmetic to reduce facial furrows?
See Table 58-4.

Table 58-4. Muscles Treated with Botox Cosmetic

Glabella	Corrugator supercilii and procerus
Forehead	Frontalis
Crow's feet	Lateral orbicularis oculi
Nasolabial folds	Levator labii superioris alaeque nasi
Upper lip	Orbicularis oris
Chin	Mentalis
Neck	Platysma

15. How can upper lid ptosis be prevented with Botox?
Botox can diffuse to the levator palpebral superioris causing upper eyelid ptosis; this can be prevented by injecting at least 1 cm away from the orbital rim.

16. What is the difference between dermal fillers and subcutaneous fillers?
Particle size is a determinant of placement of a filler. Fine-particle products will degrade faster if placed deeply. Large-particle fillers would produce lumpy results if placed too superficially.

17. What are the common available facial fillers?
Facial fillers can be categorized into hyaluronic acid and nonhyaluronic acid. Commonly used hyaluronic acid fillers include Juvederm, Restylane, and Perlane. Nonhyaluronic acid fillers include Radiesse, which is composed of calcium hydroxylapatite, whereas Sculptra Aesthetic is composed of poly-L-lactic acid. Only hyaluronic acid filler is reversible with injection of hyaluronidase.

18. What are the two most common lasers used for cosmetic skin resurfacing?
Because of their high affinity for tissue water found in the epidermis and dermis, the CO_2 and Er:YAG lasers are the most common lasers used for skin resurfacing techniques.

19. What is a chromophore?
A chromophore is a target tissue for a specific laser wavelength. The primary chromophore for the CO_2 and Er:YAG lasers is water.

20. What is thermal relaxation time?
Thermal relaxation time is the time required for a given tissue to dissipate 50% of the heat absorbed from the laser pulse. This process is important to avoid unwanted destruction in the surrounding tissue (coagulation necrosis). Hereof, high energy of short duration (microseconds) protects the remaining tissue. At the time of vaporization, the surrounding tissues are immediately cooled to 60 to 70 °C. At this temperature, one can visualize the initial collagen shrinking and tightening of the skin.

21. Describe how laser light interacts with tissue, and how does re-epithelialization occur during laser skin resurfacing?
On contact with tissue, a small amount of light is reflected; some is scattered or transmitted though the tissue. The majority of the light will be absorbed. Once it is absorbed, the imparted kinetic energy from the light will convert into heat, which coagulates, ablates, or cuts the tissue.
Re-epithelialization occurs because the progenitor cells are protected deep within the hair follicles and sweat glands at the time of laser resurfacing. Migration, reproduction, and coalescence of these progenitor epidermal cells re-epithelialize the skin.

BIBLIOGRAPHY

Alster TS: Erbium:YAG cutaneous laser resurfacing, *Dermatol Clin* 19:453–466, 2001.
Baker TJ, Gordon HL, Stuzin JM: *Surgical rejuvenation of the face*, St Louis, 1995, Mosby.
Knobloch K, Gohritz A, Reuss E, et al.: Nicotine in plastic surgery: a review, *Chirurg* 79:956–962, 2008.
Koch RJ: Microdermabrasion, *Facial Plast Surg Clin North Am* 9:377–382, 2001.
Mendelson JE: Update on chemical peels, *Otolaryngol Clin North Am* 35:55–72, 2002.

Niamtu J: *Cosmetic facial surgery*, 2011.

Obagi S: Autologous fat augmentation for addressing facial volume loss, *Oral Maxillofac Surg Clin North Am* 17:99–109, 2005.

Papel ID: *Facial and plastic reconstructive surgery*, ed 3, 2009.

Resnik SS, Resnick BI: Complications of chemical peeling, *Dermatol Clin* 13:309–311, 1995.

Thorne CH: *Grabb & Smith's plastic surgery*, ed 6, 2007.

INDEX

Note: Page numbers followed by "b," "f," and "t" indicate boxes, figures, and tables, respectively.